Recent Results in Cancer Research 84

Fortschritte der Krebsforschung
Progrès dans les recherches sur le cancer

Editor in Chief: P. Rentchnick, Genève
Co-editor: H. J. Senn, St. Gallen

Modified Nucleosides and Cancer

Edited by Gisela Nass

With 217 Figures and 89 Tables

Springer-Verlag
Berlin Heidelberg New York 1983

Contents

*List of Authors**

* The address of each mentioned authors is indicated below the according contribution heading

1 Page, on which contribution commences

Organization and Expression of tRNA Genes in Drosophila Melanogaster

S. Sharp, L. Cooley, D. DeFranco, T. Dingermann, and D. Söll*

Department of Molecular Biophysics and Biochemistry, Yale University, New Haven, CT 06511, USA

Introduction

Transfer RNA molecules are an integral component of the cellular protein-synthesizing machinery responsible for matching a codon in an RNA with the appropriate anticodon so that the correct amino acid is inserted into the growing polypeptide chain. In addition, tRNA species have also been implicated in various regulatory processes (for review, see LaRossa and Söll 1978). All tRNAs possess similar general structural features which allow for efficient recognition by the ribosome or by some nucleases involved in tRNA maturation. They also contain specific recognition features for interaction with cognate aminoacyl-tRNA synthetases and tRNA modifying enzymes. Thus tRNA, with its relatively small size but diverse structural and functional characteristics, provides a potentially useful molecule for the study of macromolecular structure-function relationships.

The maintenance of tRNA levels in a given cell requires the coordinate regulation of related yet diverse gene families. A general transcription control signal may exist within all tRNA genes, leading to very similar basal levels of transcription. Differential accumulation within the cell could result from differential stabilities of the gene products, which may be manifested in transport (nucleus to cytoplasm) or processing of precursors, or from variations in gene copy number and arrangement. Conversely, individual tRNA genes may be differentially expressed due to structural variations within gene regions which influence transcription efficiency. The components of this process may be either specific for individual tRNA genes or related families, or possess enormous flexibility in their recognition and functional properties.

The mechanisms by which tRNA levels are regulated to meet cellular demands for efficient translation are still poorly understood. The level of individual acceptor RNA species generally remains constant throughout *Drosophila* development (White et al. 1973). The only significant changes in the observed profile of tRNA species have been attributed to differences in the extent of base modification of existing tRNAs (White et al. 1973). More recent results have demonstrated that unique tRNA species which accumulate in transformed mammalian cells result from differences in nucleotide

* The work performed in the authors' laboratory has been supported by grants from the National Institutes of Health and the National Science Foundation. Theodor Dingermann is a Postdoctoral Fellow of the Deutsche Forschungsgemeinschaft

modification of the same basic sequences (Okada et al. 1978; Raba et al. 1979). Presently, the only documented example of developmental regulation of tRNA gene expression occurs in *Bombyx mori* silk glands. The predominant $tRNA^{Ala}$ species present in the posterior silk gland is a unique species ($tRNA^{Ala}_{2b}$) which is underrepresented in other tissues (Meza et al. 1977; Sprague et al. 1977). The tRNA pool is adjusted to allow efficient translation of the fibroin mRNA, which contains a relatively large percentage of alanine, as well as serine and glycine codons (Meza et al. 1977; Sprague et al. 1977; Chavancy et al. 1981). Species of $tRNA^{Gly}$ and $tRNA^{Ser}$ are accumulated in the posterior silk gland as therefore expected. Studies in these laboratories are focused on further characterizing the genes for $tRNA^{Gly}$ and $tRNA^{Ser}$.

Recent advances in recombinant DNA technology and DNA sequencing methods have greatly facilitated the study of tRNA gene expression. In this paper we summarize the present knowledge on the arrangement, structure, and in vitro expression of tRNA genes in *Drosophila*.

Number and Complexity of tRNA Genes

Several approaches have been used to determine the complexity of tRNA genes in *Drosophila*. By saturation hybridization of unfractionated radioactive tRNA to *Drosophila* DNA, Ritossa et al. (1966) estimated that there are about 750 genes for all species of tRNA. A similar value was independently determined by Tartof and Perry (1970). From a kinetic analysis of tRNA hybridization to *Drosophila* DNA, Weber and Berger (1976) estimated the presence of about 590 tRNA genes with about 59 families of genes per genome.

Unfractionated tRNA from *Drosophila* can be resolved into 99 different tRNA species (63 major and 36 minor) by reversed-phase (RPC-5) chromatography (White et al. 1973). The kinetic complexity of tRNA hybridization suggests that there are fewer than 99 tRNA species (Weber and Berger 1976). This observation is consistent with the interpretation that many chromatographically distinct forms of tRNA arise from post-transcriptional modifications of a smaller number of basic tRNA sequences (White et al. 1973; Grigliatti et al. 1974). In this respect the estimates of 60 and 59 tRNA species by Ritossa et al. (1966) and Weber and Berger (1976) respectively correspond well to the 63 major tRNA species observed by White et al. (1973).

A better way to determine the number of tRNA genes for an individual isoacceptor is by hybridization to individual DNA fragments generated by cleavage with restriction endonucleases and visualization by Southern blot analysis (Southern 1975). Using this approach with pure tRNA species, Tener et al. (1980) determined that there are 18 copies of the gene coding for $tRNA^{Lys}_{2}$. DNA probes prepared from hybrid plasmids which contain the tRNA gene of interest have also been used in this fashion. With this approach five $tRNA^{Glu}$ (Hosbach et al. 1980) and eight $tRNA^{Met}_{1}$ (Sharp et al. 1981a) genes have been visualized. These experimental approaches give more reliable estimates for tRNA gene numbers within the *Drosophila* genome (Tener et al. 1980).

Because tRNA gene arrangements in invert repeat structure are hard to detect (see below) and because pseudogenes give positive responses, the results of saturation hybridization studies may not give a true estimate of the number of tRNA genes. However, it is clear that the tRNA genes of *Drosophila* are redundant with an average reiteration frequency of 12.5 for each of the approximately 60 different kinds of tRNA genes (Ritossa et al. 1966). It seems that this redundancy is in the mitotic chromosomes and does not result from selective amplification of tRNA genes. The function of this redundancy is not known, but may be related to a requirement at certain times for a peak rate of tRNA synthesis that exceeds the maximum possible transcription rate of a single template. Concurrent transcription of an appropriate number of templates would meet such a requirement. Studies of tRNA gene localization in the *Drosophila* chromosomes indicate that this view is too simplistic. Not only are tRNA genes dispersed throughout most of the genome, but also the genes for any given isoacceptor are located at more than one chromosomal locus.

Localization of tRNA Genes

The localization of tRNA genes in the *Drosophila* genome has been determined by in situ hybridization of radioactive RNA or DNA to the DNA contained in salivary gland polytene chromosomes (Gall and Pardue 1969). The linear order of bands can be equated with the linear array of genes.

Cytological hybridization studies using unfractionated tRNA as a radioactive probe have revealed that the *Drosophila melanogaster* genome contains at least 50 different sites which code for tRNA (Steffensen and Wimber 1971; Elder et al. 1980). The tRNA genes appear to be distributed over the entire genome. However, the X chromosome contains significantly fewer sites of hybridization than chromosomes 2 and 3. Regions of tRNA hybridization have not been observed on chromosome 4.

At present the location of the genes for about 25 individual tRNA species is known (G. M. Tener, personal communication). Different, apparently unrelated tRNAs hybridized to the same sites on the genome, and also particular tRNA species hybridized to different chromosomal regions. From such studies it has become clear that although tRNA genes are distributed throughout the genome, there is marked clustering at particular loci (Elder et al. 1980; Kubli et al. 1980; Tener et al. 1980). Thus while there does not appear to be a regularity in the organization of *Drosophila* tRNA genes, such observations imply that tRNA gene expression in *Drosophila* is not an all-or-none mechanism. It is enticing to speculate that a gene for a given isoaccepting tRNA at one region is expressed at a different time during development, or differentiation, than is a gene copy located at another region.

It has not been possible to define tRNA gene loci genetically in *Drosophila.* Attwood has suggested that mutations of the *Minute* class result from mutations in tRNA genes (Ritossa et al. 1966; and see Lindsley and Grell 1968). However, at present the *Minute* class cannot be considered to be solely mutations in tRNA genes, since there is no apparent correlation between the sites of tRNA genes and sites of known *Minute* mutants (Tener et al. 1980). Similarly, it has not been possible to assign tRNA genes genetically as informational suppressor mutations in *Drosophila* (Bienz et al. 1979; Kiger 1974; Kubli 1982). This lack of mutant tRNA phenotypes will hamper studies of in vivo expression of tRNA genes.

Two independent studies have elegantly demonstrated the combined use of cytological methods and genetic methods. Dunn et al. (1979) studied two stocks of mutant flies. One, a deficiency mutant, has a deletion which includes region 84B1,2 and 84D12. This gap includes the $tRNA^{Val}_{3b}$ gene cluster at 84D3,4. In the second stock the DNA from 84B2 through 84D12 is duplicated. When the presence of $tRNA^{Val}$ was measured, the deficiency mutant showed essentially wild type levels. Since some of the $tRNA^{Val}_{3b}$ genes were missing in the deletion mutant, the organism apparently compensated for this loss by producing more $tRNA^{Val}$. The duplication mutant showed an increased level of $tRNA^{Val}$ which was greater than that expected if the amount of $tRNA^{Val}$ was directly related to the number of genes present (Dunn et al. 1979). A similar study involving $tRNA^{Glu}$ genes was performed in an embryonic lethal mutant (*1*(2)*me*). Kubli and Schmidt (1978) localized genes for $tRNA^{Glu}_{4}$ in the region 52F, which includes the *1me* locus. Compared to wild type, the $tRNA^{Glu}$ level was only slightly lowered in the mutant (Kubli and Schmidt 1978; Kubli et al. 1980). Analysis of the $tRNA^{Glu}$ isoacceptor pattern of homozygotes of this mutant revealed that the concentration of $tRNA^{Glu}_{4}$ is decreased in the mutant while there is a compensatory increase in the levels of $tRNA^{Glu}_{2}$ (E. Kubli and G. Kutzer, unpublished work). These studies indicate that the extent of tRNA gene expression in *Drosophila* is not strictly related to gene dosage.

Detailed Anatomy of tRNA Genes

Molecular cloning and DNA sequencing methods have allowed the determination of the chromosomal arrangement of some tRNA genes. With this information it may now be possible to define the nature of the transcriptional unit of a tRNA gene and identify putative regulatory signals within the DNA.

The chromosomal region 42A was the single most prominent site of tRNA hybridization in the experiments of Steffensen and Wimber (1971). This region is puffed throughout the larval third instar and most of the prepupal period (Ashburner 1969) and therefore may have some general significance for the pattern of development in *D. melanogaster*.

In the first study a hybrid Col E1 plasmid, pCIT12, was constructed which contained a 9.34 kb *Drosophila* DNA fragment from region 42A on chromosome 2R (Yen et al. 1977). Electron-microscopic and hybridization studies showed that this DNA contains four tRNA genes. Later experiments (Schmidt et al. 1978; Hovemann et al. 1980), involving purified or partially purified tRNAs as hybridization probes and extensive DNA sequence analysis, showed that pCIT12 contains eight tRNA genes: one $tRNA^{Arg}_{2}$, three $tRNA^{Asn}$, three $tRNA^{Lys}_{2}$, and one $tRNA^{Ile}$. The individual tRNA genes are irregularly spaced in the DNA. One strand contains the coding sequences for five genes and the other strand contains sequences for three genes. The genes are separated by DNA regions of varying length which seem to be transcriptionally "silent" (Schmidt et al. 1978). The direction of transcription is different for the various genes of the same isoacceptor tRNA (Fig. 1). The difficulty in determining the exact number of tRNA genes by hybridization was easily explained by the arrangement of many of the genes in perfect invert repeat structures (Hovemann et al. 1980). This fact may make impossible the determination of the number and location of all tRNA genes in the *Drosophila* genome by hybridization experiments.

A set of overlapping inserts of *Drosophila* DNA cloned in a lambdoid vector and extending in both directions from the *Drosophila* DNA fragment of plasmid pCIT12 were isolated by the procedure of "chromosomal walking" (Yen and Davidson 1980). The region isolated, which therefore includes the pCIT12 region, has a total length of

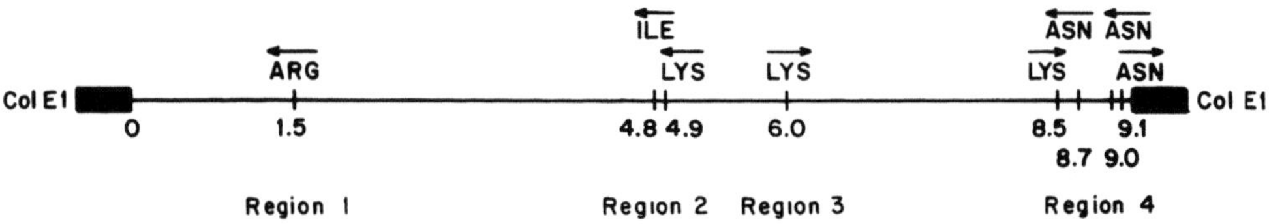

Fig. 1. Scheme of tRNA gene arrangement on the 9.34-kb *Drosophila* DNA fragment in pCIT12. Col E1 represents the ends of the plasmid DNA, the *numbers* refer to the position (in kilobase pairs) in the *Drosophila* DNA. The *arrows* indicate the transcription direction of the tRNA genes

94 kb. The central 46-kb region contains a total of eight $tRNA^{Asn}$ genes, four $tRNA_2^{Arg}$ genes, five $tRNA_2^{Lys}$ genes, and one $tRNA^{Ile}$ gene.

The irregular arrangement of tRNA genes located within the 42A tRNA gene cluster has been shown in general to be representative of the tRNA gene organization in *Drosophila.* Additional tRNA gene regions have been analyzed by DNA sequencing and restriction enzyme mapping combined with hybridization. These DNA segments include the genes which code for $tRNA^{Gly}$ (Hershey and Davidson 1980), $tRNA^{Glu}$ (Hosbach et al. 1980), $tRNA^{Leu}$ and $tRNA^{Ile}$ (Robinson and Davidson 1981), $tRNA_5^{Lys}$ (D. Cribbs, D. DeFranco, S. Hayashi, R. Miller, D. Söll and G. M. Tener, unpublished work), $tRNA_4^{Val}$ (Addison et al. 1982), $tRNA^{Ser}$ and $tRNA^{Phe}$ (W. R. Addison and G. M. Tener, unpublished work), $tRNA^{His}$ (see below), and initiator $tRNA^{Met}$ (Sharp et al. 1983a).

Structure of tRNA Genes

All the genes contained within the 42A region have coding sequences colinear with the tRNA sequence in that none of these genes contain intervening sequences (Hovemann et al. 1980; Yen and Davidson 1980). To date the only characterized *Drosophila* tRNA genes containing intervening sequences are two $tRNA^{Leu}$ genes (Robinson and Davidson 1981). Although these two genes encode the same $tRNA^{Leu}$ sequence, they have different intervening sequence (Robinson and Davidson 1981). No *Drosophila* tRNA genes sequenced so far encode the 3′-terminal trinucleotide C-C-A of the mature tRNAs.

The 3′-flanking sequences of all tRNA genes in pCIT12 are highly AT-rich. As is well known, oligothymidylate stretches serve as termination signals for RNA polymerase III directed transcription (Korn and Brown 1978; Tekamp et al. 1979; Bogenhagen and Brown 1981; Silverman et al. 1979; Hagenbüchle et al. 1979).

Such sequence similarities are not observed in regions 5′-flanking tRNA genes. There is no general sequence conservation within 5′-flanking regions that can be attributed to defining a transcriptional control sequence. An exception to this is the presence of the undecanucleotide sequence G-G-C-A-G-T-T-T-T-T-G in well-conserved form in the 5′-flanking region of four of five sequenced $tRNA_2^{Lys}$ genes (Fig. 2) (Hovemann et al. 1980; DeFranco et al. 1980; Yen and Davidson 1980).

The sequences surrounding members of the $tRNA_4^{Glu}$ gene family are highly homologous (Hosbach et al. 1980). In other instances, for example the $tRNA^{Gly}$ and initiator tRNA gene families, the sequences flanking the individual members are

```
                 -30       -20       -10        1
                  '         '         '         '
Lys 2:1    5'-AGCTTAGGTCCGTTTTAATATGGGTCATTCA GCCC-3'

Lys 2:2    5'-AATTTTGCGGCAGTTTTTGGCTCATCAAGTG GCCC-3'

Lys 2:3    5'-TGTGGTGTGGCAGTTTTTTCCACACCAAGAG GCCC-3'

Lys 2:4    5'-ATGTGAGCTTTTATCGGCGATCTTCACAAGT GCCC-3'

Lys 2:5    5'-GTATGCTCTATTCTCGGCTGTTGCGGCAACT GCCC-3'
```

Fig. 2. The 5′-flanking sequences of *Drosophila* $tRNA_2^{Lys}$ genes. They are aligned according to the mature-tRNA coding sequence (*boxed*). The *single underlined nucleotide* preceding the mature-tRNA coding region denotes the transcription initiation site

```
         10        20        30        40        50        60        70
AAGCTTAAAAATAAAAAATAACCCAACTCCGTGACAATGTTTATTTGAACATTGCCGTGACCAGGATTCG
TTCGAATTTTTATTTTTTATTGGGTTGAGGCACTGTTACAAATAAACTTGTAACGGCACTGGTCCTAAGC

         80        90       100       110       120       130       140
AACCTGGGTGTGGTAACCCACAACGTGGGGTCCTAACCACTAGACGATCACGGCTACATTGGATTGCGCC
TTGGACCCACACCATTGGGTGTTGCACCCCAGGATTGGTGATCTGCTAGTGCCGATGTAACCTAACGCGG
                                                    <--1

        150       160       170       180       190       200       210
CAGCAATTCCAAGATCCCACCACGTCACCTAATAAAAAAAAATTGCAGATGTAATTAGTAAACACAACCC
GTCGTTAAGGTTCTAGGGTGGTGCAGTGGATTATTTTTTTTTAACGTCTACATTAATCATTTGTGTTGGG

        220       230       240       250       260       270       280
C--110 b--AAGCTTGGTGTTTGTTTCAACATTGCCGTGACCAGGATTCGAACCTGGGTTACCACGGCC
G--110 b--TTCGAACCACAAACAAAGTTGTAACGGCACTGGTCCTAAGCTTGGACCCAATGGTGCCGG

        290       300       310       320       330       340       350
ACAACGTGGGGTCCTAACCACTAGACGATCACGGCTACATCGGGTGATGCGAGGTCTATGCCAAATGACT
TGTTGCACCCCAGGATTGGTGATCTGCTAGTGCCGATGTAGCCCACTACGCTCCAGATACGGTTTACTGA
                                 <--2
        360       370       380       390       400
AATTTTAGCAAAGTGCGCAGAAAATCATAGCAAGTAAGCAAGCAAGTCGTAAATAA-3'
TTAAAATCGTTTCACGCGTCTTTTAGTATCGTTCATTCGTTCGTTCAGCATTTATT-5'
```

Fig. 3. DNA sequences of tRNA gene regions contained on the recombinant plasmid p38B10. The *outlined* regions indicate the mature-tRNA coding region. The *dotted underline* indicates the extent of DNA sequence that varies from the sequence of $tRNA^{His}$. The first nucleotide in the mature-tRNA coding sequence is discussed in the text

almost identical for several hundred base pairs 5′- and 3′-flanking the coding sequence (Hershey and Davidson 1980; Sharp et al. 1981a).

The structure of some *Drosophila* mature tRNAs for which the gene sequence is known has not been deduced. However, the tRNA genes which have been sequenced can be arranged into the characteristic tRNA cloverleaf model of secondary structure.

When the gene sequences are compared to the sequences of the isolated tRNA species, deviations in the coding regions of the genes are sometimes found. The initiator tRNA gene, for example, which is contained on the plasmid pPW591, has a single nucleotide G→T transversion at tRNA coordinate 30 (Sharp et al. 1981a). Also, a gene for $tRNA_5^{Lys}$ has been sequenced which shows differences in the base composition at three positions compared to the known $tRNA_5^{Lys}$ sequence (D. Cribbs, D. DeFranco, S. Hayashi, R. Miller, D. Söll, and G. M. Tener, unpublished work). The tRNA resulting from transcription of such genes could be minor chromatographic species and thus not readily purified, or conversely may be rapidly degraded in the cell. Therefore it is not apparent which genes of a tRNA multigene family are actually expressed in the cell.

The single *Drosophila* $tRNA^{His}$ species is similar to all other $tRNA^{His}$ species that have been sequenced in that the 5′ stem of the acceptor arm is longer by one nucleotide than in all other tRNAs (Altwegg and Kubli 1980). The 5′-terminal nucleotide is a guanylate residue and is unpaired. A $tRNA^{His}$ gene from region 48F of the *Drosophila* chromosome does not encode this residue. Instead, an adenylate residue is found at this position in the DNA sequence (Fig. 3). This may represent another example of the gene sequence being different to the sequence of the isolated tRNA. However, this gene may represent a bona fide $tRNA^{His}$ gene in which the addition of the 5′ guanylate residue occurs post-transcriptionally.

Other Drosophila Structures Related to tRNA Genes

As discussed above, the sequence complexity within *Drosophila* tRNA genes, as determined by hybridization approaches, can only be considered an estimate. As was clearly demonstrated in studies on the region 42A tRNA gene cluster contained in pCIT12, DNA sequence analysis most clearly defines the complexity of tRNA gene numbers and the nature of the acceptor RNA coded by them for any given *Drosophila* locus.

Two examples of tRNA pseudogenes which cannot be transcribed in vitro are known. Of several recombinant plasmids that hybridized to homologous initiator tRNA, one was found that did not contain the complete tRNA coding sequence (Sharp et al. 1981a). This particular cloned DNA fragment, pYD6, hybridized strongly to initiator tRNA. DNA sequencing revealed several shorter regions to be homologous to parts of the initiator tRNA (Fig. 4). The largest region of homology corresponds to the region in the initiator tRNA between coordinates 7 and 39, which represents approximately 50% of an intact initiator tRNA sequence. This sequence may therefore be considered as a tRNA pseudogene. The *Drosophila* insert of pYD6 hybridizes to more than 30 sites on the *Drosophila* chromosome and has a pattern of hybridization characteristic of a mobile DNA element. This is especially intriguing since the 18 kb of *Drosophila* DNA that flank the pYD6 insert in the parental clone pPW568 (Gergen et al. 1981; Sharp et al. 1981a) displayed hybridization kinetics of middle-repetitive DNA (Gergen et al. 1981; Wensink 1978). In this respect it appears that the *Drosophila* DNA insert of pYD6 represents a "fragmented" initiator tRNA gene and that this fragmentation may have been brought about by repeated insertion and excision of a transposable element(s) into this tRNA gene coding region.

Another tRNA pseudogene was observed in the $tRNA^{His}$ gene family. This sequence was located on a *Drosophila* DNA fragment which contained the bona fide $tRNA^{His}$ gene in close proximity (Fig. 3). Similarly to the initiator tRNA pseudogene, the $tRNA^{His}$ pseudogene was detected by hybridization using purified homologous tRNA. The sequence of the $tRNA^{His}$ pseudogene (Fig. 3) differs from that of $tRNA^{His}$ in that the nucleotides between coordinates 79 and 88 have been replaced by a different sequence. The corresponding coding sequence of the pseudogene is of the same length as the bona fide $tRNA^{His}$ gene and also appears to have similar 3′- and 5′-flanking sequences.

```
        10        20        30        40        50        60        70        80        90       100       110       120
GAATTCGCTCAGACTCGGTTCTGCTTTCATCTTCCGTACGTAACCTCACCCGATTTTTCAGGATTAGCGCCTCAGGTTTTTTGCGCAGGCGCTGGGCTTCACCTTAGCCCATTCTTCGT
CTTAAGCGAGTCTGAGCCAAGACGAAAGTAGAAGGCATGCATTGGAGTGGGCTAAAAAGTCCTAATCGCGGAGTCCAAAAAACGCGTCCGCGACCCGAAGTGGAATCGGGTAAGAAGCA

       130       140       150       160       170       180       190       200       210       220       230       240
CTTTGTTATCGTCCTTGGCGACAGACGCATAACTTTCCGGTTTGGAGTCAGCCGTCGTGGGTACCGCCTTACCGGTGGATTTCGCGGCAGATCGATGGTGTCCGTTTTGCGGACCTGCAC
GAAACAATAGCAGGAACCGCTGTCTGCGTATTGAAAGGCCAAACCTCAGTCGGCAGCACCCATGGCGGAATGGCCACCTAAAGCGCCGTCTAGCTACCACAGGCAAAACGCCTGGACGTG

       250       260       270       280       290       300       310       320       330       340       350       360
ATTCGGTAATGCCTGTCTGGGTGGCGCCACCTGGCTGCGCTTCGTTTTTCTGCCTCAGTCTGTGTGGCAGTACTCCTTGGTGGGGCTTCTTGTTGATACCCTCCTGTAACTCAATTGT
TAAGCCATTACGGACAGACCCACCGCGGTGGACCGACGCGAAGCAAAAAGACGGAGTCAGACACACCGTCATGAGGAACCACCCCGAAGAACAACTATGGGAGGACATTGAGTTAACA

       68      +8      390       400       410       420       430       440       450       460       470  7*
ATGTATGTGCTATATGCTTATGTATGTATGTGTGTGTCGGCAATTTCACCACAGATCGAAATTTGCCATTTTAACTCTCTAGTTGATCACTATCCTTGTTCTAACTATTCTACGTGGGCG
TACATACACGATATACGAATACATACATACACACACAGCCGTTAAAGTGGTGTCTAGCTTTAAACGGTAAAATTGAGAGATCAACTAGTGATAGGAACAAGATTGATAAGATGCACCCGC

                        39       520       530       540       550       560       570       580      3
CAGTGGAAGCGTGCTGGGCCCATAACCTGTTGTAATTTTGGCTGAGTAATAGTTTTATTTGAGGTATAAGTAAATGATTGGAGTTTTACACCTTGTTGGCGATACGCACACAGGGCGAA
GTCACCTTCGCACGACCCGGGTATTGGACAACATTAAAACCGACTCATTATCAAAATAAACTCCATATTCATTTACTAACCTCAAAATGTGGAACAACCGCTATGCGTGTGTCCCGCTT

 17    610       620       630       640       650       660       670       680       690       700       710       720
GTGTACAATACGATCCGTGTGGCCACACTCTTGCAGTTGAACATGAACGGGGCGTTGCGTTTGTGCGGCTCTTTCTACCGTGATCCTTACGGTGCAAAAGGAGCTGGAGTTTGTAAATTG
CACATGTTATGCTAGGCACACCGGTGTGAGAACGTCAACTTGTACTTGCCCCGCAACGCAAACACGCCGAGAAAGATGGCACTAGGAATGCCACGTTTTCCTCGACCTCAAACATTTAAC

       730       740       750       760       770  18         30  790       800       810       820       830       840
GGCGAACCTCGTTTTTTCTAGGAGGCTTGTTTTCTGGTTCAAGCTCAATCTTGAAGAGTGGTTGGGCTGCCTGTTTCTGTTTTTGTATTGAACACGCTTTTGCCGTAAAATCCCTTTTC
CCGCTTGGAGCAAAAAAGATCCTCCGAACAAAAGACCAAGTTCGAGTTAGAACTTCTCACCAACCCGACGGACAAAGACAAAAACATAACTTGTGCGAAAACGGCATTTTAGGGAAAAG

       850       860       870       880       890       900       910       920       930       940       950       960
CTTTAGCGCCTCAGTTATCAGTAACATCAGACTCAATGCCTTTCAGGACTACTTGCAGGCCCTTGCTGCTTTTAAGCTGGTAGGTGTAGAAGCCTATTTTTTGTGCGGTAAAATAGTTTG
GAAATCGCGGAGTCAATAGTCATTGTAGTCTGAGTTACGGAAAGTCCTGATGAACGTCCGGGAACGACGAAAATTCGACCATCCACATCTTCGGATAAAAAACACGCCATTTTATCAAAC

       970       980       990      1000      1010      1020      1030      1040      1050      1060      1070      1080
TGACTTTTCTGAAGTTGTCCTCCGTTTTCGTCTGAAGTTTGATTTTCATTGATAGTACTTCTTACGAGGGGAATTATATGAAAGCTATCTTTTCCAATAGGGCCAATCAAAGTATTTACA
ACTGAAAAGACTTCAACAGGAGGCAAAAGCAGACTTCAAACTAAAAGTAACTATCATGAAGAATGCTCCCCTTAATATACTTTCGATAGAAAAGGTTATCCCGGTTAGTTTCATAAATGT

      1090      1100      1110      1120      1130      1140      1150
AAACCGCTTGTGCTCTTCTCGCGGATGTATATTGGCGGAGGCTTTGTTTTCTTCGGTTCGATATCAACGGATCC-3'
TTTGGCGAACACGAGAAGAGCGCCTACATATAACCGCCTCCGAAACAAAAGAAGCCAAGCTATAGTTGCCTAGG-5'
```

Fig. 4. The sequence of the *Drosophila* DNA insert of recombinant plasmid pYD6. The sequences homologous to *Drosophila* initiator tRNA are *boxed*. The nucleotide at coordinate 476, marked with an *asterisk*, is not found in initiator tRNA. *Bold-printed numbers* are coordinates from the initiator tRNA gene sequence (Sharp et al. 1981a)

The discovery of tRNA pseudogenes in the *Drosophila* genome and the presence of tRNA gene sequences that differ from the isolated tRNA sequence raise questions on the maintenance of multigene families in the *Drosophila* genome. Whether such genes are temporalintermediates in the evolution of a "new" tRNA gene or represent relics or mistakes in the evolutionary mechanism has yet to be examined. Perhaps, as for other tRNA genes in *Drosophila,* such questions are best examined by developing approaches which test biological function and expression of these genes. Neither the initiator tRNA nor the $tRNA^{His}$ pseudogenes can be transcribed in vitro (Sharp et al. 1981a; L. Cooley and D. Söll, unpublished work). Determination of whether such pseudogenes are expressed in the cell must await further investigation.

Synthesis of Eukaryotic tRNA

It is now well established that RNA polymerase III is responsible for the formation of tRNAs in eukaryotic cells. The same enzyme also transcribes the genes for 5S RNA, adenovirus-associated RNA (VA RNA), and some other small RNAs (Roeder 1976). A general scheme for the eukaryotic tRNA biosynthetic pathway has been developed (Fig. 5). Although all steps within this pathway have not been elucidated, it is clear that tRNA genes are transcribed into precursor molecules which are larger than the mature-size tRNA. These precursors are subsequently cleaved, probably within the nucleus, into mature-size tRNA molecules by 5′- and 3′-processing nucleases and splicing enzymes which excise intervening sequences. Further maturation of the transcript into a functional tRNA occurs by the addition of the 3′ terminal C-C-A and by an extensive variety of specific nucleotide modifications.

The availability of cloned tRNA genes emphasized the need for routine tests of their biological function. The *Xenopus* oocyte has proved to be an excellent system for such studies. Cloned homologous and heterologous tRNA genes (Kressmann et al. 1978; Cortese et al. 1978; DeRobertis and Olson 1979) have been faithfully transcribed in

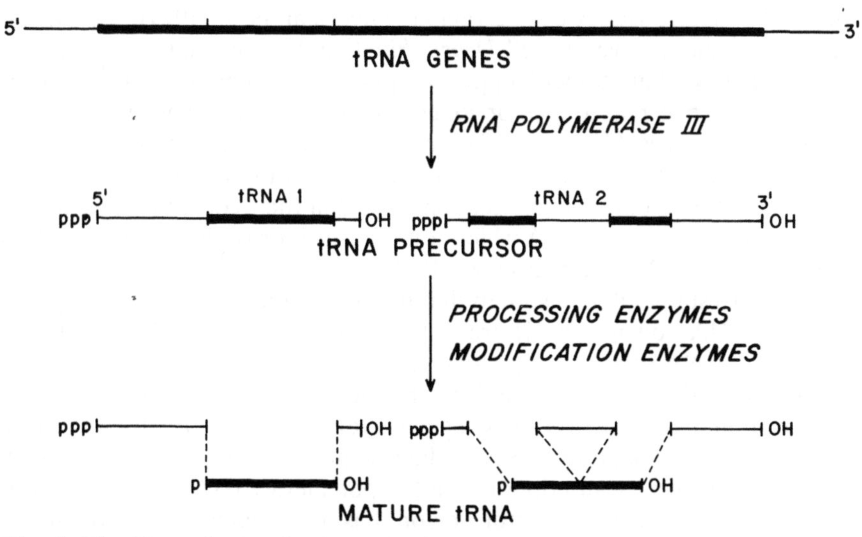

Fig. 5. The biosynthesis of eukaryotic tRNA

vivo into their mature product by injection into the *Xenopus* oocyte nucleus. Extracts prepared from *Xenopus* germinal vesicles or from *Drosophila* cell cultures allow efficient in vitro transcription of tRNA genes from a variety of sources (Schmidt et al. 1978; Dingermann et al. 1981). These extracts therefore contain all components necessary for specific transcription of isolated tRNA genes.

Purified RNA polymerase III is not able specifically to transcribe purified gene templates. This indicates that additional factors are required to ensure specificity of gene transciption. Column chromatography of an extract prepared from human KB cells led to the fractionation of multiple transcription factors. Two fractions, when added to purified RNA polymerase III, supported faithful synthesis of tRNA and VA RNA (Segall et al. 1980). Three fractions (not necessarily the same) were necessary to support the specific synthesis of 5S RNA (Segall et al. 1980). A similar factor, specific only for 5S genes, has since been purified from *Xenopus laevis* oocytes (Engelke et al. 1980). As yet the factor(s) which specifically support tRNA gene transcription have not been characterized and therefore unfractionated extracts must be used to study the transcription of tRNA genes.

Transcription of Drosophila tRNA Genes

Although most tRNA genes of *Drosophila* are clustered, transcription studies revealed the formation of tRNA precursor products in the size range of 80–100 nucleotides (Schmidt et al. 1978). Therefore the clustering of tRNA genes does not appear to result in a transcriptional unit which consists of a large precursor containing several tRNA moieties. This was later confirmed when it was shown that genes cloned individually supported formation of monomeric precursor tRNA (Silverman et al. 1979). The in vitro transcription of the single $tRNA_2^{Arg}$ gene contained on pCIT12 led to formation of a precursor tRNA 83–86 nucleotides long. The transcript began with pppG, seven nucleotides preceding the 5′ end of the mature-tRNA coding sequence, and terminated specifically within a stretch of seven oligothymidylate residues which follow the mature tRNA coding region (Silverman et al. 1979). This transcriptional trend has been observed for all *Drosophila* tRNA genes that have been transcribed. Precursor tRNA initiates with pppA or pppG and terminates within oligothymidylate sequences of five nucleotides or longer. In vitro RNA transcription can terminate within T_4 sequences. However, this probably does not occur in the cell, since a number of eukaryotic tRNAs contain U_4 sequences within the mature-tRNA coding region. Genes that contain intervening sequences within their coding regions are transcribed in vitro into a precursor tRNA which contains the intervening sequence (Robinson and Davidson 1981; Dingermann et al. 1981).

Thus in vitro studies demonstrated that the signals required for transcription of tRNA genes by RNA polymerase III are in the vicinity of the tRNA gene. Deletion of all *Drosophila* DNA sequences upstream of the mature-tRNA coding region of $tRNA_2^{Lys}$ genes revealed that the 5′-flanking region was unnecessary per se for faithful transcription of a eukaryotic tRNA gene (DeFranco et al. 1980). An internal control region within the mature-tRNA coding sequence was shown to be sufficient for accurate tRNA gene transcription by RNA polymerase III (DeFranco et al. 1980). The identity of the internal control region has now been more precisely identified (Hofstetter et al. 1981; Sharp et al. 1981b).

Internal Transcriptional Control Sequences of tRNA Genes

Two series of deletion mutations were constructed in the tRNA$_2^{Arg}$ gene which had been subcloned from pCIT12. The mutations were constructed in vitro with the aid of the processive nuclease BAL-31. In the resultant mutants successively larger sequences of *Drosophila* DNA from either the 5′ or the 3′ side of the tRNA gene have been replaced by plasmid DNA. By analyzing the ability of the 5′- and 3′-deletion templates to direct the synthesis of RNA in vitro, we have defined the outside borders of the internal control regions required for tRNA gene transcription. These results (Fig. 6) show that there are two transcriptional control regions within the mature-tRNA coding sequence (Sharp et al. 1981a). One control region, bounded by nucleotides 8 and 25, encodes the D-stem and D-loop (D-control) and the invariant U at position 8 found in all tRNAs. The second control region is bounded by nucleotides 50 and 58 and encodes the semi-invariant sequence of GTψC in loop IV of tRNA (T-control).

The D-control region of the gene displayed "classical" gene-promoter qualities in that removal of the single nucleotide thymidylate at position 8, and similarly nucleotide 25, a cytidine residue, resulted in complete loss of transcriptional activity. For in vitro transcription of this tRNA^{Arg} gene the presence of the T-control region was not an absolute requirement. Templates devoid of the T-control were still transcribed, albeit at a much-reduced capacity (approx. 10%) compared to wild type gene transcription. A comparison of all known tRNA sequences shows that the D-stem, U$_8$, and th GTψC sequence are highly conserved in eukaryotic tRNAs. Many invariant nucleotides contained within all eukaryotic tRNAs lie within the sequences which comprise the transcriptional control regions (boxed areas in Fig. 6).

From this analysis we can conclude that the D-control and T-control regions are the essential control sequences for tRNA gene transcription.

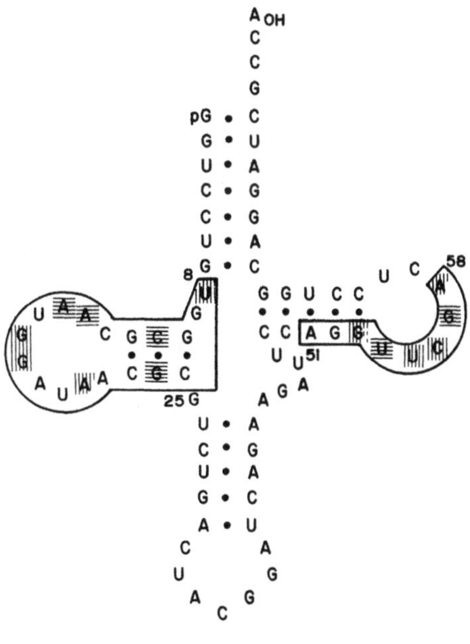

Fig. 6. Internal transcription control regions (*boxed*) drawn into the cloverleaf structure of *Drosophila* tRNA$_2^{Arg}$. *Crosshatched* nucleotides represent the invariant or semi-invariant nucleotides contained within these regions

External Control Regions of Drosophila tRNA Genes

From the studies which involved 5′-deletion templates it became clearer that while the 5′-flanking region is not required per se for tRNA gene transcription, it can markedly affect overall transcription. De Franco et al. (1980) observed earlier that two members of the $tRNA_2^{Lys}$ gene family were transcribed with different efficiencies. "Switching" the 5′-flanking region of one with the other resulted in a transfer of the transcription properties from one to the other. These studies showed that the efficiencies of transcription of these two $tRNA_2^{Lys}$ genes were a direct result of their 5′-flanking regions (DeFranco et al. 1980). The BAL-31 procedure was used to produce 5′-deletion templates within the inefficiently transcribed $tRNA_2^{Lys}$ gene. Subsequent in vitro transcription of these deletion templates showed that the sequence G-G-C-A-G-T-T-T-T-T-G was responsible for this negative transcription effect. Additional experiments (DeFranco et al. 1981) show that this sequence, when put in front of genes for other isoacceptor tRNAs, also causes inefficient in vitro transcription. However, its position relative to the mature coding sequence is extremely important for exerting its maximum effect (DeFranco et al. 1981). Independent studies from different laboratories (Hofstetter et al. 1981; Koski et al. 1980; Sharp et al. 1981b) suggest that the crucial tRNA transcriptional control region is contained within the mature-tRNA coding sequence and that this internal control region constitutes a split promoter. The relationship of this control region to the described 5′-flanking control sequence is as yet not understood. Progress in understanding the mechanism of transcriptional repression may give insight into those proteins which are involved in initiation of tRNA gene transcription. Related studies are focused on the tertiary structure of the transcription initiation complex.

References

Addison WR, Astell CR, Delaney AD, Gillam IC, Hayashi S, Miller RC, Rajput B, Smith M, Taylor DM, Tener GM (1982) The structures of genes hybridizing with $tRNA_4^{Val}$ from *Drosophila melanogaster.* J Biol Chem 257: 670–73

Altwegg M, Kubli E (1980) The nucleotide sequence of histidine tRNA of *Drosophila melanogaster.* Nucleic Acids Res 8: 3259–3262

Ashburner M (1969) Patterns of puffing activity in the salivary gland chromosomes of *Drosophila* IV. Variability of puffing patterns. Chromosoma 27: 156–177

Bienz M, Zublin E, Kubli E (1979) Transfer RNA mediated suppression in *Drosophila melanogaster.* Experientia 35: 956

Bogenhagen DF, Brown DD (1981) Nucleotide sequences in *Xenopus* 5S DNA required for transcription termination. Cell 24: 261–270

Chavancy G, Marbaix G, Huez G, Cleuter Y (1981) Effect of tRNA pool balance on rate and uniformity of elongation during translation of fibron mRNA in reticulocyte cell-free system. Biochimie 63: 611–618

Cortese R, Melton D, Tranquilla T, Smith JD (1978) Cloning of nematode tRNA genes and their expression in the frog oocyte. Nucleic Acids Res 5: 4593–4611

DeFranco D, Schmidt O, Söll D (1980) Two control regions for eukaryotic tRNA gene transcription. Proc Natl Acad Sci USA 77: 3365–3368

DeFranco D, Sharp S, Söll D (1981) Identification of regulatory sequences contained in the 5′-flanking region of *Drosophila* lysine $tRNA_2$. J Biol Chem 256: 12424–12429

DeRobertis EM, Olson MV (1979) Transcription and processing of yeast tyrosine tRNA genes microinjected into frog oocytes. Nature 278: 137–143
Dingermann T, Sharp S, Appel B, DeFranco D, Mount S, Heiermann R, Pongs O, Söll D (1981) Transcription of cloned tRNA and 5S RNA genes in a *Drosophila* cell-free extract. Nucleic Acids Res 9: 3907–3917
Dunn R, Hayashi S, Gillam IC, Delaney AD, Tener GM, Grigliatti TA, Kaufman TC, Suzuki DT (1979) Genes coding for valine transfer ribonucleic acid-3b in *Drosophila melanogaster*. J Mol Biol 128: 277–287
Elder RT, Uhlenbeck OC, Szabo P (1980) 4S RNA gene organization in *Drosophila melanogaster*. In: Söll D, Abelson J, Schimmel PR (eds) tRNA: Biological aspects. Cold Spring Harbor Laboratory, Cold Spring Harbor, New York, pp 317–323
Engelke DR, Ng SY, Shastry BS, Roeder RG (1980) Specific interaction of a purified transcription factor with an internal control region of 5S RNA genes. Cell 19: 717–728
Gall JG, Pardue ML (1969) Formation and detection of RNA-DNA hybrid molecules in cytological preparations. Proc Natl Acad Sci USA 63: 378–383
Gergen JP, Loewenberg JY, Wensink PC (1981) $tRNA_2^{Lys}$ gene clusters in *Drosophila*. J Mol Biol 147: 475–499
Grigliatti TA, White BN, Tener GM, Kaufman TC, Holden JJ, Suzuki DT (1974) Studies on the transfer RNA genes of *Drosophila*. Cold Spring Harbor Symp Quant Biol 38: 461–474
Hagenbüchle O, Larson D, Hall GI, Sprague KU (1979) The primary transcription product of a silkworm alanine tRNA gene: Identification of in vitro sites of initiation, termination and processing. Cell 18: 1217–1229
Hershey ND, Davidson N (1980) Two *Drosophila melanogaster* $tRNA^{Gly}$ genes are contained in a direct duplication at chromosomal locus 56F. Nucleic Acids Res 8: 4899–4910
Hofstetter H, Kressmann A, Birnstiel ML (1981) A split promoter for a eukaryotic tRNA gene. Cell 24: 573–585
Hosbach HA, Silberklang M, McCarthy BJ (1980) Evolution of a *D. melanogaster* glutamate tRNA gene cluster. Cell 21: 169–178
Hovemann B, Sharp S, Yamada H, Söll D (1980) Analysis of a *Drosophila* tRNA gene cluster. Cell 19: 889–895
Kiger JA Jr (1974) Participation by *Drosophila* transfer RNA in protein synthesis in an *E. coli* protein synthesizing system. Nucleic Acids Res 1: 1269–1277
Korn LJ, Brown DD (1978) Nucleotide sequence of *Xenopus borealis* oocyte 5S DNA: Comparison of sequences that flank several related eukaryotic genes. Cell 15: 1145–1156
Koski AR, Clarkson SG, Kurjan J, Hall BD, Smith M (1980) Mutations of the yeast SUP4 $tRNA^{Tys}$ locus: Transcription of mutant genes in vitro. Cell 22: 415–425
Kressman A, Clarkson SG, Pirotta V, Birnstiel ML (1978) Transcription of cloned tRNA gene fragments and subfragments injected into the oocyte nucleus of *Xenopus laevis*. Proc Natl Acad Sci USA 75: 1186–1190
Kubli E (1982) The genetics of transfer RNA in *Drosophila*. Adv Genet 21: 123–172
Kubli E, Schmidt T (1978) The localization of $tRNA_4^{Glu}$ genes from *Drosophila melanogaster* by "in situ" hybridization. Nucleic Acids Res 5: 1465–1478
Kubli E, Schmidt T, Egg AH (1980) The localization of the genes for $tRNA_4^{Glu}$ and $tRNA_2^{Asp}$ in *Drosophila melanogaster* by in situ hybridization. In: Söll D, Abelson J, Schimmel PR (eds) tRNA: Biological aspects. Cold Spring Harbor Laboratory, Cold Spring Harbor, New York, pp 309–315
LaRossa R, Söll D (1978) Other roles of tRNA In: Altman S (ed) Transfer RNA. MIT Press, Cambridge, Massachusetts, pp 136–167
Lindsley D, Grell EH (1968) Genetic variations in *Drosophila melanogaster*. Carnegie Inst Wash Publ 627: 152
Meza L, Araya A, Leon G, Krauskopf M, Siddiqui MAQ, Garel JP (1977) Specific alanine-tRNA species associated with fibroin biosynthesis in the posterior silk gland of *Bombyx Mori* L., FEBS Lett 77: 255–260

Okada N, Shindo-Okada N, Sata S, Itoh YH, Oda KI, Nishimura S (1978) Detection of unique tRNA species in tumor tissues by *Escherichia coli* guanine insertion enzyme. Proc Natl Acad Sci USA 75: 4247–4251

Raba M, Limburg K, Burghagen M, Katze JR, Simsek M, Heckman JE, RajBhandary UL, Gross HL (1979) Nucleotide sequence of three isoaccepting Lysine tRNAs from rabbit liver and SV40-transformed mouse fibroblasts. Eur J Biochem 97: 305–318

Ritossa FM, Atwood KC, Spiegelman S (1966) On the redundancy of DNA complementary to amino acid transfer RNA and its absence from the nucleolar organizer region of *Drosophila melanogaster*. Genetics 54: 663–676

Robinson RR, Davidson N (1981) Analysis of a *Drosophila* tRNA gene cluster: Two $tRNA^{Leu}$ genes containing intervening sequences. Cell 23: 251–259

Roeder RG (1976) Eukaryotic nuclear RNA polymerases. In: Losick R, Chamberlin M (eds) RNA Polymerase. Cold Spring Harbor Laboratory, Cold Spring Harbor, New York, pp 285–329

Schmidt O, Mao J, Silverman S, Hovemann B, Söll D (1978) Specific transcription of eukaryotic tRNA genes in *Xenopus* germinal vesicle extracts. Proc Natl Acad Sci USA 75: 4819–4823

Segall J, Matsui T, Roeder RG (1980) Multiple factors are required for the acurate transcription of purified genes by RNA polymerase III. J Biol Chem 225: 11986–11991

Sharp S, DeFranco D, Silberklang M, Hosbach HA, Schmidt T, Kubli E, Gergen JP, Wensink PC, Söll D (1981a) The initiator tRNA genes of *Drosophila melanogaster:* Evidence for a tRNA pseudogene. Nucleic Acids Res 9: 5867–5882

Sharp S, DeFranco D, Dingermann T, Farrell P, Söll D (1981b) Internal control regions for transcription of eukaryotic tRNA genes. Proc Natl Acad Sci USA 78: 6657–6661

Silverman S, Schmidt O, Söll D, Hovemann B (1979) The nucleotide sequence of a cloned *Drosophila* arginine tRNA gene and its in vitro transcription in *Xenopus* germinal vesicle extract. J Biol Chem 254: 10290–10294

Southern EM (1975) Detection of specific sequences among DNA fragments separated by gel electrophoresis. J Mol Biol 98: 503–517

Sprague KU, Hagenbüchle O, Zuniga M (1977) The nucleotide sequence of two silk gland alanine tRNAs: Implications for fibroin synthesis and for initiator tRNA structure. Cell 11: 561–570

Steffensen DM, Wimber DE (1971) Localization of tRNA genes in the salivary chromosomes of *Drosophila* by RNA:DNA hybridization. Genetics 69: 163–178

Tartof KD, Perry RP (1970) The 5S RNA genes of *Drosophila melanogaster.* J Mol Biol 51: 171–183

Tekamp PA, Valenzuela P, Maynard T, Bell GI, Rutter WJ (1979) Specific gene transcription in yeast nuclei and chromatin by added homologous RNA polymerase I and III. J Biol Chem 254: 959–963

Tener GM, Hayashi S, Dunn R, Delaney A, Gillam IC, Grigliatti TA, Kaufman TC, Suzuki DT (1980) tRNA genes in *Drosophila.* In: Söll D, Abelson J, Schimmel PR (eds) tRNA: Biological Aspects. Cold Spring Harbor Laboratory, Cold Spring Harbor, New York, pp 295–307

Weber L, Berger E (1976) Base sequence complexity of the stable RNA species of *Drosophila melanogaster*. Biochemistry 15: 5511–5519

Wensink PC (1978) Sequence homologies within families of *Drosophila melanogaster* middle repetitive DNA. Cold Spring Harbor Symp Quant Biol 42: 1033–1039

White BN, Tener GM, Holden J, Suzuki DT (1973) Analysis of tRNAs during the development of *Drosophila.* Dev Biol 33: 185–195

Yen PH, Davidson N (1980) The gross anatomy of a tRNA gene cluster at region 42A of the *Drosophila melanogaster* chromosome. Cell 22: 137–148

Yen PH, Sodja A, Cohen M Jr, Conrad SE, Wu M, Davidson N, Ilgen C (1977) Sequence arrangement of tRNA genes on a fragment of *Drosophila melanogaster* DNA cloned in *E. coli.* Cell 11: 763–777

Chemical Nature, Properties, Location, and Physiological and Pathological Variations of Modified Nucleosides in tRNAs

G. Dirheimer*

Institut de Biologie Moléculaire et Cellulaire du CNRS, 15 rue Descartes, 67084 Strasbourg, France

Introduction

One of the characteristics of tRNAs is that they contain a variety of atypical (also called modified or rare) nucleosides. Modified nucleosides also occur in other RNAs – mRNAs, rRNAs, small nuclear RNAs (snRNAs) – and even in DNAs, but never in such high proportions. For example, 15 of the total 75 nucleosides in beef liver $tRNA^{Trp}$ are modified (Fournier et al. 1978). Furthermore, the modified nucleosides found in tRNA exhibit a wide range of structural variations: more than 50 have been isolated and characterized. Some are modified by a single methylation of the base or on the 2′ hydroxyl of the ribose moiety, but there are also a number of so-called hypermodified nucleosides with more complex modifications.

General reviews on modified nucleosides have been published (Söll 1971; Hall 1971; Nishimura 1972; Dunn and Hall 1975; Hall and Dunn 1975; McCloskey and Nishimura 1977; Agris and Söll 1977; Feldman 1977; Nishimura 1978a, b; 1979a, b; Dirheimer et al. 1979). Agris edited a book in 1980 which gives a bibliography of biochemical and biophysical studies on modified nucleosides from 1970 to 1979. Reviews on tRNA methylation were published by Borek and Srinivasan in 1966 and Nau in 1976.

In this chapter we try to review the modified nucleosides now known and give their structure, properties, and location in the tRNA molecule. We also describe the variations of the modified nucleosides under different conditions described in the literature.

Chemical Nature of Modified Nucleosides in tRNAs

The most common modified nucleoside is pseudouridine or 5-β-ribofuranosyl uracil (ψ). It was discovered in the 1950s by Cohn (1957, 1960) and Davis and Allen (1957). It does not fit the usual definition of a modified nucleoside because neither the base

* I am grateful to Dr. S. Nishimura, Dr. G. Keith, and Dr. R.P. Martin for critical reading of the manuscript. I thank Dr. K. Randerath and Dr. S. Nishimura and Dr. R. Gupta who made unpublished data available. Some of the results quoted in this paper were obtained during work supported by grants from the Institut National de la Santé et de la Recherche Médicale (Action Thématique 58 and Contrat de Recherche Libre 79.1.154.3)

Recent Results in Cancer Research. Vol. 84

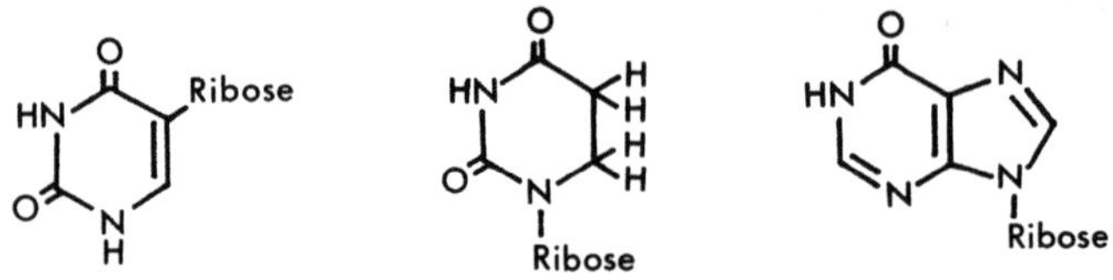

Pseudouridine (Ψ) Dihydrouridine (D or hU) Inosine (I)

Fig. 1. Structures of ψ, D, and I

nor the ribose are substituted, but the usual N-ribosyl linkage is replaced by a carbon-carbon one (Fig. 1) (Cohn 1960). It can represent up to 5.5 mol/100 mol nucleosides (Hall and Dunn 1975). The corresponding 2′-(3′)phosphate was first noticed by Cohn and Volkin (1951) during ion-exchange chromatography of an RNA hydrolysate.

The second most common modified nucleoside is 5,6-dihydrouridine (hU, or better D) (Fig. 1). It was discovered in the first tRNA sequenced (yeast $tRNA^{Ala}$) by Madison and Holley (1957). It has been detected in most specific tRNAs, up to six D residues being present in some tRNAs. However, some tRNAs, such as *Escherichia coli* tyrosine tRNA, do not have D. It does not absorb in the 260 nm region, but does absorb at 230 nm. It is hydrolyzed in alkali with opening of the ring to N^3-ribosyl-2-ureidopropionic acid, which causes loss of absorption at 230 nm. This decrease in absorption can be used (in the absence of other alkali-labile nucleosides) to detect and estimate the amount of D.

The deaminated nucleoside corresponding to adenosine (A), the so-called inosine (I), was also first found in yeast $tRNA^{Ala}$. The corresponding base, hypoxanthine, had previously been isolated from total yeast tRNA (Hall 1963). Inosine is a common degradation product of the purine nucleotides, and therefore very small amounts in tRNA hydrolysates could always come from either biological or alkaline degradation. In tRNAs inosine arises from adenosine as a result of a specific enzymatic deamination. It is widely distributed in eukaryotic tRNAs. Only one sequenced E. coli tRNA contains inosine ($tRNA_1^{Arg}$; Murao et al. 1972). Yeast mitochondrial $tRNA^{Arg}$ may also contain it in the wobble position.

The first family of modified nucleosides are the methylated ones, which differ from their parent nucleosides by one or two methyl groups. As a whole the methylated nucleosides account for 30%–70% of the modified nucleosides in tRNAs. Figure 2 gives the structures of the base methylated nucleosides found in tRNAs. They are: one type of methylated uridine, 5-methyluridine or ribothymidine (T); two methylated cytidines, 3-methylcytidine (m^3C) and 5-methylcytidine (m^5C); one methylated pseudouridine ($m^1\psi$); three methylated adenosines, 1-methyladenosine (m^1A), 2-methyladenosine (m^2A), and N^6-methyladenosine (m^6A); and four methylated guanosines, 1-methylguanosine (m^1G), N^2-methylguanosine (m^2G), $N^{2'}$-N^2-dimethylguanosine (m_2^2G), and 7-methylguanosine (m^7G). A methylated inosine has also been found in several tRNAs.

The tRNAs of almost all organisms contain 5-methyluridine (ribothymidine, = T), although it is absent from several species of plant or mammalian tRNAs. Finally, some species of microorganisms almost completely lack T on their tRNA (for a review see Nishimura 1979a). Mammalian mitochondrial tRNAs have a very low T content, whereas fungi or insect mitochondrial tRNAs have a normal T content (Dirheimer et al. 1979). $m^1\psi$ (first called xU) has very recently been found in several archaebacteria (Gupta and Woese 1980; R. C. Gupta, personal communication).

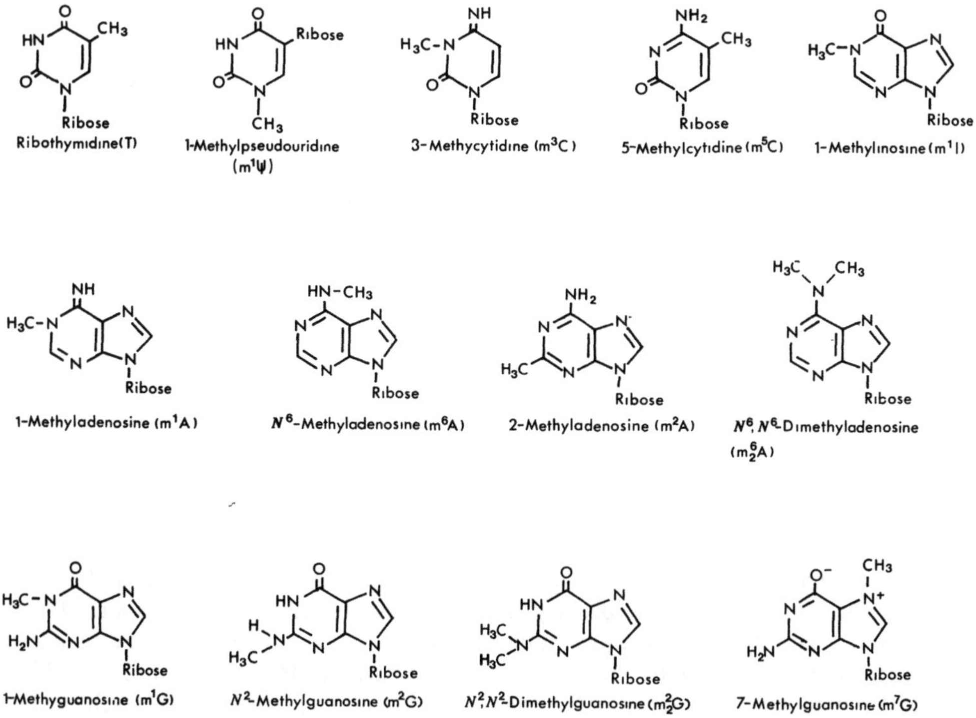

Fig. 2. Structures of the base methylated nucleosides found in tRNAs

5-Methylcytidine occurs in comparatively large amounts in tRNA, and is also found in mammalian DNA. m^3C is unstable in alkali and is converted into a non-ultraviolet-absorbing compound under the conditions normally used for alkaline hydrolysis of tRNAs. Under mild alkaline conditions it is partially converted to 3-methyluridine, and can therefore be overlooked or underestimated in total hydrolysates. These two modified nucleosides were only found in eukaryotic tRNAs.

Of the four methylated derivatives of adenosine, only m^1A is alkali-unstable. It rearranges into m^6A in alkaline solution, but can easily be obtained after acidic or enzymatic hydrolysis. m^6A itself is present in prokaryotic tRNAs, but is much less frequent than m^1A. The corresponding deoxynucleoside occurs naturally in the DNA of several microorganisms. m^2A is relatively abundant in E. coli and also in plant tRNAs. It has not yet been found in a sequenced tRNA from eukaryotes. N^6, N^6-Dimethyladenosine, which occurs in the small subunit ribosomal RNA as a dinucleotide m^6_2A-m^6_2A, has also been found in total tRNA from mammalian tissue by Gross (1975). It came from a contaminating rRNA fragment (Alberty et al. 1978).

1-Methylinosine, first localized in yeast $tRNA^{Ala}$ (Holley et al. 1965) and subsequently in other $tRNAs^{Ala}$, has also been detected in several total tRNAs from plants but not yet in prokaryotic tRNAs.

Of the four methylated derivatives of guanosine found in tRNAs, m^2G and m^2_2G have been found only in eukaryotic tRNAs, whereas m^1G is found in both eukaryotic and prokaryotic tRNAs. m^7G is also present in chloroplastic tRNAs but absent from at least yeast and Neurospora crassa mitochondrial tRNAs (Dirheimer et al. 1979). m^7G

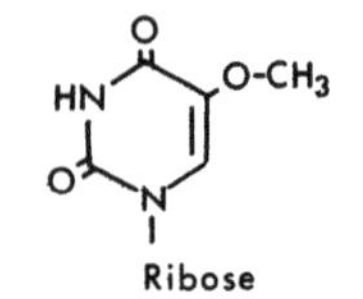

5-Methoxyuridine (mo^5U)

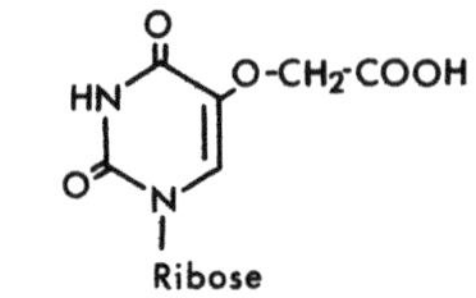

Uridin-5-oxyacetic acid
5-Carboxymethoxyuridine (cmo^5U or o^5U)

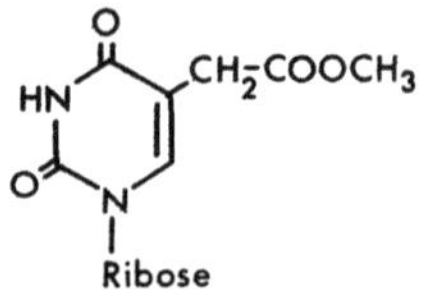

5-(Methoxycarbonylmethyl) uridine (mcm^5U)

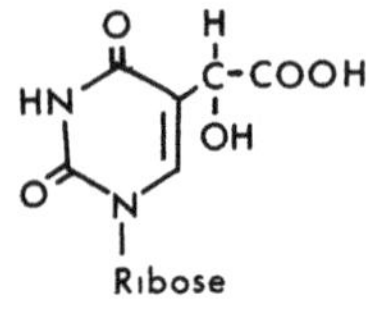

5-(Carboxy-hydroxy-methyl)uridine (chm^5U)

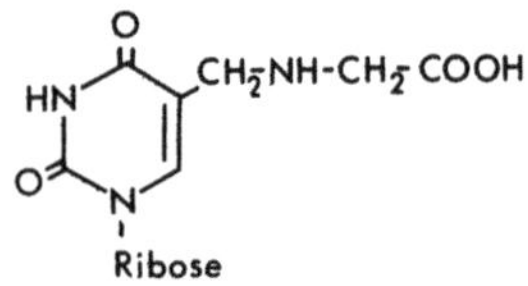

5-Carboxymethyl-aminomethyl uridine ($cmnm^5U$)

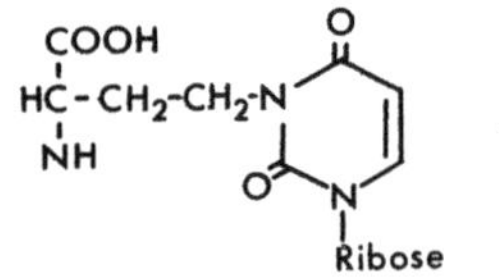

3-(3-Amino-3-carboxypropyl) uridine (acp^3U)

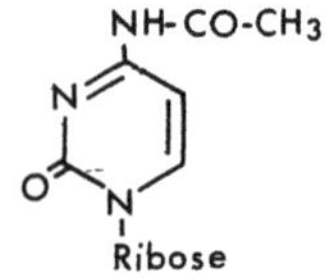

N^4-Acetylcytidine (ac^4C)

Fig. 3. The non-methylated derivatives of U and of C

has a quaternary ammonium and is unstable at alkaline and neutral pH. The corresponding nucleotide is rapidly degraded on Dowex-1 resin at pH 7.5 and 20° C (Dunn and Flack 1970). Therefore it has sometimes been overlooked even after enzymatic hydrolysis (Bonnet et al. 1974). A trimethylated guanosine, N^2, N^2, 7-trimethylguanosine, found in snRNAs (U_1, U_2, U_3, and U_5) (Reddy and Busch 1981) has never been found in tRNAs.

Ribose methylated nucleosides called $O^{2'}$-methylated nucleosides, corresponding to the four major ribonucleosides, to ψ, and to T, have been found in tRNAs, the latter so far only in a rabbit liver $tRNA^{Lys}$ (Gross et al. 1974). Let us recall that the $O^{2'}$-methylnucleoside 3′ phosphate → 5′ bond is alkaline- and ribonuclease-resistant.

Another family of modified nucleosides is formed by the derivatives of U in position 5. Seven of them have been described (Fig. 3). Although 5-hydroxyuridine has not yet been found in a sequenced tRNA, it was shown by Singhal and Vold (1976) to be present in a tRNA of Bacillus subtilis. It has also been seen in a submethylated $tRNA^{Val}$ from E. coli (Murao et al. 1978). This is not surprising, as this nucleoside is the precursor of two derivatives which have been well characterized in prokaryotic tRNAs. They are 5-methoxyuridine (mo^5U) and 5-carboxymethoxyuridine, which is also called uridine-5-oxyacetic acid, was first designated as V (cmo^5U or o^5U), and has a free carboxyl group (Murao et al. 1970).

As pointed out by Yamada et al. (1981), the carboxylation or decarboxylation patterns of some substituents at the 5 position of the uracil ring are completely opposite in tRNAs from B. subtilis and those from E. coli (Table 1). The meaning of this interesting finding must await further elucidation.

The four other uridine derivatives substituted by a carbon-carbon linkage in position 5 are:

1. 5-Methoxycarbonylmethyluridine (mcm^5U), also called 5-methylcarboxymethyl-uridine, which is the methyl ester of 5-carboxymethyluridylic acid. It is very labile in both alkali and acid.

2. The amide of 5-carboxymethyluridylic acid, isolated by Dunn and Trigg (1972, 1973) from cold acid hydrolysates of tRNA from yeast, wheat embryo, and bean

Table 1. Modified nucleosides in the wobble position of B. subtilis and E. coli tRNAs

	B. subtilis tRNAs	E. coli tRNAs
mo^5U	Val, Ala, Thr	
cmo^5U		Val, Ala, Ser
$cmnm^5s^2U$	Lys	
mnm^5s^2U		Lys, Glu, Gln

leaves. In yeast the ester and the amide are both present, whereas in wheat embryos only the latter was found.
3. 5-Carboxymethylaminomethyluridine ($cmnm^5U$ or $cmam^5U$), found in B.subtilis $tRNA^{Gly}$ (Ishikura et al. 1980). The corresponding 5-methylaminomethyluridine has not yet been found in a sequenced tRNA, although its 2-thiolated derivative has been found in several bacterial tRNAs.
4. 5-Carboxyhydroxymethyluridine (chm^5U), recently found in $tRNA_2^{Gly}$ from Bombyx mori.
The first two and the last are found in eukaryotes only, the third in prokaryotes.
Finally, there is another derivative of U, called X before being characterized by Ohashi et al. (1974). It is 3-(3-amino-3-carboxypropyl)uridine (acp^3U), and occurs in both prokaryotes and eukaryotes.
There are fewer nonmethylated derivatives of cytidine than of uridine. Only N^4-acetylcytidine (ac^4C), first characterized by Zachau et al. (1966) in yeast $tRNA^{Ser}$, has been found both in prokaryotes and in eukaryotes. It is localized at different places in the tRNA molecule.
Several thioderivatives of the different pyrimidic nucleosides mentioned above have been characterized in tRNAs (Fig. 4). 4-Thiouridine (s^4U) is very common in prokaryotic tRNA but has not been found in eukaryotic or mitochondrial tRNAs (Martin et al. 1976). This nucleoside is very sensitive to irradiation with light of wavelength 300–380 nm. It is also sensitive to hot acid or ammonia. 2-Thiouridine (s^2U) was recently located in Drosophila $tRNA^{Glu}$ (Altweg and Kubli 1980), whereas 2-thiocytidine (s^2C) was located in several prokaryotic tRNAs.
Several more complex 2-thioderivatives of U were also found. First 5-methyl-2-thiouridine, a 2-thioderivative of T (s^2T), was found in $tRNA^{Glu}$ and $tRNA^{Lys}$ of rat liver (Kimura-Harada et al. 1971), but this deserves further investigation. It was also characterized in Thermus thermophilus $tRNA_1^{Met}$ (Watanabe et al. 1979). Three other 2-thioderivatives were found: 5-(methoxycarbonylmethyl)2-thiouridine (mcm^5s^2U), which was found only in Saccharomyces cerevisiae or Schizosaccharomyces pombe, and 5-(methylaminomethyl)-2-thiouridine (mnm^5s^2U) and 5-(carboxymethylaminomethyl)-2-thiouridine ($cmnm^5s^2U$) (Yamada et al. 1981), which were found only in prokaryotes, as already pointed out.
An unknown derivative of uridine exists in the wobble position of yeast (Sibler et al. 1980; our unpublished results) and N.crassa mitochondrial tRNAs (Heckman et al. 1980) and in rat liver mitochondrial tRNAs (K. Randerath, H.P. Agrawal, and E. Randerath, personal communication), restricting in these organelles the wobble of U

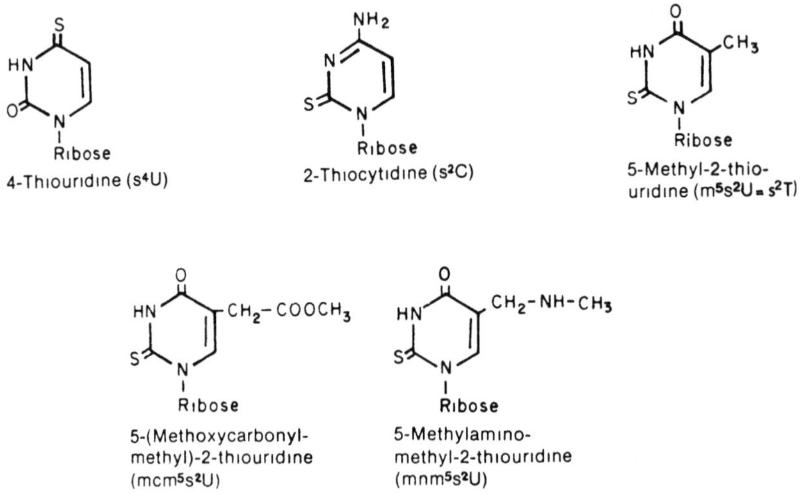

Fig. 4. Some thioderivatives of pyrimidic nucleosides

to A and G, whereas the unmodified U in these same organelles pairs with all four typical nucleosides A, G, U, and C.

The different substituents on the four typical nucleosides we have seen up to now were straight chains or single S atoms. However, more complex substitutions occur on purine nucleosides, the first family of these being N^6-threoninocarbonyladenosine (t^6A) (Fig. 5), which is also called *N*-[9-(*β*-D-ribofuranosyl)purin-6-ylcarbamoyl]threonine. It is not detected in alkaline hydrolysates of tRNAs because of its conversion to adenosine, but can be isolated by using acid or enzymatic hydrolysis. It is widely distributed in prokaryotic and eukaryotic cellular tRNAs and in mitochondrial tRNAs. The corresponding glycine derivative has been detected in yeast tRNA (Schweizer et al. 1970), but not yet in a sequenced tRNA. Other amino acid analogs may also exist in tRNAs (Hall 1964). Related compounds lacking a free carboxyl group have been detected in tRNA of E.coli, yeast, and plant tRNA (Dunn and Trigg 1973; Dunn and Flack 1970). The methylthioderivative of t^6A (ms^2t^6A) was recently detected in B.subtilis $tRNA^{Lys}_{1}$ (Yamada and Ishikura 1981) and rabbit liver $tRNA^{Lys}_{3}$ (Yamaizumi et al. 1979; Raba et al. 1979). The N^6-methylated derivative of t^6A (mt^6A) (N^6-methyl-N^6-threoninocarbonyladenosine) was also found first in E.coli by Kimura-Harada et al. (1971) and subsequently in hydrolysates of wheat embryo. It has been localized in rat liver $tRNA^{Ser}_{3}$ and in E.coli and spinach chloroplast $tRNAs^{Thr}$.

Finally, a derivative of t^6A having an aminotriol moiety attached to the carboxyl group of threonine by an amide linkage was found in E.coli $tRNA^{Met}_{2}$. However, this was demonstrated to be an artifact coming from the Tris buffer of the suspension medium used when E.coli cells were harvested, the substitution of tris(hydroxymethyl)aminomethane onto t^6A having occurred biologically in intact E.coli cells (Kasai et al. 1976a).

Another family of adenosine derivatives has a N^6-isopentenyl substitution (Fig. 6). It is N^6-(Δ^2-isopentenyl)adenosine, more commonly called N^6-isopentenyladenosine (i^6A), which is very soluble in organic solvents and has been found predominantly in cellular eukaryotic and mitochondrial tRNA, but also in small quantities in prokaryotes. Its

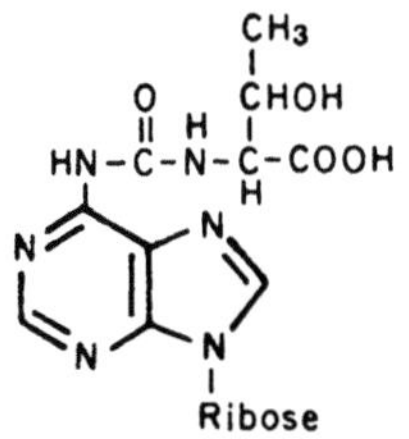

N-[N-(9-β-D-Ribofuranosylpurin-6-yl) carbamoyl]threonine (t6A)

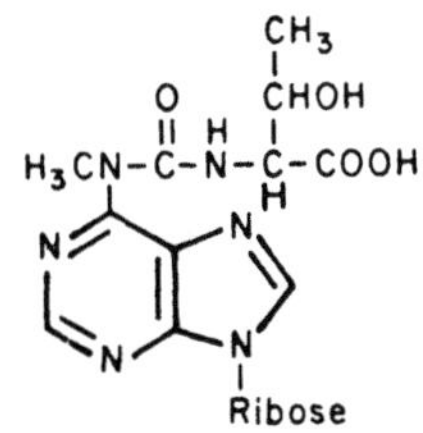

N-[N-(9-β-D-Ribofuranosylpurin-6-yl) N-methylcarbamoyl] threonine (mt6A)

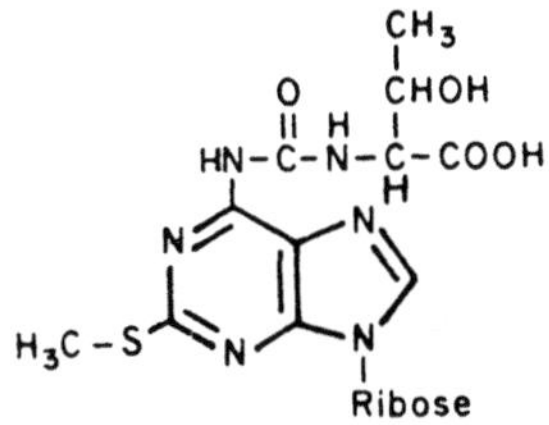

N-[N-(9-β-D-Ribofuranosyl 2-methylthiopurin-6-yl) carbamoyl] threonine (ms2t6A)

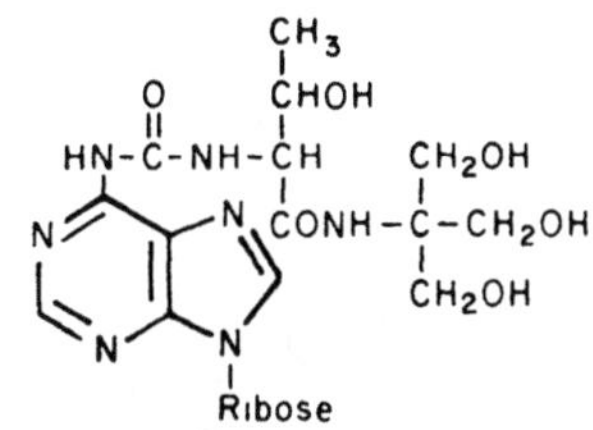

N-[N-[(9-β-D-Ribofuranosylpurin-6-yl) carbamoyl]threonyl] 2-amido-2-hydroxymethylpropane-1, 3-diol

Fig. 5. The t^{6}A family of purine nucleosides

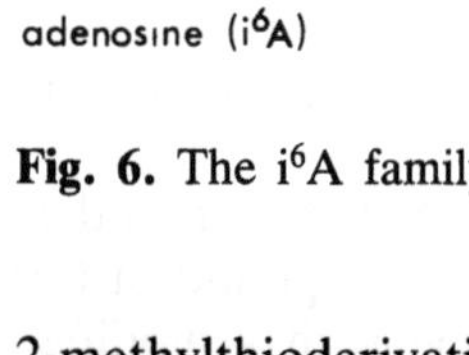

N^6 Isopentenyl adenosine (i^{6}A)

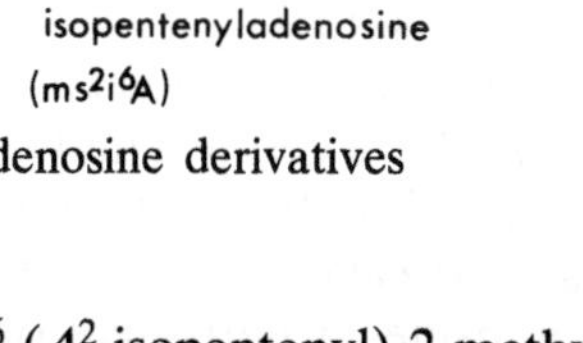

2-Methylthio-N^6-isopentenyladenosine (ms^{2}i^{6}A)

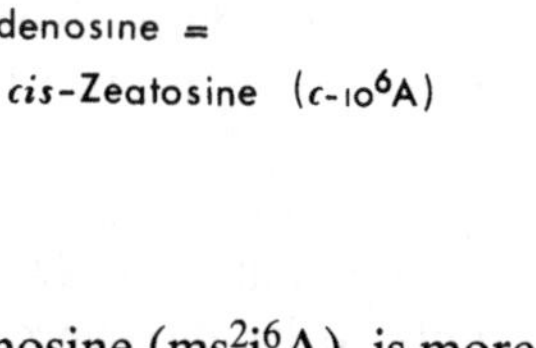

N^6-(*cis*-4-Hydroxyisopentenyl) adenosine = *cis*-Zeatosine (*c*-io^{6}A)

Fig. 6. The i^{6}A family of adenosine derivatives

2-methylthioderivative, N^6-(Δ^2-isopentenyl)-2-methylthioadenosine (ms^{2}i^{6}A), is more often found in bacteria, although small amounts of the nonthiolated compounds are sometimes present. In wheat embryo tRNAs it seems largely replaced by a hydroxyderivative N^6-(cis-4-hydroxyisopentenyl) adenosine, also called 6-(cis-4-hydroxy-3-methylbutyl-2-enyl)adenosine or cis-zeatosine (*cis*-io^{6}A) and the corresponding methylthio compound (ms^{2}io^{6}A) (Hall et al. 1967; Hecht et al. 1969; Burrows et al. 1970). Some evidence (Thimmappaya and Cherayil 1974) suggests that Pseudomonas aeruginosa tRNA contains 2-methylthiozeatosine. It has not yet been located in a sequenced tRNA. Cis-zeatosine has also been identified in tRNA from Corynebac-

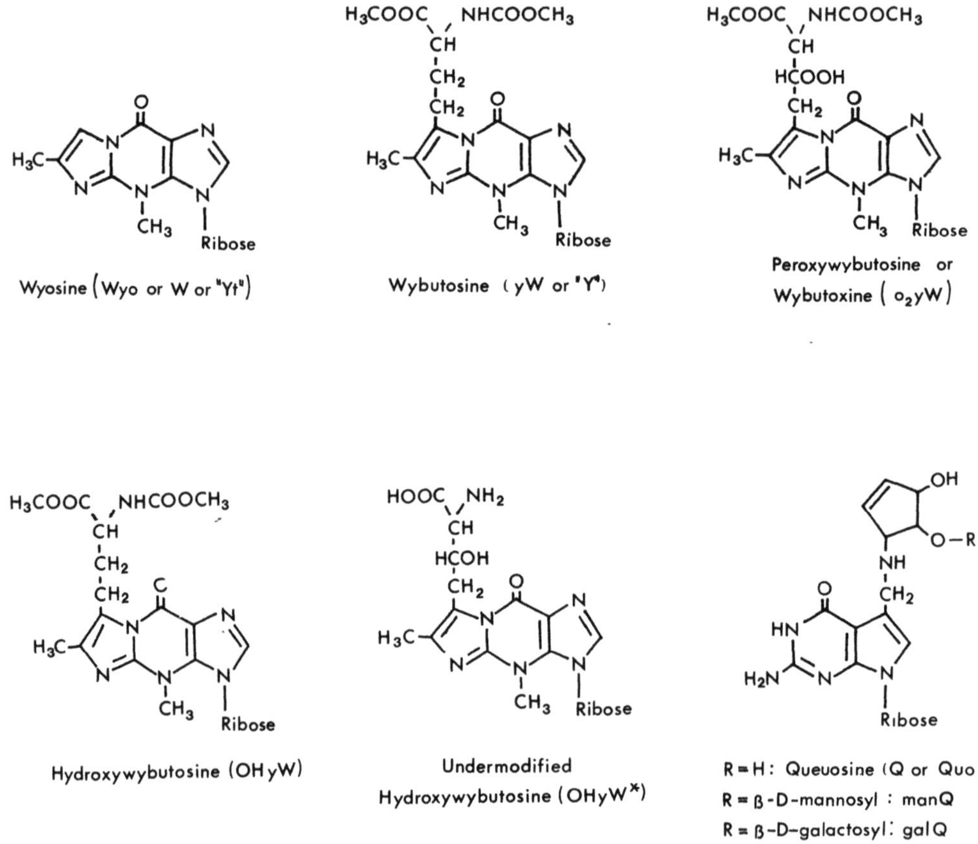

Fig. 7. The W and Q family of hypermodified nucleosides

terium fascians (Einset and Skoog 1977), and trans-zeatosine has been found in the soluble fraction of plant tissue and also in a tRNA hydrolysate of a plant pathogenic bacterium Agrobacter tumefasciens (Chapman et al. 1976). According to Vrejman (1973), the ratio of cis-io^6A to trans-io^6A is 97.5 : 2.5 and that of cis-ms^2io^6A to trans-ms^2io^6A is 47 : 53 in 7-day-old pea shoots. In field-grown pea shoots the ratio of cis- to trans-derivatives of ms^2io^6A is 80 : 20.

Finally, there are two families of hypermodified nucleosides more or less related to guanosine (Fig. 7). The first one is the wyosine family.

Wyosine (or W) is a 1-N^2-isopropeno-3-methylguanosine (Fig. 7). It was found in Torulopsis utilis $tRNA^{Phe}$ and was first called Yt. In fact the first compound of this family to be discovered was wybutosine, a derivative of wyosine with a modified aminobutyric side chain. It was first designated Y and is now abbreviated $(MeO)_2$FnBtoWyo (for [7-3-(methoxycarbonyl)-3-(methoxyformamido)propyl]wyosine), or more simply yW. It was found in yeast $tRNA^{Phe}$. This is also the case for the hydroperoxy derivative of wybutosine, named peroxywybutosine (o_2yW) which was found in wheat germ, Lupinus luteus, chicken, and rat $tRNA^{Phe}$ (Nakanishi et al. 1971; Feinberg et al. 1974). This o_2yW could be an artifact coming from hydroxywybutosine OHyW originally present in the $tRNA^{Phe}$ (Kasai et al. 1979). Very recently a unmodified wybutosine lacking a methoxy and a acetyl moiety on the side chain (Fig.

7) was detected in tumor specific $tRNA^{Phe}$ (Kuchino et al. 1981b). All these derivatives are fluorescent.

The last family of modified nucleosides is that of queuosine (Q or Quo). Its purine skeleton is itself modified to a 7-deaza structure and it has a cyclopentenediol as a side chain (Kasai et al. 1975a) (Fig. 7). Their relative stereochemistries have been determined as 3,4-trans and 4,5-cis on the basis of NMR comparison with synthetic models. In addition, absolute configuration was determined by X-ray analysis of 5′-phosphate of Q (Yokoyama et al. 1979). Q was originally isolated from E.coli but is widely distributed in various organisms (Kasai et al. 1975b). Kasai et al. (1976b) have shown that the tRNAs of various animals contain a new nucleotide Q*, which was isolated from rabbit liver. It consists of a mixture of β-D-mamosyl Q(~ 75%) and β-D-galactosyl Q (~ 25%) in which the sugar is linked through a glycosidic bond to the 4-OH of the cyclopentenediol (Fig. 7).

Several other modified nucleosides will probably be found when more mammalian or plant tRNA sequences are known, since these tRNAs are very rich in modified bases. Even in published sequences there are nucleosides for which the structures were not determined (for a compilation see Gauss and Sprinzl 1981). This is often the case with tRNAs whose primary sequences were determined by radioactive methods, like T_4-coded or E.coli tRNAs. They are mostly derivatives of uridine. These unknown compounds are generally located in the anticodon region, and it is therefore of special interest to establish their structure in order to understand the mechanism of codon-anticodon interactions.

In some eukaryotic tRNAs also, several modified nucleosides have not yet been identified, for example a nucleoside Z which replaces T in loop 4. According to Chen and Roe (1978), it is not identical to any reported E.coli or mammalian nucleoside as judged by mobility in several solvents on cellulose, PEI cellulose, or silica gel TLC.

Localization of Modified Nucleosides

In the cloverleaf model of tRNA the modified nucleosides are located in specific regions depending on their structure rather than at random in the polynucleotide chain. The numbering system used is given in Fig. 8.

Twenty different places can be occupied by ψ in the different loops and stems of the tRNA molecule, with the exception of the variable loop, loop 3 (Fig. 9). The localization is not exactly the same in eukaryotes and prokaryotes; that is in eukaryotic tRNAs only it is found at positions 1,20 : 1, 25, 26, 27, 28, 31, 35, and 57. In yeast $tRNA^{Trp}$ there is even a sequence of three ψ in positions 26–28 (Keith et al. 1972). Position 55 is almost always occupied by ψ preceded by T, which has been found only at position 54 (for exceptions see Dirheimer et al. 1979).

Dihydrouridine is located essentially in the so-called D-loop (loop 1) and sometimes in loop 3 (often after m^7G). Loop 1 can contain up to five Ds with a sequence of three Ds in tyrosine tRNAs from various yeasts (Fig. 9).

Inosine was found only in the wobble position of the anticodon, where it is believed to pair with U, C, or A in the third position of the codon, according to the wobble hypothesis of Crick (1966). However, very recently Munz et al. (1981) using a genetic approach and under in vivo conditions, showed that a I-containing $tRNA^{Ser}_{IGA}$ cannot read UCA, which rules out a I · A pairing.

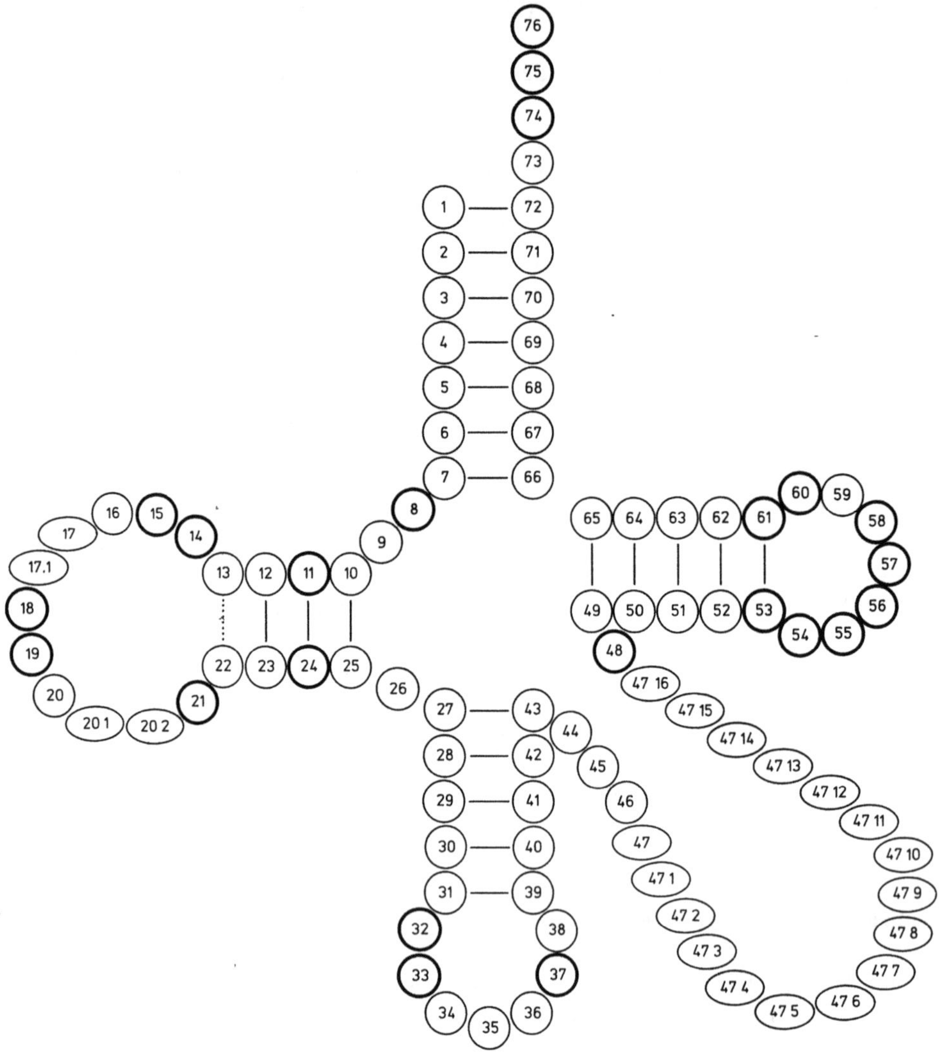

Fig. 8. Numbering system of nucleosides in tRNAs based on yeast $tRNA^{Phe}$. At the positions where the number of nucleosides varies, i.e., before and after the two constant GMP residues (18,19) in the D-loop and in the extra arm, nucleosides can be inserted or omitted as required; 17 and 17 : 1, 20 : 1 and 20 : 2, 47 : 1 to 47 : 16

The localization of the methylated nucleosides is as follows (Fig. 9): m^3C is located in loop 2 and 3, whereas m^5C has been found in the wobble position but also at positions 38, 39, and 40 and between loop 3 and the Tψ stem, sometimes as a sequence of two or even three contiguous m^5Cs in wheat germ, Bombyx mori, and human placenta $tRNA^{Gly}$ (Marcu et al. 1977; Garel and Keith 1977; Gupta et al. 1979). T is only located in loop 4.

1-Methyladenosine is found in eukaryotes essentially in loop 4 at position 58 [there is one exception, $tRNA_1^{Met}$ of the bacteria Thermus thermophilus (Watanabe et al. 1979)], also sometimes in eukaryotes at position 14 and in prokaryotes at position 22 in loop 1.

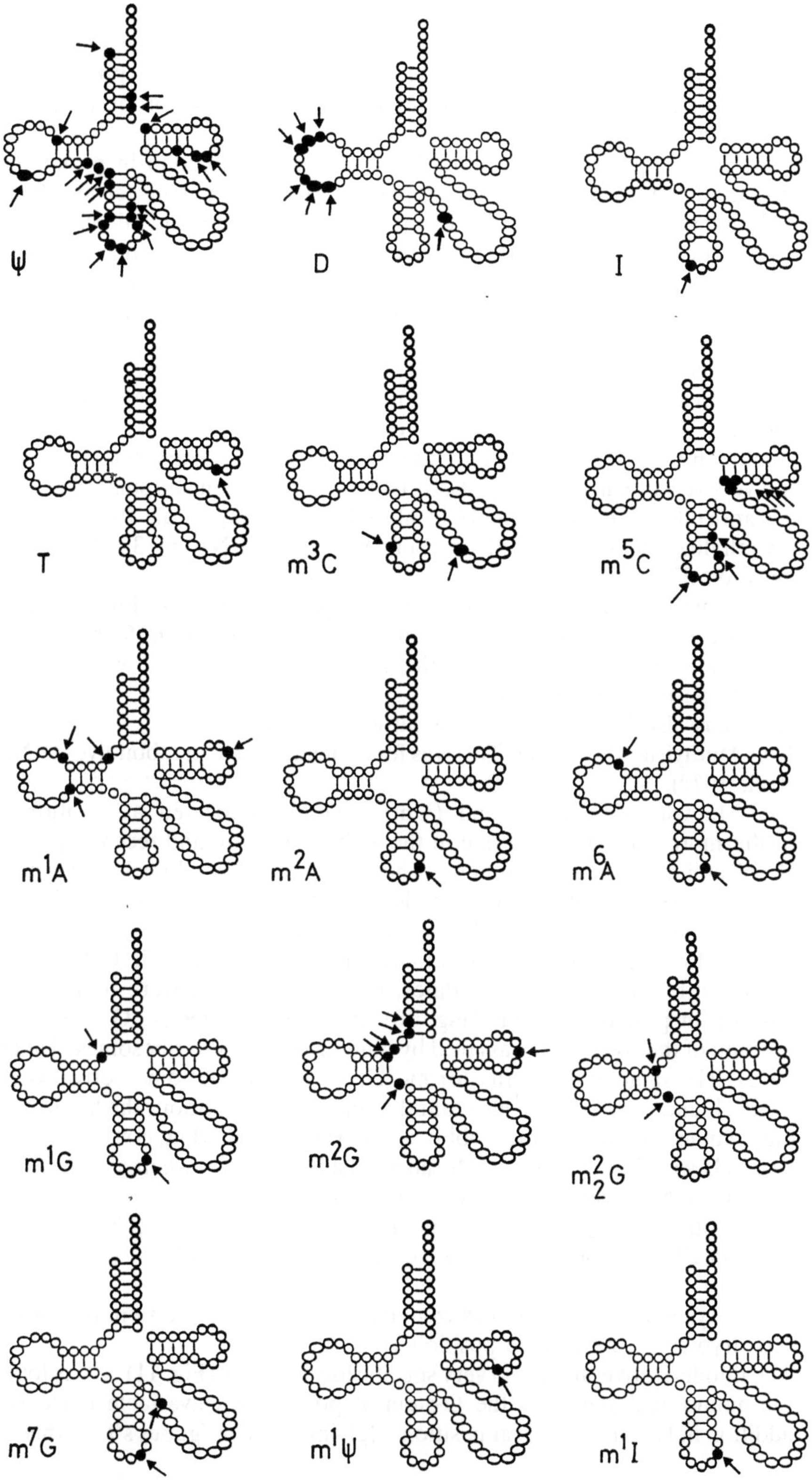

Fig. 9. Positions occupied by various modified nucleosides

m^1A has also been localized recently in position 9 in rat mitochondrial $tRNA^{Leu}$, $tRNA^{Asp}$, $tRNA^{Arg}$, $tRNA^{Val}$, $tRNA^{Trp}$, $tRNA^{Phe}$, $tRNA^{Gly}$, and $tRNA^{Lys}$ (Agrawal et al. 1981a, b; K. Randerath et al. 1981 and see this vol., pp. 103–120).
2-Methyladenosine is found only in prokaryotes and chloroplasts in 3′ after the anticodon.
*N*⁶-Methyladenosine is also found in 3′ after the anticodon in prokaryotes and at position 14 in Euglena gracilis cytoplasmic $tRNA^{Phe}$ (Chang et al. 1976).
1-Methylguanosine was found in eukaryotic, prokaryotic, and mitochondrial tRNA in 3′ after the anticodon. It was also found in position 9 between the aminoacyl stem and the D-arm, whereas m^2G has been located at five positions in the same area (positions 6, 7, 9, 10, and 26). Thus position 9 can be occupied either by m^1G or by m^2G.
$N^{2'}$-N^2-Dimethylguanosine was located at position 26 between the D-arm and the anticodon arm and very recently at position 10 in several tRNAs from Halobacterium volcanii (R. C. Gupta, personal communication).
Finally, m^7G has been found in both prokaryotes and eukaryotes in the variable loop and very recently in the chloroplastic $tRNA_3^{Leu}$ from bean and spinach at position 36 in the anticodon (Osorio-Almeida et al. 1980; Canaday et al. 1980).
1-Methylinosine was located only in eukaryotic tRNA in 3′ after the anticodon (position 37).
Ribose methylated nucleosides have also specific positions (Fig. 10). 2′-*O*-Methylguanosine (Gm) occurs in loop 1 (positions 18 and 19, position 19 only in prokaryotes). In position 18 it represents one of the invariant nucleosides. It was also located in the wobble position and at position 39.
(ψm) has also been found in this latter position.
2′-O-Methylribothymidine (Tm) was found instead of T in rabbit liver $tRNA^{Lys}$ (Raba et al. 1979).
2′-*O*-Methylcytidine (Cm) and (Um) have been located at positions 4 and 32 furthermore Cm was also found in the wobble position and recently at position 56 in H.volcanii and Um at position 44. These 2′-*O*-methylated nucleosides are located in the most exposed regions of the molecule, suggesting that these methyl groups may well be there for protection from ribonuclease attack.
2′-*O*-Methyladenosine has not yet been located in a specific tRNA.
Of the different substituted uridines, mo^5U and cmo^5U were found at the wobble position in prokaryotes only (Fig. 10). mo^5U recognizes A, G and U in the third position of the codon when assayed by binding of tRNA to ribosomes (Takemoto et al. 1973). The same may be true for mo^5U. Three other uridine derivatives, $cmnm^5U$, mcm^5U, and chm^5U, were also found at the wobble position, the latter in eukaryotes only. $cmnm^5U$ enlarges the wobble and permits the binding not only to A and G but also to U with 50% efficiency (Murao and Ishikura 1978), whereas mcm^5U restricts the pairing to A (Weissenbach and Dirheimer 1978).
On the other hand, acp^3U was found in mammalian $tRNA^{Asn}$ (Chen and Roe 1978) at position 20 : 1 in loop 1 and in several prokaryotic tRNAs at position 47 in loop 3 (Fig. 10).
*N*⁴-Acetylcytidine (ac^4C) is localized in eukaryotes in the D-stem (position 12) and in prokaryotes in the wobble position (Fig. 10).
The thioderivatives have also very specific localizations (Fig. 11): s^4U is found between the amino acid stem and the D-stem at position 8 (invariable nucleoside) and in addition in E.coli $tRNA^{Tyr}$ at position 9 (giving two contiguous s^4U in this tRNA). s^2U

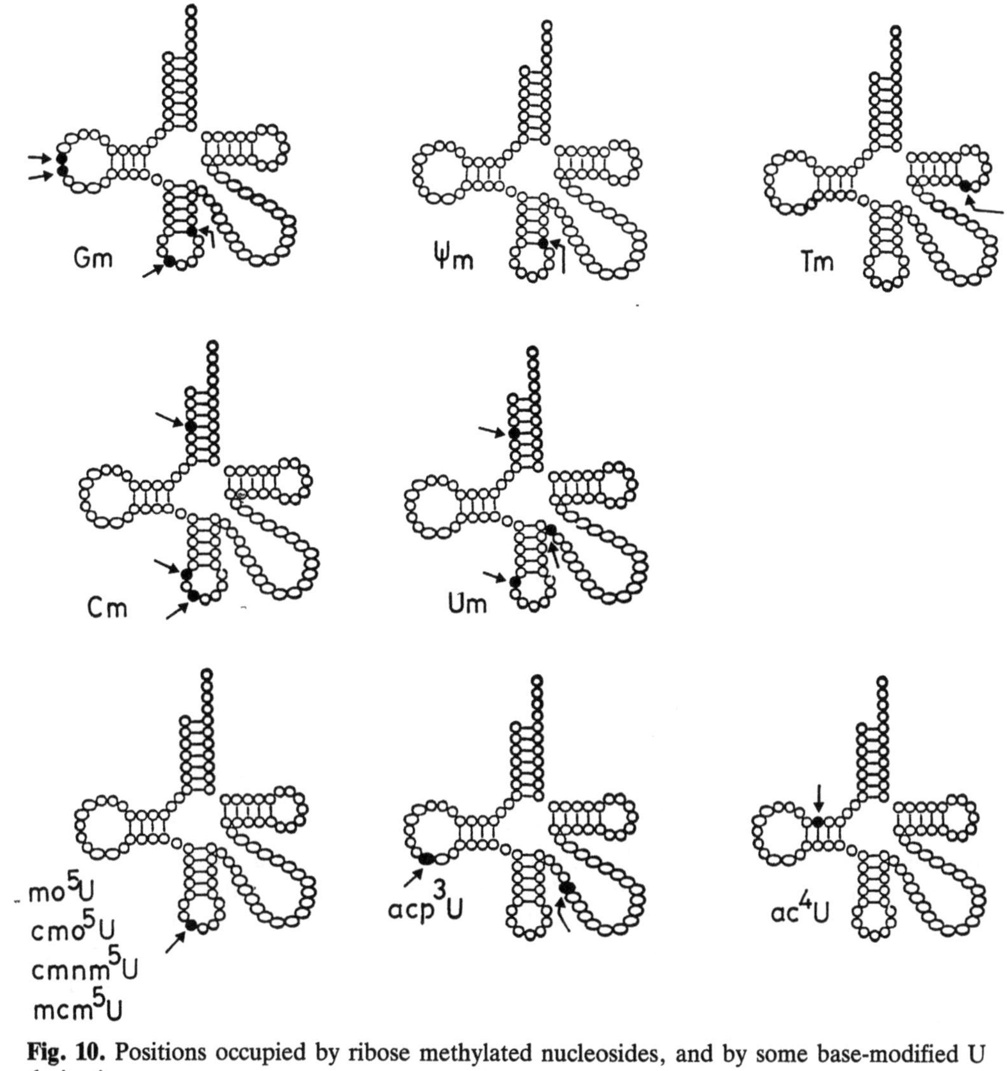

Fig. 10. Positions occupied by ribose methylated nucleosides, and by some base-modified U derivatives

was recently located in the wobble position of Drosophila tRNA$_4^{Glu}$ (Altweg and Kubli 1980). s^{2}T is found in place of T in Thermus thermophilus tRNA$_1^{Met}$ (Watanabe et al. 1979). On the basis of the restricted coding properties of tRNA^{Glu} and tRNA^{Lys} of rat liver, Kimura-Harada et al. (1971) suggested that s^{2}T may even occur in the anticodon of these tRNAs, but this has not yet been demonstrated. s^{2}C is found at the 5′ end of the anticodon loop (position 32) in prokaryotic tRNAs. The other thioderivatives of U, mcm^{5}s^{2}U and cmnm^{5}s^{2}U, are located in the wobble position and restrict codon recognition, only being able to pair with A.

N^6-Isopentenyladenosine and t^{6}A, as well as their thioderivatives and mt^{6}A, have been found adjacent to the 3′ site of the anticodon. i^{6}A or its derivatives are almost always found in tRNA that recognize codons starting with U, whereas most tRNAs that

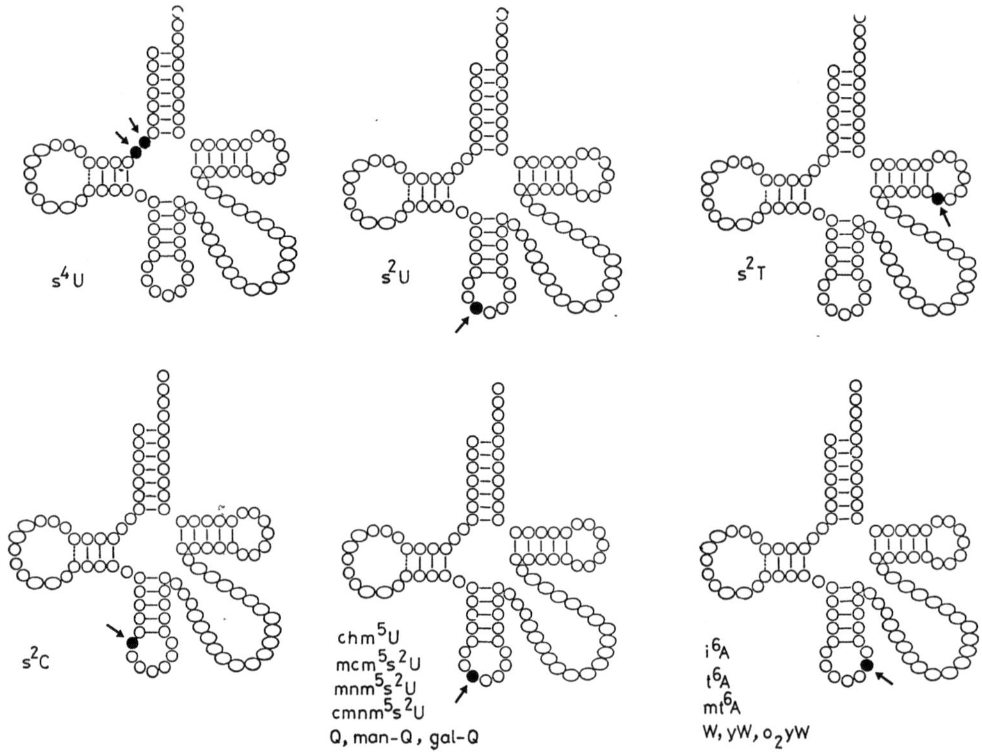

Fig. 11. Positions occupied by thioderivatives, and by some hypermodified nucleosides

recognize codons starting with A contain hydrophilic modified nucleosides such as t^6A or its derivatives (for the relationship between the nucleosides located adjacent to the anticodon and codon recognition of tRNAs see Nishimura 1979a + b). As recently shown, t^6A plays a role in the stabilization of the U · A and U · G base pairs adjacent to the 5′ side of the modified nucleoside, most probably by stacking (Weissenbach and Grosjean 1981).

The wyosine nucleosides have also been found adjacent to the 3′ side of the anticodon. They are characteristic of eukaryotic $tRNAs^{Phe}$, although Drosophila and Bombyx mori $tRNAs^{Phe}$ have m^1G in this position (Altweg and Kubli 1979; Keith and Dirheimer 1980).

Finally, the Q nucleosides have been found at the wobble position of tRNAs, Q being found in both eukaryotic and prokaryotic tRNAs whereas the mannosyl- and galactosylderivatives are found only in various animal tRNAs.

In conclusion, post-transcriptional modifications were found in 43 of the 76 positions shown in Fig. 8 (positions 17 : 1, 20 : 1, 20 : 2, etc. were not taken into account). Thus more than half of the positions can be modified. However, their localization is not uniform along the tRNA molecule, as only a very small number of tRNAs are modified in the last quarter of the molecule (nucleotides 59–76). In 32 of 41 positions only one type of modification has been found. Thus three-quarters of the positions are "reserved" for one type of modification. Five positions can present two types of modifications, but in three cases these modifications are similar: Um or Cm in position 4, m^2G or m^2_2G in position 10, m^6A or m^1A in position 14. Two positions (9 and 16) can have three modifications. Finally five postions (32, 34, 37, 39, and 54), of which four are in the anticodon loop, can be modified in four or more different ways. Let us however emphasize that in two of these "hot spots" (positions 32 and 54) only modified pyrimidines are found, whereas in the wobble position and in the position located on the 3′ side of the anticodon (positions 34 and 37) numerous modifications are observed.

The localization of the nucleosides given in this paper applies to the published structures (for a review see Gauss and Sprinzl 1981) and will certainly be modified when new structures are published. Supporting evidence for this prediction comes from the study of specificity of tRNA-modifying enzymes. For example, the existence of an enzyme methylating A22 in B. subtilis was demonstrated (Raettig et al. 1977) before the corresponding modification was found in that position in tRNA (Menichi et al. 1980). Furthermore, plant mitochondrial or chloroplastic methyltransferases methylate an A on a cytoplasmic tRNA at position 7 for which no methylation has yet been found (Dubois et al. 1974).

Variations of Modified Nucleosides in tRNA

Evidence for changing patterns of isoaccepting tRNA species under a variety of different conditions have been obtained with prokaryotes, mitochondria, plants, and animals. They may occur through variations in the biosynthesis of the different isoacceptors, lack of their 3′-terminal nucleotides, changes in tertiary structure, denaturation, limited digestion, or different post-transcriptional modification. The isoacceptors belonging to this last class of tRNAs are sometimes easy to separate, since the presence or absence of a particular modified nucleoside may greatly change the chromatographic or electrophoretic mobility of tRNAs. For example, brewer's yeast contains two forms of $tRNA_3^{Arg}$ with identical nucleotide sequences, except that one form has t^6A in position 37 and the other an unmodified A in this position (Weissenbach 1977). They are separated by reversed-phase column chromatography. On the other hand, isoaccepting species with other modifications like replacement of U by ψ, D, or T or 2′-*O*-methylations are difficult to separate and can only be detected by sequence studies. For example, beef liver $tRNA^{Trp}$, which has several incompletely modified nucleosides (m^2G, Cm, m^7G) and three differences in the major nucleotides (two $C \rightarrow D$ and one $G \rightarrow A$) (Fournier et al. 1978) is composed of at least three tRNAs but can be a mixture of many more different molecules. Two-dimensional polyacrylamide-gel-electrophoresis gives five different spots, but we have not yet determined which modification or sequence belongs to each of these spots.

Let us now focus our attention, first in prokaryotes and then in eukaryotes, on the variations of the isoaccepting tRNAs which differ from each other in their modified nucleosides.

Prokaryotic tRNAs

Alterations of the tRNA chromatographic pattern during growth and sporulation of B. subtilis have been known for a long time (Kaneko and Doi 1966; Lazzarini 1966). Vold (1973) made an extensive study of these differences for tRNAs corresponding to

19 amino acids. These changes were studied in detail for lysine, valine, tyrosine, and phenylalanine tRNAs.

Lazzarini (1966) showed the existence of one major peak of $tRNA_2^{Lys}$ in vegetative cells of B. subtilis, whereas two peaks were present in sporulating preparations. Contradictory results were obtained by Chuang et al. (1971), Chuang and Doï (1972), and Vold (1970, 1975, 1978). According to Vold, four $tRNAs^{Lys}$ exist; a change in the ratio of the two major species occurs during the growth cycle. The predominant species in spore tRNA is thought to be preferentially bound to ribosomes. The variations observed by these authors could come from different post-transcriptional modifications.

In the case of $tRNA^{Val}$, contradictory results were also obtained by Doï and co-workers (Kaneko and Doï 1966; Doï et al. 1968 and Heyman et al. 1967, 1970). A reversal in the ratio of two forms of $tRNA^{Val}$ separated by chromatography on methylated serum albumin was observed by Doï et al. during the early stationary phase. However, analysis of charging kinetics by Heyman et al. showed that form I, separated by chromatography, has a lower affinity for the valyl-tRNA synthetase than form II. Therefore an apparent variation in the ratio of the two species could be observed in the case of low valine concentration, form I not being aminoacylated to a fully saturated level.

Heyman et al. concluded that form II remains constant throughout the growth cycle. Form I always exists as the predominant species, although it decreases slightly in stationary phase. According to kinetic studies this variation might be due to the disappearance of one minor constituent in stationary phase. However, no relationship was established between this variation and sporulation.

A third tRNA from B. subtilis which shows modification of chromatographic profiles is $tRNA^{Tyr}$. This was first demonstrated by Arceneaux and Sueoka (1969) who found that there was a balance between two tyrosine tRNAs, one ($tRNA_1^{Tyr}$) being predominant during logarithmic growth and the other ($tRNA_2^{Tyr}$) during stationary phase and in spores, the total of the two tRNAs being constant. Working with asporogenic bacteria, McMillian and Arceneaux (1975) later showed that there was no direct correlation between these modifications and sporulation. The question was resolved by Keith et al. (1976) and Menichi et al. (1980), who isolated and sequenced the two forms of $tRNA^{Tyr}$. The two forms differ only in the modification state of the nucleoside in 3′ after the anticodon, $tRNA_1^{Tyr}$ having i^6A and $tRNA_2^{Tyr}$ ms^2i^6A in this position. Again, the thiomethylation can take place when there is only a small amount of sporulation. Moreover, sporulation and thiomethylation should share a common regulation process, since both phenomena are induced in a wild type strain by a lack of glucose or phosphate (Bun et al. 1981). On the other hand, certain asporogenic mutants are also deficient in thiomethylation. Although there is not a strict correlation between sporulation and thiomethylation, a tRNA having a thiomethylated i^6A is more efficient in protein synthesis than a tRNA with i^6A. As Spotts and Szulmajster (1962) have shown that protein synthesis ist two to ten times more rapid in the stationary phase of a sporulating bacteria than in an asporogenic mutant, the thiomethylation of tRNAs could represent a selective advantage for the sporulation of bacteria.

Finally, the chromatographic profiles of B. subtilis $tRNA^{Phe}$ isoacceptors also change as a function of growth conditions. In complete medium with any degree of aeration or in normally aerated minimal medium there exists only one species, $tRNA_2^{Phe}$: an additional $tRNA_1^{Phe}$ appears only in cells grown in vigorously aerated minimal medium.

This $tRNA_1^{Phe}$ also appears in cells treated with pactamycin (Arnold et al. 1976). Both species of $tRNA^{Phe}$ were isolated and analyzed, and differ only in two modifications. $tRNA_2^{Phe}$ has Gm in the wobble position and ms^2i^6A next to the 3′ end of the anticodon. The early eluting $tRNA^{Phe}$ lacks the ribose-methylation and the 2-thiomethylgroup at i^6A (Arnold et al. 1977; Arnold and Keith 1977). Hoburg et al. (1979) have shown that this undermodified $tRNA^{Phe}$ is less efficient in peptide bond formation in AUGUUU-directed synthesis of fMet-Phe with initiation and elongation factors and E. coli ribosomes.

The variations of the modifications of B. subtilis tRNAs have been treated in more detail here to emphasize the difficulties encountered in interpreting such studies when they do not include isolation and structural determinations of tRNAs. Pairing of tRNA with codons can be influenced by post-transcriptional modifications. Chromatographic peaks can represent mixtures of tRNAs which are more or less well charged by the aminoacylating enzymes; some peaks can even be artifacts due to saline concentration or absence of magnesium (Heyman et al. 1973). However, the bidimensional gel technique of Fradin et al. (1975) now represents a good tool for checking the purity of a tRNA.

Variations of E.coli tRNA isoacceptor modification in different growth conditions have also been described. An alteration in the ratio of $tRNA_1^{Tyr}$ and $tRNA_2^{Tyr}$ was found in this bacteria during early and late exponential growth (Gross and Raab 1972). An increase in the minor species of $tRNA^{Phe}$ and $tRNA^{Trp}$ of Rhodopseudomonas spheroïdes was also observed when the tRNA was extracted from aerobic, dark-grown cells as compared with anaerobic photosynthetic cells (Dejesus and Gray 1971).

Another condition affecting post-transcriptional modifications is amino acid starvation. During leucine deprivation in relaxed-control (rel^-) E. coli a number of qualitative and quantitative changes occur in the tRNAs (Fournier and Peterkofsky 1975). Kitchingman and Fournier (1976a) later showed that the major $tRNA^{Leu}$ which appears in these conditions is deficient in the formation of D at positions 16 and 17, ψ at position 38 and 55, and a modified G at position 37 after the anticodon. Another unique species of $tRNA^{Phe}$ appears in the same conditions. It is also deficient in D at position 16 and in ψ at position 39, but in addition in acp^3U and in the thiomethyl moiety of ms^2i^6A (Kitchingman and Fournier 1976b; Kitchingman et al. 1976).

The $tRNA^{Leu}$ mentioned above is also observed in rel^- cells starved of arginine and in cells treated with chloramphenicol. Other observations using this antibiotic have also been made. D- and thiouridine-lacking tRNA was obtained from chloramphenicol-treated E. coli (Waters 1969; Jacobson and Hedgcoth 1970; Waters et al. 1973).

Other species of $tRNA^{Phe}$ which appear in chloramphenicol-treated E. coli are related and can become fully modified during the period of recovery from this treatment (Mann and Huang 1973) by maturation of A to i^6A and ms^2i^6A (Juarez et al. 1975). Arnold et al. (1976) showed that B. subtilis treated with chloramphenicol, trimethoprim, or pactamycin accumulates incomplete modified tRNAs.

E. coli cells grown in low-iron medium synthesize $tRNA^{Phe}$ (Wettstein and Stent 1968), $tRNA^{Tyr}$, $tRNA^{Leu}$, $tRNA^{Ser}$, and $tRNA^{Cys}$ (Rosenberg and Gefter 1969) with an altered chromatographic profile. In the case of $tRNA^{Tyr}$, iron deficiency specifically affects the 2-methylthiolation of i^6A adjacent to the anticodon (Rosenberg and Gefter 1969). Juarez et al. (1975) showed that for $tRNA^{Phe}$ the A to ms^2i^6A modification is also incomplete after iron starvation. A ψ deficiency has been obtained in tRNAs from E. coli treated with 2-thiouracil. This compound was not incorporated in the tRNA.

The levels of D, T, and s^{4}U were unchanged (Gurchinoff and Kaiser 1973). Mevalonic acid limitation gives tRNA deficient in i^{6}A (Litwack and Peterkofsky 1971). Many studies have shown the appearance of undermethylated tRNAs during methionine starvation of E. coli rel$^-$ mutants that are auxotrophs for methionine (review Borek and Srinivasan 1966). Methyl-deficient tRNA species for phenylalanine, leucine, valine, and methionine have been purified from their normal counterpart (review Littauer and Inouye 1973). A tRNA^{Phe} lacking the thiomethyl-moiety of ms^{2}i^{6}A was characterized by Isham and Stulberg (1974). Keisel and Vold (1976) showed that unlike the undermethylated tRNA from E. coli, the tRNA from B. subtilis has a normal amount of T, since the transmethylation reaction in this organism does not involve *S*-adenosylmethionine. Great differences in the m^{1}G content were also found.

Mitochondrial tRNA

In yeast mitochondria Baldacci et al. (1979) characterized four serine isoacceptors. Their abundance varies as a function of the physiological state of the cell. When they are isolated from cells grown to late exponential phase or stationary phase, in respiratory or fermentative conditions, tRNA$_1^{Ser}$ and tRNA$_3^{Ser}$ are almost undetectable, tRNA$_2^{Ser}$ being the only major species present. We sequenced tRNA$_1^{Ser}$, tRNA$_2^{Ser}$, and tRNA$_3^{Ser}$ (A. P. Sibler, G. Dirheimer and R. P. Martin, unpublished results) (Fig. 12). The primary sequence of tRNA$_1^{Ser}$ is very different from that of tRNA$_2^{Ser}$ and tRNA$_3^{Ser}$. These last two differ only by a single modified nucleoside, ψ_{28} which is present in tRNA$_2^{Ser}$ but not in tRNA$_3^{Ser}$.

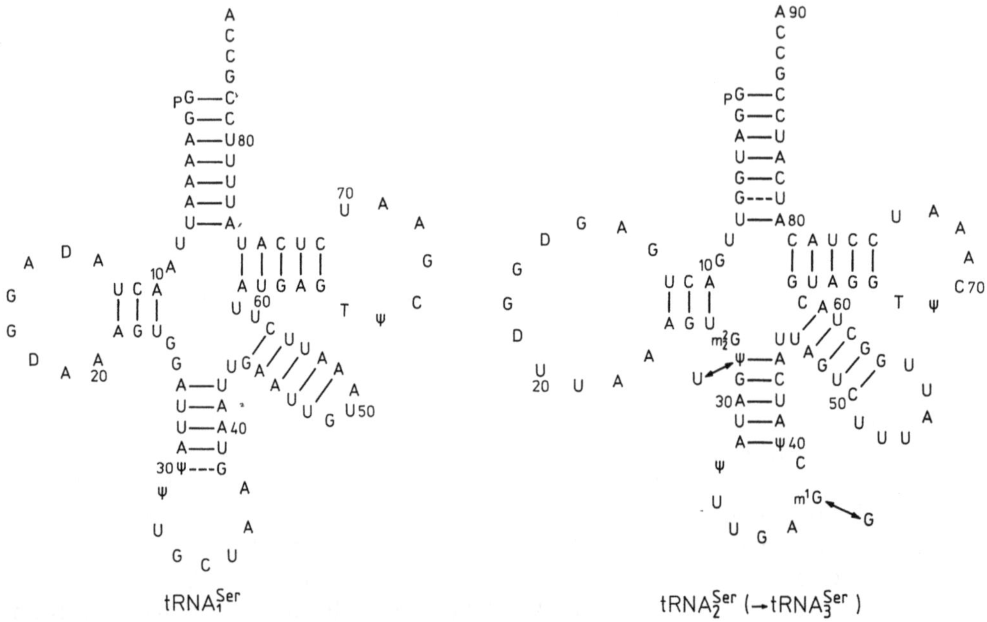

Fig. 12. Structure of yeast mitochondrial tRNAs^{Ser}

Eukaryotic tRNAs

In eukaryotes, variations in the modification level occur from organ to organ, in differentiating cells, during aging, during starvation, in response to hormones, to certain drugs, and to carcinogens, in malignant cells, and after infection with viruses. Extensive reviews describing these variations have been written by Sueoka and Kano-Sueoka (1970), Littauer and Inouye (1973), Nishimura (1978), Randerath et al. (1978), and Osterman (1979).

Although differences among the chromatographic patterns of isoaccepting tRNAs in different organs are the exception rather than the rule (Sueoka and Kano-Sueoka 1970), some variations were described but only one sequence determined. Chromatographic differences in brain and liver for rabbit liver seryl-tRNAs, first observed by Hatfield and Portugal (1970), were confirmed by structure determination. Serine tRNA from rat brain can be resolved into six isoaccepting species. Three of them show the same chromatographic behavior as the seryl-tRNAs from other rat organs, whereas the remaining species appears to be specific for brain. These latter species differ from their counterparts by the lack of G_{17} ribose-methylation (Rogg et al. 1977). The brain-specific distribution of various isoacceptor tRNAs in chromatographic systems which has been found by several authors (Hatfield et al. 1971; Murthy et al. 1974; Frazer and Yang 1972) might be due to the same specific undermethylation.

Reszelbach et al. (1977) showed that there are considerable variations in the relative amount of tRNAs lacking T from different tissues (bovine brain, kidney, liver, thymus, and testicles) from adult, newborn, and fetal stages.

In specialized tissues or organs producing specific proteins there is an extreme adaptation of the tRNA population to the amino acid composition of these proteins (for a review, see Garel 1974) and even to the codons corresponding to these amino acids (Chavancy et al. 1979). This ist the case for the posterior silk gland of Bombyx mori (Garel et al. 1970). Two $tRNAs^{Ala}$ from Bombyx mori have been sequenced (Sprague et al. 1977). One of them, $tRNA_1^{Ala}$, seem to be specific for the silk gland. It differs by having a U or ψ in position 40 (anticodon stem) instead of C in the $tRNA_2^{Ala}$. This suggests a possible activation of a new $tRNA^{Ala}$ gene. A similar case was found by Lin et al. (1980) in bovine lens, where a new species of $tRNA^{Phe}$ which accompagnies the differentiation differs from its counterpart by a G for A substitution at position 57.

Age-dependent changes at the level of tRNA modification were also seen. Wust and Rosen (1972) found that tRNA from young rats was more methylated than that from old animals. In addition the distribution of methylated isoaccepting species of tRNA from spleen of young animals was different from those from spleens of old animals, whereas there was no such qualitative difference with liver material. However, Hoffman and McCoy (1974), studying the nucleoside composition of tRNAs from "mature" and "old" adults of mosquitoes (Aedes aegypti) and of mice liver by the technique of Randerath and Randerath (1973), found neither qualitative nor significant quantitative differences during aging.

The methylation of tRNAs has been studied during regeneration of the liver (Tidwell 1970). This is an interesting model because it is a rapidly dividing normal tissue partly synchronized in cell division. Rodeh et al. (1967) showed that there was no difference in the pattern of methylation of the tRNA during regeneration. Tidwell (1970) found that the methylation of tRNA precedes tRNA synthesis by several hours during regeneration. The two activities seemed to be only weakly coupled; changing methyl content of the tRNA "pool" may regulate the rate of protein synthesis in the cell cycle at the translational level. However Shaw et al. (1978) found only a few minor statistically significant changes (2%–11%) in the base composition 18, 24, and 30 h after hepatectomy, acp^3U being slightly reduced and m^1A, m^1G, m^3C, and ψ being slightly increased. These results suggest that the process of liver regeneration is not accompagnied by a gross alteration of the modification pattern of tRNA, although the two aspartyl-tRNAs appearing in the regenerating liver and absent in control liver (Jackson et al. 1970) might differ by post-transcriptional modifications.

Variations of the modified nucleosides in tRNAs during development and differentiation have been found by the Kersten's group (Dingerman et al. 1977) in the myxamoeba Dictyostelium discoideum. They showed alterations in the T content, which is significantly lower in tRNA from developing cells and spores than in that from cells in vegetative growth. They also showed that tRNAs from undifferentiated Acetabularia mediterranea have a low T content, whereas tRNAs from vegetative stages of development have four times the amount of T. Dingerman et al. (1981) have also recently found changes in the Q content of tRNAs during the developmental cycle of D. discoideum. Two minutes after depriving vegetative amoeba of nutrients, which induces the amoeba to undergo the developmental cycle, there is an accumulation of $tRNA_3^{Asn}$ with Q at position 34, whereas the other major species, $tRNA_3^{Asn}$, has G. This $tRNA_3^{Asn}$, which predominates during vegetative growth, is totally uncharged inside the cell during this early developmental transition. During the sequence of morphogenic steps following this early change, the ratio of Q- and G-containing $tRNA^{Asn}$ continues to change (Kersten, see this vol p. 255–263). These results are in agreement with and extend the previous findings of Palatnik et al. (1977). Littauer and Inouye (1973) reviewed the features appearing during senescence of soybean cotyledons. The changes in the levels of tRNAs under different physiological conditions in plants have been reviewed more recently by Lea and Norris (1977) and Weil (1979). A change in post-transcriptional modification has up to now only been shown in $tRNA^{Phe}$ from crown gall tissue from Nicotiana tabacum, which differs from the $tRNA^{Phe}$ coming from healthy tissues by the absence of wyosine (Cornelis et al. 1975).

In *Drosophila* the Q-base-containing $tRNA^{Asp}$, $tRNA^{Asn}$, $tRNA^{His}$, and $tRNA^{Tyr}$ increase during metamorphosis (White et al. 1973a, b) and during the aging process (White et al. 1973b; Hosbach and Kubli 1979). For example, 1-day-old flies have only 5% of $tRNA^{Tyr}$ containing Q, whereas 21-day-old flies have 64% of $tRNA^{Tyr}$ containing Q (Owenby et al. (1979). These authors also showed, in agreement with earlier results (Wosnik and White 1977; Jacobson 1978), that the production of Q-containing isoacceptors is strongly favored when flies are raised on 2%–4% yeast instead of a normal diet. The chromatographic changes of the Q-containing and Q-lacking forms of the four above-mentioned tRNAs were also followed in Lucilia sericata, Musca domestica, and Tenebrio molitor during the development from larva to adult (White and Lassam 1979). Germ-free mice maintained on a chemically defined diet containing neither Q nor the corresponding base queuine had $tRNA^{Asn}$ and $tRNA^{His}$ containing only 15% Q, whereas $tRNA^{Asp}$ and $tRNA^{Tyr}$ were fully modified with respect to queuine insertion (Farkas 1980).

Agris (1975) reported changes in the tRNA population in Friend's-murine-virus-induced leukemia cells in response to dimethylsulfate-stimulated erythroid differentiation. There were changes in the modified nucleoside content of the whole cell tRNA (reduction of ψ and Y, increase of T and Gm).

Very recently Shindo-Okada et al. (1981b) showed that during erythroid differentiation of murine erythroleukemia cells into mature erythroid cells, the levels of hypomodified tRNAs containing G in place of Q decreased markedly. The decrease could be detected at an early stage of differentiation, before there was any detectable increase in the percentage of cells with hemoglobin.

In cells in culture, Q formation in $tRNA^{Asp}$ is favored not only in untransformed cells but also in cells grown to low density, as well as by medium supplemented with fetal calf serum rather than with calf serum (Katze 1975a, b). Starvation of several amino acids can lead to hypomodified tRNAs. For example, methionine starvation causes the appearance of a yW-deficient $tRNA^{Phe}$ in Vero cells (Pergolizzi et al. 1978). It seems that several modifications of tRNAs observed in cancer cells can be reversed by administration of amino acids, for example lysine and methionine for the yW base (Grunberger, see this vol., pp. 133–145).

The tRNA patterns in eukaryotes also change in certain tissues as a function of hormone administration. For example, Sharma and Borek (1970) showed that ovariectomy produces a hypomethylation of $tRNA^{Ser}$ from pig uterus. Administration of estradiol to the ovariectomized animals restores the methylation of $tRNA^{Ser}$. Estrogenic hormones given to immature hens change the levels of certain tRNAs (Beck et al. 1970) and alter the relative importance of certain isoacceptors (Busby and Hele 1970). Removal of hormone-secreting organs also affects the chromatographic profiles (for a review see Littauer and Inouye 1973). Certain drugs can also lead to inhibition of post-transcriptional modifications in animals. For example, administration of 5-fluorouracil results in reduction in the levels of m^5U, D, and ψ, and 5-azacytidine decreases m^5C in tRNA from tissues of treated animals (Tseng et al. 1978; Lu et al. 1976). However, the decrease of U modification, for example m^5U formation, is greater than the incorporation of fluorouracil into the tRNA indicating also action on the m^5U synthetase (Randerath et al., see this volume p. 103–120). The intercalating agent ellipticin preferentially inhibits in vitro methylation of adenine at low drug level and A and G at higher levels, whereas ethidium bromide and hycanthone inhibit preferentially methylation of guanine at low levels and of all tRNA nucleosides at higher levels (Liau et al. 1977). Extensive shifts in the distribution of labeled methylated nucleosides of tRNA were observed in KB cells treated with actinomycin D for 30 min prior to a 90-min pulse with $[^3H]CH_3$-methionine (Munns et al. 1973). However, to our knowledge no undermethylated tRNAs were isolated from cells or animals treated with these drugs. Ethionine produces a hypomethylation of tRNAs with quantitative differences between the modified nucleosides. It causes for example a 26% inhibition of m^1A and a 55% inhibition of m^2_2G formation (Randerath et al., see this volume, pp. 103–120).

Numerous examples have been reported in the literature of altered column-chromatographic profiles of aminoacylated tRNAs of a number of hepatoma and other tumor tissues as compared with those of normal control tissues. They have been extensively reviewed by Randerath et al. (1978) and Nishimura (1978). Most frequently these changes affect $tRNA^{Phe}$, $tRNA^{Asp}$, $tRNA^{Asn}$, $tRNA^{Tyr}$, $tRNA^{His}$, and $tRNA^{Ser}$. Several structural studies have recently defined for some tRNAs the chemical basis for these chromatographic alterations. Some of them are due to post-transcriptional modifications. These alterations were to be expected; for example, base composition analysis showed hepatoma bulk tRNA to be slightly hypomethylated and hypomodified, although the activity of tRNA methyltransferase

Table 2. Differences in post-transcriptional modifications in sequenced cytoplasmic tRNAs between normal and tumor cells and in SV40-transformed cells

tRNA	Normal tissue	Tumor tissue	Type of tumor	Authors
$tRNA^{Phe}$	O_2yW_{37}	No O_2yW_{37}	Morris hepatoma 7777	Grünberger et al. 1975
	O_2yW_{37}	No O_2yW_{37}	Mouse neuroblastoma or N-18 tumor	Salomon et al. 1976
	yW or deriv.	No yW or deriv.	Human malignant trophoblastic cells (BeWo line)	Kuchino and Borek 1978
$tRNA^{Phe}$	Cm_{32} Gm_{34} $OHyW_{37}$	Either { C_{32}, G_{34}, m^1G_{37} } or { Cm_{32}, Gm_{34}, $OHyW^{b}_{37}$ }	Ehrlich ascites tumor or neuroblastoma N18/6TC	Kuchino et al. 1981b
$tRNA^{Asn}$	Q_{34}	G_{34}	Walker 256 carcinoma	Roe et al. 1979
$tRNA_2^{Lys}$	$D_{20:1}$[a] t^6A_{37} Tm_{54}	$U_{20:1}$ A_{37}[c] U_{54}, T_{54} or ψ_{54}	SV40-transformed mouse fibroblasts	Raba et al. 1979
$tRNA^{Asp}$	$manQ_{34}$	G_{34}	Rat ascites hepatoma	Kuchino et al. 1981a
$tRNA^{Ser}_{IGA}$	Gm_{17}	G_{17}	Morris hepatoma 5123D	E. Randerath et al. 1981
$tRNA_2^{Val}$	Gm_{18} C_{32} N_{34}	G_{18} Cm_{32} I_{34}	Rat ascites	Shindo-Okada et al. 1981[a, b]

[a] Rabbit liver
[b] Under-modified OHyU
[c] May be a precursor of t^6A

was increased when compared with liver tRNA. Hepatoma mitochondrial tRNA is also undermodified (Randerath et al. 1978).

The first structural change in a sequenced tRNA from a tumor was characterized by Grunberger et al. (1975). They showed that an additional species of $tRNA^{Phe}$ in Morris hepatoma 7777 differs from normal liver $tRNA^{Phe}$ by the absence of the peroxy-Y base. A deficiency of peroxy-Y base has also been reported for mouse neuroblastoma (Salomon et al. 1976). Kuchino and Borek (1978) showed more recently that Novikoff hepatoma and Ehrlich ascites cells $tRNA^{Phe}$ have increased levels of m^5C and D as compared to $tRNA^{Phe}$ from normal rat or mouse tissue and an m^1G that is not present at all in $tRNA^{Phe}$ in the normal tissue. These results were partially confirmed by Kuchino et al. (1981b), who compared the nucleotide sequences of $tRNAs^{Phe}$ isolated from Ehrlich ascites tumor and neuroblastoma cells to normal mouse liver $tRNA^{Phe}$. This last contains Cm_{32}, Gm_{34}, and $OHyW_{37}$, whereas tumor-specific $tRNAs^{Phe}$ contain either Cm_{32}, Gm_{34}, and undermodified $OHyW_{37}$ (OHyW*) or C_{32}, G_{34}, and m^1G_{37}. The ratio of OHyW*- to m^1G-containing $tRNA^{Phe}$ is greater in Ehrlich ascites tumor $tRNA^{Phe}$ than in neuroblastoma $tRNA^{Phe}$.

Not only Y but also Q and Q* are affected by changes associated with neoplasia. They occur in $tRNA^{Asp}$, $tRNA^{Asn}$, $tRNA^{Tyr}$, and $tRNA^{His}$ (Katze 1975b; Kasai et al. 1975a, b, 1976a, b), four of the tRNAs whose chromatographic profiles change most often in tumor tissues (for a review see Randerath et al. 1978). In fact it was recently shown that Walker 256 carcinoma $tRNA^{Asn}$ contains G instead of Q (Roe et al. 1979) and that $tRNA^{Asp}$ also contains G instead of manQ (Kuchino et al. 1981a, b).

Very recently changes in hypomodified nucleosides were also found to occur in tumor tissues. Randerath et al. (1981) showed that the Gm_{17} of $tRNA^{Ser\,1}_{IGA}$ was not methylated in Morris hepatoma 5123D and Shindo-Okada et al. (1981a, b) found in rat ascites that both hypo- and hypermodification take place in the $tRNA^{Val}_{2}$ molecule, depending on the location of the nucleotide residues (Table 2).

K. Randerath et al. (1981a, and this volume p. 103–120, and Agrawal et al. 1981a, b) have recently sequenced 16 mitochondrial Morris hepatoma tRNAs. Six of them were compared to the corresponding mitochondrial rat liver tRNAs. As shown in their chapter in this volume (K. Randerath et al., p. 103–120), the differences in the post-transcriptional levels of normal and tumor tRNAs are greater in the mitochondria than in the cytoplasm. Furthermore, tumor-specific tRNAs differing from normal by changes in one basic nucleoside have also been found by these authors, possibly signifying tumor-specific point mutations in mitochondrial DNA.

Finally, there can be virally induced changes in the tRNA modification pattern. Alterations in isoaccepting tRNA patterns have been observed after infection or transformation of mammalian cells with DNA-containing viruses such as type 2 adenovirus (Raska et al. 1970), vaccinia virus (Clarkson and Runner 1971), polyoma virus (Callagher et al. 1972) and SV40 (Sekiya and Oda 1972; Callagher et al. 1972). Only one structural study has been done so far, by Raba et al. (1979), who sequenced a $tRNA^{Lys}_{2}$ which appears in SV40-transformed mouse fibroblasts. It was hypomodified compared to the corresponding rabbit liver $tRNA^{Lys}$: $U_{20:1}$ instead of $D_{20:1}$, A_{37} instead of t^6A_{37}, and U, T, or ψ_{54} instead of T_m (Table 2).

Further sequence analysis will be necessary to obtain a complete view of the problem of changes in nucleoside modification in cell transformation, neoplasia, and carcinogenesis.

References

Agrawal HP, Randerath K, Randerath E (1981a) Tumor mitochondrial tRNAs: The nucleotide sequence of Morris hepatoma 5123D mitochondrial tRNA$^{Asp}_{GUC}$. Nucleic Acids Res 9: 2535–2541

Agrawal HP, Gupta RC, Randerath K, Randerath E (1981b) The sequence of mitochondrial arginine tRNA (anticodon UCG from a transplantable rat tumor Morris hepatoma 5123D. FEBS Lett 130: 287–290

Agris PF (1975) Alterations of tRNA during erythroid differentiation of murine virus-induced leukemia cells. Arch Biochem Biophys 170: 114–123

Agris PF (1980) The modified nucleosides of tRNA. A bibliography of biochemical and biophysical studies from 1970 to 1979. Alan R Liss, New York

Agris PF, Söll D (1977) The modified nucleosides in tRNA. In: Vogel HJ (ed) Nucleic acid-protein recognition. Academic Press, New York, pp 321–344

Alberty H, Raba M, Gross HJ (1978) Isolation from rat liver and sequence of a RNA fragment containing 32 nucleotides from position 5 to 36 from the 3′ end of ribosomal 18S RNA. Nucleic Acids Res 5: 425–434

Altweg M, Kubli E (1979) The nucleotide sequence of phenylalanine tRNA$_2$ of *Drosophila melanogaster*: four isoacceptors with one basic sequence. Nucleic Acids Res 7: 93–105

Altweg M, Kubli E (1980) The nucleotide sequence of glutamate tRNA$_4$ of *Drosophila melanogaster*. Nucleic Acids Res 8: 215–223

Arceneaux JL, Sueoka N (1969) Two species of *Bacillus subtilis* tyrosine tRNA. J Biol Chem 244: 5959–5966

Arnold HH, Keith G (1977) The nucleotide sequence of phenylalanine tRNA from *Bacillus subtilis*. Nucleic Acids Res 4: 2821–2829

Arnold HH, Schmidt H, Raettig R, Sandig H, Domdey H, Kersten H (1976) 5-adenosylmethionine and tetrahydrofolate-dependant methylation of tRNA in *Bacillus subtilis*. Incomplete methylations caused by trimethoprim, pactamycin or chloramphenicol. Arch Biochem Biophys 176: 12–20

Arnold HH, Raettig R, Keith G (1977) Isoaccepting phenylalanine tRNAs from *Bacillus subtilis* as a function of growth conditions. FEBS Lett 73: 210–214

Baldacci G, Falcone C, Francisci S, Frontali L, Palleschi C (1979) Mitochondrial protein-synthesizing machinery in *Saccharomycs cerevisiae* grown in different metabolic conditions. Eur J Biochem 98: 181–186

Beck G, Hentzen D, Ebel JP (1970) Essais de mise en évidence d'une régulation hormonale au niveau des RNA de transfert. 1. Etude comparative des RNA de transfert de foie de poules immatures et de poules en ponte. Biochim Biophys Acta 213: 55–67

Bonnet J, Ebel JP, Dirheimer G, Shershneva LP, Krutilina AI, Venkstern TV, Bayev AA (1974) The corrected nucleotide sequence of valine tRNA from baker's yeast. Biochimie 56: 1211–1213

Borek E, Srinivasan PR (1966) The methylation of nucleic acids. Ann Rev Biochem 35: 275–298

Bun A, Menichi B, Heyman T (1981) Thio-methylation of tyrosine tRNA is associated with initiation of sporulation in *Bacillus subtilis:* Effect of phosphate concentration. J Bacteriol 146: 819–822

Burrows WJ, Armstrong DJ, Kaminek M, Skoog F, Bock RM, Hecht SM, Dammann LG, Leonard NJ, Occolowitz J (1970) Isolation of four and identification of four cytokinins from wheat germ tRNA. Biochemistry 9: 1867–1872

Busby WF Jr, Hele P (1970) Oestrogen-induced variation of lysine tRNA isoacceptors in chicken liver. Biochim Biophys Acta 224: 413–422

Callagher RE, Tin RC, Gallo RC (1972) A common change of aspartyl-tRNA in polyoma- and SV40 transformed cells. Biochim Biophys Acta 272: 568–582

Canaday J, Guillemaut P, Gloeckler R, Weil JH (1980) Comparison of the nucleotide sequences of chloroplast tRNAs^{Phe} and tRNAS$_3^{Leu}$ from spinach and bean. Plant Sci Lett 20: 57–62

Cedergren RJ, Cordeau JR (1973) The distribution of modified nucleosides in tRNAs. J Theor Biol 39: 477–480
Chang SH, Hecker L, Silberklang M, Brum CK, Barnett WE, RajBhandary UL (1976) The first nucleotide sequence of an organelle tRNA: chloroplastic $tRNA^{Phe}$. Cell 9: 717–724
Chapman RW, Morris RO, Zaerr JB (1976) Occurence of trans-ribosylzeatin in *Agrobacterium tumefaciens* tRNA. Nature 262: 153–154
Chavancy G, Chevallier A, Fournier A, Garel JP (1979) Adaptation of iso-tRNA concentration to mRNA codon frequency in the eukaryote cell. Biochimie 61: 71–78
Chen EY, Roe BA (1978) The nucleotide sequence of rat liver tRNA. Biochem Biophys Res Commun 82: 235–246
Chuang R, Doi RH (1972) Characterization of lysine tRNA from vegetative cells and spores of *Bacillus subtilis*. J Biol Chem 247: 3476–3484
Chuang R, Yamakawa T, Doi RH (1971) Identification of two lysine tRNA cistrons in *Bacillus subtilis* by hybridisation of lysyl-tRNA with DNA. Biochem Biophys Res Commun 43: 710–716
Clarkson SG, Runner MN (1971) Transfer RNA changes in Hela cells after *vaccinia* virus infection. Biochim Biophys Acta 238: 498–502
Cohn WE (1957) Minor constituents of RNAs. Fed Proc 16: 166
Cohn WE (1960) Pseudouridine, a carbon-carbon linked ribonucleoside in RNAs, isolation structure and chemical characteristics. J Biol Chem 235: 1488–1498
Cohn WE, Volkin, F (1951) Nucleoside-5′-phosphates from ribonucleic acids. Nature 167: 483–484
Cornelis P, Claessen E, Claessen J (1975) Reversed phase chromatography from healthy and crown-gall tissues from *Nicotiana tabacum*. Nucleic Acids Res 2: 1153–1162
Crick FHC (1966) Codon-anticodon pairing: the wobble hypothesis. J Mol Biol 19: 548–555
Davis FF, Allen FW (1957) Ribonucleic acids from yeast which contain a fifth nucleotide. J Biol Chem 227: 907–915
Dejesus TGS, Gray ED (1971) Isoaccepting tRNA species in differing morphogenetic states in *Rhodopseudomonas spheroïdes*. Biochim Biophys Acta 254: 419–428
Dingermann T, Schmidt W, Kersten H (1977) Modified bases in tRNA of *Dictyostelium discoideum*: Alterations in the ribothymidine content during development. FEBS Lett 80: 205–208
Dingermann T, Ogilvie A, Pistel F, Mühlhofer W, Kersten H (1981) Reduced aminoacylation of asparagine-tRNA early in the developmental cycle of *Dictyostelium discoideum*: Modification pattern and possible significance of the unchanged isoacceptor $tRNA_3^{Asn}$. Hoppe Seylers Z Physiol Chem 362: 763–773
Dirheimer G, Keith G, Sibler AP, Martin RP (1979) The primary structure of tRNAs and their rare nucleosides. In: Schimmel PR, Söll D, Abelson JN (eds) Transfer RNA: Structure, properties and recognition. Cold Spring Harbor Lab, Cold Spring Harbor, New York, pp 19–41
Doi RH, Kaneko I, Igaraci RT (1968) Patterns of valine tRNA of *Bacillus subtilis* under different growth conditions. J Biol Chem 243: 945–951
Dubois EG, Dirheimer G, Weil JH (1974) Methylation of yeast $tRNA^{Asp}$ by enzymes from cytoplasm, chloroplasts and mitochondria of *Phaseolus vulgaris*. Biochim Biophys Acta 374: 332–341
Dunn DB, Flack IH (1970) Minor nucleotides in RNA. John Innes Inst Ann Rep 76
Dunn DB, Hall RH (1975) Purines, pyrimidines, nucleosides and nucleotides: physical constants and spectral properties. In: Fasman GD (ed) Nucleic Acids. (Handbook of Biochemistry and Molecular Biology, 3rd ed, vol 1, CRC Press, Cleveland, Ohio pp 65–215)
Dunn DB, Trigg MDM (1972) Minor nucleotides in leaf tRNA. John Innes Inst Ann Rep 142
Dunn DB, Trigg MDM (1973) Minor nucleotides in tRNA. John Innes Inst Ann Rep 147

Einset JW, Skoog FK (1977) Isolation and identification of ribosyl-*cis*-zeatin from transfer RNA of *Corynebacterium fascians*. Biochem Biophys Res Comm 79: 1117–1121

Farkas WR (1980) Effect of diet on the queunosine family of tRNAs of germ-free mice. J Biol Chem 255: 6832–6835

Feinberg AM, Nakanishi K, Barciszewski J, Rafalski AJ, Augustyniak H, Wiewiorowski M (1974) Isolation and characterization of peroxy-y-base from $tRNA^{Phe}$ of the plant *Lupinus luteus*. J Am Chem Soc 96: 7797–7800

Feldman MY (1977) Minor components in tRNA: The location-function relationship. Prog Biophys Mol Biol 32: 83–102

Fleissner E, Borek E (1962) A new enzyme of RNA synthesis: RNA methylase. Proc Natl Acad Sci USA 48: 1199–1203

Fournier MJ, Peterkofsky A (1975) Formation of chromatographically unique species of tRNA during aminoacid starvation of relaxed-control *E. coli*. J Bacteriol 122: 538–548

Fournier M, Labouesse J, Dirheimer G, Fix C, Keith G (1978) Primary structure of bovine liver $tRNA^{Trp}$. Biochim Biophys Acta 521: 198–208

Fradin A, Grühl H, Feldmann H (1975) Mapping of yeast tRNAs by two-dimensional electrophoresis on polyacrylamide gels. FEBS Lett 50: 185–189

Frazer JM, Yang WK (1972) Isoaccepting tRNAs in liver and brain of young and old BC_3F_1 Mice. Arch Biochem Biophys 153: 610–618

Garel JP (1974) Functional adaptation of tRNA population. J Theor Biol 43: 211–225

Garel JP, Keith G (1977) Nucleotide sequence of *Bombyx mori* L.$tRNA_1^{Gly}$. Nature 269: 350–352

Garel JP, Mandel P, Chavancy G, Daillie J (1970) Functional adaptation of tRNA to fibroin biosynthesis in the silkgland of *Bombyx mori* L. FEBS Lett 7: 327–329

Gauss DH, Sprinzl M (1981) Compilation of tRNA sequences. Nucleic Acids Res 9: r1–r23

Gross HJ (1975) Natural modified nucleosides and chemical carcinogenesis: L-ethionine-dependent inhibition of N^6 – dimethyladenosine and 5-methylcytidine synthesis on the tRNA level *in vivo*. Ann NY Acad Sci 255: 564–566

Gross HJ, Raab C (1972) *In vivo* synthesis of $tRNA_1^{Tyr}$ and $tRNA_2^{Tyr}$: Differences in "early" and "late log" *E.coli* MRE 600. Biochem Biophys Res Commun 46: 2006–2011

Gross HJ, Simsek M, Raba M, Limburg K, Heckman J, RajBhandary UL (1974) 2′-O-Methylribothymidine: a component of rabbit liver lysine transfer RNA. Nucleic Acids Res 1: 35–43

Grunberger D, Weinstein IB, Mushinski JF (1975) Deficiency of the Y base in a hepatoma phenylalanine tRNA. Nature 253: 66–67

Gupta RC, Woese CR (1980) Unusual modification patterns in the tRNAs of Archaebacteria. Curr Microbiol 4: 245–249

Gupta RC, Roe BA, Randerath K (1979) The nucleotide sequence of human $tRNA^{Gly}$ (anticodon GCC). Nucleic Acids Res 7: 959–970

Gurchinoff S, Kaiser II (1973) Pseudouridine deficiency in tRNAs from *E. coli* treated with 2-thiouracil. Biochemistry 12: 3236–3241

Hall RH (1963) Isolation of 1-methylinosine and inosine from yeast soluble RNA. Biochem Biophys Res Commun 13: 394–398

Hall RH (1964) Isolation of N^6-(aminoacyl)adenosine from yeast ribonucleic acid. Biochemistry 3: 769–773

Hall RH (1971) The modified nucleosides in nucleic acids. Columbia University Press, New York

Hall RH, Dunn DB (1975) Natural occurence of the modified nucleotides. In: Fasman GD (ed) Nucleic acids. (Handbook of Biochemistry and Molecular Biology, 3rd ed, CRC Press, Cleveland, Ohio vol 1, pp 216–250)

Hall RH, Csonka L, David H, McLennan B (1967) Cytokinins in soluble RNA of plant tissues. Science 156: 69–71

Harris CL, Marashi F, Titchener EB (1976) Increased isoleucine acceptance by sulfur-deficient tRNA from *E. coli.* Nucleic Acids Res 3: 2129–2142

Hatfield D, Portugal FH (1970) Seryl-tRNA in mammalian tissues: chromatographic differences in brain and liver and a specific response to the codon UGA. Proc Natl Acad Sci USA 67: 1200–1206

Hatfield D, Portugal FH, Caicuts M (1971) Transfer RNA specificity in mammalian tissues and codon response of seryl tRNA. Cancer Res 31: 697–700

Hecht SM, Leonard NJ, Burrows WJ, Armstrong DJ, Skoog F, Occolowitz J (1969) Cytokinin of wheat germ tRNA: 6-(4-hydroxy-3-methyl-2-butenylamino)-2-methylthio-9-β-D-ribofuranosyl-purine. Science 166: 1272–1274

Heckman JE, Sarnoff J, Alzner-Deweerd B, Yin S, RajBhandary UL (1980) Novel features in the genetic code and codon reading patterns in *Neurospora crassa mitochondria* based on sequences of six mitochondrial tRNAs. Proc Natl Acad Sci USA 77: 3159–3163

Heyman T, Seror S, Desseaux B, Legault-Demare J (1967) Valine tRNA, I Chromatographic study of valine tRNA modifications during *Bacillus subtilis* growth. Biochim Biophys Acta 145: 596–604

Heyman T, Menichi-Desseaux B, Legault-Demare J (1970) Valine tRNA, II Kinetics of aminoacylation of the different species of valine tRNA in *Bacillus subtilis.* Biochim Biophys Acta 199: 71–78

Heyman T, Leidner J, Menichi-Desseaux B (1973) Chromatographic separation of two ionic strengh dependant conformations of valine tRNA of *Bacillus subtilis.* Biochimie 55: 127–134

Hoburg A, Aschhoff HJ, Kersten H, Mandershied U, Gassen HG (1979) Function of modified nucleosides 7-methylguanosine, ribothymidine and 2-thiomethyl-N^6-(isopentenyl)adenosine in procaryotic tRNA. J Bacteriol 140: 408–414

Hoffman JL, McCoy MT (1974) Stability of the nucleoside composition of tRNA during biological ageing of mice and mosquitoes. Nature 249: 558–559

Holley RW, Apgar J, Everett GA, Madison JT, Marquisee M, Merril SH, Penswick JR, Zamir A (1965) Structure of ribonucleic acid. Science 147: 1462–1465

Hosbach HA, Kubli E (1979) Transfer RNA in aging *Drosophila* II. Isoaccepting patterns. Mech Ageing Dev 10: 141–149

Huang PC, Mann MB (1974) Comparative fingerprint and composition analysis of the three forms of ^{32}P labeled phenylalanine tRNA from chloramphenicol treated *E. coli.* Biochemistry 13: 4704–4710

Isham KR, Stulberg MP (1974) Modified nucleosides in undermethylated phenylalanine tRNA from *E. coli.* Biochim Biophys Acta 340: 177–182

Ishikura H, Murao K, Yamada Y (1980) Primary structures of several tRNAs from *Bacillus subtilis.* EMBO-FEBS tRNA Workshop, Strasbourg

Jackson CD, Lowing CC, Sells BH (1970) Studies on transfer RNA population during liver regeneration in rat. Biochim Biophys Acta 224: 259–262

Jacobson KB (1978) Mechanism of suppression in Drosophila VII. Correlation between disappearance of an isoacceptor of tyrosine tRNA and activation of the vermilion locus. Nucleic Acids Res 5: 2391–2404

Jacobson M, Hedgcoth C (1970) Levels of 5,6-dihydrouridine in relaxed and chloramphenicol tRNA. Biochemistry 9: 2513–2519

Juarez H, Skjold AC, Hedgcoth C (1975) Precursor relationship of phenylalanin tRNA from *E.coli* treated with chloramphenicol or starved for iron, methionine or cysteine. J Bacteriol 121: 44–54

Kaneko I, Doi RH (1966) Alteration of valine-sRNA during sporulation of *Bacillus subtilis.* Proc Natl Acad Sci USA 55: 564–571

Kasai H, Ohashi Z, Harada F, Nishimura S, Oppenheimer NJ, Crain PF, Liehr JG, von Minden DL, McCloskey JA (1975a) Structure of the modified nucleoside isolated from *Escherichia coli* transfer ribonucleic acid. 7-(4,5-*cis*-dihydroxy-1-cyclopenten-3-ylaminomethyl)-7-deazaguanosine. Biochemistry 14: 4198–4208

Kasai H, Kuchino Y, Nihei K, Nishimura S (1975b) Distribution of the modified Q and its derivatives in animal and plant tRNAs. Nucleic Acids Res 2: 1931–1939

Kasai H, Murao K, Nishimura S, Liehr JG, Crain PF, McCloskey JM (1976a) Structure determination of a modified nucleoside isolated from *E.coli* tRNA. N- [N-[9-β-D-Ribofuranosylpurin-6-yl)carbamoyl]threonyl]2-amido-2-hydroxymethylpropane-1,3-diol. Eur J Biochem 69: 435–443

Kasai H, Nakanishi K, McFarlane RD, Togerson DF, Ohashi Z, McCloskey JA, Gross HJ, Nishimura S (1976b) The structure of Q* nucleoside isolated from rabbit liver tRNA. J Am Chem Soc 98: 5044–5045

Kasai H, Yamaizumi Z, Kuchino Y, Nishimura S (1979) Isolation of hydroxy-Y base from rat liver $tRNA^{Phe}$. Nucleic Acids Res 6: 993–999

Katze JR (1975a) Relation of cell type and cell density to the degree of posttranscriptional modification of $tRNA^{Lys}$ and $tRNA^{Phe}$. Biochim Biophys Acta 407: 392–398

Katze JR (1975b) Alterations in SVT2 cell tRNAs in response to cell density and serum type. Biochim Biophys Acta 383: 131–139

Kawakami M, Nishio K, Takemura S, Kondo T, Goto T (1979) 5-(Carboxy-hydroxymethyl) uridine a new modified nucleoside located in the anticodon of $tRNA_2^{Gly}$ from posterior silk gland of *Bombyx mori*. Nucleic Acids Res Symp Ser 6: s53–s55

Keisel N, Vold B (1976) Undermethylated RNA from a relaxed strain of *Bacillus subtilis:* construction of the strain and analysis of the tRNA. J Bacteriol 1976: 294–299

Keith G, Dirheimer G (1980) Primary sequence of *Bombyx mori* posterior silkgland $tRNA^{Phe}$. Biochem Biophys Res Commun 92: 109–115

Keith G, Roy A, Ebel JP, Dirheimer G (1972) The primary structure of $tRNA^{Trp}$ from brewer's yeast I. Complete digestion with pancreatic ribonuclease and T_1 ribonuclease. Biochimie 54: 1405–1426

Keith G, Rogg H, Dirheimer G, Menichi B, Heyman T (1976) Post-transcriptional modification of tyrosine tRNA as a function of growth in *Bacillus subtilis*. FEBS Lett 61: 120–123

Kimura-Harada F, Saneyoshi M, Nishimura S (1971) 5-Methyl-2-thiouridine: a new sulfur-containing minor constituent from rat liver glutamic and lysine tRNAs. FEBS Lett 13: 335–338

Kitchingman GR, Fournier MJ (1976a) *In vivo* maturation of an undermodified *E. coli* leucine tRNA. Biochem Biophys Res Commun 73: 314–322

Kitchingman GR, Fournier MJ (1976b) Structures of modification-deficient leucine- and phenylalanine-tRNAs produced during leucine starvation of relaxed control *E. coli*. Fed Proc 35: 1615

Kitchingman GR, Webb E, Fournier MJ (1976) Unique phenylalanine tRNA in relaxed control *E. coli*: Genetic origin and some functional properties. Biochemistry 15: 1848–1857

Kuchino Y, Borek E (1978) Tumor-specific phenylalanine tRNA contains two supernumerary methylated bases. Nature 271: 126–129

Kuchino Y, Shindo-Okada N, Ando N, Watanabe S, Nishimura S (1981a) Nucleotide sequences of two aspartic acid tRNAs from rat liver and rat ascites hepatoma. J Biol Chem 256: 9059–9062

Kuchino Y, Borek E, Grunberger D, Muchinski JF, Nishimura S (1981b) Changes of post-transcriptional modification of wye base in tumor-specific $tRNA^{Phe}$. J Biol Chem 256: 9059–9062

Lazzarini RA (1966) Differences in lysine-sRNA from spore and vegetative cells of *Bacillus subtilis*. Proc Natl Acad Sci USA 56: 185–190

Lea PJ, Norris ND (1977) tRNA and aminoacyl-tRNA synthetases from higher plants. Prog Phytochem 4: 121–167

Liau MC, Lin GW, Knight CA, Hurlbert RB (1977) Inhibition of tRNA methylation by intercalating agents. Cancer Res 37: 4202–4210

Lin FK, Furr TD, Chang SH, Horwitz J, Agris PF, Orthwerth BJ (1980) The nucleotide sequence of two bovine lens $tRNA^{Phe}$. J Biol Chem 255: 6020–6023

Littauer VZ, Inouye H (1973) Regulation of tRNA. Ann Rev Biochem 42: 439–470

Litwack MD, Peterkofsky A (1971) tRNA deficient in N^6-(Δ^2-isopentenyl) adenosine due to mevalonic acid limitation. Biochemistry 10: 994–1000

Lu LW, Chiang GH, Medina D, Randerath K (1976) Drug effects on nucleic acid modification I A specific effect of 5-azacytidine on mammalian tRNA methylation in vivo. Biochem Biophys Res Commun 68: 1094–1101

Madison JT, Holley RW (1957) The presence of 5,6-dihydrouridylic acid in yeast "soluble" RNA. Biochem Biophys Res Commun 18: 153–157

Mann MB, Huang PC (1973) Behavior of chloramphenicol-induced phenylalanine tRNA during recovery from chloramphenicol treatment in *E. coli*. Biochemistry 12: 5289–5294

Marcu KB, Mignery RE, Dudok BS (1977) Complete nucleotide sequence and properties of the major species of glycine tRNA from wheat germ. Biochemistry 16: 797–806

Marmor JB, Dickerman HW, Peterkofsky A (1971) Studies on methyl-deficient methionine tRNA from *E. coli*. J Biol Chem 246: 3464–3473

Martin RP, Schneller JM, Stahl AJC, Dirheimer G (1976) Studies of odd bases in yeast mitochondrial tRNA II Characterization of rare nucleotides. Biochem Biophys Res Commun 70: 997–1002

Martin RP, Schneller JM, Stahl AJC, Dirheimer G (1977) Study on yeast mitochondrial tRNA by two-dimensional poly-acrylamide gel electrophoresis: Characterization of isoaccepting species and search for imported cytoplasmic tRNAs. Nucleic Acids Res 4: 3497–3510

McCloskey JA, Nishimura S (1977) Modified nucleosides in tRNA. Acc Chem Res 11: 403–410

McMillian RA, Arceneaux JL (1975) Alteration of tyrosine accepting tRNA species in wildtype and asporogenous strains of *Bacillus subtilis*. J Bacteriol 122: 526–531

Menichi B, Heyman T (1976) Study of tyrosine tRNA modification in relation to sporulation in *Bacillus subtilis*. J Bacteriol 127: 268–280

Menichi B, Arnold HH, Heyman T, Dirheimer G, Keith G (1980) Primary structure of *Bacillus subtilis* $tRNA^{Tyr}$. Biochem Biophys Res Commun 95: 461–467

Munns TW, Katzman PA (1973) The methylation of tRNA in KB cells after treatment with actinomycin D. Biochem Biophys Res Commun 53: 119–125

Munz P, Leupold U, Agris P, Kohli J (1981) *In vivo* decoding rules in *Schizosaccharomyces pombe* which are at variance with in vitro data. Nature 294: 187–188

Murao K, Ishikura H (1978) A new uridine derivative located in the anticodon of $tRNA_1^{Gly}$ from *Bacillus subtilis*. Nucleic Acids Res (special publication) 5: s333

Murao K, Sanegoshi M, Harada F, Nishimura S (1970) Uridine-5-oxyacetic acid: A new minor constituent from *E. coli* valine tRNA 1. Biochem Biophys Res Commun 38: 657–662

Murao K, Tanabe T, Ishii F, Namiki M, Nishimura S (1972) Primary sequence of arginine tRNA from *E. coli*. Biochem Biophys Res Commun 47: 1332–1337

Murao K, Ishikura H, Albani M, Kersten H (1978) On the biosynthesis of 5-methoxyuridine and uridine-5-oxyacetic acid in specific procaryotic tRNAs. Nucleic Acids Res 5: 1273–1387

Murthy MRV, Roux H, Thenot JP (1974) Isoacceptor tRNAs for glutamate, glutamine, aspartate and asparagine in calf brain. J Neurochem 22: 19–22

Nakanishi K, Blobstein S, Funamizu M, Furutachi N, Van Lear G, Grunberger D, Lanks K, Weinstein IB (1971) Structure of the peroxy-Y base from liver $tRNA^{Phe}$. Nature (NB) 234: 107–109

Nau F (1976) The methylation of tRNA. Biochimie 58: 629–645

Nishimura S (1972) Minor components in tRNA: Their caracterization, location and function. Prog Nucleic Acid Res Mol Biol 12: 49–85

Nishimura S (1978) Modified nucleosides and isoaccepting tRNA. In: Altman S (ed) Transfer RNA. MIT Press, Cambridge, MA, pp 168–195

Nishimura S (1979a) Modified nucleosides in tRNA. In: Schimmel PR, Söll D, Abelson JN (eds) Transfer RNA: structure, properties, and recognition. Cold Spring Harbor Lab, Cold Spring Harbor, pp 59–79

Nishimura S (1979b) Structures of modified nucleosides found in tRNA. In: Schimmel PR, Söll D, Abelson JN (eds) Transfer RNA: structure, properties, and recognition. Cold Spring Harbor Lab, Cold Spring Harbor, pp 547–549

Ohashi Z, Maeda M, McCloskey JA, Nishimura S (1974) 3-(3-Amino-3-carboxypropyl) uridine: a novel modified nucleoside isolated from *E. coli* phenylalanine tRNA. Biochemistry 13: 2620–2625

Osorio-Almeida L, Guillemaut P, Keith G, Canaday J, Weil JH (1980) Primary structure of three leucine tRNAs from bean chloroplasts. Biochem Biophys Res Commun 92: 102–108

Osterman LA (1979) Participation of tRNA in regulation of protein biosynthesis at the translational level in eukaryotes. Biochimie 61: 323–342

Owenby RK, Stulberg MP, Jacobson KB (1979) Alteration of the Q family of tRNAs in adult *Drosophila melanogaster* as a function of age, nutrition and genotype. Mech Ageing Dev 11: 91–103

Palantnik CM, Katz ER, Brenner M (1977) Isolation and characterization of tRNAs from *Dictyostelium discoideum* during growth and development. J Biol Chem 252: 694–703

Pergolizzi RG, Engelhardt DT, Grunberger D (1978) Formation of phenylalanine tRNA lacking the Wye base in Vero cells during methionine starvation. J Biol Chem 253: 6341–6343

Raba M, Limburg K, Burghagen M, Katze JR, Simsek M, Heckman JE, RajBhandary UL, Gross HJ (1979) Nucleotide sequence of three isoaccepting lysine tRNAs from rabbit liver and SV40-transformed mouse fibroblasts. Eur J Biochem 97: 305–318

Raettig R, Kersten H, Weissenbach J, Dirheimer G (1977) Methylation of an adenosine in the D-loop of specific tRNAs from yeast by a procaryotic tRNA (adenosine-1) methyltransferase. Nucleic Acids Res 4: 1769–1782

Randerath E, Gopalakrishnan AS, Randerath K (1978) Transfer RNA in hepatomas. In: Morris HP, Criss WE (eds) Morris hepatomas, mechanisms of regulation. Plenum, New York London, pp 517–564

Randerath K, Randerath E (1973) Chemical post-labeling methods for the base composition and sequence analysis of RNA. J Chromatogr 82: 59–74

Randerath K, Agrawal HP, Randerath E (1981) Tumor mitochondrial tRNAs: The nucleotide sequence of mitochondrial $tRNA^{Leu}_{UAG}$ from Morris hepatoma 5123 D. Biochem Biophys Res Commun 100: 732–737

Randerath E, Gopalakrishnan AS, Gupta RC, Agrawal HP, Randerath K (1981) Lack of specific ribose methylation at guanosine 17 in Morris hepatoma 5123 D $tRNA^{Ser}_{IGA}$. Cancer Res 41: 2863–2867

Raska K Jr, Frohwirth DH, Schlessinger RW (1970) Transfer RNA in KB cells infected with adenovirus type 2. J Virol 5: 464–69

Reddy R, Busch H (1981) U snRNAs of nuclear snRNP's In: Busch H (ed) The cell Nucleus, vol 8. Academic Press, New York London, pp 261–306

Reszelbach R, Greenberg R, Pirtle R, Prasad R, Marcu K, Dudock B (1977) Isolation and comparison of ribothymidine-lacking tRNAs of fetal, newborn and adult bovine tissues. Biochim Biophys Acta 475: 383–392

Rodeh R, Feldman M, Littauer UZ (1967) Properties of soluble ribonucleic acid methylases from rat liver. Biochemistry 6: 451–460

Roe BA, Stankiewicz AF, Rizi HL, Weisz C, Di Lauro MN, Pike D, Chen CY, Chen EY (1979) Comparison of rat liver and Walker 256 carcinosarcoma tRNA. Nucleic Acids Res 6: 673–688

Rogg H, Müller P, Keith G, Staehelin M (1977) Chemical basis for brain-specific serine tRNA. Proc Natl Acad Sci USA 74: 4243–4247

Rosenberg AH, Gefter ML (1969) An iron dependant modification of several tRNA species in *E. coli*. J Mol Biol 46: 581–584

Salomon R, Giveon D, Kimhi Y, Littauer UZ (1976) Abundance of $tRNA^{Phe}$ lacking the peroxy Y-base in mouse. Biochemistry 15: 5258–5262

Schweizer MP, McGrath K, Baczynskyj L (1970) The isolation and characterization of N-[9-β-D-ribofuranosyl)-purin-6-ylcarbamoyl] glycine from yeast tRNA. Biochem Biophys Res Commun 40: 1046–1052

Sekiya T, Oda K (1972) The altered pattern of tRNA in SV 40-infected and transformed cells. Virology 47: 168–180

Sharma OK, Borek E (1970) Hormonal effect on tRNA methylases and on serine tRNA. Biochemistry 9: 2507–2519

Shaw PA, Tidwell JT, Chia LLSY, Randerath E, Randerath K (1978) Base composition studies on transfer RNA from normal and regenerating rat liver. Biochim Biophys Acta 518: 457–463

Shindo-Okada N, Kuchino Y, Harada F, Okada N, Nishimura S (1981a) Biological and structural differences between $tRNA^{Val}$ species isolated from rat ascite hepatoma cells and normal rat liver. J Biochem 90: 535–544

Shindo-Okada N, Terada M, Nishimura S (1981b) Changes in amount of hypo-modified tRNA having guanine in place of queuine during erythroid differentiation of murine erythroleukemia cells. Eur J Biochem 115: 423–428

Sibler AP, Bordonné R, Dirheimer G, Martin RP (1980) Structure primaire d'un tryptophane-tRNA de mitochondrie de levure capable de traduire le codon de terminaison UGA. C R Acad Sci [D] (Paris) 290: 595–598

Singhal RP, Vold B (1976) Changes in tRNA of *Bacillus subtilis* during different growth phases. Nucl Acids Res 5: 1249–1261

Söll D (1971) Enzymatic modification of tRNA. Science 173: 293–299

Sprague KU, Hagenbuechle O, Zuniga MC (1977) The nucleotide sequence of two silk gland alanine tRNAs: implication for fibroin synthesis and for initiator tRNA structure. Cell 11: 561–570

Spotts CR, Szulmajster S (1962) Synthèse de l'acide ribonucléique et des protéines dans *Bacillus subtilis* sporogène et asporogène. Biochim Biophys Acta 61: 635–638

Sueoka N, Kano-Sueoka T (1964) A specific modification of leucyl-sRNA of *E. coli* after phage T_2 infection. Proc Natl Acad Sci USA 52: 1535–1540

Sueoka N, Kano-Sueoka T (1970) Transfer RNA and cell differentiation. Prog Nucleic Acid Res Mol Biol 10: 23–55

Takemoto T, Takeishi F, Nishimura S, Ukito T (1973) Transfer of valine into rabbit haemoglobin from various isoaccepting species of valyl-tRNA differing in codon recognition. Eur J Biochem 38: 489–496

Tidwell T (1970) The methylation of tRNA during regeneration of the liver. J Cell Biol 46: 370–378

Thimmapaya B, Cherayil JD (1974) Unique presence of 2-methylthio-ribosylzeatin in the tRNA of bacterium *Pseudomonas aeruginosa*. Biochem Biophys Res Commun 60: 665–672

Tseng WC, Medina D, Randerath K (1978) Specific inhibition of tRNA methylation and modification in tissues of mice treated with 5-fluorouracil. Cancer Res 38: 1250–1257

Vold BS (1970) Comparison of lysyl-tRNA species from vegetative cells and spores of *Bacillus subtilis* by methylated albumin kieselguhr and reversed phase chromatography. J Bacteriol 102: 711–715

Vold BS (1973) Analysis of isoaccepting tRNA species of *Bacillus subtilis*: chromatographic differences between tRNAs from spores and cells in exponential growth. J Bacteriol 113: 825–833

Vold BS (1975) In: Gerhard P, Costilow R, Sadoff H (eds) Spores VI. AMS, Washington DC, pp 282–289

Vold BS (1978) Post-transcriptional modification of the anticodon loop region: Alteration in isoaccepting species of tRNAs during development in *Bacillus subtilis*. J Bacteriol 135: 124–132

Vrejman HJ (1973) Isolation of *cis* and *trans* isomers of ribosylzeatin and 2-methylthio-ribosylzeatin from plant tRNA preparation. Diss Abstr Int [B] 34: 5842–5843

Watanabe K, Kuchino Y, Yamaizumi Z, Kato M, Oshima T, Nishimura S (1979) Nucleotide sequence of formylmethionine tRNA from an extreme thermophile *Thermus thermophilus* HB8. J Biochem 86: 893–905

Waters LC (1969) Altered chromatographic properties of tRNA from chloramphenicol treated *E. coli*. Biochem Biophys Res Commun 37: 296–304

Waters LC, Shugart L, Yang WK, Best AN (1973) Some physical and biological properties of 4-thiouridine- and dihydrouridine deficient tRNA from chloramphenicol treated *E. coli*. Arch Biochem Biophys 156: 780–793

Weissenbach J (1977) Purification et structure primaire des $tRNA_2^{Arg}$, $tRNA_3^{Arg}$ et $tRNA_{Ia\ et\ b}^{Thr}$ de levure de bière. Etude des propriétés codantes des $tRNA^{Arg}$ de levure de biere. Ph. D. dissertation, Université Louis Pasteur, Strasbourg

Weissenbach J, Dirheimer G (1978) Pairing properties of the methylester of 5-carboxymethyl uridine in the wobble position of yeast $tRNA_3^{Arg}$. Biochim Biophys Acta 518: 350–354

Weissenbach J, Grosjean H (1981) Effect of threonylcarbamoyl modification (t^6A) in yeast $tRNA_3^{Arg}$ on codon – anticodon and anticodon-anticodon interaction. A thermodynamic and kinetic evaluation. Eur J Biochem 116: 207–213

Weil JH (1979) Cytoplasmic and organellar tRNAs in plants. In: Hall TC, Devis JW (eds) Nucleic acids in plants. CRC, Boca Raton, FL, pp 143–192

Wettsteim FO, Stent GS (1968) Physiologically induced changes in the property of phenylalanine tRNA in *E. coli*. J Mol Biol 38: 25–40

White BN, Lassam NJ (1979) An analysis of Q and Q* containing tRNAs during the development of *Lucilia sericata*, *Musca domestica* and *Tenebrio molitor*. Insect Biochem 9: 375–378

White BN, Tener GM, Holden J, Suzuki DT (1973a) Activity of tRNA modifying enzyme during the development of *Drosophila* and its relationship in the su(s) locus. J Mol Biol 74: 635–651

White BN, Tener GM, Holden J, Suzuki DT (1973b) Analysis of tRNAs during the development of *Drosophila*. Dev Biol 33: 185

Wosnick MA, White BN (1977) A doubtful relationship between tyrosine tRNA and suppression of the vermilion mutant in *Drosophila*. Nucleic Acids Res 4: 3919–3930

Wosnick MA, White BN (1978) Purification and nucleotide composition of a Q*-containing aspartic acid tRNA from *Drosophila*. Biochem Biophys Res Commun 81: 1131–1138

Wust CJ, Rosen L (1972) Aminoacylation and methylation of tRNA as a function of age in the rat. Exp Gerontol 7: 331–343

Yamada Y, Ishikura H (1981) The presence of N-[(9-β-D-ribofuranosyl-2-methylthiopurin 6-yl)carbamoyl] threonine in lysine $tRNA_1$ from *Bacillus subtilis*. J Biochem 89: 1589–1591

Yamada Y, Murao K, Ishikura H (1981) 5-(carboxymethylaminomethyl)-thiouridine, a new modified nucleoside found at the first letter position of the anticodon. Nucleic Acids Res 9: 1933–1938

Yamaizumi Z, Nishimura S, Limburg K, Raba M, Gross HJ, Crain PF, McCloskey JA (1979) Structure elucidation by high resolution mass spectrometry of a highly modified nucleoside from mammalian tRNA N-[(9-β-D-ribofuranosyl-2-methylthiopurin-6-yl) carbamoyl] threonine. J Am Chem Soc 101: 2224–2225

Yokoyama S, Miyazawa T, Iitaka Y, Yamaizumi Z, Kasai H, Nishimura S (1979) Three-dimensional structure of hyper-modified nucleoside Q located in the wobbling position of tRNA. Nature 282: 107–109

Zachau HG, Dutting D, Feldmann H (1966) The structure of two serine tRNAs. Hoppe Seylers Z Physiol Chem 347: 212–235

Session I

Modified Nucleosides in Situ in Tumors and Transformed Cells of Cell Culture

*Formation and Removal of Methylated Nucleosides in Nucleic Acids of Mammalian Cells**

A. E. Pegg

Department of Physiology and Specialized Cancer Research Center,
Milton S. Hershey Medical Center, Pennsylvania State University,
Hershey, PA 17033, USA

Introduction

This chapter compares the formation, turnover, and possible functions of methylated nucleosides present in nucleic acids under normal conditions and after exposure to alkylating agents. No attempt is made to provide a totally comprehensive review of the occurrence and biochemistry of such products. Many recent reviews have covered portions of this field, and to summarize such a broad area is probably impossible and unlikely to be useful. More relevantly, it is also outside the limited capabilities of the author. Attention, therefore, is concentrated on the methylation of DNA by certain carcinogens which may have environmental importance and on selected references to certain areas of the immense biochemical literature relating to normal cellular methylations.

The methylated nucleosides produced by the administration of carcinogens are compared to those formed by normal cellular methylation processes. The alkylation of DNA by *N*-nitroso-compounds, by related alkylating agents, and by ethionine is discussed in terms of the sites of reaction, their enzymatic repair, and the possible consequences of their persistence in DNA. Some properties of the enzyme system responsible for the removal of O^6-methylguanine by transfer of the methyl group to protein and its induction by exposure to hepatotoxins are described. Finally, there is discussion of the possible mechanism by which alkylated bases which are substrates for DNA repair enzymes can be formed in cells not exposed experimentally to exogenous alkylating agents.

Alkylated Derivatives Present in Nucleic Acids

All the major nucleic acids and most minor species present in mammalian cells appear to contain some methylated nucleosides. A selection of these is indicated in Table 1. Such methylation products range from the simple methyl-group addition to the carbon or nitrogen atoms of the purine or pyrimidine skeleton through addition to the 2′-OH group of ribose or additions on the "exo"-nitrogen groups at the N^6 or N^2 positions of

* This research was supported by grant CA 18137 from the National Cancer Institute, DHEW

Recent Results in Cancer Research. Vol. 84

Table 1. Methylation sites in mammalian nucleic acids [from Agris and Söll (1977), Pegg (1977), and Busch (1976)]

A. DNA		
	Cytosine	5-
B. mRNA		
	Adenine	N^6-
	Guanine	7-
	Ribose	2'-OH
C. rRNA		
	Adenine	N^6-, N^6,N^6-dimethyl
	Guanine	7-
	Cytosine	5-, N^4-
	Uracil	5-, 3-
	Ribose	2'-OH
D. tRNA		
	Adenine	1-, 2-, N^6-
	Guanine	1-, 7-, N^2-, N^2,N^2-dimethyl
	Cytosine	3-, 5-
	Others	1-methylinosine, Y-base, etc.
	Ribose	2'-OH
E. Other RNA species		
	Guanine	7-, N^2,N^2-trimethyl

Other methylated products are also found in some RNA species, including those in mitochondria

purines to more complex modifications involving several methyl groups or methylation in addition to other modification. Transfer RNA is the most extensively methylated species, and methylation, which occurs at particular sequences and positions, is essential to maintain normal structure and function. The methylated sequence forming the cap at the end of mRNA is essential for normal translation, and methylation is important for both processing and function of ribosomal RNA.

Mammalian DNA appears to contain only one normal methylated base, namely 5-methylcytosine. Methylation occurs predominantly but not exclusively in the sequence CpG (Razin and Riggs 1980; Razin and Friedman 1981; Ehrlich and Wang 1981). Suggestions that such methylations may be involved in differentiation and gene expression have received recent support from findings that 5-methylcytosine is present in certain genes in cells in which this gene product is not expressed but that the same sequence is unmethylated in cells in which the gene is active (Compere and Palmiter 1981; McGhee and Ginder 1979; Jones and Taylor 1980).

The source of the methyl-groups in mammalian nucleic acids is *S*-adenosylmethionine (Kerr and Borek 1972; Borek et al. 1977; Pegg 1977). Specific methyltransferase enzymes are responsible for the production of the methylated nucleosides. Some of these enzymes have been highly purified, but much remains to be accomplished in this area. A particular problem in such purification is the need to obtain an unmethylated substrate for assay. Many methylation reactions are complete in vivo and methylation of RNA takes place on a precursor which frequently requires further processing by nucleases etc. Thus a physiological substrate for methyltransferases may be very difficult to obtain. Methylation is both sequence-specific and dependent on the tertiary structure of the nucleic acid, and discrete enzymes are responsible for each methylation. Methylation of DNA may, under some circumstances, be possible at methylatable sites which are completely unmethylated. However, many theories and some experimental evidence favor the concept that methylation is maintained during DNA replication by the selective methylation by the DNA methylase of the hemimethylated sites of the type:

$$\begin{array}{l} -m^5CpG- \\ \quad -GpC- \end{array}$$

containing 5-methylcytosine in the parent strand (Razin and Riggs 1980; Drahovsky and Boehm 1980). This provides a mechanism by which methylation is conserved during cell division but can be removed for succeeding generations if the methylation process is ever inhibited. Such inhibition would generate a completely nonmethylated site which would not be recognized by the maintenance methylase. In this way, factors preventing methylation could act and produce a permanent change in methylation even though the methylase enzyme is present and active in the cells when measurements are made at later times.

Methylation of Nucleic Acids by Nitrosamines and Related Alkylating Agents

Methylation can also be brought about in the cell by exposure to a variety of chemicals which are either themselves alkylating agents or are converted within the cell to methylating species (Table 2). These include dimethyl sulfate, methyl methanesulfonate, *N*-methyl-*N*-nitrosourea, *N*-methyl-*N'*-nitro-*N*-nitrosoguanidine, and streptozotocin, which do not require enzymatic activation to generate a reactive species. Examples of those agents which do require metabolic activation are dimethylnitrosamine, 1,2-dimethylhydrazine, *N*-methyl-*N*-benzylnitrosamine, cycasin, and dimethylphenyltriazines. Since the final reactive methylating agent generated from these compounds following metabolism is too unstable to travel far from the cells in which it is generated (Pegg 1977, 1980a), much higher levels of methylation are produced in some cells than in others because these cells contain much higher levels of the activating enzymes. Methylation produced by the direct-acting alkylating agents such as methyl methanesulfonate or *N*-methyl-*N*-nitrosourea occurs more evenly throughout most tissues, because the compounds do not require enzymatic attack to generate the alkylating species and penetrate most cells to approximately the same extent. However, even agents not requiring metabolic activation may show striking tissue specificity in the extent to which methylation can occur. For example, streptozotocin preferentially alkylated the β-cells in the pancreatic islets and the kidney, but produced virtually no methylation in the brain. (Bennett and Pegg 1981). Presumably this is due to the selective uptake of the compound, which is a glucose derivative of nitrosomethylurea. The glucose moiety results in ready uptake into the pancreas but prevents passage into the brain. *N*-methyl-*N'*-nitro-*N*-nitrosoguanidine decomposes to generate the methylating species more readily in the presence of sulfhydryl groups, and intracellular methylation may reflect the presence of such catalysts (Lawley 1976).

Table 2. Carcinogenic methylating agents

Compound	[O]-Alkylation[a]	Metabolic Activation	Tissue selectivity in distribution of methylation
Dimethylnitrosamine	High	Yes	Yes
N-methyl-*N*-nitrosourea	High	No	No
1,2-Dimethylhydrazine	High	Yes	Yes
3,3-Dimethyl-1-phenyl-triazine	High	Yes	Yes
Cycasin	High	Yes	Yes
Streptozotocin	High	No	Yes
Dimethyl sulfate	Very low	No	No
Methyl methanesulfonate	Low	No	No
N-Methyl-*N'*-nitro-*N*-nitrosoguanidine	High	No	Yes
Methyl, R >N-N = O	High	Yes	Yes

[a] [O]-Alkylation refers to the ability to methylate the oxygen atoms in guanine, pyrimidines, and phosphate groups

Table 3. Methylation sites in nucleic acids subject to attack by carcinogenic alkylating agents

Cytosine	3-, O^2-
Uracil	3-, O^2-,O^4-
Thymine	3-, O^2-, O^4-
Adenine	1-, 3-, 7-
Guanine	3-, 7-, O^6-
Phosphate	

At least 12 methylation sites have been identified as the result of methylation of nucleic acids by the chemicals shown in Table 2 and related compounds under physiological conditions (Singer 1976; Lawley 1976; Pegg 1977; Margison and O'Connor 1979; Singer and Kusmierek 1982). These sites (Table 3), include methylation on phosphate groups, methylation of the nitrogen atoms at positions 1, 3, and 7 of adenine, positions 1 and 7 of guanine, and position 3 of pyrimidines. Additionally, there is methylation at the exo-oxygen atoms of guanine and the pyrimidines. Similar products are formed in RNA, although the relative amounts are somewhat different, with 3-methyladenine being a very small fraction and 1-methyladenine relatively larger. Although there have been some suggestions that such methylation of nucleic acids may not be entirely random, methylation occurs at many places within the nucleic acid sequence. Under most experimental conditions the overall degree of alkylation produced by nonlethal doses of the compounds is quite small, amounting to less than one methyl group per 1000 nucleosides. Thus, nucleic acid sequences present as many copies per cell are unlikely all to be methylated in the same sites. However, more information is needed on the distribution of methylated bases, particularly within the chromatin structure.

Different methylating species produce different relative amounts of the methylated bases in Table 3. The *N*-nitroso-compounds generate an alkylating species with properties of a methyl carbonium ion, and this produces a higher proportion of adducts on oxygens than methyl methanesulfonate or dimethylsulfate, which react more via an S_N2-type mechanism. Because the *N*-nitroso-compounds are much more potent carcinogens than the latter agents, particular attention has been focussed on the oxygen adducts as being important in tumor initiation. Most of this research has centered on O^6-methylguanine rather than on the *O*-methylpyrimidines and the methylphosphate triesters. The reasons for this are more practical than scientific; O^6-methylguanine is formed in considerably larger amounts than the pyrimidines and is easier to measure than the other *O*-methyl products. Nevertheless, quite persuasive evidence has been gathered that the persistence during cell replication of O^6-methylguanine may be able to cause a neoplastic change. (Pegg 1977; Margison and O'Connor 1979). O^6-Alkylation of guanine in a nucleic acid promotes misincorporation by nucleic acid polymerases and mutations in viruses. This is probably not the case with other alkylations of the purines at ring nitrogens, but the *O*-methylpyrimidines could also contribute (Singer 1976; Singer and Kusmierek 1982). This work suggests one possible way in which the presence of abnormal alkylation might lead to neoplastic growth, namely by producing a somatic cell mutation, but other possibilities are by no means ruled out. As discussed below, methylation by chemicals could influence normal enzymatic methylation and this could affect subsequent differentiation.

Effect of Ethionine on Nucleic Acid Alkylation

Ethionine is the ethyl analog of the amino acid methionine, and is known to be carcinogenic if fed in large quantities to rats (Farber 1963). Administration of ethionine leads to the production of *S*-adenosylethionine in the liver, since at least one of the isoenzymes of *S*-adenosylmethionine synthetase present in mammalian cells can use ethionine for this reaction. Administration of ethionine alters nucleic acid alkylation in several ways. Both DNA and RNA are ethylated, but they are also undermethylated. (Swann et al. 1971; Pegg 1972; Lu et al. 1976; Christman et al. 1977, 1980; Cox and Irving 1977; Goswami and Sharma 1980; Boehm and Drahovsky 1979). The undermethylation probably relates to the competitive inhibition of methyltransferases activities by *S*-adenosylethionine. Part of the ethylation of nucleic acid is likely to be mediated via the action of methyltransferase enzymes which are able to use *S*-adenosylethionine as a substrate, but not all the ethylation (for example, that of DNA at the 7 position of guanine) could be explained in this way, since no methyltransferase carrying out this reaction is known. Thus it is possible that a direct ethylating agent is involved in these reactions. One possible candidate is *S*-adenosylethionine itself (see this chapter, "Rationale for Presence of Enzymes Repairing Methylation Damage in DNA"), although some evidence that carcinogenicity and nucleic acid ethylation is decreased by treatment with agents which enhance the content of *S*-adenosylethionine has been published (Kamamoto et al. 1973; Brada et al. 1975; Yamane et al. 1976, 1977) and other reactive intermediates such as *S*-vinyl homocysteine have been suggested (Leopold et al. 1979).

There is no doubt that ethionine is somewhat unusual for an alkylating agent which is also carcinogenic, in that its reaction with protein and RNA is much greater than its

Table 4. Ethylation of DNA in vivo following administration of ethionine or diethylnitrosamine [From Swann et al. (1971) and Pegg and Balog (1979)]

Treatment	Ethylation of DNA (μmol 7-ethylguanine/mol guanine)
Ethionine (500 mg/kg)	4.3
Diethylnitrosamine (1 mg/kg)	4.5

reaction with DNA. However, this is not a good argument for ruling out DNA as a possible target molecule. As shown in Table 4, the interaction of ethionine with DNA compares quite well with that of diethylnitrosamine when expressed in terms of a dietary level at which tumors are obtained. Although ethionine ethylates DNA two orders of magnitude less well than diethylnitrosamine, it also requires two orders of magnitude more ethionine for a carcinogenic regime.

Other Carcinogens Producing DNA Methylation

Recent experiments from Shank's laboratory raise the possibility that DNA methylation may be a more general response to carcinogens and toxins, rather than solely due to alkylating agents of the type described in Table 2. They observed the formation of 7-methylguanine and, in some cases, O^6-methylguanine in rat liver DNA after treatment with hydrazine, carbon tetrachloride, or ethanol (Barrows and Shank 1981; Becker et al. 1981). The bases were separated by high-performance liquid chromatography (HPLC) and quantitated by ultraviolet absorption or fluorescence spectrophotometry. Independent confirmation of these findings with other methods is urgently needed. The mechanism by which the methylation occurs is unclear but experiments in which rats were treated with [methyl-^{3}H]methionine showed incorporation of the methyl group into the methylated bases (Barrows and Shank 1981). This suggest that *S*-adenosylmethionine may be involved either directly or via the reaction of methyltransferases.

Effect of Carcinogens on 5-Methylcytosine Production in DNA

Several groups have provided evidence that exposure to carcinogens reduces the methylation of DNA at the 5 position of cytosine. In addition to the results obtained with ethionine and discussed above, such inhibition was seen after reaction of the DNA substrate with acetylaminofluorene (Pfohl-Leskowicz et al. 1981; Salas et al. 1979; Lapeyre and Becker 1979), and exposure to *N*-methyl-*N'*-nitro-*N*-nitrosoguanidine or *N*-methyl-*N*-nitrosourea (Cox 1980; Boehm and Drahovsky 1981). Such inhibition may be caused by direct alkylation of the methylase in the case of the nitrosoguanidine derivative (Cox 1980), but other alkylating agents did not affect the enzyme directly (Cox 1980) and are more likely to act via alteration in the ability of the DNA to serve as substrate (Drahovsky and Boehm 1980), as is also the case with DNA modified by acetylaminofluorene (Pfohl-Leskowicz et al. 1981).

These inhibitions are of particular interest since it is known that inhibition of DNA(cytosine-5)methylase by exposure of cells to 5-azacytidine (Friedman 1979,

1981) results in reduction of methylation of DNA which persists through many generations and is associated with changes in the differentiated state (Jones and Taylor 1980; Compere and Palmiter 1981; Christman et al. 1980). This provides evidence supporting the hypothesis that the maintenance methylase described above and the level of 5-methylcytosine in DNA are important in differentiation. Ethionine can also cause persistent changes in the differentiated state, presumably by preventing methylation in this manner (Christman et al. 1977, 1980). The implications of these findings for carcinogenesis are of obvious importance and are receiving much experimental attention.

Removal of Methylated Bases from Nucleic Acids in Vivo

As yet, no specific mechanisms for the removal of methylated nucleosides from RNA are known. The methylated derivatives are, therefore, liberated as free nucleotides after degradation of the RNA as part of the normal process of RNA turnover. Methylation products formed in reaction of carcinogenic alkylating agents with cellular RNA are also lost only as the RNA is degraded (Pegg 1977; Margison and O'Connor 1979). We have tested the enzymes described below which remove 7-methylguanine and O^6-methylguanine from DNA for the ability to release these bases from RNA, and they have no activity with RNA substrates. Chemically alkylated RNA turns over at the same rate as normal RNA (Margison and O'Connor 1979). Therefore, except under conditions where massive doses are given which induce cell necrosis, methylated bases will be liberated only as a consequence of normal cellular catabolism.

There is also no known enzyme able to remove 5-methylcytosine from DNA, and reductions in methylation status at this site appear to require cell replication. In contrast, most of the methylation products produced by interaction with carcinogens decline with time in vivo (Pegg 1977; Margison and O'Connor 1979; Singer and Kusmierek 1982). Discrete enzymes have been characterized from mammalian cells for the removal of only three of these products, namely 3-methyladenine, 7-methylguanine and O^6-methylguanine. The first two of these are removed by the action of glycosylases which liberate the free base and leave behind an apurinic site (Brent 1979; Singer and Brent 1981; Margison and Pegg 1981; Cathcart and Goldthwait 1981). Similar enzymes are present in bacteria and have been purified more extensively from this source (Lindahl 1979; Lindahl et al. 1982). Since the methylation labilizes the bond between the purine and the sugar to an extent that considerable depurination occurs even at normal physiological pH, these enzymes speed up a reaction which takes place at a considerable rate in any case (Lawley 1976; Pegg 1977; Margison and O'Connor 1979). As shown in Table 5, which compares the loss of methylated bases from DNA in rat and hamster liver in vivo and in isolated DNA in vitro, the 3-methyladenine-DNA glycosylase increases this rate by a factor of 3 in both species. Rat liver contains less of the 7-methylguanine-DNA glycosylase than hamster liver and in the rat the rate of loss of this purine is about twice that in vitro, whereas in the hamster it is about five times faster. These results suggest that the enzymes responsible for these reactions are separate, but Cathcart and Goldthwait (1981) have claimed that a partially purified enzyme is able to remove both 3-methyladenine and 7-methylguanine. The presence of more than one glycosylase, at least one of which is specific, would explain this discrepancy, and evidence for such multiplicity is available for bacteria (Lindahl et al. 1982).

Table 5. Removal of 3-methyladenine and 7-methylguanine from DNA in vivo and in vitro by extracts from rat or hamster liver

Species	Half-life of purine (h)		Activity of glycosylase (units/mg protein)	
	3-methyl-adenine	7-methyl-guanine	3-methyl-adenine	7-methyl-guanine
Rat	6	70	1.23	0.47
Hamster	5	24	1.65	1.07
Incubated DNA in vitro	18	140	–	–

An enzyme removing O^6-methylguanine from DNA was present in greatest amounts in extracts from liver. Appreciable activity was also found in kidney extracts, although less than in liver, but other organs were much less active (Pegg 1978, 1980b). This correlates well with the persistence of O^6-methylguanine in DNA in vivo (Pegg 1977). There are also striking species differences in the activity of the enzyme system responsible for O^6-methylguanine removal. Hamster liver was less active than rat liver in removing O^6-methylguanine from DNA after dimethylnitrosamine, which correlates with the greater sensitivity of the hamster to liver tumor induction by single doses of this carcinogen (Stumpf et al. 1979). Recently, we have observed that human liver extracts are six to ten times more active than those from rats in catalyzing O^6-methylguanine removal, which raises the possibility than human liver may be relatively resistant to carcinogenesis by methylating agents (Pegg et al. 1982 b).

The mechanism by which O^6-methylguanine is removed from DNA is depicted in Fig. 1 and is similar in some respects to that pertaining in certain bacteria *(Escherichia coli)* in that the methyl group is removed directly, regenerating the guanine residue in the DNA (Foote et al. 1980; Pegg and Perry 1981). The methyl group is transferred to a protein acceptor molecule which in *E. coli* forms an *S*-methylcysteine residue and prevents the acceptor from being used again (Olsson and Lindahl 1980). In rat liver it may be that the reaction is catalytic rather than stoichiometric, but we have also identified *S*-methylcysteine as a product (unpublished observations) and recently Bogden et al. (1981) have also found this with mouse liver extracts. The mechanism of regeneration of the acceptor, which could be the rate-limiting step in this reaction, remains unclear.

The *E. coli* enzyme responsible for demethylation of O^6-methylguanine in DNA is inducible in response to exposure to certain alkylating agents which bring about a manyfold increase in activity. This phenomenon protects against mutagenesis by alkylating agents and has been termed the adaptive response (Cairns et al. 1981). The possibility that mammalian cells might also show such induction was supported by the findings of several groups showing that chronic treatment with dimethylnitrosamine, 3,3-dimethyl-1-phenyltriazine, or diethylnitrosamine increased the rate of O^6-methylguanine loss in vivo (Montesano and Margison 1980; Pegg 1980b). Such an increase can also be demonstrated by assay of the enzyme in vitro (Pegg 1980b), but as shown in Table 6 more recent studies have shown that increases are produced by many

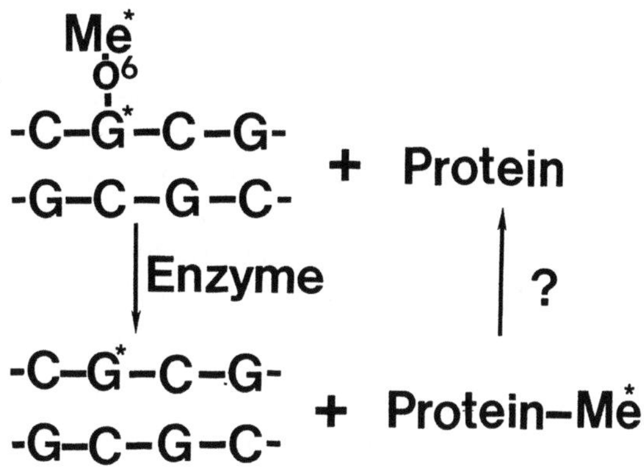

Fig. 1. Mechanism of removal of O^6-methylguanine from DNA by rat liver extracts. The experiment was carried out with a synthetic DNA substrate containing O^6-methylguanine labeled in both the purine and the methyl group as shown. After incubation with an extract purified 200-fold from regenerating rat liver, stoichiometric amounts of labeled guanine in DNA and labeled protein were formed. It is not known whether the protein acceptor is the enzyme itself or the methyl acceptor can be regenerated as shown (A. E. Pegg, unpublished results)

Table 6. Enhancement of O^6-methylguanine removal from DNA in vivo and in vitro

Treatment	Stimulation of O^6-methylguanine removal	
	In vivo	In vitro by isolated enzyme
Dimethylnitrosamine[a, b]	+	+
Diethylnitrosamine[a, b]	+	+
3,3-Dimethyl-1-phenyltriazine[a]	+	Not tested
Acetylaminofluorene[a]	+	Not tested
Aflatoxin[c]	+	Not tested
Streptozotocin[b]	Not tested	−
N-methyl-*N*-nitrosourea[b, d]	−	−
1,2-Dimethylhydrazine[b, d]	+	+
Carbon tetrachloride[b]	Not tested	+
Thioacetamide[b]	Not tested	+
Phenobarbital[b]	−	−
3-Methylcholanthrene[b]	−	−

[a] See reviews by Pegg (1980b) and Montesano and Margison (1980)
[b] Pegg and Perry (1981)
[c] Chu et al. (1981)
[d] Margison (1981)

hepatotoxins or carcinogens which are not alkylating agents (Chu et al. 1981; Pegg and Perry 1981). Furthermore, direct alkylating agents such as *N*-methyl-*N*-nitrosourea and streptozotocin did not induce activity (Pegg and Perry 1981; Margison 1981). Therefore alkylation alone does not induce the liver enzyme. A possible explanation of the induction by nitrosamines and other hepatotoxins was provided by our finding that partial hepatectomy increases the activity (Pegg et al. 1981). It is possible that a substantial part of the increase brought about by chemicals is due to tissue damage and restorative growth. Whether all of the increase can be explained in this way remains to be determined.

Excretion of Methylated Nucleosides and Bases

Methylated nucleosides or bases derived from nucleic acids by degradation or repair are not reutilized, but are either metabolized further or excreted unchanged. Numerous methylation products derived from RNA are found in the urine (Pegg 1977; Gehrke et al. 1978). The appearance of elevated amounts of these products has been suggested as a screening method for neoplastic disease, since increased cell turnover and possibly a more rapid degradation of some tRNAs in tumors could lead to such elevation (Borek et al. 1977). The appearance of the methylation products in the urine is a consequence of the resistance conferred by methylation of nucleosides to many of the reactions by which they are degraded or salvaged and reincorporated. This is also the case for some of the products of alkylating agents. There is particular interest in the quantitation of such products by ultrasensitive methods such as radioimmunoassay or other coupled immunological techniques, because it might then be possible to measure environmental or occupational exposure to such agents. Although 7-methylguanine is a major product of such exposure and is excreted completely (Pegg 1977; Margison and O'Connor 1979), either unchanged or with the minor modification of 8-hydroxylation, it is not useful for such a purpose because of its occurrence as a normal product in tRNA and mRNA. There is no way to distinguish the small amount which will be generated by low levels of exposure to alkylating agents from the higher background produced by RNA metabolism. O^6-Methylguanine is also not suitable for such purposes, even though it may be a critical product for carcinogenesis. As discussed above, the DNA repair reaction responsible for the loss of this product involves transfer of the methyl group, and the free base or nucleoside is not formed. Degradation of alkylated RNA presumably generates the nucleoside, but O^6-methylguanosine is a good substrate for adenosine deaminase which demethylates it (Pegg and Swann 1979). Thus no O^6-methylguanine or its nucleoside would be expected in the urine of rats treated with nitrosamines, and none has been found. The most viable candidate for such screening would appear to be 3-methyladenine, since this is rapidly removed as the base from DNA, is not metabolized further, and is excreted quantitatively (Pegg 1977; Margison and O'Connor 1979). However, antibodies to this base are not available at present and it is formed to only a small extent in RNA, which may limit the sensitivity of detection.

Rationale for Presence of Enzymes Repairing Methylation Damage in DNA

It is interesting to speculate why mammalian cells contain DNA-repairing enzymes specific for removal of alkylation damage. It is still remotely possible that the enzymes described above have other substrates, but at present only methylated or ethylated bases in DNA are known to be attacked. The energy and resources devoted to making these enzymes would presumably not be expended without a good reason, which may be taken as evidence that alkylation is not a rare occurrence. Although the O^6-methylguanine removal system is inducible to a small extent and there is a recent report that the 3-methyladenine-DNA glycosylase is also inducible (Gombar et al. 1981), a significant fraction of these activities is present in uninduced cells. [In *E. coli,* both the O^6- and the 7-methylguanine removal enzymes are inducible, as is one minor form of the 3-methyladenine-DNA glycosylase (Cairns et al. 1981; Lindahl et al. 1982)].

These results may be indicative of a continued alkylation of DNA, but at present the mechanism of such methylation is unknown. Three obvious possibilities are (a) the ingestion of small amounts of nitrosamine in the diet and the probable synthesis endogenously of larger amounts through the reaction of nitrite and secondary amines in the gastrointestinal tract; (b) the formation of methylation products by the as yet uncharacterized reactions responsible for such methylation in the presence of hepatotoxins seen by Shank and co-workers (see this chapter, "Other Carcinogens Producing DNA Methylation"); and (c) *S*-adenosylmethionine acting as a chemical methylating agent and producing a low level of methylation without enzymatic catalysis. This third possibility has been considered in the past by a number of workers, particularly those interested in the pathobiochemistry of ethionine, since *S*-adenosylethionine accumulates in some organs and chemical ethylation by this agent could account for the presence of 7-ethylguanine in DNA (Swann et al. 1971). More recently, Lindahl et al. (1982) reported the formation of 7-methylguanine and 3-methyladenine in DNA after incubation for 6 h with *S*-adenosylmethionine. We have also observed the production of material cochromatographing with 7-methylguanine on HPLC when DNA is incubated with *S*-adenosylmethionine (R. A. Bennett and A. E. Pegg, unpublished observations), although the amount formed (one 7-methylguanine per 50,000,000 guanine molecules after 4 h exposure to 50 μM *S*-adenosylmethionine) was somewhat less than that seen by Lindahl et al. (1982). These results provide preliminary evidence that chemical methylation by *S*-adenosylmethionine may take place, but more rigorous product identification and proof that no impurities are responsible for this very small amount of reaction are needed. Evidence that this reaction does take place in the cell may be quite difficult to obtain, but one possible approach is based on another potential alkylating agent present in mammalian cells. This is decarboxylated *S*-adenosylmethionine, which is used as the aminopropyl donor for polyamine synthesis (Williams-Ashman and Pegg 1981). Normally decarboxylated *S*-adenosylmethionine concentrations are very low, 20–100 times less than those of *S*-adenosylmethionine itself (Hibasami et al. 1980), but when the cell is prevented from forming putrescine by administration of inhibitors of ornithine decarboxylase, the acceptor for the aminopropyl group is not present and decarboxylated *S*-adenosylmethionine accumulates. Therefore, increases of more than 500-fold in the content of decarboxylated *S*-adenosylmethionine take place in cells treated with α-difluoromethylornithine (Pegg et al. 1982). Under these circumstances the total cellular content of the putative alkylating agents, *S*-adenosylmethionine and its decarboxylated derivative, is five to ten times higher than normal. Unlike the small increase in *S*-adenosylmethionine produced by excess methionine, which is very transient, such conditions can be maintained over a long period of time. It will, therefore, be of particular interest to test whether any methylation of DNA at sites attacked by alkylating agents occurs under these circumstances. These experiments are in progress, but it may be relevant that Hung et al. (1981) have very recently reported that exposure to α-difluoromethylornithine renders rat brain tumor cells more sensitive to the toxicity of certain nitrosourea derivatives known to be alkylating agents.

References

Agris P, Söll D (1977) The modified nucleosides in transfer RNA. In: Vogel HJ (ed) Nucleic acid-protein recognition. Academic Press, New York, pp 321–344

Barrows LR, Shank RC (1981) Aberrant methylation of liver DNA in rats during hepatotoxicity. Toxicol Appl Pharmacol 60:334–345

Becker RA, Barrows LR, Shank RC (1981) Methylation of liver DNA guanine in hydrazine hepatotoxicity: dose response and kinetic characteristics of 7-methylguanine and O^6-methylguanine formation and persistence in rats. Carcinogenesis 2:1181–1188

Bennett RA, Pegg AE (1981) Alkylation of DNA in rat tissues following administration of streptozotocin. Cancer Res 41:2786–2790

Boehm TLJ, Drahovsky D (1979) Effect of carcinogen ethionine on enzymatic methylation of DNA sequences with various degrees of repetitiveness. Eur J Cancer 15:1167–1175

Boehm TLJ, Drahovsky D (1981) Hypomethylation of DNA in Raji cells after treatment with *N*-methyl-*N*-nitrosourea. Carcinogenesis 2:39–42

Bogden JM, Eastman A, Bresnick E (1981) A system in mouse liver for the repair of O^6-methylguanine lesions in methylated DNA. Nucleic Acids Res 9:3089–3103

Borek E, Baliga BS, Gehrke CW, Kuo CW, Belman S, Troll W, Waalkes TP (1977) Higher turnover rate of transfer RNA in tumor tissue. Cancer Res 37:3362–3366

Brada Z, Altman NH, Bulba S (1975) The effect of cupric acetate on ethionine metabolism. Cancer Res 35:3172–3180

Brent TP (1979) Partial purification and characterization of human 3-methyladenine-DNA glycosylase. Biochemistry 18:911–916

Busch H (1976) The function of the 5′CAP of mRNA and nuclear RNA species. Perspect Biol Med 19:549–567

Cairns J, Robins P, Sedgwick B, Talmud P (1981) The inducible repair of alkylated DNA. Prog Nucleic Acid Res Mol Biol 26:237–246

Cathcart R, Goldthwait DA (1981) Enzymatic excision of 3-methyladenine and 7-methylguanine by a rat liver nuclear fraction. Biochemistry 20:273–280

Christman JK, Price P, Pedrinan L, Acs G (1977) Correlation between hypomethylation of DNA and expression of globin genes in friend erythroleukemia cells. Eur J Biochem 81:366–370

Christman JK, Weich N, Schoenbrun B, Schneiderman N, Acs G (1980) Hypomethylation of DNA during differentiation of friend erythroleukemia cells. J Cell Biol 86:366–370

Chu Y-H, Craig AW, O'Connor PJ (1981) Repair of O^6-methylguanine in rat liver DNA is enhanced by pretreatment with single or multiple doses of aflatoxin B_1. Br J Cancer 43:850–855

Compere SJ, Palmiter RD (1981) DNA methylation controls the inducibility of the mouse metallothionine-1 gene in lymphoid cells. Cell 25:233–240

Cox R (1980) DNA methylation inhibition *in vitro* by *N*-methyl-*N*′-nitro-*N*-nitrosoguanidine. Cancer Res 40:61–63

Cox R, Irving CC (1977) Inhibition of DNA methylation by S-adenosylethionine with the production of methyl-deficient DNA in regenerating rat liver. Cancer Res 37:222–225

Drahovsky D, Boehm TLJ (1980) Enzymatic DNA methylation in higher eukaryotes. Int J Biochem 12:523–528

Ehrlich M, Wang RY-H (1981) 5-methylcytosine in eukaryotic DNA. Science 212:1350–1357

Farber E (1963) Ethionine carcinogenesis. Adv Cancer Res 7:383–474

Foote RS, Mitra S, Pal BC (1980) Demethylation of O^6-methylguanine in a synthetic DNA polymer by an inducible activity in *Escherichia coli*. Biochem Biophys Res Commun 97:654–659

Friedman S (1979) The effect of 5-azacytidine on *E. coli* DNA methylase. 89:1328–1333

Friedman S (1981) The inhibition of DNA(cytosine-5)methylases by 5-azacytidine. The effect of azacytosine-containing DNA. Mol Pharmacol 19:314–320

Gehrke CW, Kuo KC, Davis GE, Suits RD, Waalkes TP, Borek E (1978) Quantitative high-performance liquid chromatography of nucleosides in biological materials. J Chromatogr 150: 455–476

Gombar CT, Katz EJ, Magee PN, Sirover MA (1981) Induction of the DNA repair enzymes uracil DNA glycosylase and 3-methyladenine DNA glycosylase in regenerating rat liver. Carcinogenesis 2: 595–599

Goswami BB, Sharma OK (1980) Accumulation of methyl-deficient rat liver messenger ribonucleic acid on ethionine administration. Biochemistry 19: 2101–2108

Hibasami H, Hoffman JL, Pegg AE (1980) Decarboxylated S-adenosylmethionine in mammalian cells. J Biol Chem 255: 6675–6678

Hung DT, Deen DF, Seidenfeld J, Marton LJ (1981) Sensitization of 9L rat brain gliosarcoma cells to 1,3-bis(2-chloroethyl)-1-nitrosourea by α-difluoromethylornithine, an ornithine decarboxylase inhibitor. Cancer Res 41: 2783–2785

Jones PA, Taylor SM (1980) Cellular differentiation, cytidine analogs and DNA methylation. Cell 20: 85–93

Kamamoto Y, Makiura S, Sugihara S, Hiasa Y, Masayuki A, Ito N (1973) The inhibitory effect of copper on DL-ethionine carcinogenesis in rats. Cancer Res 33: 1129–1135

Kerr SJ, Borek E (1972) The tRNA methyltransferases. Adv Enzymol 36: 1–28

Lapeyre J-N, Becker FF (1979) 5-methylcytosine content of nuclear DNA during chemical hepatocarcinogenesis and in carcinomas which result. Biochem Biophys Res Commun 87: 698–705

Lawley PD (1976) Methylation of DNA by carcinogens. In: Montesano R, Bartsch H, Tomatis L (eds) Screening tests in chemical carcinogenesis. IARC Sci Publ 12: 181–210

Leopold WR, Miller JA, Miller EC (1979) S-vinyl homocysteine, an analog of ethionine that is highly mutagenic for *S. typhimurium* TA100. Biochem Biophys Res Commun 88: 395–401

Lindahl T (1979) DNA glycosylases, endonucleases for apurinic/apyrimidinic sites and base excision repair. Prog Nucleic Acid Res Mol Biol 22: 135–192

Lindahl T, Rydberg B, Hjelmgren T, Olsson M, Jacobsson A (1982) Cellular defense mechanisms against alkylation of DNA. In: Lemon HJF, Generoso WM (eds) Molecular and cellular mechanisms of mutagenesis. Plenum Press. New York, pp 89–102

Lu WL, Chiang GH, Randerath K (1976) Effects of DL-ethionine on mouse liver tRNA base composition. Nucleic Acids Res 3: 2243–2253

Margison GP (1981) Effect of pretreatment of rats with *N*-methyl-*N*-nitrosourea on the repair of O^6-methylguanine in liver DNA. Carcinogenesis 2: 431–434

Margison GP, O'Connor PJ (1979) Nucleic acid modification by *N*-nitrosocompounds. In: Grover PL (ed) Chemical carcinogenesis and DNA. CRC Press, West Palm Beach, FL, pp 111–159

Margison GP, Pegg AE (1981) Enzymatic release of 7-methylguanine from methylated DNA by rodent liver extracts. Proc Natl Acad Sci USA 78: 861–865

McGhee JD, Ginder GD (1979) Specific DNA methylation sites in the vicinity of the chicken β-globin genes. Nature 280: 419–420

Montesano R, Margison GP (1980) Modulation of repair of DNA damages induced by nitrosamines. In: Pullman B, Ts'o POP, Gelboin H (eds) Carcinogenesis: Fundamental mechanisms and environmental effects. Reidel, Dordrecht, Holland, pp 441–451

Olsson M, Lindahl T (1980) Repair of alkylated DNA in Escherichia coli. J Biol Chem 255: 10569–10571

Pegg AE (1972) Studies of the ethylation of rat liver transfer ribonucleic acid after administration of L-ethionine. Biochem J 128: 59–68

Pegg AE (1977) Formation and metabolism of alkylated nucleosides: possible role in carcinogenesis by nitroso compounds and alkylating agents. Adv Cancer Res 25: 195–269

Pegg AE (1978) Enzymatic removal of O^6-methylguanine from DNA by mammalian cell extracts. Biochem Biophys Res Commun 84: 166–173

Pegg AE (1980a) Metabolism of N-nitrosodimethylamine. In: Montesano R, Bartsch H, Tomatis L (eds) Molecular and cellular aspects of carcinogen screening tests. IARC Sci Publ 27: 3–22

Pegg AE (1980b) Formation and subsequent repair of alkylation lesions in tissues of rodents treated with nitrosamines. Arch Toxicol [Suppl 3] 5: 55–68

Pegg AE, Balog B (1979) Formation and subsequent excision of O^6-ethylguanine from DNA of rat liver following administration of diethylnitrosamine. Cancer Res 39: 5003–5009

Pegg AE, Perry W (1981) Stimulation of transfer of methyl groups from O^6-methylguanine in DNA to protein by rat liver extracts in response to hepatotoxins. Carcinogenesis 2: 1195–1200

Pegg AE, Swann PF (1979) Metabolism of O^6-alkyldeoxyguanosines and their effect on removal of O^6-methylguanine from rat liver DNA. Biochim Biophys Acta 565: 241–252

Pegg AE, Perry W, Bennett RA (1981) Effect of partial hepatectomy on removal of O^6-methylguanine from alkylated DNA by rat liver extracts. Biochem J 197: 195–201

Pegg AE, Pösö H, Shuttleworth K, Bennett RA (1982a) Effect of inhibition of polyamine synthesis on the content of decarboxylated *S*-adenosylmethionine. Biochem J 202: 519–526

Pegg AE, Roberfroid H, Bresil H, Likhachev A, Montesano R (1982b) Removal of O^6-methylguanine from DNA by human liver extracts. Proc Natl Acad Sci USA 79: 5162–5165

Pfohl-Leszkowicz A, Salas C, Fuchs RPP, Dirheimer G (1981) Mechanism of inhibition of enzymatic deoxyribonucleic acid methylation by 2-(acetylamino)fluorene bound to deoxyribonucleic acid. Biochemistry 20: 3020–3024

Razin A, Friedman J (1981) DNA methylation and its possible biological roles. Prog Nucleic Acid Res Mol Biol 25: 33–52

Razin A, Riggs AD (1980) DNA methylation and gene function. Science 210: 604–610

Salas CE, Pfohl-Leszkowicz A, Lang MC, Dirheimer G (1979) Effect of modification by N-acetoxy-N-2-acetylaminofluorene on the level of DNA methylation. Nature 278: 71–72

Singer B (1976) All oxygens in nucleic acids react with carcinogenic ethylating agents. Nature 264: 333–339

Singer B, Brent TP (1981) Human lymphoblasts contain DNA glycosylase activity excising N-3 and N-7 methyl and ethyl purines but not O^6-alkylguanines or 1-alkyladenines. Proc Natl Acad Sci USA 78: 856–860

Singer B, Kusmierek JT (1982) Chemical mutagenesis. Annu Rev Biochem 51: 655–693

Singer B, Spengler S, Bodell WJ (1981) Tissue-dependent enzyme-mediated repair or removal of O-ethyl pyrimidines and ethyl purines in carcinogentreated rats. Carcinogenesis 2: 1069–1073

Stumpf R, Margison GP, Montesano R, Pegg AE (1979) Formation and loss of alkylated purines from DNA of hamster liver after administration of dimethylnitrosamine. Cancer Res 39: 50–54

Swann PF, Pegg AE, Hawks A, Farber A, McGee PN (1971) Evidence for ethylation of rat liver deoxyribonucleic acid after administration of ethionine. Biochem J 123: 175–181

Williams-Ashman HG, Pegg AE (1981) Aminopropyl group transfers in polyamine biosynthesis In: Morris DR, Marton LJ (eds) Polyamines in biology and medicine. Dekker, New York, pp 43–74

Yamane Y, Sakai K, Kojima S (1976) Mechanism of suppressive effect of basic cupric acetate on rat liver carcinogenesis by ethionine. Gan 67: 295–302

Yamane Y, Sakai K, Shibata M, Chiba K (1977) Suppressive effect of copper on ethylation of rat liver DNA with ethionine *in vivo*. Gann 68: 713

*Structural Modifications and Repair of DNA in Neuro-Oncogenesis by N-Ethyl-N-nitrosourea**

M. F. Rajewsky

Institut für Zellbiologie (Tumorforschung), Universität Essen (GH), Hufelandstrasse 55, 4300 Essen 1, FRG

Introduction and General Considerations

Structural alterations of DNA in the chromatin of target cells are primary events in the multistep process of malignant transformation and tumorigenesis by most chemical carcinogens (Lawley 1976; Pegg 1977; Weinstein 1977; Grover 1979; Singer 1979; Pullman et al. 1980; Rajewsky 1980a). In general, covalent binding occurs between nucleophilic centers (electron-rich nitrogen and oxygen atoms) in cellular DNA and highly reactive, electrophilic derivatives (ultimate carcinogens) generated from the respective parent compounds (precarcinogens), either by enzyme-catalyzed "metabolic activation" or via nonenzymatic decomposition (Miller and Miller 1976, 1979). As a consequence of their reaction with DNA, most chemical carcinogens are also mutagenic (McCann et al. 1975; Nagao et al. 1978; Hollstein et al. 1979). The strong correlation of carcinogenicity and mutagenicity does not, however, constitute proof for an obligatory requirement of mutation (nor even of modification of DNA structure in general) for malignant tranformation. Cellular macromolecules other than DNA also contain multiple nucleophilic sites which can, and indeed do, react with carcinogen-generated electrophiles. In spite of this proviso, the central importance of DNA structure and conformation for the expression of genetic information provides a strong argument for a critical role of DNA alterations as a prerequisite for the initiation of carcinogenesis by chemical agents.

Besides leading to local alterations of nucleotide sequence (mutations) and helical distortions, or possibly facilitating transition of the B form of the double helix to a left-handed conformation (Z-DNA: Wang et al. 1979; Sage and Leng 1980; Santella et al. 1981; Nordheim et al. 1981), carcinogen-modified DNA structures could, for example, interfere with the patterns of mRNA processing (splicing) or DNA methylation, affect the precision of DNA rearrangements (note that transpositional events in the genome may be associated with development/differentiation in mammalian cell systems), cause inappropriate gene amplification and rearrangements at the chromosomal level, and perhaps induce error-prone DNA repair (Radman et al. 1977; Grunberger and Weinstein 1979; Crick 1979; Lapeyre and Becker 1979; Rajewsky 1980a; Boehm and Drahovsky 1981; Cairns 1981; Ehrlich and Wang 1981;

* Experimental studies in the author's laboratory were supported by the Deutsche Forschungsgemeinschaft (SFB 102) and by the Fritz Thyssen Stiftung (1980/2/41)

Fuchs et al. 1976, 1981; Lavi 1981; Pfohl-Leszkowicz et al. 1981). Whether one or several (and if so, which) of these mechanisms are of predominant importance in terms of malignant transformation is at present a matter of speculation. There can, however, be little doubt that the common denominator is interference with the genetic programmes of target cells. More information is therefore needed on the molecular basis of eukaryotic gene expression, on the mechanisms controlling phenotypic differentiation and cell proliferation in developing and mature cell systems, and on the particular combinations of genes involved in these processes.

The phenotypes of cancer cells vary not only between different tumors but also within the same tumor cell population. The wide spectrum of differing tumor cell phenotypes may not merely reflect the expression of different combinations of genes characteristic of the type of the corresponding normal cells of origin and their developmental and differentiation stage; it could also indicate that qualitatively different phenotypic alterations may share the property of resulting in a malignant behavior of cells in their respective tissue environments. The DNA transfection approach recently introduced to define animal and human genes involved in malignant transformation may soon shed further light on this problem (Lane et al. 1981; Weinberg 1981).

The late stages of the maturation of cells from the stem cell level to a terminally differentiated state are generally accompanied by a cessation of proliferative activity (Fig. 1). In mature cells, the nonproliferative state can either be of an apparently irreversible nature (e.g., neurons, granulocytes) or be reversible ("G_0-cells") under special physiological conditions, such as the requirement for reparative or functional hyperplasia (e.g., hepatocytes, astrocytes in the brain). Temporary nonproliferative states of part of a cell population are, however, also characteristic of stem cells, and probably of "precursor" cells at more advanced stages of maturation (Lajtha 1979).

Analogous to UV-induced photoproducts in DNA (Hanawalt et al. 1979), certain carcinogen-DNA adducts can be specifically recognized, removed, and repaired by cellular enzymes (Rajewsky et al. 1977; Lindahl 1979; Margison and O'Connor 1979; Lehmann and Karran 1981; Seeberg and Kleppe 1981). The majority of nonrepaired, persistent modifications introduced into DNA by carcinogens are likely to be localized in transcriptionally silent parts of the genome, and will become effective only when the functional integrity of the respective DNA sequences is "put to the test" in the course of gene activation, e.g., by the further progression of cells along the developmental/differentiation pathway, or by inducing cells to express specialized functions and to enter the cell cycle from a G_0 state (e.g., by the action of tumor promoters). No evidence is available which would indicate that cells can undergo malignant transformation after having reached a terminally differentiated, irreversibly nonproliferative state (Rajewsky 1972, 1974, 1980b). Instead, it appears that the expression of malignant phenotypes is much more readily induced in cells exposed to carcinogenic agents, either during earlier proliferation-linked stages of their differentiation pathway or in a G_0 state (Rajewsky 1972; Saunders 1978). Of particular interest is the question of whether along the differentiation pathway of a given cell lineage specific stem cell and precursor cell stages exist where by interaction with a carcinogen the gene programme can be shifted to the expression of malignant phenotypes with above-random probability (Rajewsky et al. 1977; Graf and Beug 1978; Jaenisch 1980; Rudland et al. 1980).

The molecular and cellular mechanisms of carcinogenesis can probably be best studied in so-called pulse carcinogenesis systems, i.e., systems where, after a single dose of a

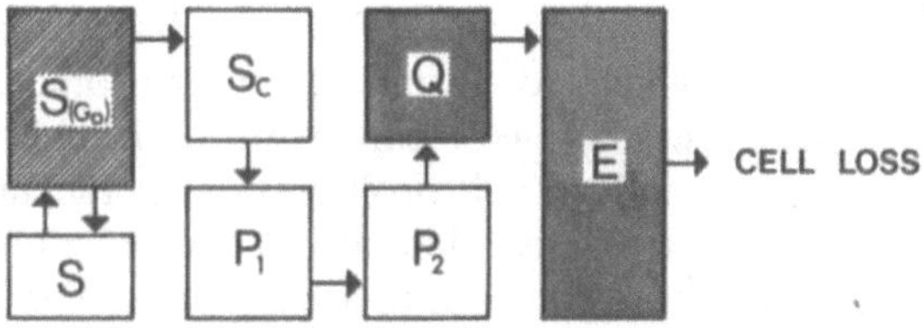

Fig. 1. Differentiating (developing) mammalian cell system. *S,* stem cells (proliferative + G_0); *Sc,* committed stem cells (proliferative); *P,* proliferative precursor cells (amplification of cell population size); *Q,* nonproliferative precursor cells; *E,* terminally differentiated, nonproliferative "end cells" (sometimes G_0)

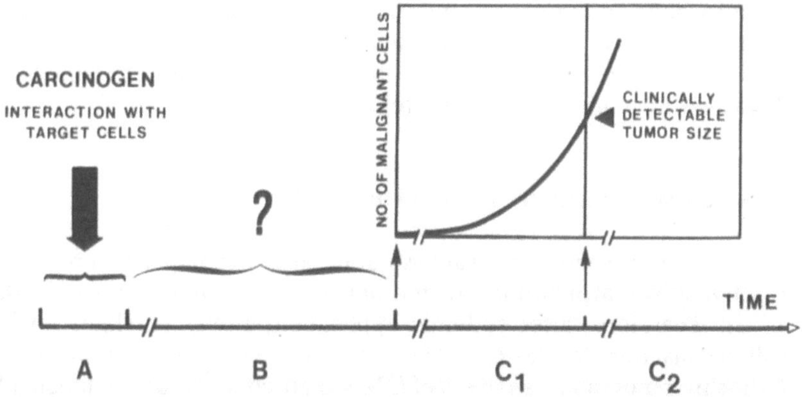

Fig. 2. Sequential phases in the process of pulse carcinogenesis. *Phase A:* Carcinogen-target cell interactions. *Phase B:* Various possible genetic consequences of persisting (unrepaired) DNA alterations in proliferative target cells. Probability of malignant transformation of target cells varies with their stage of development/differentiation and their proliferative activity (stem cells, proliferative precursors, terminally differentiated cells) at the time of carcinogen exposure. Gradual expression of malignant phenotypes. Epigenetic "second mechanisms" (altered patterns of gene expression, stimulation of cell proliferation) probably required (promotion). Host-mediated processes can influence the number of resulting tumorigenic cells and the duration of phase B. *Phase C:* (1) Onset of clonal proliferation of tumorigenic cells ("microtumors"). Host-mediated control involved: selection processes (tumor progression). (2) Tumors clinically detectable ($\geqq 10^9$ tumor cells). More rapid tumor growth. Invasion and metastasis. Host-mediated control increasingly ineffective

short-lived carcinogen sufficient to produce a high tumorigenic effect, the process proceeds autonomously without the complication of continued interaction of the target cell population(s) with the carcinogen (Rajewsky et al. 1977; Rajewsky 1980b). In such systems one can operationally separate the process of carcinogenesis into three stages: phase A, period of carcinogen interaction with target cells; phase B, interval between phase A and phase C; and phase C, period of tumor growth, beginning with the onset of (clonal) proliferation of tumorigenic cells (Fig. 2). More or less synonymous terms are "initiation" for phase A and (gradual) "expression" (of malignant phenotypes) for phase B. In spite of its obvious importance, least is presently known about phase B, which is often the longest of the three phases. Phase B appears to encompass a sequence of phenotypic changes (including acquisition of the capacity for continuous proliferation) in the cells which ultimately become tumorigenic (Laerum and

Rajewsky 1975; Barrett and Ts'o 1978; Kakunaga et al. 1980), and represents the period during which, for instance, tumor promoters (Berenblum 1975; Slaga et al. 1978; Hecker et al. 1982) can exert their pleiotropic effects, i.e., modify gene expression and induce cell proliferation in the target cell population.

In terms of their reactive derivatives and reaction products with cellular DNA, the alkylating *N*-nitroso compounds are at present the best-characterized class of chemical carcinogens (Lawley 1976; Pegg 1977; Grover 1979; O'Connor et al. 1979; Singer 1979; Rajewsky 1980a). They include the alkylnitrosamines (which require enzymatic activation) and the alkylnitrosoureas and alkylnitro-nitrosoguanidines (which undergo rapid, nonenzymatic decomposition). The resulting electrophilic alkyl substituents are very small in comparison with the bulky adducts derived from, e.g., carcinogenic hydrocarbons or aromatic amines. We have used one of the alkylnitrosoureas, *N*-ethyl-*N*-nitrosourea (EtNU; Ivankovic and Druckrey 1968), as a model "pulse carcinogen" in the BDIX rat, and the properties of this experimental system will be described in more detail in the following.

Pulse Carcinogenesis by EtNU in the Rat

N-ethyl-*N*-nitrosourea is water-soluble and decomposes nonenzymatically to a reactive ethyldiazonium ion with a half-life of < 8 min in vivo (Goth and Rajewsky 1972). Therefore, after systemic application, EtNU ethylates nucleophilic sites in cellular macromolecules (e.g., DNA) to a similar extent in all tissues, as shown by radiochromatographic analyses of DNA exposed to ^{3}H- or ^{14}C-labeled EtNU in vivo or by radioimmunoassay (RIA), and also by whole-body autoradiography (Goth and Rajewsky 1974a, b; Johansson-Brittebo and Tjälve 1979; Müller and Rajewsky 1980, and 1982 unpublished work). In spite of the similar initial degree of ethylation in all cells of the organism (phase A in the process of carcinogenesis; Fig. 2), a single dose (pulse) or EtNU applied to fetal or newborn rats results in the death of a very high proportion of the animals from malignant neuroectodermal tumors, while tumors in tissues other than the brain and peripheral nervous system (PNS) are rarely detected (neural tissue tropism of the carcinogenic effect). Following transplacental exposure to EtNU and subsequent transfer to a long-term culture system, fetal BDIX rat brain cells undergo malignant transformation in vitro after a period similar to that required for tumor formation in vivo after the same carcinogen dose (Laerum and Rajewsky 1975; Rajewsky et al. 1977; Laerum et al. 1979). Tumor yield and latency period are dose-dependent (Druckrey et al. 1970b; Rajewsky et al. 1977) and strain-dependent (Druckrey et al. 1970a).

The tumorigenic effect is, however, also a function of the developmental stage of the nervous system at the time of the carcinogen pulse (developmental/differentiation stage dependence of the carcinogenic effect; Fig. 3). The carcinogenic effect is highest after an EtNU pulse during late prenatal or early postnatal development, but decreases strongly in animals exposed to the same dose of EtNU at a later age. The carcinogenic effect is thus inversely correlated with the developmental/differentiation stage of the neural cell populations, and appears to require the presence of proliferative neural (precursor) cells at the time of exposure to the carcinogen. However, the carcinogenic effect apparently also decreases when the EtNU pulse is applied at developmental stages prior to the 15th day of gestation, and no neuroectodermal tumors were observed (in limited numbers of experimental animals;

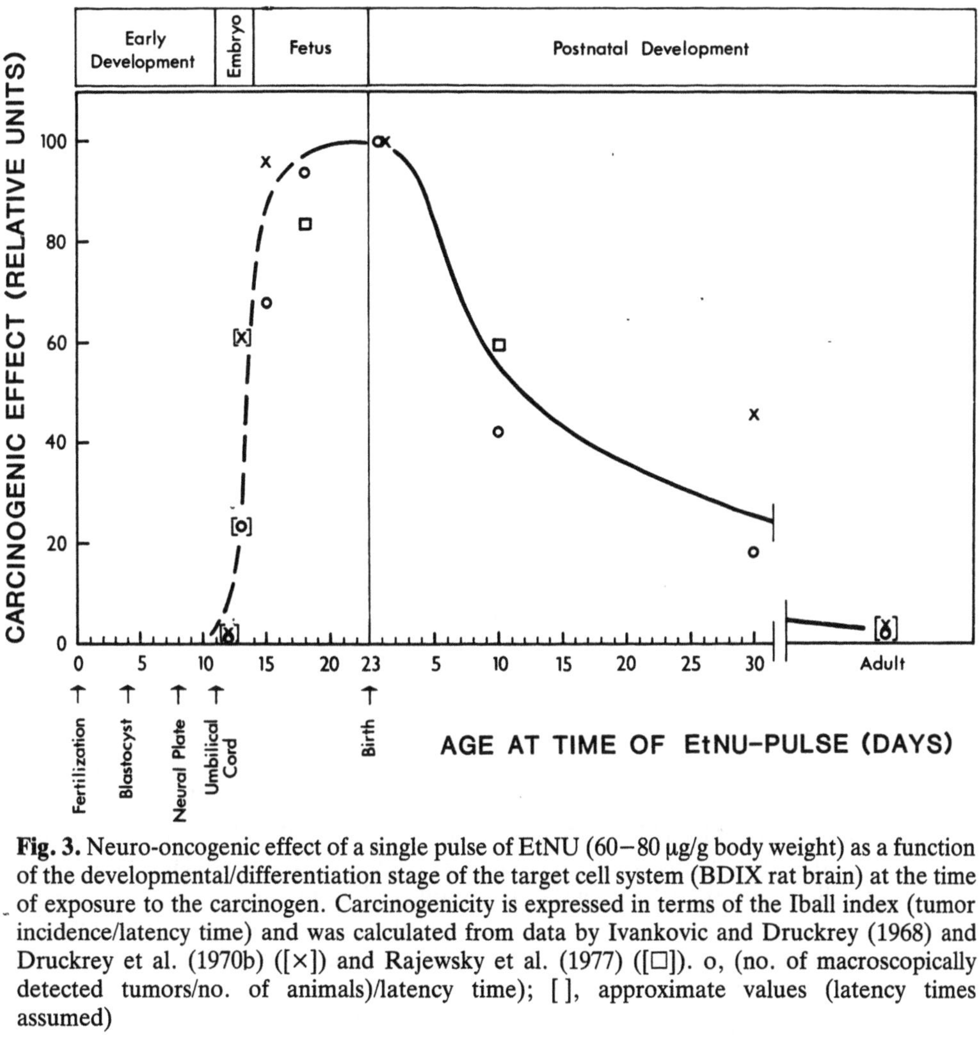

Fig. 3. Neuro-oncogenic effect of a single pulse of EtNU (60–80 μg/g body weight) as a function of the developmental/differentiation stage of the target cell system (BDIX rat brain) at the time of exposure to the carcinogen. Carcinogenicity is expressed in terms of the Iball index (tumor incidence/latency time) and was calculated from data by Ivankovic and Druckrey (1968) and Druckrey et al. (1970b) ([×]) and Rajewsky et al. (1977) ([□]). o, (no. of macroscopically detected tumors/no. of animals)/latency time); [ ], approximate values (latency times assumed)

Ivankovic and Druckrey 1968) after exposure to EtNU before the 11th day of gestation (Fig. 3). On day 11 of prenatal development the total number of cells in BDIX rat brain (probably almost all proliferating) has reached a value of approximately 10^5 (R. Müller and M. F. Rajewsky 1982, unpublished work). Thus in an experiment with ~20 rat embryos (Ivankovic and Druckrey 1968) the total neural target cell population amounts to $\sim 2 \times 10^6$ cells.

Interestingly, the developmental period of maximum sensitivity in terms of the neuro-oncogenic effect of EtNU appears to vary in different species. Only a low incidence of neural tumors has been observed in a number of mouse strains after late prenatal and neonatal administration of EtNU (Denlinger et al. 1974; Jones et al. 1976), and early postnatal application of EtNU to Mongolian gerbils has resulted in malignant transformation of (neural-crest-derived) cutaneous melanocytes but not in tumors of the brain or PNS (Kleihues et al. 1978). However, Stutman (1979) observed mainly brain tumors (besides kidney and ovary tumors) when immunologically competent (nu/+) or incompetent nu/nu mice (CBA/H or Balb/c) were treated with EtNU on days 12–14 of prenatal development, while in animals treated on days 16–18 most tumors were found in lung, liver (males), and kidney. Similarly, EtNU caused predominantly neural tumors in rabbits when applied during early phases of prenatal development, whereas exposure to EtNU during later fetal stages led mainly to kidney tumors (Stavrou et al. 1975, 1977; Fox et al. 1975). Careful analyses are therefore required in order to localize phases of increased carcinogenic risk during development/differentiation of a given cell system in different species.

The detection of alkylation products in the DNA of target tissues and cells requires highly sensitive analytical methods. The sensitivity of radiochromatographic techniques commonly used to quantitate alkylation products in DNA (Baird 1979) is limited mainly by the specific radioactivity of the respective ^{3}H- or ^{14}C-labeled carcinogens. These procedures will, under favorable conditions, detect one alkylated base in $\sim 10^6$ molecules of the corresponding normal base, and relatively large amounts of DNA (i.e., large numbers of cells) are necessary for analysis. Since radiochromatography requires the use of radioactively labeled, synthetic carcinogens, analysis of DNA from (e.g., human) tissues and cells exposed to low doses of nonradioactive (e.g., environmental) agents is not possible. In this respect, recently developed immunoanalytical procedures using high-affinity "conventional" and monoclonal antibodies (antibody affinity constants, 10^9 to $> 10^{10}$ l/mol) directed specifically against defined alkylation products in DNA have opened new possibilities (Rajewsky et al. 1980; Müller and Rajewsky 1981). Thus Müller and Rajewsky (1978, 1980) have developed a sensitive competitive RIA for the quantification of the ethylation product O^6-ethyldeoxyguanosine (O^6-EtdGuo) in DNA exposed to EtNU in vivo or in vitro. At present 0.04 pmol O^6-EtdGuo can be detected by RIA at 50% tracer-antibody binding, thus permitting quantification of O^6-EtdGuo at an O^6-EtdGuo/deoxyguanosine molar ratio of $\sim 3 \times 10^{-7}$ in a hydrolysate of 100 μg ethylated DNA (corresponding to $\sim 10^7$ diploid cells). The detection limit can be lowered even further if the alkyl-deoxynucleosides to be quantitated are separated from the DNA hydrolysate by high-performance liquid chromatography (HPLC) prior to the RIA. The spectrum of high-affinity monoclonal antibodies specific for different DNA alkylation products is presently being expanded (Adamkiewicz et al. 1981; Müller et al. 1982; Saffhill and Boyle 1981; J. Adamkiewicz and M. F. Rajewsky 1982, unpublished work), and their application is extended to the use of immunostaining techniques for detection and quantification of alkylation products in the DNA of individual cells (J. Adamkiewicz, G. Ahrens and M. F. Rajewsky, in preparation), and in isolated DNA molecules (P. Nehls, J. Adamkiewicz, H. Spiess, and M. F. Rajewsky, in preparation).

A comparison of different alkylating carcinogens indicates a positive correlation between their carcinogenicity and the relative extent of alkylation on oxygen (e.g., O^6-EtdGuo) versus nitrogen atoms [e.g., 7-ethyldeoxyguanosine (7-EtdGuo)] in DNA. Thus for the potent carcinogen EtNU the initial O^6-EtdGuo/7-EtdGuo ratio lies between 0.63 and 0.72 (Goth and Rajewsky 1974b; Singer et al. 1978), while the corresponding value for the weakly carcinogenic diethylsulfate is ~ 0.003 (Sun and Singer 1975). The relative extent of alkylation on oxygen atoms in DNA is a function of the reaction mechanism of the respective agent, in the sense that a bimolecular nucleophilic substitution (SN2) reaction will result in a lower O/N alkylation ratio than an SN2 mechanism with a tendency towards a unimolecular (SN1) reaction (Ingold 1953; Lawley 1976).

The different ethylation products formed in DNA after exposure to EtNU have been carefully analyzed (Loveless 1969; Lawley 1976; Singer et al. 1978; O'Connor et al. 1979; Singer 1979; Singer and Kröger 1979; Rajewsky 1980a). They are produced with equal relative frequencies, regardless of whether the reaction with EtNU occurs in vivo, in cell culture, or with purified DNA in vitro (Goth and Rajewsky 1974a, b; Singer et al. 1978). The following ethylation products have been detected in DNA: (a) ethylation on oxygen atoms (~80% of all ethylation products in DNA): O^6-EtdGuo (~10%), O^2-ethyldeoxythymidine (O^2-EtdThd; ~7%), O^2-ethyldeoxycytidine (O^2-EtdCyd; ~4%), O^4-ethyldeoxythymidine (O^4-EtdThD; ~3%), and ethylphosphotriesters (~56%); (b) ethylation on nitrogen atoms: 7-EtdGuo (~14%), 3-ethyldeoxyadenosine (3-EtdAdo; ~5%), 7-ethyldeoxyadenosine (7-EtdAdo; ~0.4%), 1-ethyldeoxyadenosine (1-EtdAdo; ~0.3%), 3-ethyldeoxycytidine (3-EtdCyd; ~0.2%), 3-ethyldeoxyguanosine (3-EtdGuo; ~0.1%), and 3-ethyldeoxythymidine (3-EtdThd; <0.1%).

In the case of O^6-EtdGuo, O^2-EtdCyd, O^4-EtdThd, 3-EtdThd, 3-EtdCyd, and 1-EtdAdo, the alkyl groups are localized on atoms normally involved in Watson-Crick base pairing. With the use of a competitive RIA (Müller and Rajewsky 1978, 1980), the relative O^6-EtdGuo content in DNA has been determined in chromatin of different folding levels, isolated from fetal rat brain cells and briefly exposed to EtNU in vitro (Nehls and Rajewsky 1981 and 1982, unpublished work). Compared with naked DNA (1.0), the degree of O^6-deoxyguanosine ethylation decreases from the DNA of extended (histone-H1-free) chromatin fibers (~0.6) to the DNA in nucleosomes (core particles; ~0.5), and is lowest (~0.4) in the DNA of condensed chromatin fibers ("superbeads"; Renz et al. 1977). Independent of the chromatin folding level, nucleophilic sites located in the major and minor groove and in base-pairing regions of the DNA double helix are equally accessible to the reactive ethyldiazonium ion (or equally protected by the basic structural proteins) (Nehls and Rajewsky 1981 and 1982, unpublished work). Chromosomal DNA preferentially digested with DNase I (transcribable conformation; Garel and Axel 1976; Weintraub and Groudine 1976) was found to have a higher O^6-EtdGuo content than chromosomal DNA less susceptible to this enzyme (nontranscribable genome regions) (Nehls and Rajewsky 1981 and 1982, unpublished work).

As indicated above, the initial degree of ethylation by EtNU in the DNA of pre- and postnatal rat brain (high carcinogenic risk) is not significantly different from that found in the DNA of other "low-risk" tissues (Goth and Rajewsky 1972, 1974a, b; Müller and Rajewsky 1982, unpublished work). However, as shown by kinetic analyses after a pulse of 1-^{14}C-labeled EtNU to 10-day-old BDIX rats, the content of O^6-EtdGuo decreases very rapidly in liver DNA (and less rapidly in the DNA of other tissues), but much more slowly in brain DNA. The difference in the elimination rates of O^6-EtdGuo from brain and, e.g., liver DNA is so dramatic that a specific enzymatic recognition and elimination mechanism had to be assumed for this particular alkylation product (Goth and Rajewsky 1974a; Rajewsky et al. 1977). In contrast, ethylation products such as 3-EtdAdo and 7-EtdGuo disappear from the DNA of brain and other tissues at much faster rates than does O^6-EtdGuo from brain DNA, and significant differences in tissue-specific elimination rates are not apparent. These results have recently been confirmed for an EtNU-pulse applied to Fisher rats on the 20th day of prenatal development (Chang et al. 1980). In a semilogarithmic plot, the elimination kinetics of O^6-EtdGuo have a bi- or multicomponential appearance. The reasons for this phenomenon have thus far not been definitively clarified, but several mechanisms, alone or in combination, could account for it: (a) an enzyme – or (one of) several enzymes – initially present in excess (long-lived mRNA?), consumed upon reaction, and synthesized at relatively low rate; (b) differential accessibility of O^6-EtdGuo in the DNA of chromatin of different folding levels (see above); and (c) the tissue composed of subpopulations of cells with different capacities for enzymatic elimination of O^6-EtdGuo.

O^6-ethyldeoxyguanosine not eliminated from DNA prior to a subsequent round of DNA replication can, like O^4-EtdThd (Abbott and Saffhill 1977), lead to anomalous base pairing (Loveless 1969; Abbott and Saffhill 1979), i.e., cause an alteration of nucleotide sequence in the daughter strand. Note that EtNU is presently considered the most potent point mutagen in eukaryotic systems (Russel et al. 1979; Vogel and Natarajan 1979a, b; Johnson and Lewis 1981). It is possible that persistence of O^6-EtdGuo in brain DNA and the high rate of DNA replication of the neural precursor cells during the transformation-sensitive period of brain development are among the factors reponsible for the neural tissue tropism of the carcinogenic effect of EtNU in the rat.

In spite of considerable efforts by various research groups, the search for the enzyme(s) responsible for the removal of O^6-alkylguanine from DNA has taken a surprisingly long time. In *Escherichia coli* an "adaptive response" has been discovered which can be induced by low concentrations of simple methylating agents (Samson and Cairns 1977; Jeggo et al. 1977). This response involves the expression of a system capable of transferring a methyl group (possibly also an ethyl group) from the O^6-deoxyguanosine in DNA to a cysteine residue in an acceptor protein, which is thereby apparently inactivated (Karran et al. 1979; Foote et al. 1980; Olsson and Lindahl 1980; Lindahl 1982). Although it is not excluded that an intermediate methyltransferase may be involved, it seems likely that the alkyl group is bound directly to the acceptor protein, which would then itself have the properties of a DNA methyltransferase. Interestingly, similar enzyme activities, with transfer of methyl and ethyl groups from the O^6-deoxyguanosine in DNA to cysteine residues in acceptor proteins, have recently been described for mouse and rat liver (Bogden et al. 1981; Mehta et al. 1981). Previously an active fraction specifically reducing the O^6-alkyl-deoxyguanosine content of DNA had been isolated from rodent and human liver homogenates (Pegg and Hui 1978; Pegg and Balog 1979; Pegg et al. 1982). Furthermore, evidence has been obtained indicating that the enzyme system reducing the O^6-methyldeoxyguanosine content of rat liver DNA has an elevated activity during the S phase (and possibly the G_2-M phase) of the cell cycle as compared to the G_1 phase and to the G_0 state (Rabes et al. 1979; Pegg et al. 1981). Finally, it is now well established that the enzymatic elimination of O^6-alkylguanine from liver DNA is less efficient after high carcinogen doses ("saturation" of the enzyme system; Kleihues and Margison 1976), and that in different species this saturation effect occurs at different carcinogen dose levels. Thus the liver of the Syrian golden hamster has a much lower "saturation threshold" than rat liver (Margison et al. 1976; Stumpf et al. 1979; Montesano 1981). Correspondingly, hamster liver is sensitive to the induction of hepatocellular cancer by a single dose of, e.g., dimethylnitrosamine, but rat liver is not (Tomatis and Cefis 1967; IARC 1978).

It is not yet clear whether in addition to a constitutive O^6-alkylguanine eliminating enzyme(s), there is also an inducible enzyme activity in mammalian systems, analogous to the "adaptive" DNA methyltransferase in *E. coli*. An elevated elimination capacity has been observed in rat liver in response to pretreatment with low doses of dimethylnitrosamine, diethylnitrosamine, 1,2-dimethylhydrazine, *N*-acetylaminofluorene, and 3,3-dimethyl-1-phenyltriazene (reviewed by Montesano 1981). However, the relatively low increase in elimination activity appears equally compatible with an increased fraction of proliferating hepatocytes in S phase (Rabes et al. 1979; Pegg et al. 1981), i.e., a regenerative hyperplasia in response to the carcinogen pretreatment (Rajewsky 1972). The question of cell-type and developmental/differentiation stage-dependent differences in the capacity for enzymatic elimination of critical alkylation products from DNA has not yet been investigated, except for the case of parenchymal vs nonparenchymal rat liver cells after treatment with 1,2-dimethylhydrazine, which induces hemangiosarcomas but not hepatocellular carcinomas in rats (Lewis and Swenberg 1980). It was found that O^6-methyldeoxyguanosine accumulated selectively in the nonparenchymal cells. This approach will in the future be facilitated considerably by the use of high-affinity monoclonal antibodies in conjunction with sensitive immunostaining techniques. Moreover, these techniques will permit the study of enzymatic repair processes in small numbers of cells, e.g., during prenatal stages of development. In the EtNU rat brain system, it will be important to investigate whether in the early stages of prenatal development (i.e., prior to day 15 of gestation; Fig. 3) the enzyme(s) responsible for the elimination of O^6-EtdGuo from neural precursor cells shows activity as low as or higher than during later development (Müller and Rajewsky 1982, unpublished work).

Conclusion

The formation of specifically structured, persistent carcinogen-DNA adducts (e.g., O^6-alkyldeoxyguanosine) may be a prerequisite for the initiation of the process of carcinogenesis, and (via mechanisms which remain to be clarified) lead to those alterations in the cellular genome that ultimately result in the expression of malignant phenotypes. Enzyme systems for the specific recognition, elimination, and repair of critical DNA lesions appear to be differentially expressed in different cell types, tissues, and species. The capacity of cells to repair carcinogen-modified DNA may thus constitute one of the determinants for the probability of malignant transformation, no less important than the expression of enzymes required for the metabolic "activation" of many carcinogens to their ultimate reactive forms.

References

Abbott PJ, Saffhill R (1977) DNA synthesis with methylated poly (dA-dT) templates: possible role of O^4-methylthymine as a pro-mutagenic base. Nucleic Acids Res 4: 761–769

Abbott PJ, Saffhill R (1979) DNA synthesis with methylated poly (dC-dG) templates. Evidence for a competitive nature of miscoding by O^6-methylguanine. Biochim Biophys Acta 562: 51–61

Adamkiewicz J, Eberhardt W, Langenberg U, Müller R, Rajewsky MF (1981) Monoclonal antibodies for the specific detection and quantification of DNA components structurally modified by alkylating carcinogens. Proc. Sect. Exp. Cancer Res. German Cancer Soc. J Cancer Res Clin Oncol 99: A21

Baird WM (1979) The use of radioactive carcinogens to detect DNA modifications. In: Grover PL (ed) Chemical carcinogens and DNA. CRC Press, Boca Raton, pp 59–83

Barrett JC, Ts'o POP (1978) Evidence for the progressive nature of neoplastic transformation in vitro. Proc Natl Acad Sci USA 75: 3761–3765

Berenblum I (1975) Sequential aspects of chemical carcinogenesis: Skin. In: Becker FF (ed) Cancer: A comprehensive treatise, vol 1. Plenum Press, New York, pp 323–344

Boehm TL, Drahovsky D (1981) Hypomethylation of DNA in Raji cells after treatment with N-methyl-N-nitrosourea. Carcinogenesis 2: 39–42

Bogden JM, Eastman A, Bresnick E (1981) A system in mouse liver for the repair of O^6-methylguanine lesions in methylated DNA. Nucleic Acids Res 9: 3089–3102

Cairns J (1981) The origin of human cancers. Nature 289: 353–357

Chang MJW, Hart RW, Koestner A (1980) Retention of promutagenic O^6-ethylguanine in the DNA of various rat tissues following transplacental inoculation with ethylnitrosourea. Cancer Lett 9: 199–205

Crick F (1979) Split genes and RNA splicing. Science 204: 264–271

Denlinger RH, Koestner A, Wechsler W (1974) Induction of neurogenic tumors in C3HeB/FeJ mice by nitrosourea derivatives: Observations by light microscopy, tissue culture, and electron microscopy. Int J Cancer 13: 559–571

Druckrey H, Landschütz C, Ivankovic S (1970a) Transplacentare Erzeugung maligner Tumoren des Nervensystems. II. Äthyl-nitrosoharnstoff an 10 genetisch definierten Rattenstämmen. Z Krebsforsch 73: 371–386

Druckrey H, Schagen B, Ivankovic S (1970b) Erzeugung neurogener Malignome durch einmalige Gabe von Äthyl-nitrosoharnstoff (ÄNH) an neugeborene und junge BDIX-Ratten. Z Krebsforsch 74: 141–161

Ehrlich M, Wang RY-H (1981) 5-Methylcytosine in eukaryotic DNA. Science 212: 1350–1357

Foote RS, Mitra S, Pal BC (1980) Demethylation of O^6-methylguanine in a synthetic DNA polymer by an inducible activity in Escherichia coli. Biochem Biophys Res Commun 97: 654–659

Fox RR, Diwan BA, Meier H (1975) Transplacental induction of primary renal tumors in rabbits treated with 1-ethyl-1-nitrosourea. J Natl Cancer Inst 54: 1439–1448

Fuchs RPP, Lefévre JF, Pouyet J, Daune MP (1976) Comparative orientation of the fluorene residue in native DNA modified by N-acetoxy-N-2-acetylaminofluorene and two 7-halogeno derivatives. Biochemistry 15: 3347–4451

Fuchs RPP, Schwartz N, Daune MP (1981) Hot spots of frameshift mutations induced by the ultimate carcinogen N-acetoxy-N-2-acetylaminofluorene. Nature 294: 657–659

Garel A, Axel R (1976) Selective digestion of transcriptionally active ovalbumin genes from oviduct nuclei. Proc Natl Acad Sci USA 73: 3966–3970

Goth R, Rajewsky MF (1972) Ethylation of nucleic acids by ethylnitrosourea-1-^{14}C in the fetal and adult rat. Cancer Res 32: 1501–1505

Goth R, Rajewsky MF (1974a) Persistence of O^6-ethylguanine in rat brain DNA: Correlation with nervous system specific carcinogenesis by ethylnitrosourea. Proc Natl Acad Sci USA 71: 639–653

Goth R, Rajewsky MF (1974b) Molecular and cellular mechanisms associated with pulse-carcinogenesis in the rat nervous system by ethylnitrosourea: Ethylation of nucleic acids and elimination rates of ethylated bases from the DNA of different tissues. Z Krebsforsch 82: 37–64

Graf T, Beug H (1978) Avian leukemia viruses: interaction with their target cells in vivo and in vitro. Biochim Biophys Acta 516: 269–299

Grover PL (ed) (1979) Chemical carcinogens and DNA. CRC Press, Boca Raton

Grunberger D, Weinstein IB (1979) Conformational changes in nucleic acids modified by chemical carcinogens. In: Grover PL (ed) Chemical carcinogens and DNA. CRC Press, Boca Raton, pp 59–93

Hanawalt PC, Cooper PK, Ganesan AK, Smith CA (1979) DNA repair in bacteria and mammalian cells. Annu Rev Biochem 48: 783–836

Hecker E, Fusenig NE, Kunz W, Marks F, Thielmann HW (eds) Cocarcinogenesis and biological effects of tumor promoters. Raven Press, New York

Hollstein M, McCann J, Angelosanto FA (1979) Short-term tests for carcinogens and mutagens. Mutat Res 65:133–226

IARC (1978) IARC Monographs on the evaluation of the carcinogenic risk of chemicals to humans, vol 17, some N-nitroso compounds. International Agency for Research on Cancer, Lyon

Ingold CK (1953) Structure and mechanism in organic chemistry, Chapter 7. Cornell University Press, Ithaca, New York

Ivankovic S, Druckrey H (1968) Transplacentare Erzeugung maligner Tumoren des Nervensystems. I. Äthylnitrosoharnstoff (ÄNH) an BDIX-Ratten. Z Krebsforsch 71:320–360

Jaenisch W (1980) Retroviruses and embryogenesis: Microinjection of Moloney leukemia virus into midgestation mouse embryos. Cell 19:181–188

Jeggo P, Defais M, Samson L, Schendel P (1977) An adaptive response of E. coli to low levels of alkylating agents: Comparison with previously characterised DNA repair pathways. Mol Gen Genet 157:1–9

Johansson-Brittebo EJ, Tjälve H (1979) Studies on the tissue-disposition and fate of N-(^{14}C)ethyl-N-nitrosourea in mice. Toxicology 13:275–285

Johnson FM, Lewis SE (1981) Electrophoretically detected germinal mutations induced in the mouse by ethylnitrosourea. Proc Natl Acad Sci USA 78:3138–3141

Jones EL, Searle CE, Smith TW (1976) Medulloblastomas and other neural tumours in mice treated neonatally with N-ethyl-N-nitrosourea. Acta Neuropathol 36:57–70

Kakunaga T, Lo K-Y, Leavitt J, Ikenaga M (1980) Relationship between transformation and mutation in mammalian cells. In: Pullman B, Ts'o POP, Gelboin H (eds) Carcinogenesis: Fundamental mechanisms and environmental effects. Reidel, Dordrecht Boston London, pp 527–541

Karran P, Lindahl T, Griffin B (1979) Adaptive response to alkylating agents involves alteration in situ of O^6-methylguanine residues in DNA. Nature 280:76–77

Kleihues P, Margison GP (1976) Exhaustion and recovery of repair excision of O^6-methylguanine from rat liver DNA. Nature 259:153–155

Kleihues P, Bücheler J, Riede UN (1978) Selective induction of melanomas in gerbils (meriones unguiculatus) following postnatal administration of N-ethyl-N-nitrosourea. J Natl Cancer Inst 61:859–863

Laerum OD, Rajewsky MF (1975) Neoplastic transformation of fetal rat brain cells in culture following exposure to ethylnitrosourea in vivo. J Natl Cancer Inst 55:1177–1187

Laerum OD, Haugen Å, Rajewsky MF (1979) Neoplastic transformation of foetal rat brain cells in culture after exposure to ethylnitrosourea in vivo. In: Franks LM, Wigley CB (eds) Neoplastic transformation in differentiated epithelial cell systems in vitro. Academic Press, London, New York, pp 190–201

Lajtha L (1979) Stem cell concepts. Differentiation 14:23–34

Lane M-A, Sainten A, Cooper GM (1981) Activity of related transforming genes in mouse and human mammary carcinomas. Proc Natl Acad Sci USA 78:5185–5189

Lapeyre JN, Becker FF (1979) 5-Methylcytosine content of nuclear DNA during chemical hepatocarcinogenesis and in carcinomas which result. Biochem Biophys Res Commun 87:698–705

Lavi S (1981) Carcinogen-mediated amplification of viral DNA sequences in simian virus 40-transformed Chinese hamster embryo cells. Proc Natl Acad Sci USA 78:6144–6148

Lawley PD (1976) Carcinogenesis by alkylating agents. In: Searle CE (ed) Chemical carcinogens. ACS Monograph No. 173. American Chemical Society, Washington, D.C., pp 83–244

Lehmann AR, Karran P (1981) DNA repair. Int Rev Cytol 72:101–146

Lewis JG, Swenberg JA (1980) Differential repair of O^6-methylguanine in DNA in rat hepatocytes and non-parenchymal cells. Nature 288:185–187

Lindahl T (1979) DNA glycosylases, endonucleases for apurinic/apyrimidinic sites, and base excision repair. Progr Nucleic Acid Res Mol Biol 22:135–192
Lindahl T (1982) DNA repair enzymes. Annu Rv Biochem 51:59–85
Loveless A (1969) Possible relevance of O^6-alkylation of deoxyguanosine to the mutagenicity and carcinogenicity of nitrosamines and nitrosamides. Nature 223:206–207
Margison GP, O'Connor PJ (1979) Nucleic acid modification by N-nitroso compounds. In: Grover PL (ed) Chemical carcinogens and DNA, vol 1. CRC Press, Boca Raton, pp 111–159
Margison GP, Margison JM, Montesano R (1976) Methylated purines in the deoxyribonucleic acid of various Syrian-golden-hamster tissues after administration of a hepatocarcinogenic dose of dimethylnitrosamine. Biochem J 157:627–634
McCann J, Choi E, Yamasaki E, Ames BN (1975) Detection of carcinogens as mutagens in the Salmonella/microsome test: Assay of 300 chemicals. Proc Natl Acad Sci USA 72:5135–5139
Mehta JR, Ludlum DB, Renard A, Verly WG (1981) Repair of O^6-ethylguanine in DNA by a chromatin fraction from rat liver: Transfer of the ethyl group to an acceptor protein. Proc Natl Acad Sci USA 78:6766–6770
Miller EC, Miller JA (1976) The metabolism of chemical carcinogens to reactive electrophiles and their possible mechanisms of action in carcinogenesis. In: Searle CE (ed) Chemical carcinogens. ACS Monograph 173. American Chemical Society, Washington, D.C., pp 737–762
Miller JA, Miller EC (1979) Perspectives on the metabolism of chemical carcinogens. In: Emmelot P, Kriek E (eds) Environmental carcinogenesis. Elsevier/North-Holland Biomedical Press, Amsterdam, pp 25–50
Montesano R (1981) Alkylation of DNA and tissue specificity in nitrosamine carcinogenesis. J Supramolec Struct Cell Biochem 17:259–273
Müller R, Rajewsky MF (1978) Sensitive radioimmunoassay for detection of O^6-ethyldeoxyguanosine in DNA exposed to the carcinogen ethylnitrosourea in vivo or in vitro. Z Naturforsch 33c:897–901
Müller R, Rajewsky MF (1980) Immunological quantification by high affinity antibodies of O^6-ethyldeoxyguanosine in DNA exposed to N-ethyl-N-nitrosourea. Cancer Res 40:887–896
Müller R, Rajewsky MF (1981) Antibodies specific for DNA components structurally modified by chemical carcinogens. J Cancer Res Clin Oncol 102:99–113
Müller R, Adamkiewicz J, Rajewsky MF (1982) Immunological detection and quantification of carcinogen-modified DNA components. In: Bartsch H, Armstrong B (eds) Host factors in human carcinogenesis. IARC Scientific Publications No. 39. International Agency for Research on Cancer, Lyon, pp 443–459
Nagao M, Sugimura T, Matsushima T (1978) Environmental mutagens and carcinogens. Annu Rev Genet 12:117–159
Nehls P, Rajewsky MF (1981) Ethylation of fetal rat brain chromosomal DNA by ethylnitrosourea. Proc. Sect. Exp. Cancer Res. German Cancer Soc. J Cancer Res Clin Oncol 99:A38
Nordheim A, Pardue ML, Lafer EM, Möller A, Stollar BD, Rich A (1981) Antibodies to left-handed Z-DNA bind to interband regions of Drosophilia polytene chromosomes. Nature 294:417–423
O'Connor P, Saffhill R, Margison GP (1979) N-nitroso compounds: Biochemical mechanisms of action. In: Emmelot P, Kriek E (eds) Environmental carcinogenesis. Elsevier/North Holland Biomedical Press, Amsterdam, pp 73–96
Olsson M, Lindahl T (1980) Repair of alkylated DNA in E. coli: Methyl group transfer from O^6-methylguanine to a protein cysteine residue. J Biol Chem 255:10569–10572
Pegg AE (1977) Formation and metabolism of alkylated nucleosides: Possible role in carcinogenesis by nitroso compounds and alkylating agents. Adv Cancer Res 25:195–269

Pegg AE, Balog B (1979) Formation and subsequent excision of O^6-ethylguanine from DNA of rat liver following administration of diethylnitrosamine. Cancer Res 39: 5003–5009

Pegg AE, Hui G (1978) Formation and subsequent removal of O^6-methylguanine from DNA in rat liver and kidney after small doses of dimethylnitrosamine. Biochem J 173: 739–748

Pegg AE, Perry W, Bennett RA (1981) Effect of partial hepatectomy on removal of O^6-methylguanine from alkylated DNA by rat liver extracts. Biochem J 197: 195–201

Pegg AE, Roberfroid M, von Bahr C, Foote RS, Mitra S, Bresil H, Likhachev A, Montesano R (1982) Removal O^6-methylguanine from DNA by human liver fractions. Proc Natl Acad Sci USA 79: 5162–5165

Pfohl-Leszkowicz A, Salas C, Fuchs RPP, Dirheimer G (1981) Mechanism of inhibition of enzymatic deoxyribonucleic acid methylation by 2-(acetylamino)fluorene bound to deoxyribonucleic acid. Biochemistry 20: 3020–3024

Pullman B, Ts'o POP, Gelboin H (eds) (1980) Carcinogenesis: Fundamental mechanisms and environmental effects. Reidel, Dordrecht Boston London

Rabes HM, Kerler R, Wilhelm R, Rode G, Riess H (1979) Alkylation of DNA and RNA by [^{14}C] dimethylnitrosamine in hydroxyureasynchronized regenerating rat liver. Cancer Res 39: 4228–4236

Radman M, Villani G, Boiteux S, Defais M, Caillet-Fauquet P (1977) On the mechanism and genetic control of mutagenesis induced by carcinogenic mutagens. In: Hiatt HH, Watson JD, Winston JA (eds) Origins of human cancer. Book B: Mechanisms of carcinogenesis. Cold Spring Harbor Laboratory, Cold Spring Harbor, N.Y., pp 903–922

Rajewsky MF (1972) Proliferative parameters of mammalian cell systems and their role in tumour growth and carcinogenesis. Z Krebsforsch 78: 12–30

Rajewsky MF (1974) Proliferative properties of malignant cell systems. In: Altmann H et al. (eds) Geschwülste / Tumors I. Springer, Berlin Heidelberg New York (Handbuch der allgemeinen Pathologie, vol VI/5, pp 289–325)

Rajewsky MF (1980a) Specificity of DNA damage in chemical carcinogenesis. In: Montesano R, Bartsch H, Tomatis L (eds) Molecular and cellular aspects of carcinogen screening tests. IARC Scientific Publications No. 27. International Agency for Research on Cancer, Lyon, pp 41–54

Rajewsky MF (1980b) Possible determinants for the differential susceptibility of mammalian cells and tissues to chemical carcinogens. Arch Toxicol [Suppl] 3: 229–236

Rajewsky MF, Augenlicht LH, Biessmann H, Goth R, Hülser DF, Laerum OD, Lomakina LYa (1977) Nervous system-specific carcinogenesis by ethylnitrosourea in the rat: Molecular and cellular mechanisms. In: Hiatt HH, Watson JD, Winsten JA (eds) Origins of human cancer. Book B: Mechanisms of carcinogenesis. Cold Spring Harbor Laboratory, Cold Spring Harbor, N.Y., pp 709–726

Rajewsky MF, Müller R, Adamkiewicz J, Drosdziok W (1980) Immunological detection and quantification of DNA components structurally modified by alkylating carcinogens (ethylnitrosourea). In: Pullman B, Ts'o POP, Gelboin H (eds) Carcinogenesis: Fundamental mechanisms and environmental effects. Reidel, Dordrecht Boston London, pp 207–218

Renz M, Nehls P, Hozier J (1977) Involvement of histone H1 in the organization of the chromosome fiber. Proc Natl Acad Sci USA 74: 1879–1883

Rudland PS, Ormerod EJ, Paterson FC (1980) Stem cells in rat mammary development and cancer: a review. J R Soc Med 73: 437–442

Russel WL, Kelly EM, Hunsicker PR, Bangham JW, Maddux SC, Phipps EL (1979) Specific-locus test shows ethylnitrosourea to be the most potent mutagen in the mouse. Proc Natl Acad Sci USA 76: 5818–5819

Saffhill R, Boyle JM (1981) Detection of carcinogen-DNA adducts by radio-immunoassay. Abstr. Proc. 22nd Ann. Gen. Meeting Brit. Assoc. Cancer Res. Br J Cancer 44: 275

Sage E, Leng M (1980) Conformation of poly (dG-dC) · poly (dG-dC) modified by the carcinogens N-acetoxy-N-acetyl-2-aminofluorene and N-hydroxy-N-2-aminofluorene. Proc Natl Acad Sci USA 77: 4597–4601

Samson L, Cairns J (1977) A new pathway for DNA repair in Escherichia coli. Nature 267: 281–283

Santella RM, Grunberger D, Weinstein IB, Rich A (1981) Induction of the Z conformation in poly (dG-dC) · poly (dG-dC) by binding of N-2-acetylaminofluorene to guanine residues. Proc Natl Acad Sci USA 78: 1451–1455

Saunders GF (ed) (1978) Cell differentiation and neoplasia. Raven, New York

Seeberg E, Kleppe K (eds) (1981) Chromosome damage and repair. Plenum, New York

Singer B (1979) N-nitroso alkylating agents: Formation and persistence of alkyl derivatives in mammalian nucleic acids as contributing factors in carcinogenesis. J Natl Cancer Inst 62: 1329–1339

Singer B, Kröger M (1979) Participation of modified nucleosides in translation and transcription. Prog Nucleic Acid Res Mol Biol 23: 151–194

Singer B, Bodell WJ, Cleaver JE, Thomas EH, Rajewsky MF, Thon W (1978) Oxygens in DNA are main targets for ethylnitrosourea in normal and Xeroderma pigmentosum fibroblasts and fetal rat brain cells. Nature 276: 85–88

Slaga TJ, Sivak A, Boutwell RK (eds) (1978) Carcinogenesis., A comprehensive survey, vol 2. Mechanisms of tumor promotion and cocarcinogenesis. Raven, New York

Stavrou D, Hänichen T, Wriedt-Lübbe I (1975) Onkogene Wirkung von Äthylnitrosoharnstoff beim Kaninchen während der pränatalen Periode. Z Krebsforsch 84: 207–215

Stavrou D, Dahme E, Schröder B (1977) Transplacentare neuroonkogene Wirkung von Äthylnitrosoharnstoff beim Kaninchen während der frühen Graviditätsphase. Z Krebsforsch 89: 331–339

Stumpf R, Margison GP, Montesano R, Pegg AE (1979) Formation and loss of alkylated purines from DNA of hamster liver after administration of dimethylnitrosamine. Cancer Res 39: 50–54

Stutman O (1979) Transplacental carcinogenesis in athymic nude mice. Pathol Res Pract 165: 170

Sun L, Singer B (1975) The specificity of different classes of ethylating agents toward various sites of HeLa cell DNA in vitro and in vivo. Biochemistry 14: 1795–1802

Tomatis L, Cefis F (1967) The effects of multiple and single administration of dimethylnitrosamine to hamsters. Tumori 53: 447–452

Vogel E, Natarajan AT (1979a) The relation between reaction kinetics and mutagenic action of mono-functional alkylating agents in higher eukaryotic system. I. Recessive lethal mutations and translocations in Drosophilia. Mutat Res 62: 51–100

Vogel E, Natarajan AG (1979b) The relation between reaction kinetics and mutagenic action of mono-functional alkylating agents in higher eukaryotic systems. II. Total and partial sex-chromosome loss in Drosophilia. Mutat Res 62: 101–123

Wang AH, Quigley GJ, Kolpak FJ, Cranford JL, Van Boom JA, Van der Macel G, Rich A (1979) Molecular structure of a left-handed double helical DNA fragment at atomic resolution. Nature 282: 680–686

Weinberg RA (1981) Use of transfection to analyze genetic information and malignant transformation. Biochim Biophys Acta 651: 25–35

Weinstein IB (1977) Types of interaction between carcinogens and nucleic acids. In: Méchanismes d'alteration et de réparation du DNA, relations avec la mutagenèse et la cancerogenèse chimique. Colloques Internationaux du CNRS No. 256. Centre National de la Recherche Scientifique, Paris, pp 2–40

Weintraub H, Groudine M (1976) Chromosomal subunits in active genes have an altered conformation. Science 193: 848–856

*Role of Extent and Persistence of DNA Modifications in Chemical Carcinogenesis by Aromatic Amines**

H.-G. Neumann

Institut für Pharmakologie und Toxikologie, Universität Würzburg,
Versbacherstrasse 9, 8700 Würzburg, FRG

Introduction

Numerous known and suspected human carcinogens belong to the chemical class of aromatic amines, among them many compounds used extensively in industrial processes and in the manufacture of drugs, pesticides, and plastics. Industrial bladder cancer has been attributed primarily to exposure to aromatic amines; this group of compounds has therefore received considerable attention. Particular problems are the wide variety of species and the tissue specificity elicited by these compounds in experimental systems, and much effort has been devoted in the past to identifying the common properties of aromatic amines and explaining specific effects.

Since the pioneering work of the Millers and their collaborators (Miller and Miller 1969), it is widely accepted that metabolic *N*-oxidation is the first step in producing intermediates which after a second activation step may lead to ultimate reactive forms capable of reacting with cellular macromolecules. The reaction with DNA is considered to result in a genotoxic lesion, which is a prime prerequisite for the transformation of somatic cells into initiated cells which may then grow into a tumor. The effective tissue concentration of reactive metabolites is largely determined by many inactivating metabolic pathways and the reaction with noncritical target molecules. The extent of the primary DNA lesions obtained with different aromatic amines should therefore depend on the compound's overall metabolism and the chemical reactivity of the ultimate metabolite. Furthermore, when the reaction products with DNA have been formed, they may be recognized by repair enzymes and eliminated before any genetic consequences are realized.

From these considerations, a working hypothesis has evolved which postulates that the extent of the formation of DNA adducts and their persistence should correlate with the biological effect. Accordingly, attempts have been made in many laboratories to find quantitative differences in DNA binding and in persistence of specific DNA adducts between susceptible and nonsusceptible species and between target and nontarget tissues.

In this laboratory, we investigate aminostilbene derivatives as model compounds for aromatic amines. The parent compound, *trans*-DAS, is acutely toxic and highly

* Work carried out in the author's laboratory was supported by the Deutsche Forschungsgemeinschaft

carcinogenic. It produces ear duct tumors in the rat quite specifically after repeated administration of nontoxic doses. In a number of recent experiments, we have collected data which appear not to support the tissue burden concept outlined above. I would therefore like to (1) briefly summarize those results; (2) compare them with those obtained with other aromatic amines, which will demonstrate that aminostilbenes are not an exception in this class of compounds; and (3) discuss the necessity of extending the working hypothesis to include secondary effects of the compounds which influence later stages in tumor induction, for an improved understanding of the specific activities of aromatic amines.

Extent and Persistence of DNA Lesions from Aminostilbenes

After oral administration of *trans*-DAS or *trans*-AAS to female Wistar rats, the parent compounds are rapidly metabolized and reactive metabolites bind to cellular macromolecules in all tissues. A maximum is reached within 24 h. The level of nucleic acid binding in different tissues varies by a factor of 20 (Table 1). Tissue exposure in liver is obviously highest, kidney and lung follow, and an additional group of tissues usually shows still lower binding values. Among the tissues in the latter group are glandular stomach, the target for acute toxicity (Marquardt et al., to be published), and Zymbal gland, from which the ear duct tumors arise (Haddow et al. 1948). The pattern of nucleic acid adducts in liver, kidney, lung, and glandular stomach is very similar, as shown by elution profiles obtained from DNA hydrolysates on Sephadex LH 20 columns (Baur and Neumann 1980). The different tissues appear therefore to be exposed to the same reactive metabolites, and it is not very promising to search for a tissue-specific metabolite. However, the possibility that such specificity exists cannot be excluded for Zymbal gland at the present time.

If the initial lesion does not correlate with tissue susceptibility, tissue-specific elimination could modulate the persistence of DNA adducts. Elimination of total metabolites bound to macromolecules, predominantly proteins, however, is very

Table 1. Binding to cellular macromolecules

Tissue	Binding index (24 h)		
	Proteins	rRNA	DNA
Liver	786	293	321
Kidney	110	42	99
Lung	96	11	21
Glandular stomach	50	26	41
Bladder	44	16	9
Zymbal gland	27	21	53
Mammary tissue	2	16	16

[^{3}H]*trans*-AAS was administered to female Wistar rats, and macromolecules were isolated from the different tissues after 24 h. Values represent averages from one to three isolations. In some cases tissues from four to eight animals were pooled. Binding index: μmol metabolite bound/mol nucleotide or amino acid (MG 120), divided by dose in mmol/kg body weight. (Baur and Neumann 1980)

similar in all tissues within the first 4 weeks (Neumann 1981). Liver is an exception, presumably because more proteins, labeled during their synthesis, are secreted into the circulation. There are, on the other hand, persistant DNA adducts in all tissues studied. Some of the adducts in liver are undoubtedly eliminated, but some of the major in vivo reaction products persist at least 4 weeks (Fig. 1). Similarly, DNA

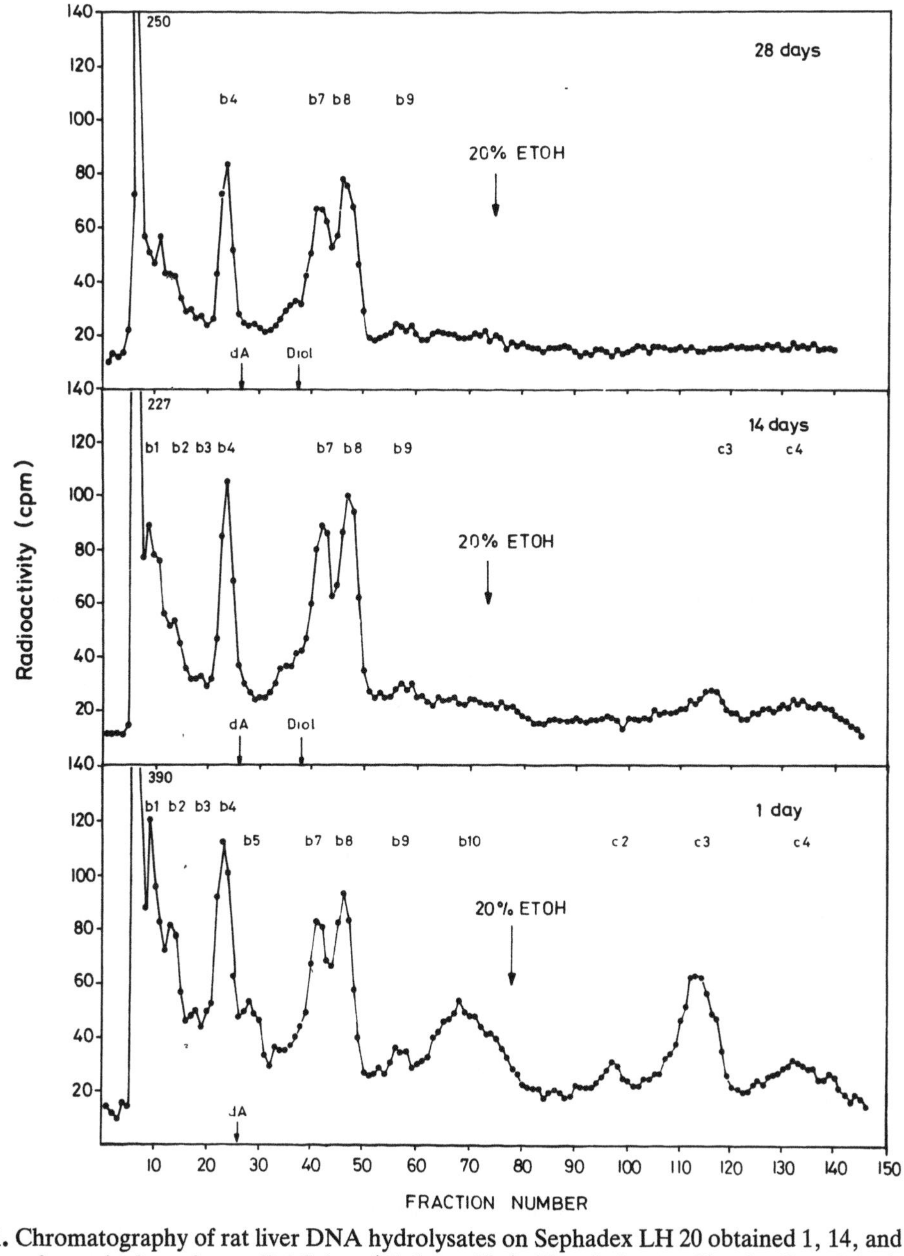

Fig. 1. Chromatography of rat liver DNA hydrolysates on Sephadex LH 20 obtained 1, 14, and 28 days after a single oral *trans*-DAS dose (10.5 μmol/kg). The elution profile of radioactivity is shown (Baur and Neumann 1980)

binding in kidney remains high over this period of time (Neumann 1981; see also Table 3). Although repair has not yet been studied with the desirable precision on the level of individual, identified adducts, it appears unlikely that differential repair of critical DNA adducts will explain the nonsusceptibility of the tissues studied. Support for the working hypothesis would also come from demonstration of differential cumulation with repeated doses using a regimen also applied for tumor induction. Either metabolic activation could be altered by enzyme induction under these circumstances, such that the fraction of subsequent doses binding to DNA is reduced in nonsusceptible tissues, or repair processes could be induced. We have tested this by administering 12 labeled doses of *trans*-AAS, distributed over 6 weeks, and measuring the cumulation of DNA binding during that time (Table 2). Tissue exposure does not change, and the tissue burden is still highest in liver and kidney. In another experiment only the last of 1, 4, 8, or 12 doses was labeled, and DNA binding was measured 17 days after that last dose. The same binding levels were found after different feeding periods, indicating no changes in the elimination rates (Table 3).

Table 2. Macromolecular binding after repeated dosing

Tissue	Total tissue binding		DNA binding
	First dose	Twelve doses	Twelve doses
Liver	2.4	7.2	24.4
Kidney	1.8	7.0	17.1
Lung	0.7	3.0	1.9
Glandular stomach	0.3	1.3	3.9
Zymbal gland	0.4	1.4	n.d.
Mammary tissue	0.2	0.8	n.d.

[^{3}H]*trans*-AAS (5 μmol/kg) was administered to female Wistar rats twice a week for up to 6 weeks, and radioactivity was determined 3 days after the last dose. Data are given in pmol/mg and represent averages from three animals. *n.d.*, not determined. (G. Hilpert and H.-G. Neumann, unpublished work)

Table 3. Elimination of DNA binding after repeated dosing

Tissue	Binding to DNA (pmol/mg) 17 days after labeled last dose				Half-life (days)	
	First	Fourth	Eighth	Twelfth	DNA label	Protein label
Liver	2.6	3.4	3.0	2.8	22	5.1
Kidney	0.7	0.7	0.7	1.0	Persistent	8.7
Lung	0.14	0.13	0.14	0.18	18	7.3
Glandular stomach	0.11	0.12	0.15	0.16	9	6.5

trans-AAS (5 μmol/kg) was administered to female Wistar rats twice a week for up to 6 weeks. The final dose was ^{3}H-labeled, and radioactivity was determined 3 days (not shown) and 17 days after the last dose. From the decrease between day 3 and day 17, half-life was calculated (G. Hilpert and H.-G. Neumann, unpublished work)

In summary, none of the parameters measured (total initial DNA binding, initial pattern of DNA adducts, persistence of DNA adducts, accumulation of DNA binding after repeated doses, and persistence of DNA adducts after repeated doses) support the hypothesis that extent and persistence of DNA lesions determine tissue susceptibility with aminostilbenes. According to these criteria, liver, kidney, lung, and glandular stomach should be much more affected than Zymbal gland.

Comparison with Other Aromatic Amines

This raises the question of whether aminostilbenes are an exception among aromatic amines, or whether lack of correlation is a common feature in this class of compounds.

Among five typical examples of aromatic amines total DNA binding in rat liver varies somewhat, but the binding indices are not different enough to explain why three of them do not induce liver tumors (Table 4). However, recent work identifying the molecular structure of some of these adducts showed that quite different types of reaction products are formed and a direct comparison neglects the possibility that some of these adducts could be more critical than others.

If DNA is treated in vitro with the respective *N*-acetoxy-*N*-arylacetamides, which represent one type of ultimate metabolite, then all of them react with guanine; the phenanthryl derivative reacts in addition with adenine (N^6), and the stilbenyl derivative also with adenine (*N*-1) and cytosine (*N*-3) (Kriek, 1980). The reactions with guanine are summarized in Fig. 2, which shows that substitutions at C-8 and N^2 predominate. With the stilbenyl derivative a Gua-C-8 adduct has not been found. It reacts with positions usually preferred by alkylating carcinogens, namely *N*-1 and O^6. In vivo, however, the situation is more complicated because additional activating pathways exist. Adducts lacking the *N*-acetyl group prevail (Table 5). With 2-fluorenylacetamide, Gua-C-8-AF has been identified as the major adduct. In addition, the ratio of substitution C-8/N^2 varies with different arylacetamides. It turned out that substitution at C-8 of guanine with arylamides (acetylated adducts) alters the DNA conformation much more than substitution with arylamines

Table 4. Binding of arylamides to rat liver nucleic acids

Compound administered	Binding index[a] DNA	Binding index[a] RNA	Primary target tissues	Author(s)
2-Fluorenylacetamide	300	330	Liver	Kriek 1969/70
4-Stilbenylacetamide	280	230	Ear duct	Gaugler and Neumann 1979
2-Phenanthrylacetamide	110	160	Mamma, ear duct	Scribner and Koponen 1979
4-*N*-OH-Biphenylacetamide	84	317	Mamma, ear duct	Kriek 1971
4-Methylaminoazobenzene	8	–	Liver	Beland et al. 1980b

[a] The binding index (cf. Table 1) was calculated from published data

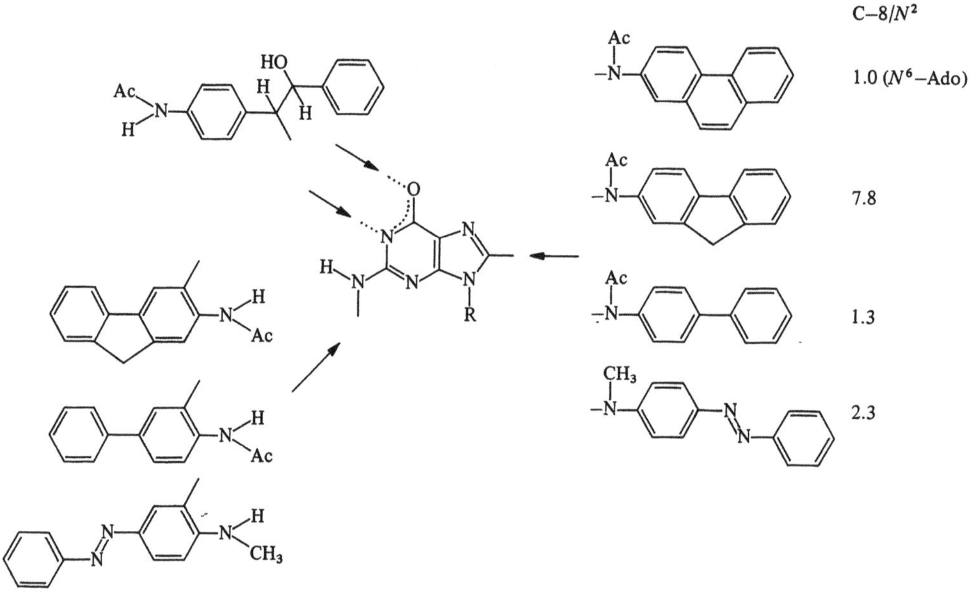

Fig. 2. Reactions of aryl hydroxamic acid esters with guanine in vitro. For those compounds reacting in the C-8 position the ratio C-8/N^2 of reaction products is given; for the phenanthryl derivative, the ratio Gua-C-8/Ade-N^6 applies

Table 5. Adducts formed with rat liver DNA in vivo

Compound administered	Acetylated adducts (%)	Non-acetylated adducts (%)	dGuo-C-8-acetamide (relative)
2-Fluorenylacetamide	30	70	100
4-*N*-OH-Biphenylacetamide	20	80	5
2-Phenanthrylacetamide	0	100	0
4-Stilbenylacetamide	Very little	?	0

(nonacetylated adducts), or with arylamides in N^2 (Grunberger and Weinstein 1979). As a consequence these lesions are recognized by repair enzymes and are eliminated with half-lives in the order of several days, whereas nonacetylated adducts in general and Gua-N^2 adducts are much more persistent (Table 6). Putting this information togehter there appears to be a correlation, if at all, between the formation of Gua-C-8-acetamides and liver tumor induction. Considerably more of this particular DNA lesion is produced with fluorenylacetamide than with the inactive arylamides (Table 5). The respective adduct is also formed with *N*-methylaminoazobenzene in vivo (Beland et al. 1980b). If this adduct were more critical than others, persistence would not be a good parameter to characterize critical DNA lesions. This conclusion is difficult to accept, because the other adducts are not only more persistent but also contain bulky molecules at positions involved in base pairing (Gua-N^2, Ade-N^6).

Table 6. Elimination of adducts from rat liver DNA

Compound administered	Acetylated (methylated)		
	dGuo-C-8-derivative (half-life in days)	dGuo-N^2-derivative	dGuo-C-8-amine
2-Fluorenylacetamide	7	Persistent	Persistent
4-*N*-OH-Biphenylacetamide	2	Persistent	–
Methylaminoazobenzene	1	Persistent	–
2-Phenanthrylacetamide	Unidentified nonacetylated persistent adducts		
4-Stilbenylacetamide	Unidentified persistent adducts		

Persistent: little elimination within 4 weeks

This conclusion is also difficult to accept because all these arylamides are good mutagens, initiators, and local carcinogens when metabolically activated. In fact, Scribner and his collaborators, using *N*-acetoxy-*N*-arylacetamides as potentially ultimate forms, have shown that the same decreasing order of efficiency (2-phenanthryl > 4-stilbenyl > 2-fluorenyl > 4-biphenyl) emerges from testing of three quite different parameters [mutagenesis in *Salmonella typhimurium* (Scribner et al. 1979), initiation on mouse skin with TPA as promotor (Scribner and Slaga 1975), and local carcinogenesis after subcutaneous injection, (Scribner et al. 1970)]. Although the pattern of adducts has not been determined in these experiments, the results would indicate that there must be more critical adducts than the one described above.

One approach in evaluating the role of different base adducts for genotoxic lesions makes use of bacterial test systems for mutagenic activity. When arylhydroxamic acid esters were tested in different strains of *S. typhimurium,* no correlation with carcinogenic potency could be found with any single strain used (TA 1535, TA 1538, TA 98, TA 100). However, the decreasing order of efficiency mentioned above was obtained when the effects in strain TA 98 and TA 100 were taken together (Table 7). *N*-Acetoxy-*N*-2-fluorenylacetamide ranks third, and frameshift mutations were observed, whereas error-prone gap-filling due to repair of lesions caused by the arrest of DNA synthesis contributed very little to the mutagenic activity. This is in line with the base displacement model (Grunberger and Weinstein 1979) for the Gua-C-8-AAF adduct in DNA. Gap-filling is quite prominent with the stilbenyl and biphenyl derivatives, however, and has been explained by the arresting effect of bulky residues attached to extranuclear base atoms. On the other hand, besides producing base-pair substitution mutations these two amines are quite active as frameshift mutagens, a property assigned to Gua-C-8-acetamides, which are not expected to contribute in these cases. Thus critical DNA lesions could not be identified from these data. The results rather indicate that all the arylamines tested are mutagenic and exert their effects in different ways.

The situation becomes even more complicated when it is realized that three different pathways are held responsible for different biological effects, and mutagenic lesions might be elicited by nonbinding metabolites. Partially purified arylhydroxamic acid acyltransferase catalyses the formation of mutagens from *N*-hydroxy-AAF, but

Table 7. Mutagenicity of aryl hydroxamic acid esters in strains of *Salmonella typhimurium* (Scribner et al. 1979)

Aryl moiety	Mutagenicity TA 98 + TA 100 (rev/nmol)	Most susceptible strain	Type of mutation	Gap-filling	Major in vitro adduct
2-Phenanthryl	18.6	TA 98	Frameshift Base-pair substitution	(+)	Ade-N^6
4-Stilbenyl	9.6	TA 100	Base-pair substitution Frameshift	+	Base-pairing sites
2-Fluorenyl	8.3	TA 98	Frameshift	–	Gua-C-8
2-Naphthym	5.1	TA 100	Base-pair substituent	–	Ade-N^6
4-Biphenyl	0.5	TA 98	Frameshift	+	Gua-N^2

binding to added tRNA may be suppressed without decreasing the mutagenic effect (Weeks et al. 1978, 1980). The major adduct formed in the acyltransferase-mediated reaction is the Gua-C-8-AF adduct, which is also found in vivo (Beland et al. 1980a). Neither this nor acetylated adducts formed in sulfotransferase-mediated reactions of hydroxamic acids appear to account for mutations in in vitro systems. Several pieces of evidence rather indicate that arylhydroxylamines originating either from direct oxidation of amines (Brouns et al. 1981) or from deacetylation of arylhydroxamic acids (Schut et al. 1978; Wirth and Thorgeirsson 1981) are closest to the mutagenic molecules which may ultimately be generated by one electron oxidation (Stout et al. 1976; Weeks et al. 1978, 1980; Glatt et al. 1980). The possible involvement of an arylnitrenium radical is underlined by the effects of ascorbic acid, which increases mutagenicity but decreases nucleic acid binding in in vitro test systems (Thorgeirsson et al. 1980). Such radicals may act by abstracting an electron from DNA rather than by covalent binding (Andrews et al. 1979). These findings may explain why correlations between specific types of mutations produced by aromatic amines and their carcinogenic activity cannot be established at the present time.

The Role of Secondary Effects

It may be too naive to expect simple relationships between primary DNA lesions and the development of overt tumors. After all, adduct formation is considered only as a first step in a multistage process progressing over an extended period of time. But very little is known about how chemical carcinogens may modulate secondary steps in tumor formation.

We touched upon this problem when we studied the acute toxicity of *trans*-DAS in rats (Marquardt et al. to be published). It turned out that even with lethal doses no substance-related morphological damage could be detected in liver. Cytotoxicity

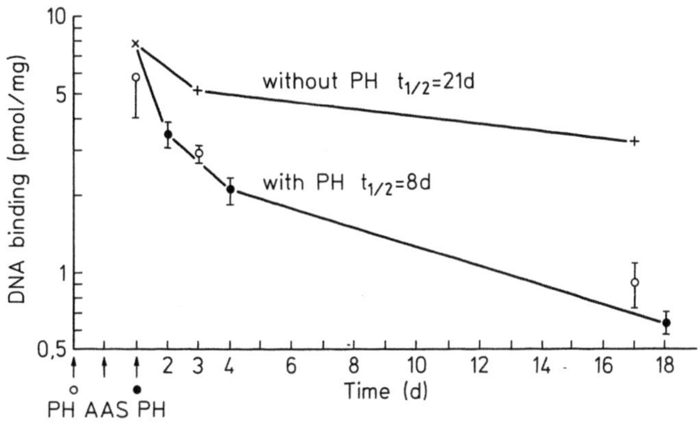

Fig. 3. The role of partial hepatectomy (*PH*) on DNA binding. [^{3}H]*trans*-AAS was administered to female Wistar rats without or with *PH* either 24 h before or 24 h after the administration of the test compound. Liver DNA was isolated and the total of bound radioactivity determined. From the decrease between day 4 and day 17, half-life was calculated (G. Hilpert and H.-G. Neumann, unpublished work)

should therefore be very low in this tissue despite the high exposure to reactive metabolites, as indicated by the binding indices (Table 4). The proliferating cells in the antrum of the glandular stomach necrotize under these circumstances. The stomach epithelium is damaged and massive bleeding causes the death of the animals. Bone marrow is also involved, and leukocyte counts decrease drastically during the latent period. Tissue exposure is certainly lower in glandular stomach than in liver, but the proliferation rate of stem cells is higher and is therefore thought to make this tissue, as well as bone marrow, more vulnerable. Surprisingly, comparable effects were not seen in the intestine with its equally rapidly proliferating epithelial cells. The role of the proliferation rate was then tested in liver by performing a partial hepatectomy before lethal doses of *trans*-DAS were administered. Even in this situation toxic effects did not occur in liver and the remaining part regenerated normally. Stomach effects were aggravated under these circumstances (Marquardt 1979; Marquardt et al., to be published).

This observation has more recently been supported on the molecular level by experiments designed to demonstrate the effects of partial hepatectomy on metabolism and primary DNA lesions. When the operation was performed 24 h prior to the administration of a nontoxic *trans*-AAS dose, DNA binding was somewhat lower in the remaining stump than in normal liver (Fig. 3). Increased binding would have been expected if better accessibility of DNA in reduplicating cells accounted for greater susceptibility. When partial hepatectomy was performed 24 h after the same *trans*-AAS dose, DNA binding after an additional 24 h was also considerably lower than in normal liver. The stimulated cell turnover, as expected, decreases specific DNA binding faster. After 17 days it was down to a quarter of that in normal liver at that time (Fig. 3).

Noncorrelations between tissue exposure and toxic effects may also arise from species comparisons. Mice are much more resistant to *trans*-DAS and do not develop liver tumors (Arcos and Argus 1974). In our hands, NMRI mice tolerated considerably higher doses of this compound, and the LD_{50} is estimated to be five times greater than in rats (Marquardt 1979). With acute toxic doses, however, liver damage prevailed in these mice but no changes were seen in stomach. With subtoxic doses, the DNA binding index in liver is 30 (H.-G. Neumann, unpublished work). This is roughly one-tenth of that in rat liver, which is less susceptible to acute toxic effects.

Two important points about the multistage process in chemical carcinogenesis emerge from the models: (1) only the fixation of primary DNA damage produces initiated cells, and (2) initiated cells acquire properties which provide them with growth advantages under certain selection conditions. This raises the question of how chemical carcinogens may modulate fixation and selection.

Any cytotoxic effects occurring concurrently with the formation of DNA adducts may lead to cell death and trigger regenerative proliferation (Ying et al. 1981). At a later stage damage to noninitiated cells may help more resistant cells to grow selectively. Evidence to support such a model has been provided by initiation-promotion experiments in rat liver. Typically, subcarcinogenic doses of AAF may produce lesions which grow into tumors only under the influence of promoters like DDT and phenobarbital (Peraino et al. 1975, 1977, 1980). It is also possible to reverse the experiment, using another initiator first and then AAF as a promoter (Columbano et al. 1981). The results indicate that AAF possesses initiating as well as promoting properties. These properties, however, are not necessarily linked, as another example of aromatic amines shows. 2-Methyl-4-dimethylaminoazobenzene induces no liver tumors in rats, but metabolites bind to liver DNA as well as with 4-dimethylaminoazobenzene, which is carcinogenic. If dosing with the former compound is followed by either partial hepatectomy or phenobarbital treatment, tumors develop (Kitagawa et al. 1979), indicating that it lacks the capability to fix the genotoxic damage and to promote the growth of initiated cells. Similarly, *N*-hydroxy-*N*-acetylaminobiphenyl becomes effective in liver when supplemented with partial hepatectomy and dietary phenobarbital (Shirai et al. 1981). Equivalent experiments with *trans*-AAS have not yet been completed, but they already show that after partial hepatectomy and subsequent treatment with promoters, not only preneoplastic lesions but also liver tumors can be induced in rats (Hilpert G. and H.-G. Neumann, unpublished work).

These results have several implications. DNA adducts should be regarded as lesions which may precipitate into tumor induction under certain circumstances and change a nonsusceptible tissue into a susceptible tissue. Persistent adducts should be considered more critical than repairable ones in this regard. Furthermore, it will be necessary to separate genotoxic and cytotoxic effects more carefully. The latter may turn out to be even more specific than the former. The possible difference in the relation of reactive metabolites to the two is quite poorly defined at the present time.

The inducing activity of AAF has been clearly demonstrated (Åström and DePierre 1981). The activity of several drug-metabolizing enzymes is increased. In contrast to the effect of phenobarbital, the endoplasmic reticulum does not proliferate concurrently. The change of enzyme activities leads to an increase of reactive metabolites at the beginning of a feeding period, sufficient to induce tumors. Thereafter the activating capacity decreases steadily. At the time when preneoplastic nodules appear, it is significantly lower than in normal liver tissue. This may be due to the low activity within the nodules, where the content of microsomal protein and accordingly metabolic activity is considerably lower than in the surrounding tissue (Stout and Becker 1978). These findings are in line with the model. At the beginning of AAF feeding, enhanced activation favors cytotoxicity and fixing of genotoxic effects by stimulating regenerative proliferation. Later on, the initiated cells are metabolically less active and therefore less exposed to cytotoxic metabolites than are the surrounding normal cells.

The model can be tested with other aromatic amines which are not carcinogenic to liver. *Trans*-DAS, for instance, appears not to induce liver enzymes. Metabolic activation remains constant over several weeks (Neumann 1973). Much more information is obviously necessary to evaluate the correlation between enzyme induction and cytotoxicity. Possibly enzyme induction is only part of a pleiotropic effect, as has been demonstrated recently for many promoters (Diamond and O'Brien 1980), and is in itself not very important. Since extrahepatic tissues are exposed to lower levels of reactive metabolites than liver, their susceptibility could be expected to depend on much more subtle effects than overt macromolecular damage. One example is inhibition of DNA methylation (Salas et al. 1979, Pfohl-Leszkowicz et al. 1981), an effect which is dealt with in great detail by Pfohl-Leszkowicz et al. (see this volume p. 193–201).

Summary

The initial step in tumor formation with aromatic amines is assumed to involve the modification of nucleic acids. Reactive metabolites bind covalently to purine and pyrimidine bases. The extent of formation of DNA adducts and their persistence is therefore expected to correlate with the biological effect. Using [^{3}H]*trans*-4-aminostilbene derivatives as model compounds, several parameters have been measured in susceptible and nonsusceptible rat tissues: total initial DNA binding, initial pattern of adducts, persistence of DNA adducts, accumulation of DNA binding after repeated doses, and persistence of DNA adducts after repeated doses. They did not correlate with tissue susceptibility. The tissue burden decreased in the order: liver > kidney > lung > glandular stomach > Zymbal gland. The latter tissue is the primary target for tumor formation. Comparison with other aromatic amines shows that aminostilbene derivatives are no exceptions. The role of specific nucleic acid modifications for mutagenic and carcinogenic effects is also difficult to evaluate in these cases. It is therefore emphasized that modulation of secondary steps in the multistage process may largely influence the final outcome. The role of cell proliferation and its stimulation as well as tumor promoting effects are discussed. Aminostilbene derivatives appear to produce primary lesions quite efficiently in rat liver but lack cytotoxic and promoting properties for this tissue.

Abbreviations

AAF, 2-*N*-acetylaminofluorene; *AF,* 2-aminofluorene; *trans-AAS, trans*-4-*N*-acetylaminostilbene; *trans-DAS, trans*-4-*N,N*-dimethylaminostilbene; *DDT,* 1,1,1,-trichloro-2,2-bis-(*p*-chlorophenyl)-ethane; *TPA,* phorbol-12-tetradecanoyl-13-acetyl-diester; *Ade-N*^{6}, adenine-N^6 derivative; *Gua-C-8,* guanine-C-8 derivative; *Gua-N*^{2}, guanine-N^2 derivative; *Gua-O*^{6}, guanine-O^6 derivative.

References

Andrews LS, Fysh JM, Hinson JA, Gilette JR (1979) Ascorbic acid inhibits covalent binding of enzymatically generated 2-acetyl-aminofluorene-N-sulfate to DNA under conditions in which it increases mutagenesis in Salmonella TA-1538. Life Sci 24: 59–64

Arcos JC, Argus MF (1974) Chemical induction of cancer, vol II B. Academic Press, New York London, pp 176–177

Åström A, DePierre JW (1981) Characterization of the induction of drug metabolizing enzymes by 2-acetylaminofluorene. Biochim Biophys Acta 673: 225–233

Baur H, Neumann H-G (1980) Correlation of nucleic acid binding by metabolites of trans-4-aminostilbene derivatives with tissue specific acute toxicity and carcinogenicity in rats. Carcinogenesis 1: 877–885

Beland FA, Allaben WT, Evans FE (1980a) Acyltransferase-mediated binding of N-hydroxy-arylamides to nucleic acids. Cancer Res 40: 834–840

Beland FA, Tullis DL, Kadlubar FF, Straub KM, Evans FE (1980b) Characterization of DNA adducts of the carcinogen N-metyhl-4-aminoazobenzene in vitro and in vivo. Chem Biol Interact 31: 1–17

Brouns RME, VanDoorn R, Bos RP, Mulleners LJS, Henderson PT (1981) Metabolic activation of 2-aminofluorene by isolated rat liver cells through different pathways leading to hepatocellular DNA-repair and bacterial mutagenesis. Toxicology 19: 67–75

Columbano A, Rajalakshmis S, Sarma R (1981) Requirement of cell proliferation for the initiation of liver carcinogenesis as assayed by three different procedures. Cancer Res 41: 2079–2083

Diamond L, O'Brien TG (1980) Tumor promoters and the mechanism of tumor promotion. Adv Cancer Res 32: 1–74

Gaugler BJM, Neumann H-G (1979) The binding of metabolites formed from aminostilbene derivatives to nucleic acids in the liver of rats. Chem Biol Interact 24: 355–372

Glatt HR, Oesch F, Neumann H-G (1980) Factors responsible for the metabolic formation and inactivation of bacterial mutagens from trans-4-acetylaminostilbene. Mutat Res 73: 237–250

Grunberger D, Weinstein IB (1979) Conformational changes in nucleic acids modified by chemical carcinogens. In: Grover PhL (ed) Chemical carcinogens and DNA. CRC Press, Boca Raton, Fl, pp 60–93

Haddow A, Harris RJC, Kon GAR, Roe EMF (1948) The growth-inhibitory and carcinogenic properties of 4-aminostilbene derivatives. Philos Trans R Soc Lond Ser A 241: 147–195

Kitagawa T, Pitot HC, Miller EC, Miller JA (1979) Promotion by dietary phenobarbital of hepatocarcinogenesis by 2-methyl-N,N-dimethyl-4-aminoazobenzene in the rat. Cancer Res 39: 112–115

Kriek E (1969/1970) On the mechanism of action of carcinogenic aromatic amines I. Binding of 2-acetylaminofluorene and N-hydroxy-2-acetylaminofluorene to rat liver nucleic acids in vivo. Chem Biol Interact 1: 3–17

Kriek E (1971) On the mechanism of action of carcinogenic aromatic amines II. Binding of N-hydroxy-N-acetyl-4-aminobiphenyl to rat liver nucleic acids in vivo. Chem Biol Interact 3: 19–28

Kriek E (1980) Modification of DNA by carcinogenic aromatic amines in vivo and in vitro with possible promutagenic consequences. In: Pullman B, Ts'o POP, Gelboin H (eds) Carcinogenesis: Fundamental mechanisms and environmental effects. Reidel, pp 103–111

Marquardt P (1979) Die akute Toxizität des carcinogenen aromatischen Amins trans-4-Dimethylaminostilben bei der Ratte. Dissertation, Universität Würzburg

Marquardt P, Neumann H-G, Romen W (to be published) Tissue specific, acute toxic effects of the carcinogen trans-4-dimethylaminostilbene. J Environ Pathol Toxicol

Miller JA, Miller EC (1969) The metabolic activation of carcinogenic aromatic amines and amides. Prog Exp Tumor Res 11: 273–301

Neumann H-G (1973) The metabolism of repeatedly administered trans-4-dimethylaminostilbene and 4-dimethylaminobibenzyl. Z Krebsforsch 79: 60–70
Neumann H-G (1981) On the significance of metabolic activation and binding to nucleic acids of aminostilbene derivatives in vivo. J Natl Cancer Inst Monographs 58: 165–171
Peraino C, Fry RJM, Staffeldt E, Christopher JP (1975) Comparative enhancing effects of phenobarbital, amobarbital, diphenylhydantoin, and dichlorodiphenyltrichloroethane on 2-acetylaminofluorene-induced hepatic tumorigenesis in the rat. Cancer Res 35: 2884–2890
Peraino C, Fry RJM, Staffeldt E, Christopher JP (1977) Enhancing effects of phenobarbitone and butylated hydroxytoluene on 2-acetylaminofluorene-induced hepatic tumorigenesis in the rat. Food Cosmet Toxicol 15: 93–96
Peraino C, Staffeldt E, Hanzen DA, Lombard LS, Stevens FI, Fry RJM (1980) Effects of varying the dietary concentration of phenobarbital on its enhancement of 2-acetylaminofluorene-induced hepatic tumorigenesis. Cancer Res 40: 3268–3273
Pfohl-Leszkowicz A, Salas C, Fuchs RPP, Dirheimer G (1981) Mechanism of inhibition of enzymatic deoxyribonucleic acid methylation by 2-(acetylamino)-fluorene bound to deoxyribonucleic acid. Biochemistry 20: 3020–3024
Salas CE, Pfohl-Leszkowicz A, Lang MC, Dirheimer G (1979) Effect of modification by N-acetoxy-N-2-acetylaminofluorene on the level of DNA methylation. Nature 278: 71–72
Schut HAJ, Wirth PJ, Thorgeirsson SS (1978) Mutagenic activation of N-hydroxy-2-acetylaminofluorene in the Salmonella test system: the role of deacetylation by liver and kidney fractions from mouse and rat. Mol Pharmacol 14: 682–692
Scribner JD, Koponen G (1979) Binding of the carcinogen 2-acetamidophenanthrene to rat liver nucleic acids: lack of correlation with carcinogenic activity, and failure of the hydroxamic acid ester model for in vivo activation. Chem Biol Interact 15: 201–209
Scribner JD, Slaga TJ (1975) Brief comm: Tumor initiation by acyloxy derivatives of piperidine and N-arylacetamides. J Natl Cancer Inst 54: 491–493
Scribner JD, Miller EC, Miller JA (1970) Nucleophilic substitution on carcinogenic N-acetoxy-N-arylacetamides. Cancer Res 30: 1570–1579
Scribner JD, Fist SR, Scribner NK (1979) Mechanisms of action of carcinogenic aromatic amines: an investigation using mutagenesis in bacteria. Chem Biol Interact 26: 11–25
Shirai T, Lee M-S, Wang CY, King CM (1981) Effects of partial hepatectomy and dietary phenobarbital on liver and mammary tumorigenesis by two N-hydroxy-N-acylaminobiphenyls in female CD rats. Cancer Res 41: 2450–2456
Stout DL, Becker FF (1978) Alteration of the ability of liver microsomes to activate N-2-fluorenylacetamide to a mutagen of Salmonella typhimurium during hepatocarcinogenesis. Cancer Res 38: 2274–2278
Stout DL, Babtist JN, Matney TS, Shaw CR (1976) N-hydroxy-2-aminofluorene: the principal mutagen produced from N-hydroxy-2-acetylaminofluorene by a mammalian supernatant enzyme preparation. Cancer Lett 1: 269–274
Thorgeirsson SS, Sakai S, Wirth PJ (1980) Effect of ascorbic acid on in vitro mutagenicity and in vivo covalent binding of N-hydroxy-2-acetylaminofluorene in the rat. Mutation Res 70: 395–398
Weeks CE, Allaben WT, Louie SC, Lazear EJ (1978) Role of arylhydroxamic acid acyltransferase in the mutagenicity of N-2-fluorenylacetamide in Salmonella typhimurium. Cancer Res 38: 613–618
Weeks CE, Allaben WT, Tresp NM, Louie SC, Lazear EJ, King CM (1980) Effects of structure of N-acyl-N-2-fluorenylhydroxylamines on arylhydroxamic acid acyltransferase, sulfotransferase, and deacylase activities, and on mutations in Salmonella typhimurium TA 1538. Cancer Res 40: 1204–1211
Wirth PJ, Thorgeirsson SS (1981) Mechanism of N-hydroxy-2-acetylaminofluorene mutagenicity in the Salmonella test system. Role of N-O acyltransferase and sulfotransferase from rat liver. Mol Pharmacol 19: 337–344
Ying TS, Sarma DSR, Farber E (1981) Role of acute hepatic necrosis in the induction of early steps in liver carcinogenesis by diethylnitrosamine. Cancer Res 41: 2096–2102

Can DNA Methylation Regulate Gene Expression?

L. Vardimon, D. Renz, and W. Doerfler*

Institut für Genetik, Universität Köln, Weyertal 121, 5000 Köln-Lindenthal, FRG

DNA Methylation

The DNA from many different animals contains 5-methyl-cytosine (m^5C) in addition to the four DNA bases (Wyatt 1951; Vanyushin et al. 1970). m^5C is predominantly found in the sequence m^5CpG (Grippo et al. 1968), and is known to arise by the direct methylation of cytosine residues in DNA (Sneider and Potter 1969; Burdon and Adams 1969). There is considerable variation in the degree of methylation in DNA from different animals (Waalwijk and Flavell 1978b; Drahovsky et al. 1979; Bird and Taggart 1980; Eden et al. 1981).

The DNAs of adenoviruses type 2 (Ad2) and type 12 (Ad12) have been found to contain low amounts of m^5C, if any. Using two-dimensional thin-layer chromatography, it has been shown (Günthert et al. 1976) that Ad2 and Ad12 contain 0,04% and 0.06% m^5C per cytosine respectively. The host cells in which these viruses are propagated contain higher amounts of m^5C (3.57% for human KB cells). Differences in the levels of DNA methylation have been found also between different Ad12-transformed hamster cell lines (HA 12/7, 3.11% m^5C; T637, 3.14% m^5C and the nonvirus untransformed hamster cells (BHK21, 2.22% m^5C).

Certain restriction endonucleases have been found to be unable to cleave at their specific recognition sequence if the cytosine within this recognition sequence is methylated (Roberts 1980, for review). The use of such restriction enzymes facilitates more detailed analyses of the presence and the location of m^5C in the DNA of specific genes (Doerfler 1981, for review).

Correlations Between DNA Methylation and Gene Expression

The two isoschizomeric restriction endonucleases *Hpa*II and *Msp*I recognize the restriction site 5′-CCGG-3′. The *Hpa*II restriction enzyme cannot cut at this site when

* We thank Armin Kressmann and Marco Maechler, Zürich, for help with the microinjection experiments, Howard Cedar, Jerusalem, for providing the HpaII DNA methyltransferase, and Gertrud Deutschländer for typing the manuscript. This research was supported by grants from the Ministry of Science and Research of the State of North Rhine-Westphalia (IIB5-FA8381) and by the Deutsche Forschungsgemeinschaft through SFB 74

the internal cytosine of the sequence 5′-CC*GG-3′ is methylated, whereas *Msp*I does cut (Waalwijk and Flavell 1978a). When the external cytosine of the 5′-C*CGG-3′ sequence is methylated, the site can be cleaved by *Hpa*II but not by *Msp*I (Sneider 1980). A comparison of the cleavage patterns obtained with the two restriction enzymes allows a more detailed analysis of the patterns of methylation in specific genes.

Using this approach in various viral and nonviral systems, an inverse correlation between the levels of DNA methylation at 5′-CCGG-3′ sites and specific gene expression has been demonstrated. In *Herpes saimiri*-transformed cells, the viral DNA in a nonproducer lymphoid cell line has been found to be methylated, whereas in the producer cell line the viral DNA has been found to be undermethylated (Desrosiers et al. 1979). In the retroviruses system it has been demonstrated that the proviral DNA sequences of avian sarcoma virus are methylated at the 5′-CCGG-3′ sites in a nonpermissive rat cell line, but not in permissive chicken cells (Guntaka et al. 1980).

In nonviral systems, tissue-specific differences in methylation patterns have been observed for the globin gene (Waalwijk and Flavell 1978b), for chicken ovalbumin (Mandel and Chambon 1979; Kuo et al. 1979), and for ribosomal DNA (Bird et al., to be published).

A correlation between methylation and gene expression could also be demonstrated by using the cytidine analog 5-azacytidine, which could not be methylated. Incorporation of 5-azacytidine into DNA led to differentiation of a certain percentage of mouse embryo cells to muscle cells (Constantinides et al. 1977; Taylor and Jones 1979) or to the activation of a specific proviral gene (Groudine et al. 1981).

Adenovirus-transformed cells are particularly suitable for studying the correlation between methylation and gene expression. In many Ad12-transformed hamster cell lines, the regions of the viral genome which encode late proteins are not expressed and have been found to be heavily methylated. The early regions are expressed and are undermethylated (Ortin et al. 1976; Sutter and Doerfler 1979; 1980). The best correlation so far has been found in Ad2-transformed hamster cell lines. An inverse correlation between DNA methylation at 5′-CCGG-3′ sites in the structural gene for the specific DNA-binding protein (DBP) of Ad2 and its expression could be demonstrated (Vardimon et al. 1980).

Expression of the DBP (E2a Region) in Ad2-Transformed Cell Lines

A detailed analysis of the integration patterns of the viral DNA in five Ad2-transformed cell lines, HE1 to HE5 (Cook and Lewis 1979), has shown that in three of the cell lines, HE1, HE2, and HE3, the structural gene for the DBP is present (Fig. 1; Vardimon and Doerfler 1981). In these cell lines, parts of the viral DNA are integrated in the cellular DNA. The cell lines HE2 and HE3 contain different numbers of genome equivalents of integrated viral DNA, although they exhibit the same patterns of integration. The viral DNA in cell line HE1 is integrated in a different fashion.

The structural gene for the DBP is located on the *Eco*RI B fragment of the Ad2 genome. It has been demonstrated that although the *Eco*RI B fragment is present in all three cell lines, only the HE1 cell line expresses the DBP (Johannsson et al. 1978; Vardimon et al. 1980; Esche, to be published). We have determined whether the DNAs of these cell lines are methylated to different extents in the sequence encoding

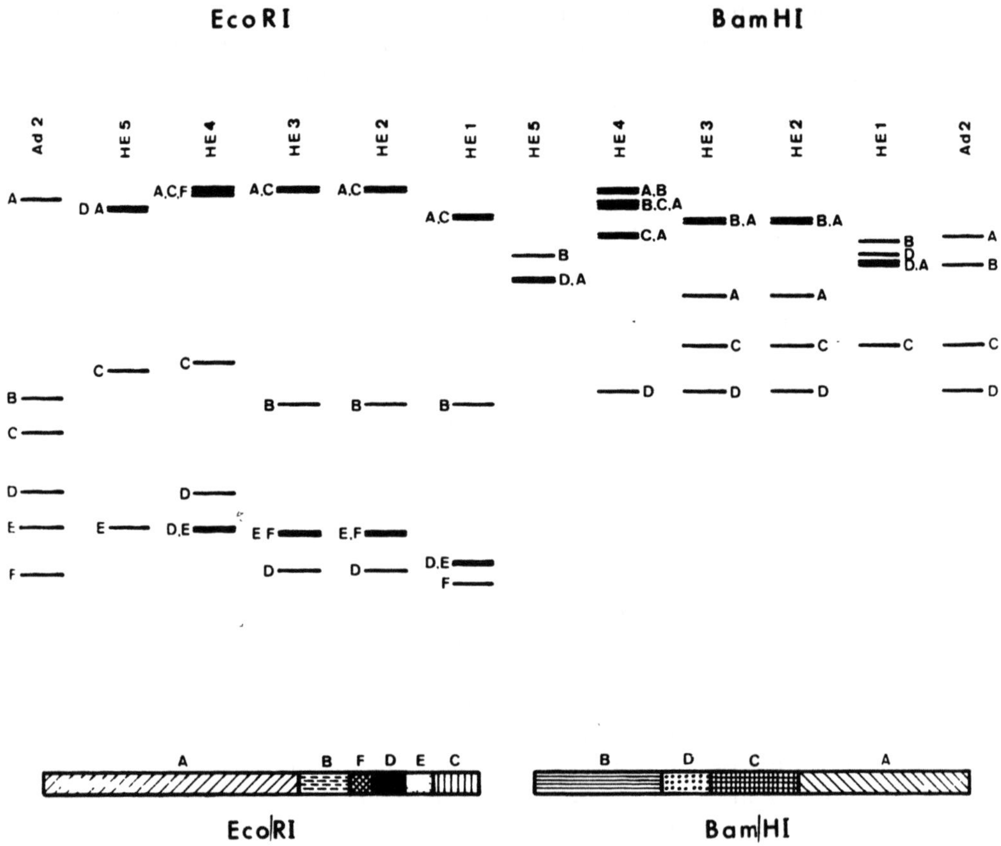

Fig. 1. Analysis of the integration patterns of the viral DNA in Ad2-transformed cell lines: schematic summary of hybridization experiments using the purified *Eco*RI or *Bam*HI fragments of Ad2 DNA as probes. The DNAs of cell lines HE1, HE2, HE3, HE4, and HE5 were cleaved with restriction endonuclease *Eco*RI *(left)* or *Bam*HI *(right)*. DNA fragments were separated by electrophoresis on 0.5% agarose slab gels and transferred to nitrocellulose filters by the Southern blotting technique. The DNA on the filters was subsequently hybridized with Ad2 DNA or restriction fragments of the Ad2 DNA labeled with ^{32}P by nick translation. Ad2-specific sequences were visualized by autoradiography. The identities of Ad2-specific DNA bands in autoradiographs are indicated by letters in the schemes presented, and the map locations of individual restriction endonuclease fragments are designated in the restriction map

for the DBP. DNA was extracted from the Ad2-transformed cell lines and was cleaved using the restriction enzyme *Hpa*II or *Msp*I. The DNA fragments generated were then analyzed for the presence of Ad2-specific DNA sequences by electrophoresis on horizontal agarose slab gels, by Southern blotting (Southern 1975), and by DNA-DNA hybridization using a nick-translated (Rigby et al. 1977) *Eco*RI B fragment of the Ad2 genome as probe. Specific DNA sequences were visualized by autoradiography. The *Eco*RI B fragment was found to be methylated in all internal cytosine residues of the 5′-CCGG-3′ sites in the cell lines HE2 and HE3, but not methylated at all at these sites in the cell line HE1, which expresses the DBP (Fig. 2; Vardimon et al. 1980).

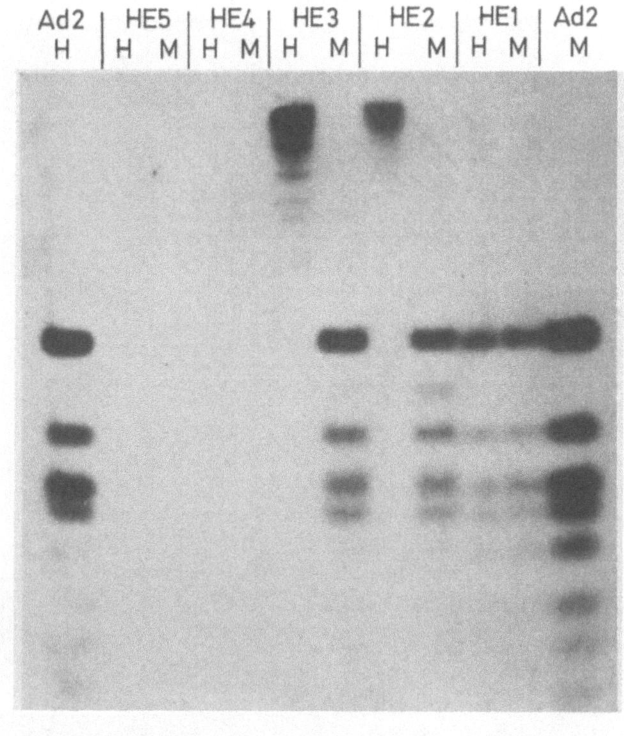

Fig. 2. Extent of methylation of *Eco*RI B fragment of the Ad2 DNA in Ad2-transformed hamster cell lines. DNA extracted from the cell lines HE1 and HE5 or from Ad2 virions was digested with the restriction endonucleases *Hpa*II *(H)* or *Msp*I *(M)*. The DNA on the Southern blot was hybridized with the ^{32}P-labeled *Eco*RI B fragment of Ad2 DNA, and the specific viral sequences were visualized by autoradiography

A Late Promoter/Leader of the DBP (E2a Region) is Used in Transformed Cells

The DBP of Ad2 is encoded in the E2a region on the leftward-transcribed strand of the viral genome. Four different leader regions have been found to be used in the productive system for transcription of the E2a region into mRNA (Fig. 4c; Chow et al. 1979). One of the four leaders is used early after infection and the other three are used late after infection (Chow et al. 1979; Baker and Ziff 1981; Goldenberg et al. 1981).

The analysis of the integration patterns of the viral DNA in the Ad2-transformed cell lines (Vardimon and Doerfler 1981) has revealed that the early leader region of the DBP is absent in the cell lines HE2 and HE3, but at least part of the late leader located at coordinate 72 on the genomic map of Ad2 is present.

In order to decide whether the absence of the early leader in the cell lines HE2 and HE3 is the immediate reason for the lack of expression of the DBP, which may raise the possibility that methylation is the consequence of the failure of gene expression rather than its cause, the following experiment was designed (Vardimon et al. 1981). The region for the late leader for the DBP was subcloned from a cloned *Hind*III A fragment, kindly provided by S.-L. Hu and D. Solnick, Cold Spring Harbor, New York. The cloned *Hind*III A fragment was cleaved with the restriction enzymes *Eco*RI and *Hind*III. DNA of plasmid pBR322 (Bolivar et al. 1977) was cleaved with the same pair of restriction enzymes. The cleaved products were mixed and ligated as described elsewhere (Deuring et al. 1981). Using standard selection procedures a clone containing the 70.7 (*Eco*RI site) to 72.8 (*Hind*III site) map units was selected

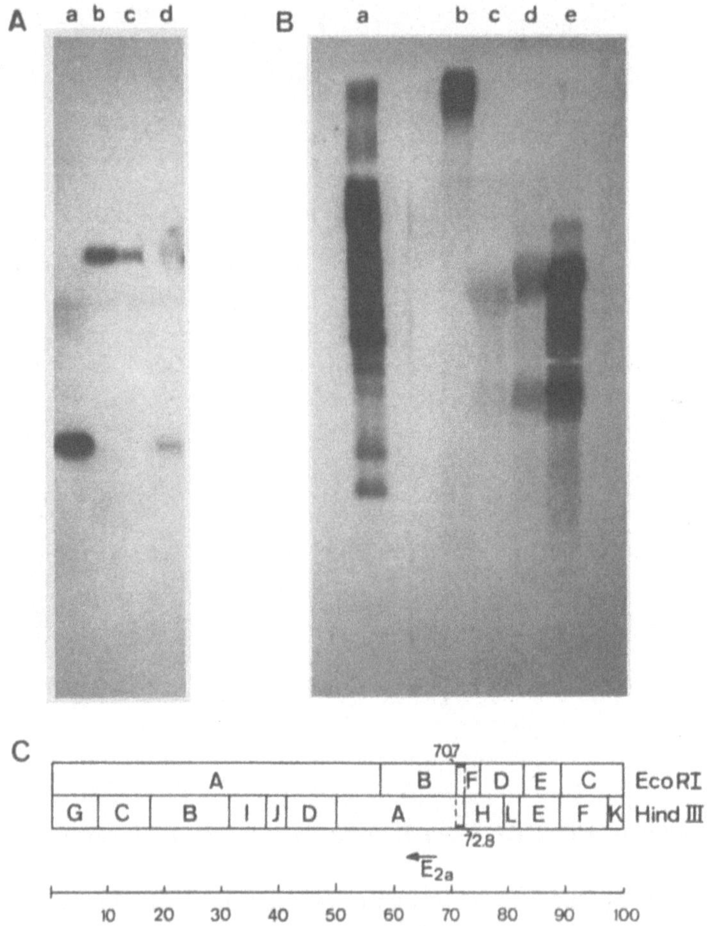

Fig. 3A–C. Persistence and expression of a late promoter/leader for the E2a region of Ad2 DNA in cell lines HE1, HE2, and HE3. **A** The DNAs from Ad2 *(a)* and cell lines HE3 *(b),* HE2 *(c),* and HE1 *(d)* were cleaved with both *Eco*RI and *Hin*dIII and the fragments were separated by electrophoresis on a horizontal 0.8% agarose slab gel. DNA was transferred to nitrocellulose paper, and the blot was hybridized with a ^{32}P-labeled Ad2 fragment (with map coordinates 70.7–72.8) cloned in pBR322. Further experimental details described in text. **B** Cytoplasmic RNA was extracted from KB cells productively infected with Ad2 at 7 h *(d)* or 21 h *(e)* postinfection or from the Ad2-transformed cell line HE1 *(c).* Cytoplasmic RNA (*c* 30 μg, *d* 10 μg, *e* 0.5 μg) was size-fractionated by electrophoresis on a horizontal 0.8% agarose slab gel as described and transferred to nitrocellulose filters. Subsequently, Ad2-specific fragments were detected by hybridization to a cloned Ad2 DNA fragment comprising map coordinates 70.7 to 72.8. The clonal fragment was ^{32}P-labeled by nick translation. In *a* and *b Hin*dIII-cleaved Ad2 DNA was coelectrophoresed as marker. After transfer, viral specific fragments were visualized by hybridization to ^{32}P-labeled Ad2 DNA and by autoradiography. **C** Map positions of the E2a region of Ad2 DNA and some of the early and late promoter regions of this segment (Chow et al. 1979; Baker and Ziff 1981). The position of the subcloned fragment with map coordinates 70.7 to 72.8 which was used as a probe in these experiments is also indicated. The schemes represent the *Eco*RI and *Hin*dIII maps of Ad2 DNA

(Fig. 3C). Cytoplasmic RNA extracted from the cell line HE1, which expresses the DBP, was analyzed as outlined elsewhere (Schirm and Doerfler 1981). RNA was fractionated by electrophoresis on 0.8% agarose slab gels containing 2.2 *M* formaldehyde, blotting to nitrocellulose filters, and DNA-RNA hybridization using the nick-translated cloned late leader region as probe. Cytoplasmic RNA from KB cells productively infected with Ad2 was isolated early (7 h) or late (21 h) after infection and was coelectrophoresed as a control. The data presented in Fig. 3B demonstrate that the late leader of the E2a region of Ad2 DNA is expressed in cytoplasmic RNA from cell line HE1 as well as both early and late in productively infected cells.

We also used the subcloned fragment (70.2–72.8 map units) to analyze in more detail the late leader region in the HE2 and HE3 cell lines. DNA extracted from these cell lines was cleaved with both the *Eco*RI and *Hin*dIII restriction endonucleases and the fragments were separated by electrophoresis on an agarose slab gel and blotted to a nitrocellulose filter. DNA-DNA hybridization experiments using the cloned 70.7–72.8 map unit fragment of Ad2 DNA as the ^{32}P-labeled probe revealed that at least part of the late leader region of the E2a region was present in the DNA of the two cell lines (Fig. 3A). In line HE1 this leader region exhibited the authentic size of virion DNA, whereas in lines HE2 and HE3 it was displaced to an off-size position.

In Vitro Methylated *Hin*dIII A Fragment of Ad2 DNA is not Expressed upon Microinjection into Oocytes of Xenopus laevis

Correlations between methylation and gene expression may indicate that methylation is involved in the regulation of gene expression or is a consequence of lacking gene expression. In order to decide whether DNA methylation constitutes a cause or the consequence of gene inactivation, an in vitro methylation system has been developed (L. Vardimon, A. Kressmann, H. Cedar, M. Maechler, W. Doerfler, 1981, The expression of a cloned adenovirus gene is unhibited by in vitro methylation, submitted for publication). The cloned *Hin*dIII A fragment of Ad2 DNA contains the sequence of the structural gene as well as the late leader region of the DBP. As was previously demonstrated (Vardimon et al. 1980), this fragment is totally methylated at the *Hpa*II sites in the HE2 and HE3 cell lines which do not express the DBP. Thus the cloned *Hin*dIII A fragment was methylated in vitro using the *Hpa*II DNA methyltransferase. The enzyme was purified from *Hemophilus parainfluenzae* according to a published procedure (Mann and Smith 1977; Quint and Cedar 1981) by Howard Cedar, Jerusalem. The in vitro methylated DNA fragment was subsequently tested for the completeness of the methylation reaction by cleavage with the *Hpa*II and *Msp*I restriction enzymes. The effect of in vitro methylation of the *Hpa*II sites on gene expression was tested in the *Xenopus laevis* oocyte system. Methylated or unmethylated cloned *Hin*dIII A fragment was microinjected into the nuclei of oocytes from *Xenopus laevis* according to a method described in detail by Kressmann and Birnstiel (1980). DNA was extracted 24 h after microinjection and was analyzed by digestion with the restriction enzymes *Hpa*II and *Msp*I, followed by gel electrophoresis, Southern blotting, and DNA-DNA hybridization to nick-translated Ad2 DNA. The data presented in Fig. 4 demonstrate that the microinjected viral DNA remained in its preinjection state (methylated or unmethylated) over the period of the experiment.

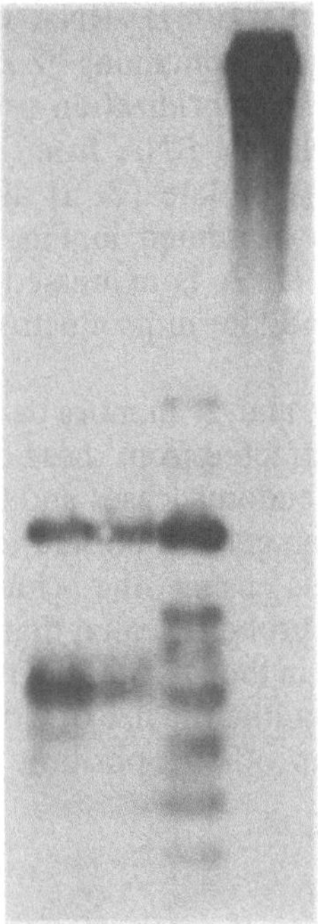

Fig. 4. Stability of the methylation pattern of the cloned *Hin*dIII A fragment of Ad2 DNA on microinjection into nuclei of *Xenopus laevis* oocytes. The cloned DNA fragment was methylated in vitro (*c, d*) by *Hpa*II DNA methyltransferase or was left unmethylated (*a, b*). The DNA preparations were then microinjected into nuclei of *Xenopus laevis* oocytes, and 24 h later the total intracellular DNA was extracted. Subsequently the DNA preparations were cleaved with the *Msp*I (*a, c*) or *Hpa*II (*b, d*) restriction endonuclease. The restriction fragments were then separated by electrophoresis on 1.5% agarose slab gels, transferred to nitrocellulose filters, and visualized by hybridization to ^{32}P-labeled Ad2 DNA followed by autoradiography. Failure of cleavage by the *Hpa*II restriction enzyme indicated methylation at the internal C of the 5′-CCGG-3′ sequence

We compared the ability of an unmethylated or a methylated cloned viral fragment to be expressed into a specific message in the oocytes of *Xenopus laevis*.

RNA was extracted at 24 h after microinjection and was analyzed by electrophoresis, blotting to a nitrocellulose filter, and RNA-DNA hybridization with a nick-translated Ad2 DNA probe. The oocytes microinjected with the unmethylated *Hin*dIII A fragment were found to express virus-specific RNA (Fig. 5A, tracks b and d; Fig. 5B, track c), whereas the oocytes microinjected with an unmethylated fragment failed to express virus-specific RNA (Fig. 5A, tracks a and c; Fig. 5B, track b). To rule out the possibility of an unspecific inhibitory factor in the methylated probe, unmethylated histone genes of the sea urchin, h22 DNA (Telford et al. 1979), were microinjected jointly with the methylated cloned *Hin*dIII A fragment of Ad2 DNA. At 24 h after microinjection, RNA was extracted and analyzed as described above. The RNA blot was hybridized with nick-translated Ad2 DNA, and Ad2-specific sequences were visualized by autoradiography and then hybridized with nick-translated h22 DNA. The oocytes microinjected with the unmethylated cloned *Hin*dIII A fragment expressed virus-specific RNA (Fig. 5B, track c), and histone-gene-specific RNA (Fig. 5C, track c). No virus-specific RNA could be detected in oocytes injected with the methylated *Hin*dIII A fragment (Fig. 5B, track b), whereas specific histone gene transcripts were readily detected (Fig. 5C, track b). These results demonstrate that the block in transcription of the methylated viral DNA is not due to an unspecific inhibitory factor.

Furthermore, we have shown (Fig. 6a) that transcription of the cloned *Hin*dIII A fragment of the Ad2 DNA initiates in the oocytes of *Xenopus laevis* exactly at the same site on the Ad2 genome as in Ad2 productively infected human cells (L. Vardimon, A. Kressmann, H. Cedar, M. Maechler, W. Doerfler, 1981, The expression of a cloned

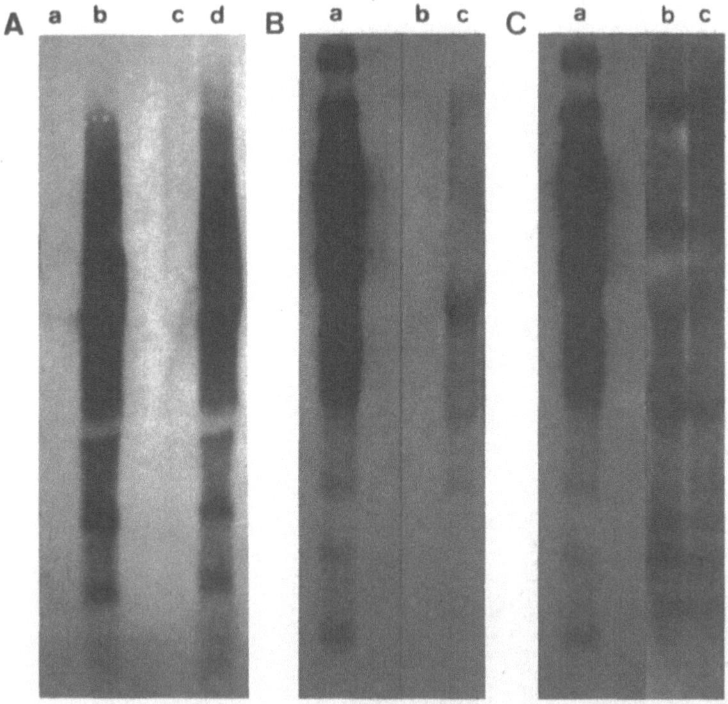

Fig. 5A–C. Test for the expression of the methylated or unmethylated cloned *Hin*dIII A fragment of Ad2 DNA or of unmethylated h22 DNA (histone gene from sea urchin) after microinjection into oocytes from *Xenopus laevis*. Some experimental detail is given in the text. At 24 h after microinjection the total intracellular RNA was extracted from *Xenopus laevis* oocytes and fractionated by electrophoresis on 0.8% agarose slab gels. The RNA was then transferred to nitrocellulose filters. Ad2-specific RNA sequences were detected by hybridization to ^{32}P-labeled Ad2 DNA (**A, B**) or to ^{32}P-labeled h22 DNA from sea urchin (**C**). **A** Experiment 1. The cloned *Hin*dIII A fragment of Ad2 DNA was in vitro methylated (*a, c*) using the *Hpa*II DNA methyltransferase or was left unmethylated (*b, d*). The RNA blot was probed with ^{32}P-labeled Ad2 DNA. The RNA preparations analyzed in *c* and *d* were treated with DNAse as described. **B** Experiment 2. Methylated, cloned *Hin*dIII A fragment (*b*) or unmethylated DNA (*c*), each mixed with unmethylated recircularized h22 DNA, was microinjected. RNA was analyzed as described above. In *a Hin*dIII-cleaved Ad2 DNA was coelectrophoresed as a size marker. The blot was probed with ^{32}P-labeled Ad2 DNA. **C** The blot obtained in experiment 2 was rehybridized after autoradiography with ^{32}P-labeled h22 DNA from sea urchin

adenovirus gene is inhibited by in vitro methylation, submitted for publication). The single-strand-specific endonuclease S_1 was used for this experiment (Berk and Sharp 1977). A fragment of 71.4 (*Kpn*I site) to 72.8 (*Hin*dIII site) map units which contains the late leader region of the DBP was prepared, ^{32}P-labeled at the 5′ termini using polynucleotide kinase (Richardson 1965), and strand-separated according to published protocols (Maxam and Gilbert 1980). RNA synthesized in *Xenopus laevis* oocytes upon microinjection of the cloned *Hin*dIII A fragment, or RNA from Ad2-infected KB cells, was hybridized to the l strand of the labeled leader DNA fragment. The reaction products were treated with the S_1 endonuclease and analyzed by electrophoresis on a sequencing gel (Maxam and Gilbert 1980) and by autoradio-

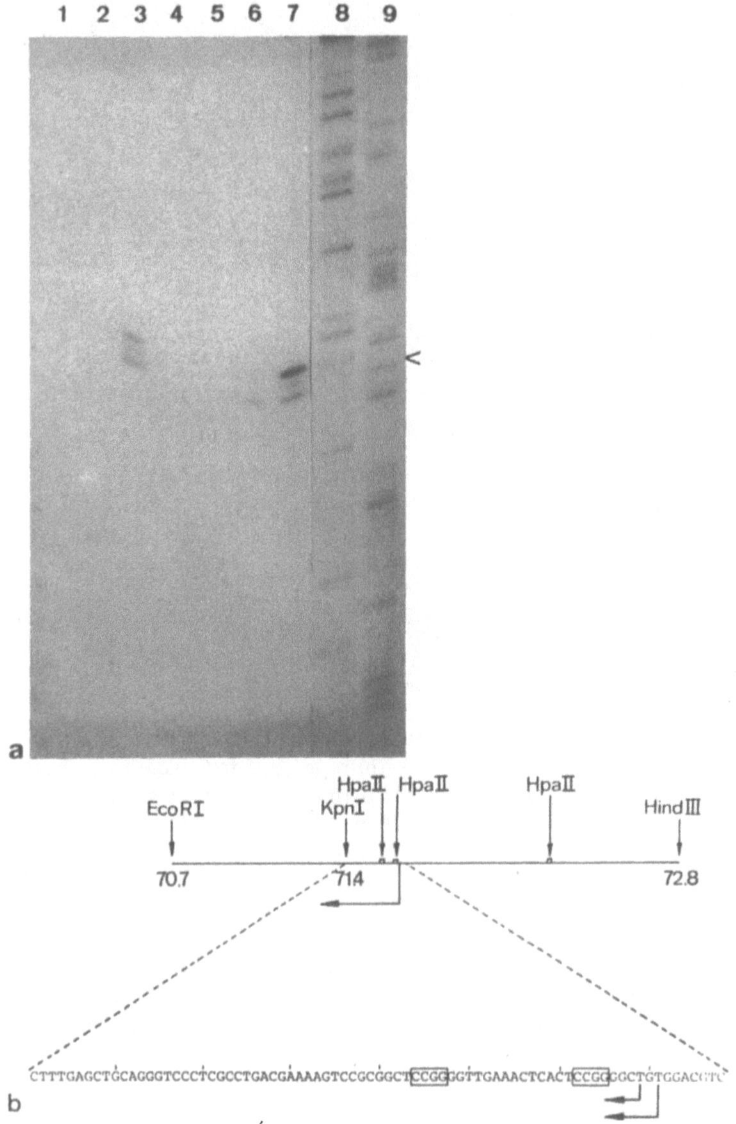

Fig. 6. a Specific initiation of Ad2-specific RNA from the E2a region in KB cells productively infected with Ad2 and in *Xenopus laevis* oocytes microinjected with the *Hin*dIII A fragment of Ad2 DNA. Most experimental details are described in the text. RNAs from sources as indicated below were annealed to the ^{32}P-labeled l strand of a 71.4–72.8 map unit fragment of Ad2 DNA. Subsequently the hybrids were treated with the single-strand-specific nuclease S_1, and the reaction products were analyzed as described in the text. *1* Nuclear RNA from KB cells isolated 12 h after infection with Ad2. The hybrids were not treated with S_1 nuclease. *2* No RNA was added. *3* Total RNA extracted from *Xenopus laevis* oocytes which were microinjected with the unmethylated, cloned *Hin*dIII A fragment of Ad2 DNA. *4* Total RNA from oocytes microinjected with *Hpa*II-methylase-treated, cloned *Hin*dIII A fragment of Ad2 DNA. *5* RNA from oocytes that had not been microinjected. *6* Nuclear RNA isolated 12 h after the infection of KB cells with Ad2. *7* Cytoplasmic RNA isolated 12 h after the infection of KB cells with Ad2. *8, 9* Size markers from a routine sequencing experiment. The *arrow* indicates a 70-nucleotide fragment. **b** Structure of the 71.4 (*Kpn*I site) to 72.8 (*Hin*dIII site) map unit fragment of Ad2 DNA. A blow-up of the initiation site of the E2a region exhibiting part of the nucleotide sequence is also presented

graphy. The data show that the RNA from oocytes microinjected with an unmethylated cloned *Hin*dIII A fragment (Fig. 6a, track 3) and RNA from Ad2 productively infected human cells protect a DNA fragment of 69–71 nucleotides in length (Fig. 6a, tracks 6, 7). DNA of this length was expected from previously published RNA sequence analyses (Baker and Ziff 1981). The RNA from oocytes microinjected with the methylated cloned *Hin*dIII A fragment did not protect the DNA from the S_1 digestion experiment (Fig. 6a, track 4).

These studies demonstrated that the cloned *Hin*dIII A fragment of the Ad2 genome in *Xenopus laevis* oocytes was faithfully transcribed. Methylation of the *Hpa*II sites in this fragment inhibited the specific initiation of viral DNA transcription.

Methylation: A Possible Signal in Gene Regulation

Analyses of the patterns of methylation at the 5′-CCGG-3′ sites of the viral DNA in Ad12-transformed (Sutter and Doerfler 1979, 1980) and Ad2-transformed (Vardimon et al. 1980, 1981) hamster cell lines showed that there was an inverse correlation between the level of DNA methylation and the extent of gene expression. The role of DNA methylation was analyzed by using an in vitro system. The gene for the DBP of Ad2, which was found to show a correlation between expression and methylation in transformed cells, was chosen. The cloned *Hin*dIII A fragment of the Ad2 genome, which encodes the DBP, was methylated in vitro by *Hpa*II DNA methyltransferase and microinjected into oocytes of *Xenopus laevis*. It was demonstrated that methylation of the *Hpa*II sites in the *Hin*dIII A fragment inhibited specific transcription of the DBP gene in oocytes of *Xenopus laevis*.

The way in which DNA methylation inhibits gene expression is not known. There are three recognition sites for the *Hpa*II DNA methyltransferase around the late promoter/leader region of the DBP in the *Hin*dIII A fragment (Fig. 6b). The location of these methylation sites (one of them is six nucleotides downstream from the initiation point of RNA synthesis) may play an important role in the ability of methylation to inhibit transcription. The involvement of highly specific sites in methylation was also emphasized by the results of preliminary studies with the *Bsu*RI DNA methyltransferase (recognition site 5′-GGC*C-3). Methylation of the cloned *Hin*dIII A fragment was found not to influence transcription in *Xenopus laevis* oocytes (L. Vardimon, U. Günthert, and W. Doerfler, manuscript in preparation). The specificity of the sites for DNA methylation should also be analyzed with respect to the location of the sites which can determine the inhibition of gene expression. Are the sites sufficient for shutting off transcription located in the leader region, in the structural gene, or upstream and downstream from either?

It has recently been demonstrated that under physiological conditions a methylated (dCdG) · (dCdG) polymer undergoes a transition from a right-handed B conformation to a left-handed Z conformation (Behe and Felsenfeld 1981). Such dramatic structural changes may affect the ability of genes to be expressed. The availability of specific antibodies against DNA with a left-handed Z conformation (Lafer et al. 1981) may facilitate a detailed analysis of the DNA conformation along silent and active parts of the genome.

Little is known about DNA methyltransferases and their recognition sites in eukaryotic cells. It is not understood what regulates de novo methylation and demethylation. It is not even clear whether demethylation can occur independently of replication.

Although a correlation between DNA methylation and gene expression was demonstrated in many viral and nonviral systems, such a clear correlation was apparently not found in all systems investigated. DNA methylation is probably only one signal in a more complicated array of regulatory mechanisms influencing gene expression.

Summary

The E2a region of the Ad2 genome encodes the Ad2-specific DBP. An inverse correlation between the level of DNA methylation at the 5′-CC*GG-3′ sites of the E2a region and the extent of expression of DBP has been demonstrated in Ad2-transformed hamster cell lines (Vardimon et al. 1980).

Four different leaders are used in the transcription of the E2a region in cells productively infected with Ad2. The leader located at coordinate 75 on the viral genome is used early after infection and the other three leaders are used late after infection (Chow et al. 1979). The analysis of the integration patterns of the viral DNA in the Ad2-transformed cell lines has revealed that the early leader is deleted in the cell lines which do not express the DBP (Vardimon and Doerfler 1981). The late leader located at coordinate 72 on the viral genome is present. The region encoding that late leader has been subcloned, and the cytoplasmic RNA from the cell line which expresses the DBP has been analyzed. It has been shown that the late leader is used in transformed cells. Hence the absence of the early leader cannot be the immediate reason for the lack of expression of the DBP.

Correlations between DNA methylation and the absence of gene expression may indicate that methylation regulates gene expression or that methylation is the consequence of lacking gene expression. In order to decide between these alternatives an in vitro system has been employed. The *Hin*dIII A fragment of the Ad2 DNA which encodes the DBP has been methylated in vitro by the *Hpa*II DNA methyltransferase. Methylated or unmethylated *Hin*dIII A fragment has been microinjected into the nuclei of *Xenopus laevis* oocytes. Unmethylated *Hin*dIII A fragment has been found to be expressed as specific viral RNA, whereas no viral RNA can be found in oocytes microinjected with methylated *Hin*dIII A fragment. The possibility of a nonspecific inhibitory factor in the methylated DNA preparation has been ruled out by the simultaneous microinjection of sea urchin histone gene DNA together with the methylated *Hin*dIII A fragment. Histone genes are expressed, while the expression of the methylated viral gene is blocked. By using the single-strand-specific endonuclease S_1 we have shown that in *Xenopus laevis* oocytes initiation of transcription of the E2a region starts exactly at the same site as in Ad2 productively infected cells.

These results provide direct evidence for the notion that DNA methylation at specific sites is involved in the regulation of gene expression.

References

Baker CC, Ziff EB (1981) Promoters and Heterogeneous 5′ termini of the messenger RNAs of adenovirus serotype 2. J Mol Biol 149: 189–221

Behe M, Felsenfeld G (1981) Effects of methylation on a snythetic polynucleotide: The B-Z transition in poly(dG-m^{5}dC) · poly(dG-m^{5}dC). Proc Natl Acad Sci USA 78: 1619–1623

Berk AJ, Sharp PA (1977) Sizing and mapping of early adenovirus mRNAs by gel electrophoresis of S-1 endonuclease-digested hybrids. Cell 12: 721–732

Bird AP, Taggart MH (1980) Variable patterns of total DNA and rDNA methylation in animals. Nucleic Acids Res 8: 1485–1497

Bird AP, Taggart MH, Gehring CA (to be published) Methylated and unmethylated ribosomal RNA genes in the mouse. Cell

Bolivar F, Rodriguez R, Greene PJ, Betlach MC, Heyneker HL, Boyer HW (1977) Construction and characterization of new cloning vehicles. II. A multipurpose cloning system. Gene 2: 95–113

Burdon RH, Adams RLP (1969) The in vivo methylation of DNA in mouse fibroblasts. Biochim Biophys Acta 174: 322–329

Chow LT, Broker TR, Lewis JB (1979) Complex splicing patterns of RNAs from the early regions of adenovirus-2. J Mol Biol 134: 265–303

Constantinides PG, Jones PA, Gevers W (1977) Functional striated muscle cells from nonmyoblast precursors following 5-azacytidine treatment. Nature 267: 364–366

Cook JL, Lewis AM (1979) Host response to adenovirus 2-transformed hamster embryo cells. Cancer Res 39: 1455–1461

Desrosiers RC, Mulder C, Fleckenstein B (1979) Methylation of Herpesvirus saimiri DNA in lymphoid tumor cell lines. Proc Natl Acad Sci USA 76: 3839–3843

Deuring R, Winterhoff U, Tamanoi F, Stabel S, Doerfler W (1981) The site linkage between adenovirus type 12 and cell DNAs in hamster tumor line CLAC3. Nature 293: 81–84

Doerfler W (1981) DNA methylation – A regulatory signal in eukaryotic gene expression. J Gen Virol 57: 1–20

Drahovsky D, Boehm TLJ, Kreis W (1979) Distribution pattern and enzymic hypermethylation of inverted repetitive DNA sequences in P815 mastocytoma cells. Biochim Biophys Acta 563: 28–35

Eden FC, Musti AM, Sobieski DA (1981) Clusters of repeated sequences of chicken DNA are extensively methylated but contain specific undermethylated regions. J Mol Biol 148: 129–151

Esche H (to be published) Viral gene products in adenovirus type 2 transformed hamster cells. J Virol

Goldenberg CJ, Rosenthal R, Bhaduri S, Raskas H (1981) Coordinate regulation of two cytoplasmic RNA species transcribed from early region 2 of the adenovirus 2 genome. J Virol 38: 932–939

Grippo P, Iaccarino M, Parisi E, Scarano E (1968) Methylation of DNA in developing sea urchin embryos. J Mol Biol 36: 195–208

Groudine M, Eisenmann R, Weintraub H (1981) Chromatin structure of endogenous retroviral genes and activation by an inhibitor of DNA methylation. Nature 292: 311–317

Guntaka RV, Rao PY, Mitsialis SA, Katz R (1980) Modification of avian sarcoma proviral DNA sequences in nonpermissive XC cells but not in permissive chicken cells. J Virol 34: 569–572

Günthert U, Schweiger M, Stupp M, Doerfler W (1976) DNA methylation in adenovirus, adenovirus-transformed cells, and host cells. Proc Natl Acad Sci USA 73: 3923–3927

Johannsson K, Persson H, Lewis AM, Pettersson U, Tibbetts C, Philipson L (1978) Viral DNA sequences and gene products in hamster cells transformed by adenovirus type 2. J Virol 27: 629–639

Kressmann A, Birnstiel ML (1980) Transfer of cell constituents into eukaryotic cells. NATO Adv Study Inst Ser 31: 383–407

Kuo MT, Mandel JL, Chambon P (1979) DNA methylation: correlation with DNase I sensitivity of chicken ovalbumin and conalbumin chromatin. Nucleic Acids Res 7: 2105–2113

Lafer EM, Möller A, Nordheim A, Stollar BD, Rich A (1981) Antibodies specific for lefthanded Z-DNA. Proc Natl Acad Sci USA 78: 3546–3550
Mandel JL, Chambon P (1979) DNA methylation: organ specific variations in the methylation pattern within and around ovalbumin and other chicken genes. Nucleic Acids Res 7: 2081–2103
Mann MB, Smith HO (1977) Specificity of HpaII and HaeIII methylases. Nucleic Acids Res 4: 4211–4221
Maxam AM, Gilbert W (1980) Sequencing endlabeled DNA with base-specific chemical cleavages. Methods Enzymol 65: 499–560
Ortin J, Scheidtmann KH, Greenberg R, Westphal M, Doerfler W (1976) Transcription of the genome of adenovirus type 12. III. Maps of stable RNA from productively infected cells and abortively infected and transformed hamster cells. J Virol 20: 355–372
Quint A, Cedar H (1981) In vitro methylation of DNA with HpaII methylase. Nucleic Acids Res 9: 633–646
Richardson CC (1965) Phosphorylation of nucleic acid by an enzyme from T-4 bacteriophage-infected Escherichia coli. Proc Natl Acad Sci USA 54: 158–165
Rigby PJW, Dieckmann M, Rhodes C, Berg P (1977) Labeling deoxyribonucleic acid to high specific activity in vitro by nick translation with DNA polymerase I. J Mol Biol 113: 237–251
Roberts RJ (1980) Restriction and modification enzymes and their recognition sequences. Nucleic Acids Res 8: r63–r80
Schirm S, Doerfler W (1981) The expression of viral DNA in adenovirus type 12-transformed cells and in revertants. J Virol 39: 694–702
Sneider TW (1980) The 5′-cytosine in CCGG is methylated in two eukaryotic DNAs and MspI is sensitive to methylation at this site. Nucleic Acids Res 8: 3829–3840
Sneider TW, Potter VR (1969) Methylation of mammalian DNA: studies on Novikoff hepatoma cells in tissue culture. J Mol Biol 42: 271–284
Southern EM (1975) Detection of specific sequences among DNA fragments separated by gel electrophoresis. J Mol Biol 98: 503–517
Sutter D, Doerfler W (1979) Methylation of integrated viral DNA sequences in hamster cells transformed by adenovirus 12. Cold Spring Harbor Symp Quant Biol 44: 565–568
Sutter D, Doerfler W (1980) Methylation of integrated adenovirus type 12 DNA sequences in transformed cells is inversely correlated with viral gene expression. Proc Natl Acad Sci USA 77: 253–256
Taylor SM, Jones PA (1979) Multiple new phenotypes induced in 10T1/2 and 3T3 cells treated with 5-azacytidine. Cell 17: 771–779
Telford JL, Kressmann A, Koski RA, Grosschedl R, Müller F, Clarkson SG, Birnstiel ML (1979) Delimitation of a promoter for RNA polymerase III by means of a functional test. Proc Natl Acad Sci USA 76: 2590–2594
Vanyushin BF, Tkacheva SG, Belozersky AN (1970) Rare bases in animal DNA. Nature 225: 948–949
Vardimon L, Doerfler W (1981) Patterns of integration of viral DNA in adenovirus type 2-transformed hamster cell lines. J Mol Biol 147: 227–246
Vardimon L, Sutter D, Neumann R, Kuhlmann I, Doerfler W (1980) Methylation of adenovirus DNA in transformed and infected cells. Nucleic Acids Res 8: 2461–2473
Vardimon L, Kuhlmann I, Cedar H, Doerfler W (1981) Methylation of adenovirus genes in transformed cells and in vitro: Influence of the regulation of gene expression? Eur J Cell Biol 25: 13–15
Waalwijk C, Flavell RA (1978a) MspI, an isoschizomer of HpaII which cleaves both unmethylated and methylated HpaII sites. Nucleic Acids Res 5: 3231–3236
Waalwijk C, Flavell RA (1978b) DNA methylation at a CCGG sequence in the large intron of the rabbit β-globin gene: tissue specific variations. Nucleic Acids Res 5: 4631–4641
Wyatt GR (1951) Recognition and estimation of 5-methylcytosine in nucleic acids. Biochem J 48: 581–584

In tRNA

*tRNA Alterations in Cancer**

K. Randerath, H. P. Agrawal, and E. Randerath

Department of Pharmacology, Baylor College of Medicine, Texas Medical Center, Houston, TX 77030, USA

Introduction

During recent years the structures of nucleic acids in cancer cells have attracted attention because their investigation will be essential in defining the biochemical lesion(s) distinguishing cancer cells from normal cells. It appears reasonable to assume that ultimately both prevention and therapy of cancer will be improved by knowledge of the structure of macromolecules involved in DNA replication, transcription, and translation in normal and neoplastic mammalian cells.

Our laboratory has been interested in tRNA ever since two of the authors (E. R. and K. R.) became members of Paul C. Zamecnik's group at Massachusetts General Hospital in Boston. He had been instrumental in elucidating the basic principles of protein synthesis (Zamecnik 1969), but it was a seminar organized by E. Borek at Harvard University about 12 years ago on the possible involvement of tRNA in neoplasia that stimulated our interest in comparative studies of tRNA from normal and neoplastic cells. Borek and co-workers (Tsutsui et al. 1966) had found that the activities of tRNA-methylating enzymes were elevated in neoplastic cells. In addition, various groups reported in the late 1960s that column-chromatographic profiles of tRNAs in neoplastic cells were altered in comparison to their normal counterparts (reviewed by Borek and Kerr 1972). Preliminary experiments had seemed to indicate that bulk tRNA in tumors might be hypermethylated (reviewed by Borek and Kerr 1972).

Radioactive Derivative Methods for Base Composition Analysis of Nucleic Acids

Analytical methods available 15 years ago for structural characterization of nonradioactive nucleic acids were not sufficiently sensitive to characterize the minute amounts of tRNAs and other nucleic acids obtainable from neoplastic mammalian tissues. Therefore in 1967 we decided to develop radioactive derivative methods for base composition and sequence analysis of RNA. We anticipated that such methods might be valuable in comparative studies of nucleic acids from normal and neoplastic

* Work supported by American Cancer Society Grant NP-315 and USPHS Grants CA 13591, CA 16840, CA 25590, and CA 10893 (P8)

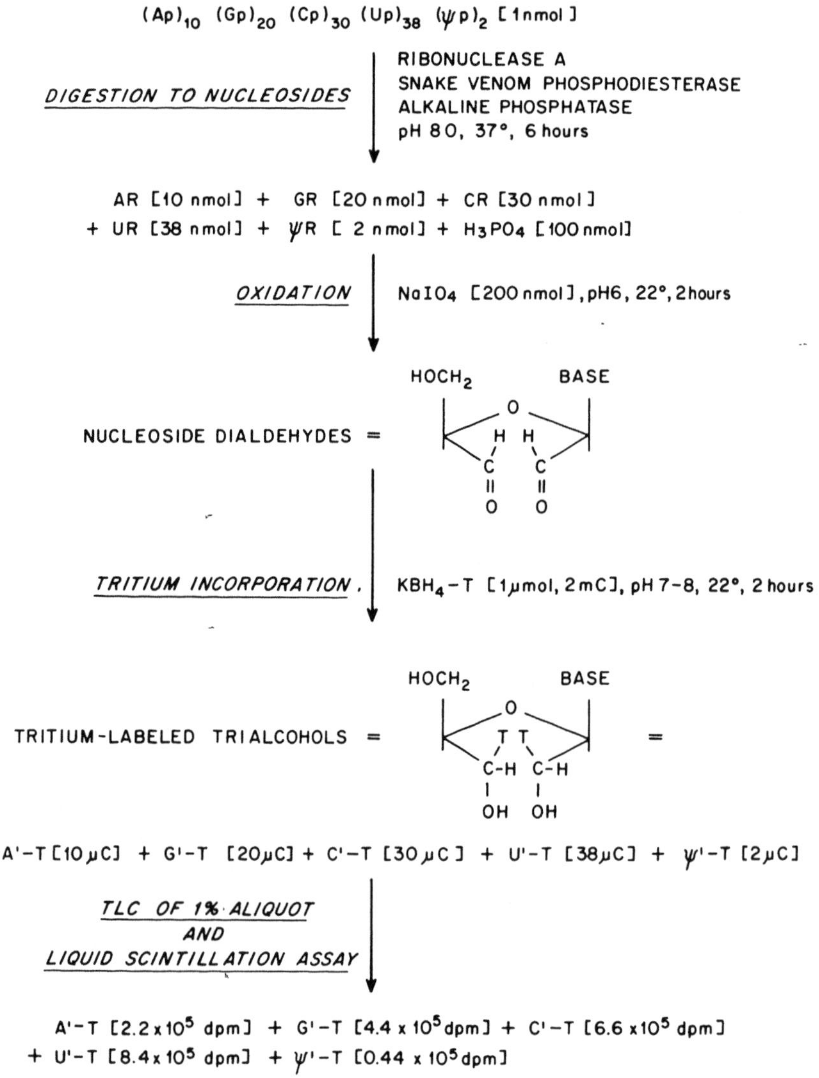

Fig. 1. Base analysis of RNA by digestion to nucleosides and chemical ^{3}H-incorporation

sources. A ^{3}H-derivative method for base composition analysis of RNA was developed (K. Randerath and E.Randerath 1968, 1969, 1971, 1973; E. Randerath et al. 1972; K. Randerath et al. 1974, 1980). As shown in Fig. 1, in this method the RNA is digested completely to the nucleoside level and the nucleosides are then oxidized with sodium periodate to dialdehydes, which are reduced subsequently with ^{3}H-labeled borohydride to ^{3}H-labeled nucleoside trialcohols. These compounds are separated by two-dimensional thin-layer chromatography (TLC) and assayed by lidquid scintillation counting. The method was standardized to afford quantitative digestion, oxidation, and labeling of the RNA constituents so that this approach was suitable for the quantitative base analysis of RNA. An application of this method to normal mouse liver tRNA is shown in Fig. 2. It can be seen that the four major nucleoside derivatives

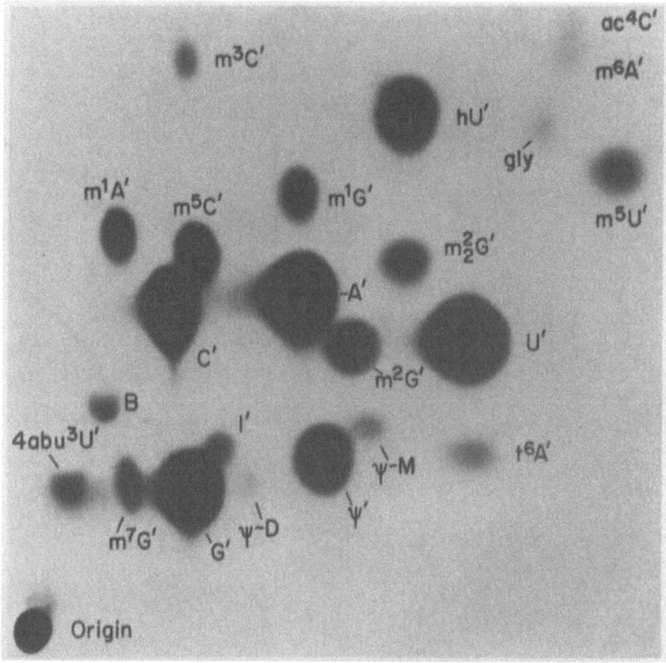

Fig. 2. Fluorogram of chemically labeled ^{3}H-digest obtained from normal mouse liver tRNA. *N'*, a nucleoside trialcohol; *B*, background spot (not from RNA); *Ψ-D*, decomposition product of pseudouridine; *gly*, glycerol; *Ψ-M*, pseudouridine monoaldehyde

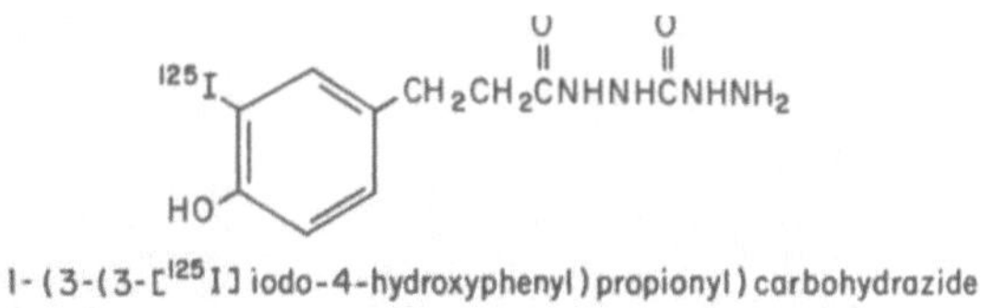

Fig. 3. 1-(3-(3-[^{125}I]iodo-4-hydroxy-phenyl)-propionyl)carbohydrazide, a radioiodination reagent for the analysis of carbonyl compounds such as nucleoside dialdehydes

Table 1. Base composition analysis of DNA containing modified nucleosides by ^{32}P-labeling

Modified DNA
↓ Digestion with micrococcal nuclease/spleen phosphodiesterase
Deoxynucleoside 3′-monophosphates
↓ ^{32}P-labeling by T_4 polynucleotide kinase/[γ-^{32}P]ATP
[5′-32P]deoxynucleoside 3′,5′-bisphosphates of normal and modified DNA constituents
↓ Purification by reversed-phase HPLC or PEI-cellulose TLC
5′-^{32}P-labeled DNA adducts
↓ (i) TLC
(ii) Autoradiography
Fingerprints

and a large number of derivatives of modified nucleosides can be separated by TLC and subsequently assayed.

In addition to ^{3}H labeling, labeling with other isotopes such as ^{125}I or ^{32}P can be used for base analysis of nucleic acids. These isotopes offer advantages particularly in terms of sensitivity, as discussed elsewhere (K. Randerath 1981; Reddy et al. 1981;

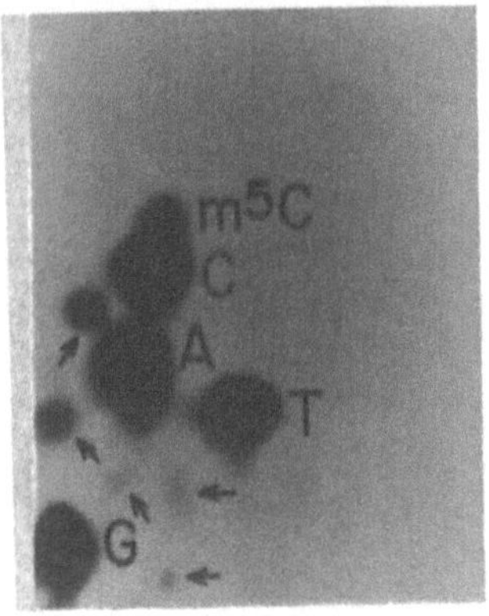

a Control

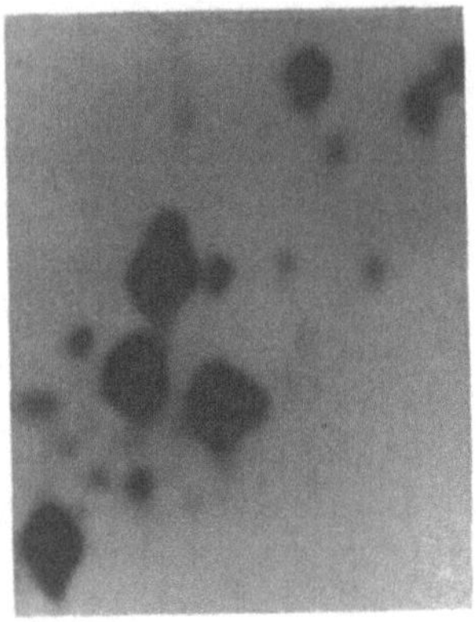
b N-Methyl-N-nitrosourea

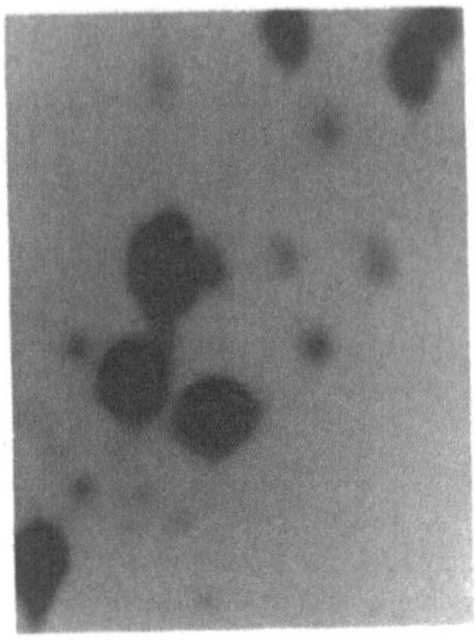
c Dimethyl sulfate

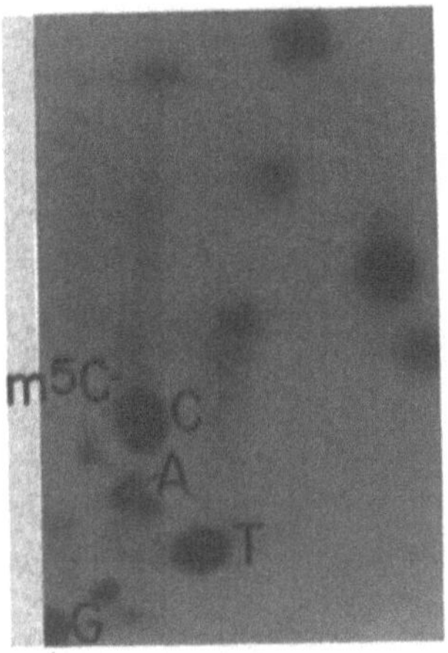

d Formaldehyde

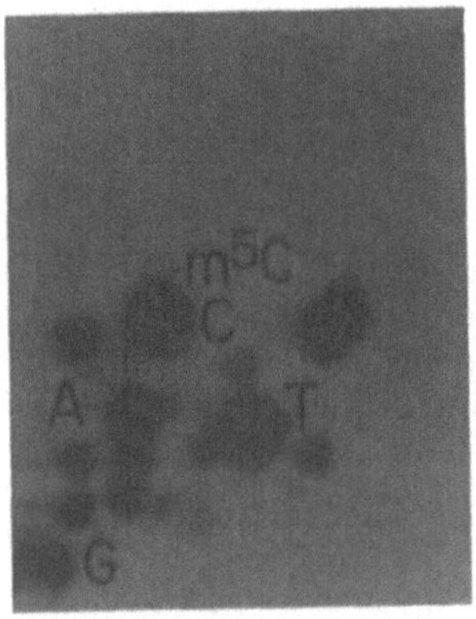

e β-Propiolactone

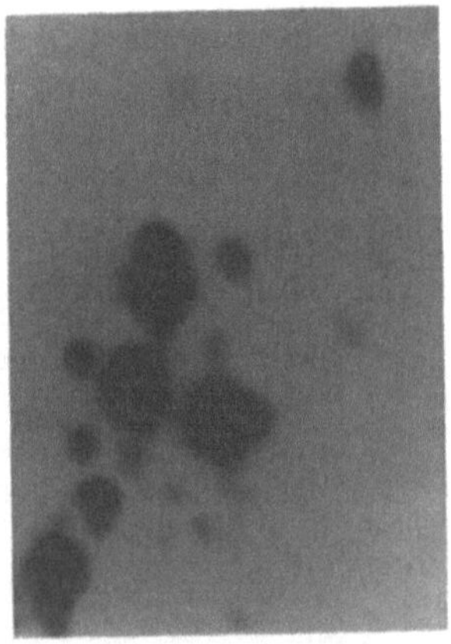
f Propylene oxide

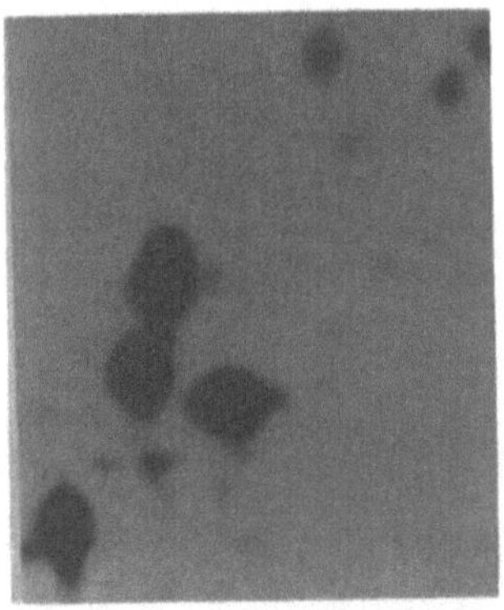
g Streptozotocin

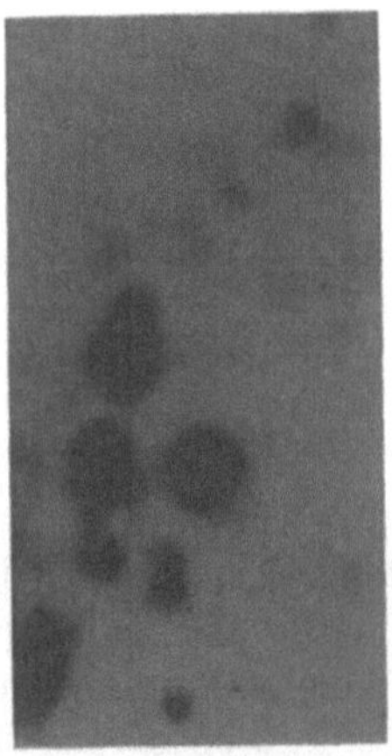
h Nitrogen mustard

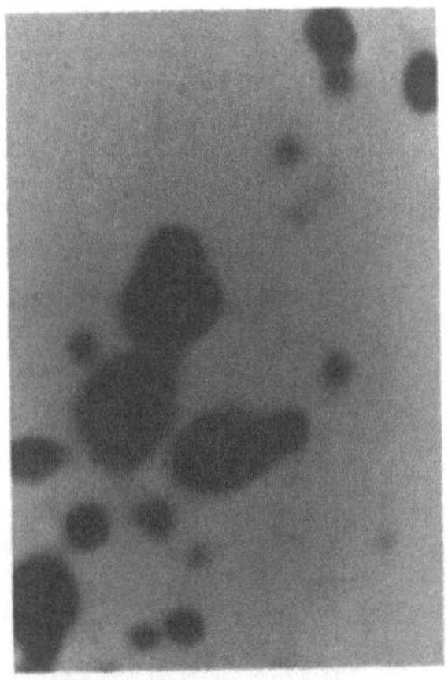
i 1,3-Bis(2-chloroethyl-1-nitrosourea

K. Randerath et al. 1981). Figure 3 shows the structure of a ^{125}I-iodination reagent recently developed in our laboratory (K. Randerath 1981); this compound reacts with nucleoside dialdehydes stoichiometrically to give ^{125}I-labeled morpholine derivatives. This reaction is also suitable for quantitative base analysis of RNA. Its application to the analysis of modified nucleosides is currently under investigation in our laboratory. In addition, ^{32}P-labeling methods can be used for base analysis of RNA (Silberklang et al. 1979) and DNA (Reddy et al. 1981; Randerath et al. 1981). Application of this method to carcinogen-modified DNA is shown in Table 1. Modified DNA is digested with a mixture of micrococcal nuclease and spleen phosphodiesterase to deoxynucleoside 3′-monophosphates. These compounds are then labeled with ^{32}P by the T_4 polynucleotide kinase-catalyzed phosphorylation reaction to give [5′-^{32}P]deoxynucleoside 3′,5′-bisphosphates of normal and modified DNA constituents. These components may then be analyzed by high-performance liquid chromatography (HPLC) or TLC. As shown in Fig. 4, maps obtained from DNA exposed to various alkylating agents exhibit patterns typical for the particular mutagen or carcinogen used for treatment of DNA (Randerath et al. 1981). Application of this approach to the detection of chemicals capable of reacting with nucleic acids in vitro or in vivo is currently being studied in our laboratory. Such radioactive derivative methods make possible the detection of trace amounts of modified constituents (1 in > 100 000 bases) in submicrogram amounts of nucleic acids.

Status of Modification of Bulk tRNA in Neoplastic Cells

Alterations of the modification patterns of tRNA in neoplastic cells, if they exist, must be regarded as highly significant deviations from the norm, because as shown in Fig. 5, the modification pattern of eukaryotic tRNA has been highly conserved during evolution. It can be seen that human $tRNA^{Gly}_{GCC}$ (Gupta et al. 1979) exhibits not only an almost identical primary structure but also an almost identical methylation and modification pattern to those in the insect *Bombyx mori* (Zuniga and Steitz 1977). The observation that the modifications of these tRNAs from two organisms that diverged about 500 million years ago have been conserved suggests very strongly that the modifications play an essential role in tRNA functions.

Our first experiments with bulk tRNA from normal human brain and various brain tumors (K. Randerath 1971; K. Randerath et al. 1971) revealed almost no base composition differences between tumor tRNAs and their normal counterpart (K. Randerath and E. Randerath 1973). However, systematic studies on bulk tRNA of normal rat liver and several minimal deviation hepatomas [Morris hepatomas (Morris and Wagner 1968)] demonstrated reproducible differences in the modified base contents of these tRNAs (Table 2). These differences persisted in different transplant generations of the tumors (E. Randerath et al. 1974). This work also showed clearly for the first time that the tumor tRNAs exhibit a trend toward undermodification and undermethylation rather than overmodification. This trend was even more pro-

◀

Fig. 4a–i. ^{32}P-Fingerprints obtained from control calf thymus DNA **(a)** and from calf thymus DNA that had been exposed to the indicated mutagens and carcinogens **(b–i)**. The nucleotides were mapped by PEI-cellulose TLC

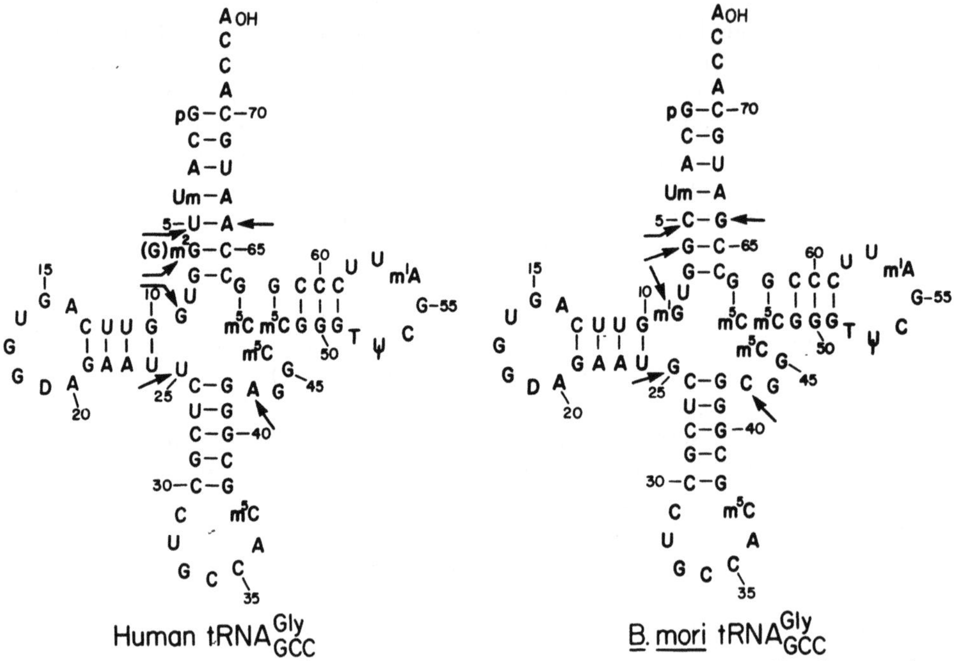

Fig. 5. Sequences of $tRNA^{Gly}_{GCC}$ from human placenta and the silkworm *Bombyx mori*

Table 2. Total base composition of 4S RNA from "pH 5 precipitates" of Morris hepatoma 7777 and host liver

Nucleosides	Hepatoma 7777 (%)	Host liver (%)	*P*	Total b.c., hepatoma compared with liver	Minor b.c., hepatoma compared with liver
U	13.983	14.232	0.001	(↓)	
A	16.618	17.377	0.001	(↓)	
C	26.568	25.762	0.001	(↑)	
G	28.460	27.860	0.001	(↑)	
m^5U	0.515	0.572	0.001	(↓)	(↓)
hU	2.868	2.887	0.4	↓	(↑)
ψ	3.455	3.605	0.001	(↓)	(↓)
m^1A	1.260	1.303	0.01	(↓)	↓
I	0.330	0.325	0.9	↑	↑
t^6A	0.388	0.403	0.4	↓	↓
m^3C	0.315	0.343	0.001	(↓)	(↓)
m^5C	1.803	1.948	0.001	(↓)	(↓)
m^2_2G	0.582	0.572	0.5	↑	↑
m^2G	1.203	1.247	0.1	↓	↓
m^1G	0.842	0.780	0.1	↑	(↑)
m^7G	0.803	0.787	0.6	↑	↑
Sum	99.993	100.003			
Modif. nucl. / Major nucl.	0.1678	0.1733	0.001	(↓)	
Methyl. nucl. / Major nucl.	0.08561	0.08862	0.01	(↓)	

nounced when bulk mitochondrial tRNAs from Morris hepatomas 5123D and 7777 were compared with mitochondrial tRNA from normal rat liver (Chia et al. 1976). Undermethylation and undermodification were found to be more prevalent in mitochondrial tRNA from the very rapidly growing, highly malignant hepatoma 7777 than in mitochondrial tRNA from the more slowly growing, less malignant hepatoma 5123D (Chia et al. 1976).

Sequence Analysis of tRNA by Postlabeling Methods

In the early part of the past decade, when the experiments described in the previous section were carried out, available methods for sequence analysis of RNA were not sufficiently sensitive to analyze the minute amounts of individual tRNAs available from neoplastic mammalian tissues. Therefore, we and others (K. Randerath et al. 1980; Silberklang et al. 1979) have developed postlabeling methods for sequence analysis of microgram and submicrogram amounts of individual nonradioactive tRNAs. The first nucleic acid to be sequenced by a radioactive derivative method was yeast $tRNA^{Leu}_{UAG}$ (Randerath et al. 1975; 1979). The method we now use most extensively was developed in 1978 (Gupta and Randerath 1979) and is illustrated in Fig. 6. The tRNA is subjected to single-hit cleavage (Stanley and Vassilenko 1978). The cleavage products are 5′-^{32}P-labeled using the [γ-^{32}P]ATP/polynucleotide kinase reaction, the fragments are separated by size on a polyacrylamide gel, and their termini are characterized by enzymatic digestion and PEI-cellulose TLC. R_F values of the four major nucleotides and numerous modified nucleotides in two solvent systems (Gupta and Randerath 1979) have been determined (Fig. 6). This thin-layer readout method enables one to read directly the sequence of most or all nucleotides in a tRNA, except for the 3′-terminal adenosine, without necessitating the use of partial chemical or enzymatic cleavages at specific sites, a technique that may present difficulties in identifying pyrimidines and modified nucleotides.

Cytoplasmic tRNAs from Normal and Neoplastic Tissues

When a cytoplasmic leucine tRNA from Morris hepatoma 5123D was compared with its counterpart from normal liver, the only difference found was a partial modification of m^2G10 (about 60%) in the tumor tRNA, while this residue was fully modified in its counterpart from liver (E. Randerath et al. 1980) (Fig. 7). Interestingly, m^2G6 was fully modified in both liver and hepatoma leucine tRNA. Volkers and Taylor (1971) had reported shifts in reversed-phase column-chromatographic profiles of serine tRNAs from Morris hepatoma 5123D. To determine the structural basis of this phenomenon, we have isolated and sequenced $tRNA^{Ser}_{IGA}$ from hepatoma 5123D and normal rat liver (E. Randerath et al. 1981a). The only difference found between these cytoplasmic serine tRNAs was a lack of a ribose methylation at guanosine 17 in the hepatoma tRNA (Fig. 8). Work by Mushinski and co-workers (Marini and Mushinski 1979) suggested that a similar alteration might exist in mouse plasmacytomas. The fact that simple lack of a ribose methylation leads to extensive changes in elution profiles of serine tRNA suggests that the tertiary structure of the tumor tRNA might depend on this specific ribose methylation. It is known that the -G(m)G-sequence is essential for

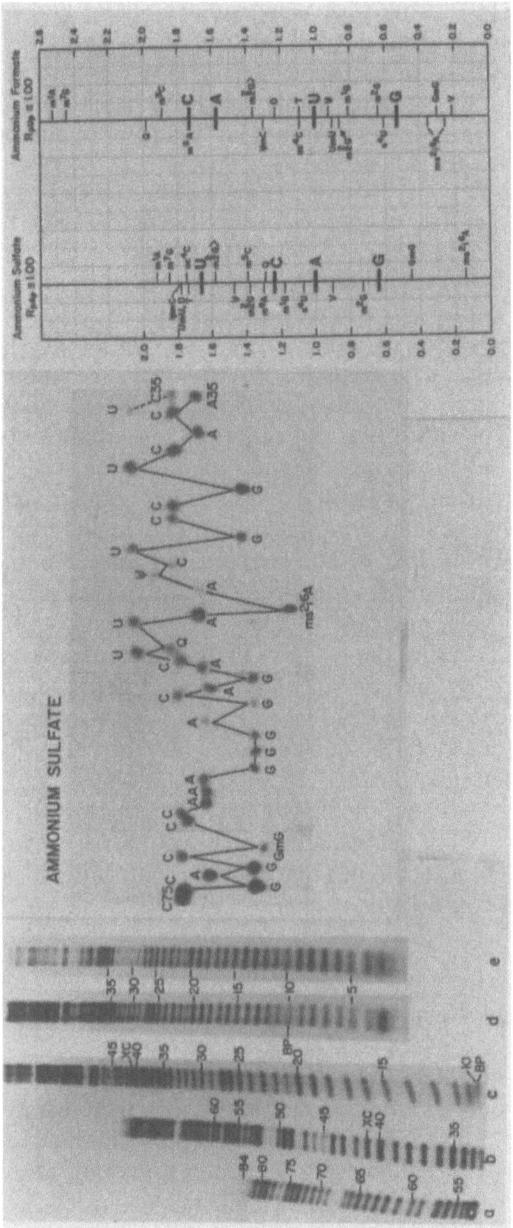

Fig. 6. Thin-layer readout procedure for sequence analysis of RNA. *Left:* separation of 5′-^{32}P-labeled fragments of a partial digest of *Escherichia coli* tRNA^{Tyr} by size on a polyacrylamide gel. "Ladders" are obtained by single-hit cleavage of the RNA and 5′-terminal ^{32}P-labeling. *Middle:* readout of the nucleotide sequence (positions 75–35) of the RNA in the 5′ → 3′ direction. *Right:* relative R_F values of pNp compounds on PEI-cellulose

the tertiary interaction between D-loop and T-loop in tRNA (Rich and RajBhandary 1976). Similar observations for serine tRNAs from brain were reported by Rogg et al. (1977).

Mitochondrial tRNAs from Hepatoma and Normal Liver

Because of the extensive base composition differences between mitochondrial tRNAs from rat liver and two transplantable rat tumors, Morris hepatomas 5123D and 7777

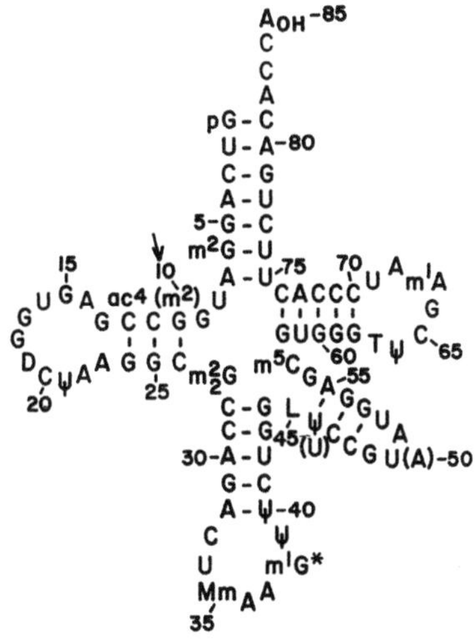

Fig. 7. The sequence of cytoplasmic $tRNA^{Leu}_{MmAA}$ from Morris hepatoma 5123D

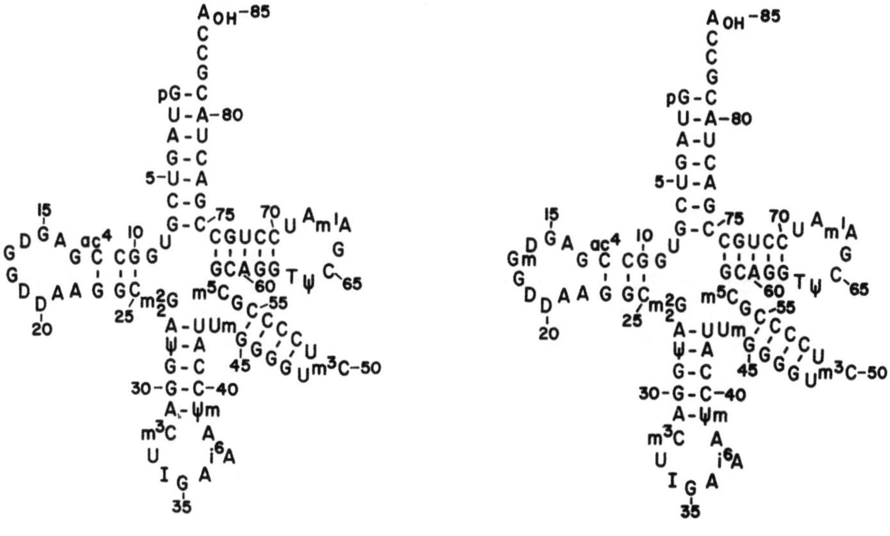

MH 5123D cyt $tRNA^{Ser}_{IGA}$ Rat liver cyt $tRNA^{Ser}_{IGA}$

Fig. 8. The sequences of $tRNA^{Ser}_{IGA}$ from Morris hepatoma 5123D and from rat liver

(Chia et al. 1976), we have recently initiated a project aimed at comparing sequences of mitochondrial tRNAs from rat liver and hepatomas of different growth rates. The fascinating subject of morphological and functional alterations of tumor mitochondria has been reviewed recently by Pedersen (1978). As early as 1939, Graffi reported that carcinogenic polycyclic aromatic hydrocarbons preferentially concentrated in mitochondria of animal cells. During the past year additional evidence has been adduced for the high susceptibility of mitochondrial DNA to chemical carcinogens (Backer and Weinstein 1980; Allen and Coombs 1980; Niranjan and Avadhani 1980), a phenomenon first reported by Wunderlich et al. (1971/1972). This and numerous other

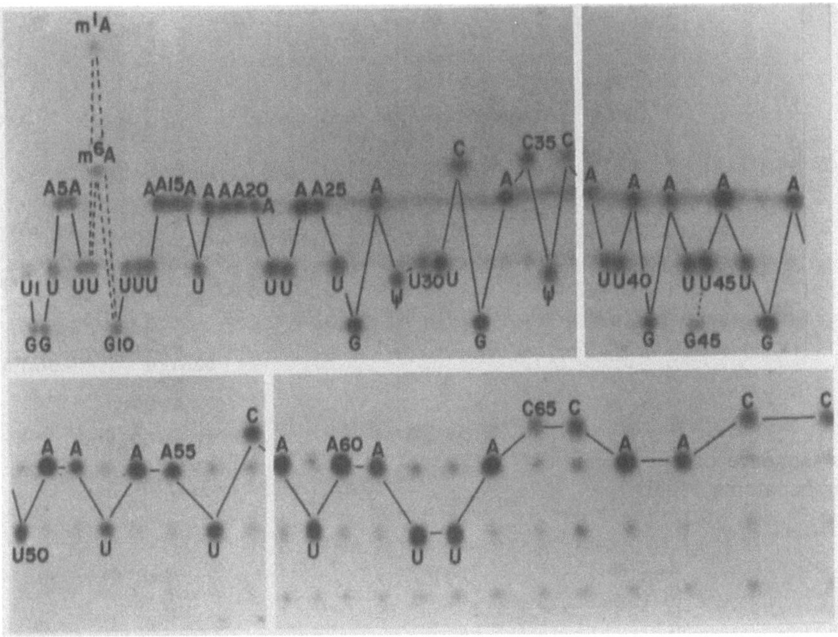

Fig. 9. PEI-cellulose thin-layer readout of the sequence of mitochondrial tRNA$^{Arg}_{UCG}$ from Morris hepatoma 5123D

observations (Pedersen 1978) suggest that alterations of mitochondria may play a pivotal role in the induction and maintenance of the neoplastic state. It is of interest therefore to search for structural alterations in neoplastic cells of mitochondrial DNA, mitochondrial RNAs, and proteins coded for by mitochondrial DNA.

We have isolated several mitochondrial tRNAs from Morris hepatoma 5123D and rat liver and determined their structures. The thin-layer readout of mitochondrial arginine tRNA of the hepatoma is shown in Fig. 9. The readout shows the presence of three modified nucleosides, m^{1}A (partially converted to m^{6}A during the experimental manipulations) and two pseudouridine residues. In position 45, two nucleosides were found, U and G. This observation was confirmed by repeated analyses under different electrophoretic and chromatographic conditions (Agrawal et al. 1981a). The structure of the mitochondrial arginine tRNA deduced from these experiments is shown in Fig. 10. Sequence analysis of tRNA$^{Arg}_{UCG}$ from liver of Buffalo rats (the tumor's host) showed the structure to be identical to the one shown in Fig. 10, except that in position 45 only a single nucleoside, U, was detected. Differences in primary structures between hepatoma 5123D and liver mitochondrial tRNAs were also found for valine and leucine tRNAs, as shown in Fig. 11. Our finding that the 5′-terminal sequence of liver mitochondrial tRNA$^{Val}_{UAC}$ predominantly reads pCAUAG- (see also Fig. 12), with a minor component having C in position 3, indicates that this tRNA consists of one major and one minor species. The hepatoma mitochondrial tRNA$^{Val}_{UAC}$ also consists of more than one species, but the predominant nucleosides in positions 3 and 5, G and U respectively (see Fig. 12), were not found at all in its normal counterpart. Thus liver mitochondrial tRNA$^{Val}_{UAC}$ has U3, while hepatoma tRNA$^{Val}_{UAC}$ has predominantly G3 and no U at all (Fig. 12). In position 5 of the tumor

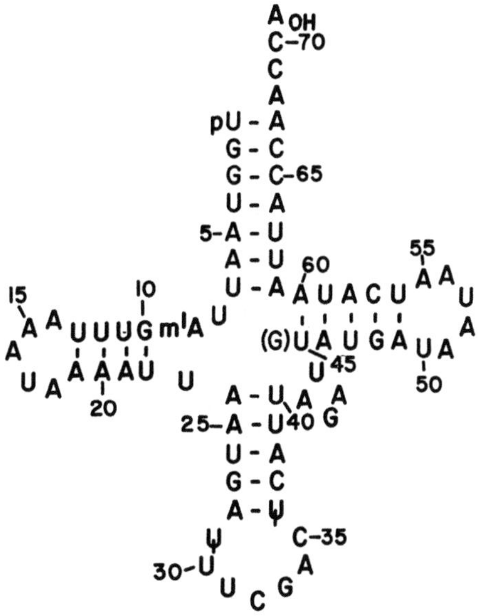

Fig. 10. The sequence of mitochondrial tRNA$^{Arg}_{UCG}$ from Morris hepatoma 5123D

mitochondrial tRNA$^{Val}_{UAC}$ we find mainly U, while the liver tRNA has onyl G5. Liver mitochondrial tRNA$^{Leu}_{UAG}$ has a single nucleotide, U, in position 5, while its counterpart from hepatoma 5123D has U + G in this position (Fig. 11). It is of particular interest that this alteration in the leucine tRNA occurs in a highly conserved region of the nucleotide chain (thus possibly having functional significance), as human placenta mitochondrial tRNA$^{Leu}_{UAG}$ (Anderson et al. 1981) and its counterpart from rat liver have the same acceptor stem sequence. As in the case of the mitochondrial arginine tRNA, we conclude that the changes in hepatoma mitochondrial valine and leucine tRNAs are due to point mutations in the mitochondrial tRNA genes rather than to transcriptional errors, which would affect more than a few positions of the nucleotide chain.

To our knowledge, this is the first demonstration of point mutations in any tumor nucleic acid. While the majority of chemical carcinogens are mutagens, most of which are electrophilic chemicals capable of covalent binding to DNA, or premutagens, i.e., chemicals requiring metabolic activation in mammalian cells to DNA-reactive chemicals (Miller 1970; Miller 1978; Miller and Miller 1981; Ames 1979; McCann and Ames 1976), the role of somatic mutations in the initiation of cancer is still controversial (Weinstein 1980; Cairns 1981; Garner and Hertzog 1981; Woodruff 1981). This is not surprising, as systematic comparisons of sequences of DNA, RNA, and protein from normal and neoplastic tissues are lacking. It is of interest that Vandekerckhove et al. (1980) have reported that a chemically transformed human cell line (HUT 14) displayed a novel actin species which had arisen by a point mutation in one of the beta-nonmuscle actin genes. Our findings of alterations of single nucleotides in hepatoma mitochondrial tRNAs may reflect an increased susceptibility of the affected DNA sites to the attack by chemical carcinogens. Hyper-reactivity of certain DNA sites would not be without precedent because this phenomenon has been observed repeatedly for nonmitochondrial DNA (e.g., Czech and Pardue 1977; Wiesehahn et al. 1977; Metzger et al. 1977; Beard et al. 1981). It has been presumed that DNA regions free of protein, or associated with less tightly bound protein,

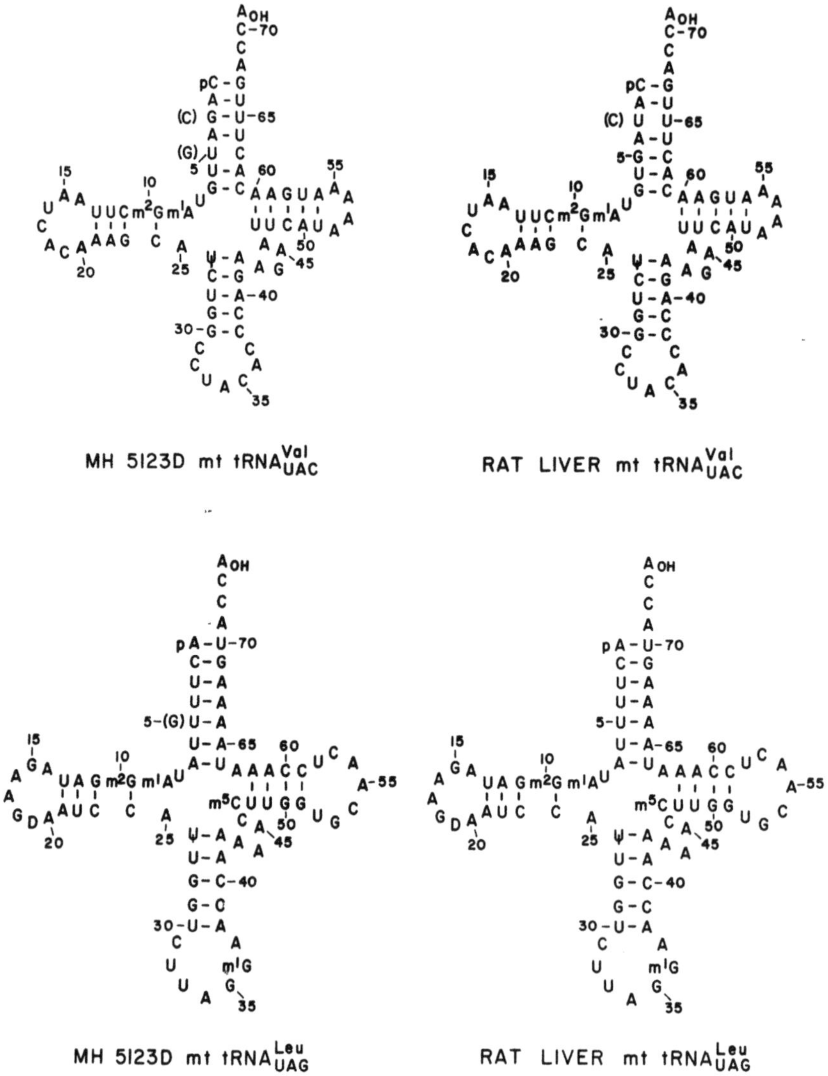

Fig. 11. Sequences of mitochondrial tRNA$^{Val}_{UAC}$ and mitochondrial tRNA$^{Leu}_{UAG}$ from Morris hepatoma 5123D and rat liver

preferentially react with electrophilic carcinogens, but in addition the structure of DNA itself as determined by its nucleotide sequence may be involved.

As shown in Fig. 13, hepatoma 5123D mitochondrial tRNA$^{Phe}_{GAA}$ and tRNA$^{Trp}_{U^*CA}$ are both deficient in m^{2}G10, an observation also made for cytoplasmic leucine tRNA from the hepatoma (see above). The corresponding liver tRNAs are fully modified with respect to m^{2}G10. We have not observed differences in primary structure between liver and hepatoma mitochondrial tRNA$^{Phe}_{GAA}$ and tRNA$^{Trp}_{U^*CA}$.

Similarly, hepatoma 5123D mitochondrial tRNA$^{Asp}_{GUC}$ (Agrawal et al. 1981b) was found to have G in the anticodon wobble position, while its counterpart from liver has queuosine (Q) (Fig. 14). Reduction in the amount of Q or lack of Q has previously

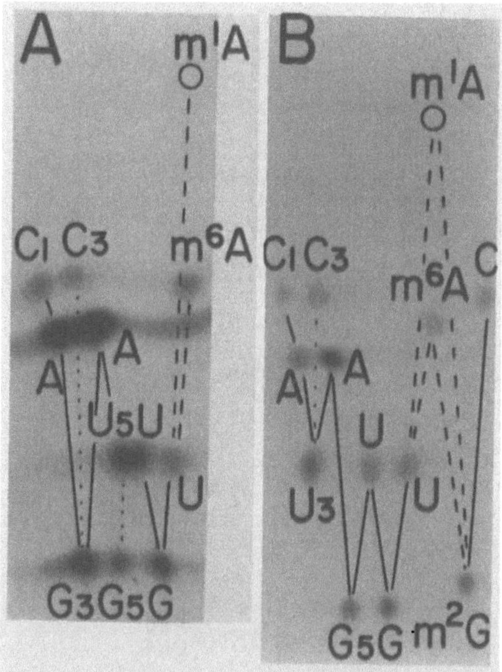

Fig. 12A, B. PEI-cellulose thin-layer readouts of the 5′-terminal regions of mitochondrial $tRNA^{Val}_{UAC}$ from Morris hepatoma 5123D **(A)** and rat liver **(B)**

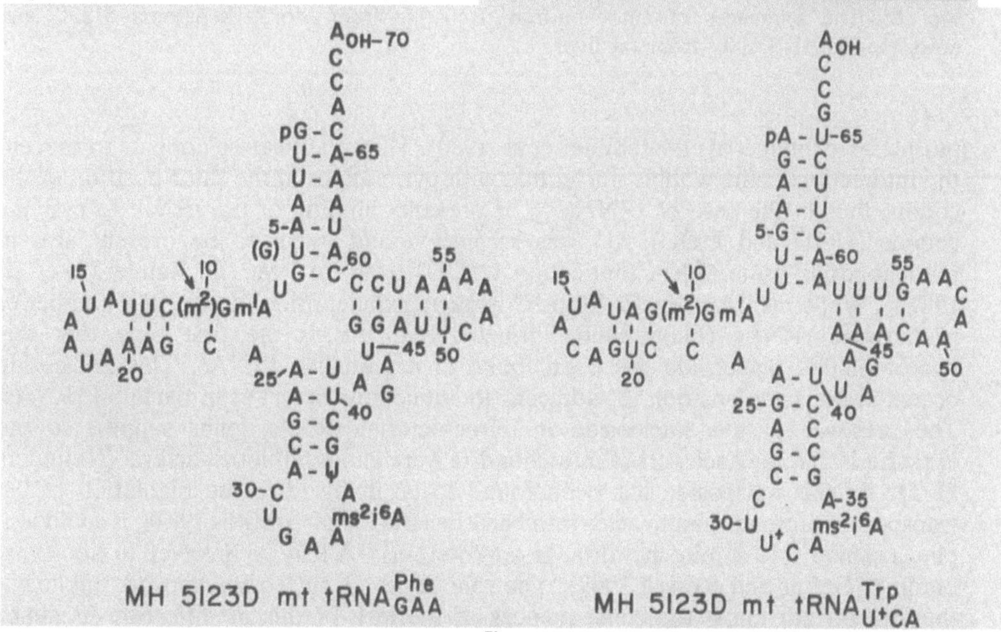

Fig. 13. The sequences of mitochondrial $tRNA^{Phe}_{GAA}$ and mitochondrial $tRNA^{Trp}_{U^*CA}$ from Morris hepatoma 5123D

been found for cytoplasmic tRNAs from various tumors (Okada et al. 1978; Roe et al. 1979).

Our work demonstrates for the first time the presence of hypermodified nucleosides in mammalian mitochondrial tRNAs. U*, an unknown derivative of U occupies the wobble position of mitochondrial tRNAs recognizing nonfamily codons ending in a

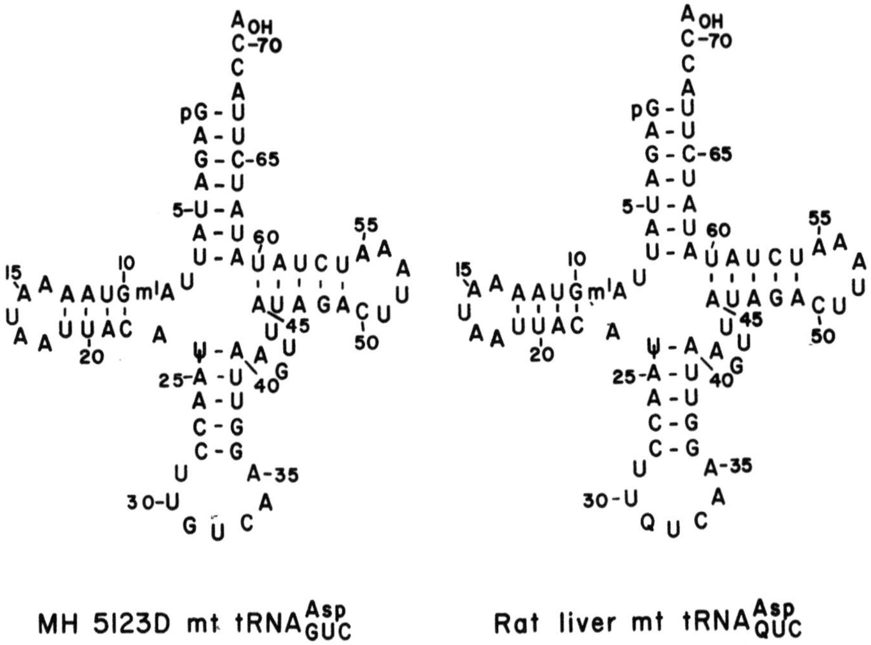

Fig. 14. The sequences of mitochondrial tRNA$^{Asp}_{GUC}$ from Morris hepatoma 5123D and mitochondrial tRNA$^{Asp}_{QUC}$ from rat liver

purine (Heckman et al. 1980; Sibler et al. 1980). This modification appears to prevent the interaction of the wobble nucleotide with pyrimidines in the third position of the codon; thus in the case of tRNA$^{Trp}_{U^*CA}$ it prevents binding of the tRNA to cysteine codons (UGU and UGC). U* was recently found by us to be present also in mitochondrial lysine tRNA (anticodon U*UU) from rat liver (E. Randerath et al. 1981b). While ms^2i^6A (2-methylthio-N^6-isopentenyladenosine) occurs in a number of prokaryotic tRNAs (Gauss and Sprinzl 1981), this is the first time that this hypermodified nucleoside has been found in mammalian tRNAs. This nucleoside occurs in the same position (3′-adjacent to anticodon triplet) as in bacterial tRNAs. The presence of this nucleoside in mitochondrial tRNAs lends support to the hypothesis that the ancestors of mitochondria were endosymbiotic bacteria (Reijnders 1975). As this nucleoside has been found to be involved in the regulation of the transport of aromatic amino acids into bacteria (Buck and Griffiths 1981), it could also play a similar role in mitochondria. In addition, ms^2i^6A may be involved in ribosomal binding (Gefter and Russell 1969). The role of the Q nucleoside appears unknown; thus we do not know the consequences of the lack of this modification in tumor tRNAs.

It appears significant that the modification patterns of mammalian mitochondrial tRNAs strongly resemble those of prokaryotic and cytoplasmic eukaryotic tRNAs, while the primary structures of the A- and U-rich mammalian mitochondrial tRNAs bear little resemblance to the primary structures of other tRNAs. This is another indication of the great importance of the modified nucleosides in tRNAs. On the basis of the results presented, we speculate that post-transcriptional modifications may play a more critical role in the proper functioning of tRNA than certain elements of primary structure. This in turn implies that alterations of tRNA modifications in cancer have to be regarded as serious deviations from the norm and thus may be crucially involved in the induction and maintenance of the neoplastic state.

Summary

1. ^{3}H-, ^{125}I-, and ^{32}P-labeling methods were developed for base composition and sequence analysis of minute amounts of nonradioactive nucleic acids containing modified constituents.
2. Base composition analysis showed tRNA from two "liver-like" minimal deviation hepatomas, Morris hepatomas 5123D and 7777, to exhibit typical alterations when compared with liver tRNA. Our observations, which were made for different transplant generations of the tumors, indicated a trend toward undermethylation and undermodification of tRNA.
3. Sequence analysis of several cytoplasmic and mitochondrial tRNAs from hepatoma 5123D showed partial lack of m^{2}G and complete lack of Gm and Q.
4. Sequence analysis of mitochondrial tRNAs from hepatoma 5123D indicated several instances of alterations of primary structure, a phenomenon not previously observed for cytoplasmic tRNAs from neoplasms.
5. Biochemical mechanisms underlying these alterations, as well as their functional implications, have yet to be investigated.
6. Modification patterns, but not primary structures, of mitochondrial tRNAs have been highly conserved when compared to prokaryotic and eukaryotic cytoplasmic tRNAs. This implies that (a) post-transcriptional modifications must play a crucial role in tRNA function, and (b) alterations of post-transcriptional modifications in tumor tRNAs have to be regarded as highly significant deviations from the norm.

References

Agrawal HP, Gupta RC, Randerath K, Randerath E (1981a) The sequence of mitochondrial arginine tRNA (anticodon UCG) from a transplantable rat tumor, Morris hepatoma 5123D. FEBS Lett 130: 287–290

Agrawal HP, Randerath K, Randerath E (1981b) Tumor mitochondrial ribonucleic acids: the nucleotide sequence of Morris hepatoma 5123D mitochondrial tRNA$^{Asp}_{GUC}$. Nucleic Acids Res 9: 2535–2541

Allen JA, Coombs MM (1980) Covalent binding of polycyclic aromatic compounds to mitochondrial and nuclear DNA. Nature 287: 244–245

Ames BN (1979) Identifying environmental chemicals causing mutations and cancer. Science 204: 587–593

Anderson S, Bankier AT, Barrell BG, de Bruijn MHL, Coulson AR, Drouin J, Eperon IC, Nierlich DP, Roe BA, Sanger F, Schreier PH, Smith AJH, Staden R, Young IG (1981) Sequence and organization of the human mitochondrial genome. Nature 290: 457–465

Backer JM, Weinstein IB (1980) Mitochondrial DNA is a major target for a dihydrodiol-epoxide derivative of benzo(a)pyrene. Science 209: 297–299

Beard P, Kaneko M, Cerutti P (1981) N-Acetoxy-acetylaminofluorene reacts preferentially with a control region of intracellular SV40 chromosome. Nature 291: 84–85

Borek E, Kerr SJ (1972) Atypical transfer RNA's and their origin in neoplastic cells. Adv Cancer Res 15: 163–190

Buck M, Griffiths E (1981) Regulation of aromatic amino acid transport by tRNA: role of 2-methylthio-N^6-(Δ^2-isopentenyl)adenosine. Nucleic Acids Res 9: 401–414

Cairns J (1981) The origin of human cancers. Nature 289: 353–357
Cech T, Pardue M (1977) Cross-linking of DNA with trimethylpsoralen is a probe for chromatin structure. Cell 11: 631–640
Chia LSY, Morris HP, Randerath K, Randerath E (1976) Base composition studies on mitochondrial 4S RNA from rat liver and Morris hepatomas 5123D and 7777. Biochim Biophys Acta 425: 49–62
Garner RC, Hertzog PJ (1981) Origin of cancer (Correspondence). Nature 289: 627
Gauss DH, Sprinzl M (1981) Compilation of tRNA sequences. Nucleic Acids Res 9: r1–r23
Gefter ML, Russell RL (1969) Role of modifications in tyrosine transfer RNA: A modified base affecting ribosome binding. J Mol Biol 39: 145–157
Graffi A (1939/40) Zelluläre Speicherung cancerogener Kohlenwasserstoffe. Z Krebsforsch 49: 447–495
Gupta RC, Randerath K (1979) Rapid print-readout technique for sequencing of RNA's containing modified nucleotides. Nucleic Acids Res 6: 3443–3458
Gupta RC, Roe BA, Randerath K (1979) The nucleotide sequence of human $tRNA^{Gly}$ (anticodon GCC). Nucleic Acids Res 7: 959–970
Heckman JE, Sarnoff J, Alzner-deWeerd B, Yin S, RajBhandary UL (1980) Novel features in the genetic code and codon reading patterns in Neurospora crassa mitochondria based on sequences of six mitochondrial tRNAs. Proc Natl Acad Sci USA 77: 3159–3163
Marini M, Mushinski JF (1979) Transfer ribonucleic acids from eleven immunoglobulin-secreting mouse plasmacytomas. Constant and variable chromatographic profiles compared with the myeloma protein sequences. Biochim Biophys Acta 562: 252–270
McCann J, Ames BN (1976) Detection of carcinogens as mutagens in the Salmonella/microsome test: Assay of 300 chemicals. Proc Natl Acad Sci USA 73: 950–954
Metzger G, Wilhelm F, Wilhelm M (1977) Non-random binding of a chemical carcinogen to the DNA in chromatin. Biochem Biophys Res Commun 75: 703–710
Miller EC (1978) Some current perspectives on chemical carcinogenesis in humans and experimental animals: Presidential address. Cancer Res 38: 1479–1496
Miller EC, Miller JA (1981) Searches for ultimate chemical carcinogens and their reactions with cellular macromolecules. Cancer 47: 2327–2345
Miller JA (1970) Carcinogenesis by chemicals: An overview – GHA Clowes memorial lecture. Cancer Res 30: 559–576
Morris HP, Wagner BP (1968) Induction and transplantation of rat hepatomas with different growth rate (including "minimal deviation" hepatomas). Methods Cancer Res 4: 125–152
Niranjan BG, Avadhani NG (1980) Activation of aflatoxin B_1 by a mono-oxygenase system localized in rat liver mitochondria. J Biol Chem 255: 6575–6578
Okada N, Shindo-Okada N, Sato S, Itoh YH, Oda K-I, Nishimura S (1978) Detection of unique tRNA species in tumor tissues by *Escherichia coli* guanine insertion enzyme. Proc Natl Acad Sci USA 75: 4247–4251
Pedersen PL (1978) Tumor mitochondria and the bioenergetics of cancer cells. Prog Exp Tumor Res 22: 190–274
Randerath E, Yu CT, Randerath K (1972) Base analysis of ribopolynucleotides by chemical tritium labeling. A methodological study with model nucleosides and purified tRNA species. Anal Biochem 48: 172–198
Randerath E, Chia LSY, Morris HP, Randerath K (1974) Transfer RNA base composition studies in Morris hepatomas and rat liver. Cancer Res 34: 643–653
Randerath E, Gupta RC, Chia LSY, Chang SH, Randerath K (1979) Yeast $tRNA^{Leu}_{UAG}$. Purification, properties, and determination of the nucleotide sequence by radioactive derivative methods. Eur J Biochem 93: 79–94
Randerath E, Gupta RC, Morris HP, Randerath K (1980) Isolation and sequence analysis of two major leucine transfer ribonucleic acids (anticodon MmAA) from a rat tumor, Morris hepatoma 5123D. Biochemistry 19: 3476–3483

Randerath E, Gopalakrishnan AS, Gupta RC, Agrawal HP, Randerath K (1981a) Lack of a specific ribose methylation at guanosine 17 in Morris hepatoma 5123D $tRNA^{Ser}_{IGA}$. Cancer Res 41: 2863–2867

Randerath E, Agrawal HP, Randerath K (1981b) Rat liver mitochondrial lysine tRNA (anticodon U*UU) contains a rudimentary D-arm and 2 hypermodified nucleotides in its anticodon loop. Biochem Biophys Res Commun 103: 739–744

Randerath K (1971) Application of a tritium derivative method to human brain and brain tumor transfer RNA analysis. Cancer Res 31: 658–661

Randerath K (1981) 3-([3-^{125}I]Iodo-4-hydroxyphenyl)propionyl carbohydrazide, a new radioiodination reagent for ultrasensitive detection and determination of periodate-oxidized nucleoside derivatives and other carbonyl compounds. Anal Biochem 115: 391–397

Randerath K, Randerath E (1968) Analysis of nucleic acid derivatives at the subnanomole level. II. Quantitative analysis of ribose derivatives by tritium labeling. Experientia 24: 1192–1193

Randerath K, Randerath E (1969) Analysis of nucleic acid derivatives at the subnanomole level. III. A tritium labeling procedure for quantitative analysis of ribose derivatives. Anal Biochem 28: 110–118

Randerath K, Randerath E (1971) A tritium derivative method for base analysis of ribonucleotides and RNA. Proc Nucl Acid Res 2: 796–812

Randerath K, Randerath E (1973) Chemical characterization of unlabeled RNA and RNA derivatives by isotope derivative methods. Methods Cancer Res 9: 3–69

Randerath K, MacKinnon SK, Randerath E (1971) An investigation of the minor base composition of transfer RNA in normal human brain and malignant brain tumors. FEBS Lett 15: 81–84

Randerath K, Randerath E, Chia LSY, Nowak BJ (1974) Base analysis of ribopolynucleotides by chemical tritium labeling: An improved mapping procedure for nucleoside trialcohols. Anal Biochem 59: 263–271

Randerath K, Chia LSY, Gupta RC, Randerath E, Hawkins ER, Brum CK, Chang SH (1975) Structural analysis of nonradioactive RNA by postlabeling: The primary structure of baker's yeast $tRNA^{Leu}_{CUA}$. Biochem Biophys Res Commun 63: 157–163

Randerath K, Gupta RC, Randerath E (1980) ^{3}H and ^{32}P derivative methods for base composition and sequence analysis of RNA. Methods Enzymol 65: 638–680

Randerath K, Reddy MV, Gupta RC (1981) ^{32}P-Labeling test for DNA damage. Proc Natl Acad Sci USA 78: 6126–6129

Reddy MV, Gupta RC, Randerath K (1981) ^{32}P-Base analysis of DNA. Anal Biochem 117: 271–279

Reijnders L (1975) The origin of mitochondria. J Mol Evol 5: 167–176

Rich A, RajBhandary UL (1976) Transfer RNA: Molecular structure, sequence, and properties. Annu Rev Biochem 45: 805–860

Roe BA, Stankiewicz AF, Rizi HL, Weisz C, DiLauro MN, Pike D, Chen CY, Chen EY (1979) Comparison of rat liver and Walker 256 carcinosarcoma tRNAs. Nucleic Acids Res 6: 673–688

Rogg H, Müller P, Keith G, Staehelin M (1977) Chemical basis for brain specific serine transfer RNAs. Proc Natl Acad Sci USA 74: 4243–4247

Sibler A-P, Bordonné R, Dirheimer G, Martin R (1980) Structure primaire d'un tryptophane-tRNA de mitochondrie de levure capable de traduire le codon de terminaison U-G-A. CR Acad Sci [D] (Paris) 290: 695–698

Silberklang M, Gillum AM, RajBhandary UL (1979) Use of in vitro ^{32}P labeling in the sequence analysis of nonradioactive tRNAs. Methods Enzymol 59: 58–109

Stanley J, Vassilenko S (1978) A different approach to RNA sequencing. Nature 274: 87–89

Tsutsui E, Srinivasan PR, Borek E (1966) tRNA methylases in tumors of animal and human origin. Proc Natl Acad Sci USA 56: 1003–1009

Vandekerckhove J, Leavitt J, Kakunaga T, Weber K (1980) Coexpression of a mutant β-actin and the two normal β- and γ-cytoplasmic actins in a stably transformed human cell line. Cell 22: 893–899
Volkers SAS, Taylor MW (1971) Chromatographic comparison of the transfer ribonucleic acids of rat liver and Morris hepatomas. Biochemistry 10: 488–497
Weinstein IB (1980) Molecular and cellular mechanisms of chemical carcinogenesis. Cancer Chemother 1: 169–196
Wiesehahn G, Hyde J, Hearst J (1977) The photoaddition of trimethylpsoralen to *Drosophila melanogaster* nuclei: A probe for chromatin substructure. Biochemistry 16: 925–932
Woodruff M (1981) Origin of cancer (Correspondence). Nature 290: 173
Wunderlich V, Tetzlaff I, Graffi A (1971/72) Studies on nitrosodimethylamine: Preferential methylation of mitochondrial DNA in rats and hamsters. Chem-Biol Interact 4: 81–89
Zamecnik PC (1969) An historical account of protein synthesis, with current overtones – A personalized view. Cold Spring Harbor Symp Quant Biol 34: 1–16
Zuniga MC, Steitz JA (1977) The nucleotide sequence of a major glycine transfer RNA from the posterior silk gland of *Bombyx mori* L. Nucleic Acids Res 4: 4175–4196

Tumor-Specific tRNA Modifications in Mouse Plasmacytomas and Other Tumors

J. F. Mushinski and M. Marini*

Laboratory of Cell Biology, National Cancer Institute, Bethesda, MD 20205, USA

Transfer RNA Variations in Mouse Plasmacytomas

We have been studying the tRNA populations in mineral-oil-induced, immunoglobulin-secreting Balb/c mouse plasmacytomas (Potter 1972) for more than a decade in an attempt to determine if these "adaptor" molecules, which are essential to protein synthesis, play a role in regulating or modulating protein synthesis or in affecting the amino acid sequence of the product of this synthesis. From the outset we were struck by the large number of isoaccepting species of aa-tRNA molecules that sensitive separation techniques revealed for each amino acid. Not only did amino acids such as tryptophan that have one code word frequently have more than one isoaccepting tRNA, but as many as nine peaks of seryl-tRNA were identified for serine, which has six code words (Mushinski 1971). This redundancy of isoaccepting tRNAs was more obvious in the plasmacytomas than in normal tissues. In addition, we found a remarkable number of differences, both quantitative and qualitative, in the aa-tRNA chromatographic patterns when different plasmacytomas were compared. The comparisons were done in pairs by separately aminoacylating tRNA from two different tissues or tumors with ^{3}H- or ^{14}C-labeled amino acid, mixing them, and cochromatographing them on reversed phase columns (RPC-2, as shown in Fig. 1, or RPC-5, as shown in Figs. 2 and 3). The chromatographic pattern of aa-tRNA was not affected by the source of enzymes, and a standard preparation of aa-tRNA synthetase from liver was used in all reactions.

Profiles of aa-tRNAs for All 20 Amino Acids Compared Among Normal Liver and Brain and 11 Plasmacytomas

We decided to investigate this system more thoroughly by determining the RPC-5 patterns of all the aa-tRNAs of normal mouse liver and of 11 plasmacytomas that

* We thank Drs. Aldo Spizzichino and James Koziol for their collaboration in computer and statistical analyses, Mr. William Muldoon for expert laboratory assistance, Drs. Dolph Hatfield and Dezider Grunberger for helpful discussions, Drs. Dolph Hatfield and Carol Thiele for a thoughtful reading of this article, and Ms. Victoria Armstrong for expert preparation of the manuscript

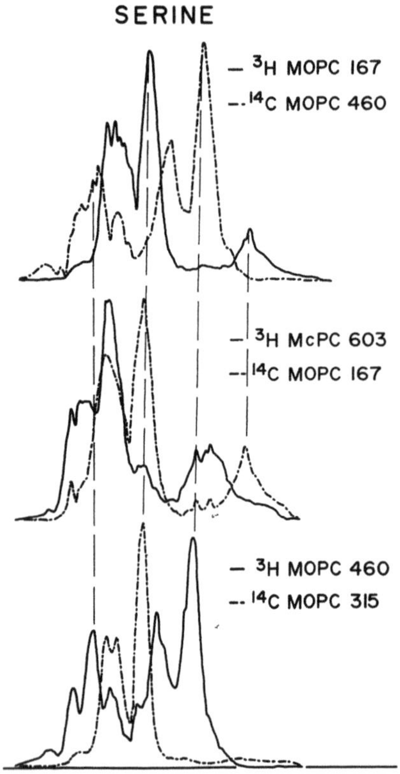

Fig. 1. RPC-2 (Weiss and Kelmers 1967) elution profiles of seryl-tRNA from 4 IgA($\varkappa$) secreting plasmacytomas. The tRNAs were separately aminoacylated with ^{3}H-serine or ^{14}C-serine, mixed in different combinations, and cochromatographed. Trichloroacetic acid precipitates of each of the 160 column fractions were counted and the dpm of each isotope were computed and normalized. The results of three such cochromatographic comparisons were plotted with reference peaks seen in more than one profile connected by *light vertical lines*

devoted a substantial percentage of their protein synthesis to production of well-characterized myeloma proteins (Marini and Mushinski 1979). Each tumor originally secreted a single light chain (ca. 23 000 daltons) and a single heavy chain (ca. 53 000 daltons), of which the amino acid sequence had been determined. Also included in the study were certain tumors and variants derived from those tumors which exhibited well-defined changes in various aspects of their myeloma protein sythesis (Table 1). In this way we hoped to be able to determine (1) which variations in tRNA profiles might be correlated with particular amino acid substitutions in very similar myeloma proteins, (2) which variations might have been influenced by or responsible for protein synthesis changes in mutants derived from a known parent tumor line, and (3) which variations might be related to the tumorous nature of the tissue under study.

Of the 20 amino acids whose aa-tRNA profiles were studied, nine were found to be virtually the same in all tumors and normal tissues: alanine, arginine, aspartic acid, cysteine, glutamine, glycine, leucine, methionine, and phenylalanine. These patterns are presented elsewhere (Marini and Mushinski 1979).

In order to examine more critically the aa-tRNA differences between tumors and normal tissues, another normal tissue besides liver was needed. Brain tRNA was added to the study, and it became clear that normal brain and normal liver had some aa-tRNA profile differences for certain amino acids (Fig. 2). Some of the plasmacytoma patterns can be seen to be similar to the brain pattern, others resemble liver more than brain, and still others resemble neither normal tissue. The amino acids

Table 1. Key to Plasmacytomas and Normal Tissues Studied by tRNA Profile Comparison

Group	Tumor	Characteristics
A. Normal	1. –	Balb/c liver
B. Four tumors derived from an IgG_{2b} (κ)-producing plasmacytoma	2. MPC11	Producer
	3. NP2	Nonproducer
	4. B47P	Producer clone from tissue culture
	5. B47L3NP1	Nonproducing clone from tissue culture
C. Two κ secretors with minimal Vκ differences		26 27 27A 27B 27C 27D 28 ... 93 94 95
	6. MOPC321	ALA *LYS* SER VAL ASN *THR* TYR ... GLX *ASX* PRO
	7. TEPC124	ALA *GLN* SER VAL ASX *TRP* TYR ... GLX ALA PRO
D. Two IgA (κ) tumors with minimal Vα differences and identical κ chains		96 97 98 99 100 101
	8. HOPC8	TYR TYR GLY *ASN* SER TYR
	9. TEPC15	TYR TYR GLY *SER* SER TYR
E. Three tumors derived from an IgA (κ)-producing plasmacytoma	10. Adj. PC 6A	Synthesizes IgA
	11. Adj. PC 6A′	Synthesizes κ-type light chains only
	12. Adj. PC 6C	Premature termination due to frame shift mutation in α chain gene
F. Another normal tissue	13. –	NIH/Swiss brains

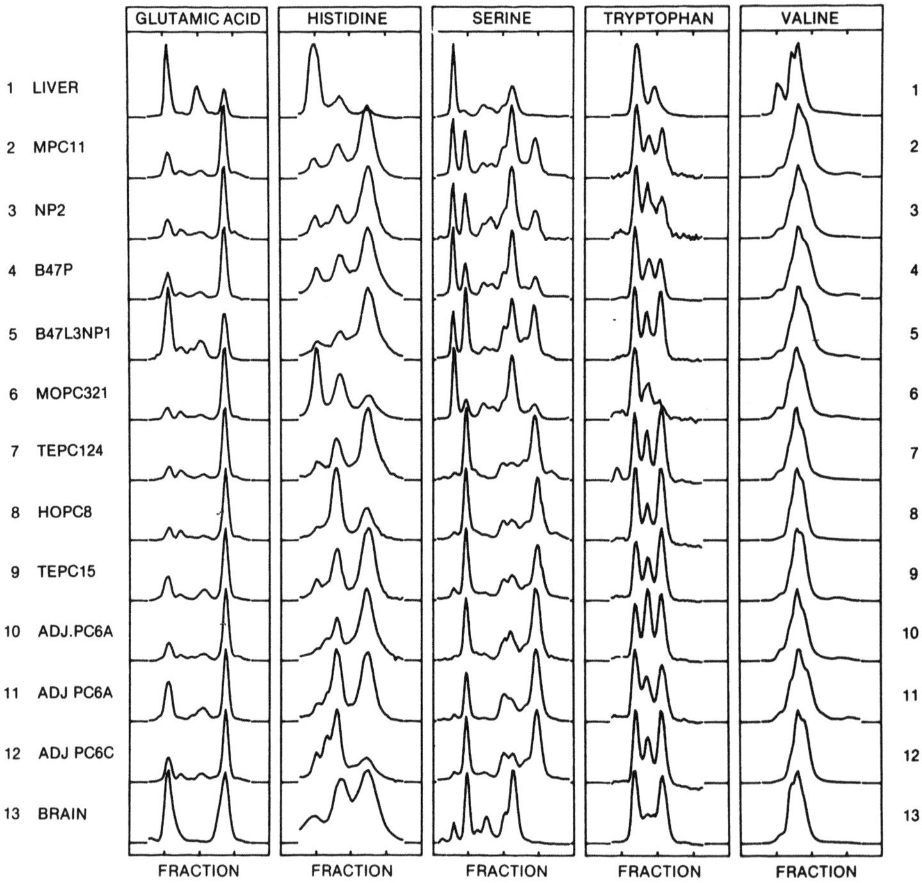

Fig. 2. Composites of RPC-5 (Kelmers and Heatherly 1971) chromatograms for five amino acids that have different aa-tRNA profiles in normal brain and liver

for which the brain and liver tRNA profiles were essentially the same are shown in Fig. 3. Comparing the 11 plasmacytoma patterns with the pattern of the normal tissues, tumor-related variations in aa-tRNA patterns can be seen for several of these amino acids. For example, the tumors contain additional peaks of asparaginyl-tRNA and lysyl-tRNA not found in liver or brain.

Computer-Assisted Statistical Comparisons of the Profiles

Variations among profiles were widespread and patterns of variation were hard to correlate with the different tumor characteristics, so a computer program was devised to normalize all profiles to the maximum peak and line up and display all the profiles in the manner shown in Figs. 2 and 3. To augment the visual comparison and to render a certain degree of objectivity to these comparisons, the computer program was also used to compare all possible pairs of the 13 profiles generated for each amino acid and to determine a DI for each pairing using a modified form of the multidimensional

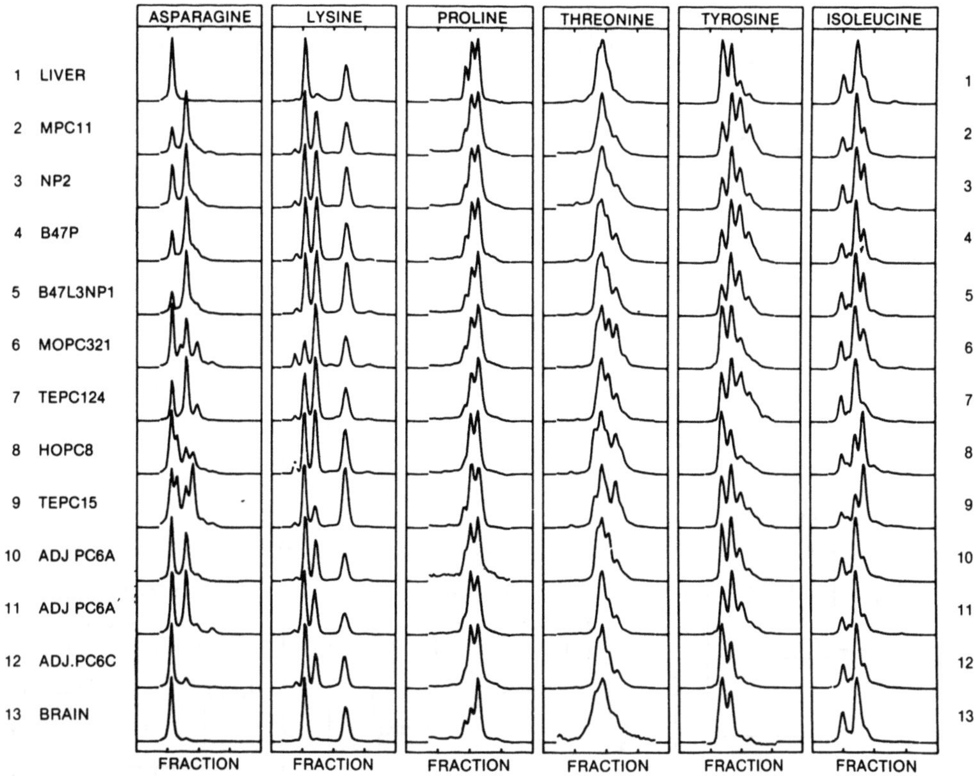

Fig. 3. Composites of RPC-5 chromatograms for six amino acids that have similar brain and liver aa-tRNA profiles

Euclidean distance metric (Mushinski et al. 1980). Cluster analysis of the DIs of all the pairs of profiles for a particular amino acid was performed. A graphical representation of the results of this process can be presented as a dendrogram wherein each tissue's aa-tRNA profile is represented by a vertical line starting at the top, where the DI is 0.0. The vertical lines are connected by horizontal lines when they reach the DI computed for that pair of profiles. This clustering process begins with the most similar profiles (those having the smallest DI) and sequentially adding single profiles or already-clustered groups of profiles. Figure 4 presents dendrograms for the 11 amino acids whose profiles are shown in Figs. 2 and 3. To save space each tissue is represented by a number from 1 to 13 as explained in Table 1. Clusters that form near the top include tissues with homogeneous profiles and clusters that form further down represent groups in which the profiles are more dissimilar.

Previous analysis of four of these dendrograms (Mushinski et al. 1980) concentrated upon the correlation of some early clustering of tumors with myeloma proteins having similar amino acid sequences. This finding is extended in the more complete study presented in Fig. 4 where tumors 8 and 9, which are clonally unrelated but make nearly identical myeloma proteins, cluster very high and very early in the serine, valine, threonine, isoleucine, and asparagine dendrograms. This analysis also reveals an early clustering of clonally related tumors, e.g., 2, 3, 4, and 5, in the serine, tyrosine, and asparagine dendrograms, and a different group of related tumors, 10, 11, and 12,

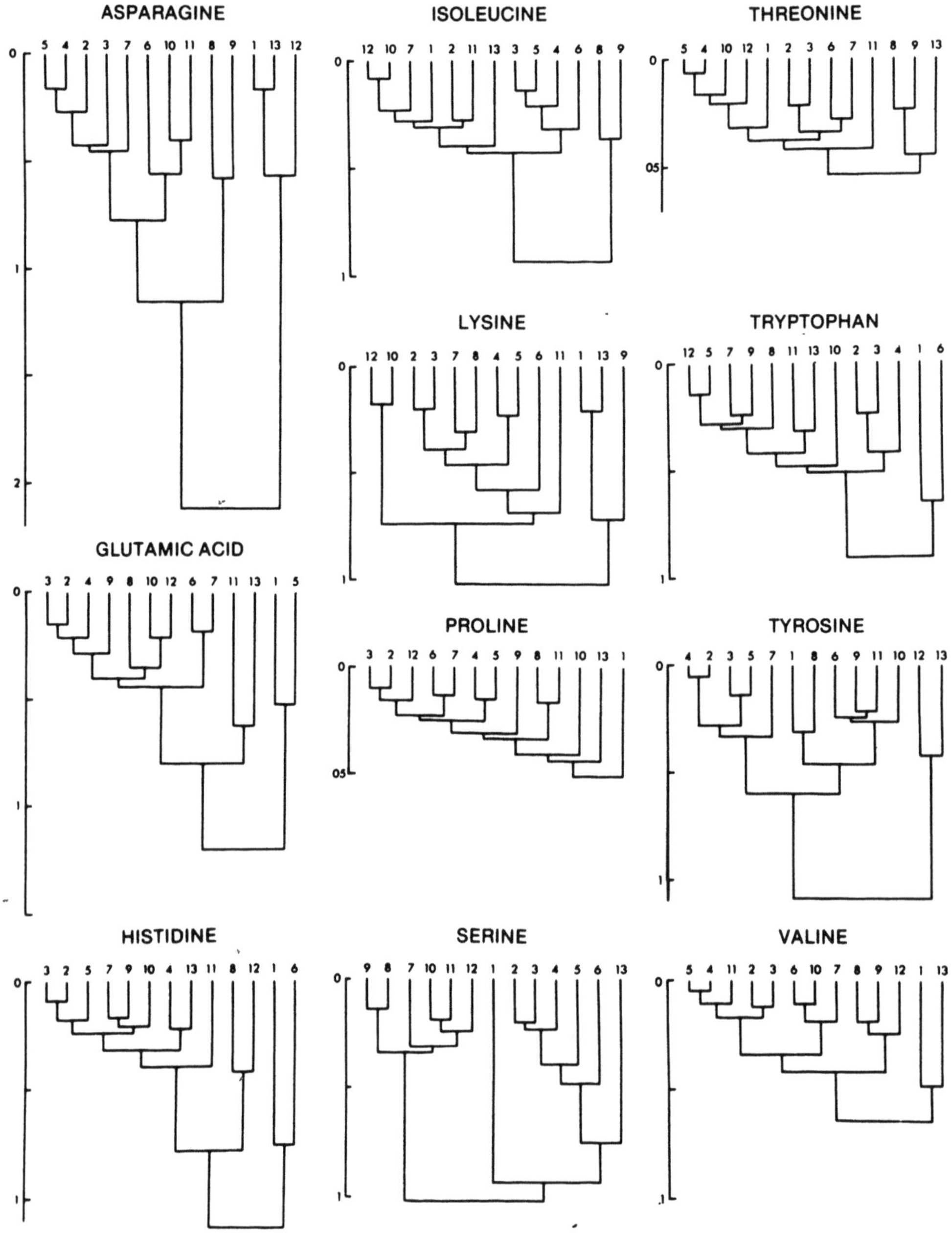

Fig. 4. Dendrograms relating the chromatographic profiles of the aa-tRNAs illustrated in Figs. 2 and 3 by increasing degree of dissimilarity. The number at the top of each vertical line indicates the source of the aa-tRNA profile represented by that line. The key to these numbers is found in Table 1. The vertical scale is in arbitrary units of dissimilarity

which cluster tightly in the serine dendrograms. This suggests that the amino acid sequence of the myeloma proteins may influence the aa-tRNA profiles. Since the codon usage in these proteins is not completely determined and the anticodon present in each isoaccepting tRNA is not known for all the tumor peaks, this kind of analysis cannot yet be made.

Plasmacytoma Patterns Statistically Compared and Contrasted with Those of Normal Tissues

Tumor related differences in the aa-tRNA patterns are particularly obvious in Fig. 3, which includes the amino acids where liver and brain have similar profiles. This composite figure shows that the plasmacytomas often contain aa-tRNA peaks not seen in either normal tissue. Cluster analysis of the more complex and variable aa-tRNA profiles shown in Fig. 2 shows that some of the aa-tRNA profiles included in this composite can be used to differentiate the normals from the plasmacytomas. For example, in the valine dendrogram (Fig. 4), liver and brain cluster very far down the scale of DI, but do not cluster with any of the tumors until even further down. This indicates that a greater dissimilarity exists between tumors and normal tissues than within either the malignant or the nonmalignant group. The asparagine and lysine dendrograms indicate a similar sort of relationship, but these two dendrograms show one plasmacytoma that for some reason clusters with the normals rather than the tumors.

A statistical analysis was brought to bear upon this dendrogram data using the Friedman rank test [see Mushinski et al. (1980) and references therein for more details of this analysis]. The DIs between each normal tissue and each of the tumor lines were ranked in ascending order. The order and magnitude of distance between ranked DIs were combined and averaged for all 11 dendrograms. This rank analysis showed a significantly more consistent pattern than would be expected if the ranks had been assigned at random ($P < 0.0001$ in each case). That is to say, tumor tissues can be distinguished from normal tissues using dendrograms derived from aa-tRNA chromatograms. Consistent with our visual impression, this statistical analysis also showed that the profiles of brain and liver were no more similar to each other than to any other single tumor profile than might be expected by chance ($P \approx 0,10$). This indicates that while plasmacytoma profiles can usually be distinguished from those of the two normal tissues, the brain and liver profiles frequently differ from one another as much as individual plasmacytomas do from each other.

Transfer RNA Variations in Rat Hepatomas

Very early in the plasmacytoma study we decided that it would be important to see if a similar degree of aa-tRNA variations would also be present in another tumor system. We chose to look at the tRNAs from a series of minimal-deviation hepatomas which had been induced by carcinogens in inbred Buffalo rats (Morris and Wagner 1968). We selected three hepatoma lines: 7777 (rapidly growing), 7800 (slowly growing), and 5123D (intermediate growth rate). As in the plasmacytoma study, quantitative and qualitative variations in RPC-2 patterns were seen, such as those shown in Fig. 5. Similar pattern differences in hepatomas were reported in studies by other groups

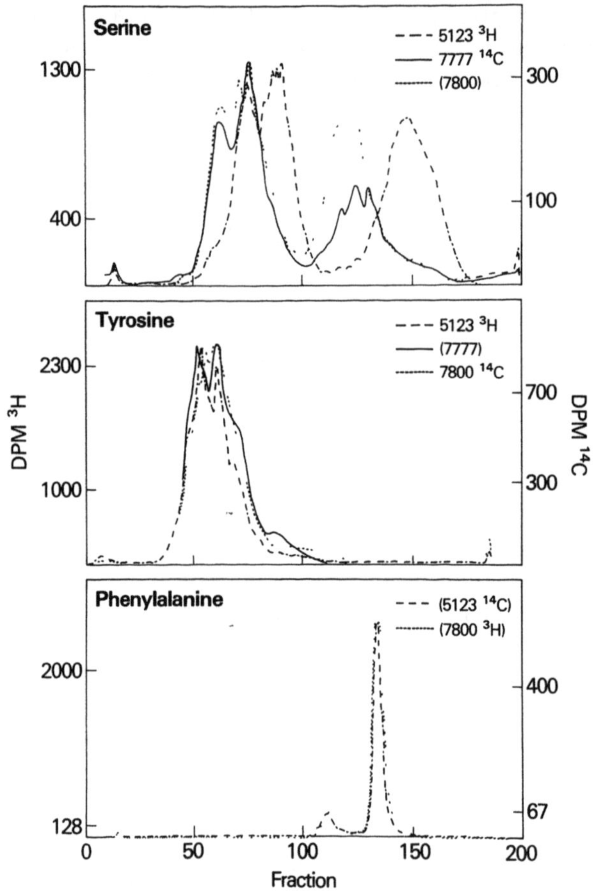

Fig. 5. RPC-2 elution profiles of seryl-tRNA, tyrosyl-tRNA, and phenylalanyl-tRNA from three minimal-deviation rat hepatomas. The composites of three profiles were generated by superimposing profiles from two cochromatographic runs which had been analyzed as indicated in the legend to Fig. 1

(Gonano et al. 1971; Volkers and Taylor 1971) and are reviewed in Borek and Kerr (1972).

The only finding from the hepatoma study that we pursued in depth was the presence of an early-eluting peak of phenylalanyl-tRNA that was not present in normal adult, fetal, or regenerating liver. It was found, however, in all three hepatomas, as well as in many other rat and mouse tumors (Mushinski and Marini 1979). Not all tumors contained this tumor-specific phenylalanyl-tRNA, but it made up virtually all the phenylalanyl-tRNA in some tumors such as mouse neuroblastoma. The results of extensive studies on the structure and modified nucleoside content of the tumor-specific phenylalanyl-tRNAs in several tumor lines are presented in the next chapter in this volume (Grunberger et al. pp. 133–145).

Structural Explanations for tRNA Pattern Variations

To date there is no evidence to suggest that new chromatographic peaks of aa-tRNA are caused by activation of new tRNA genes in tumors, although Randerath et al. (1982) demonstrate some structural changes in tRNAs from hepatoma mitochondria.

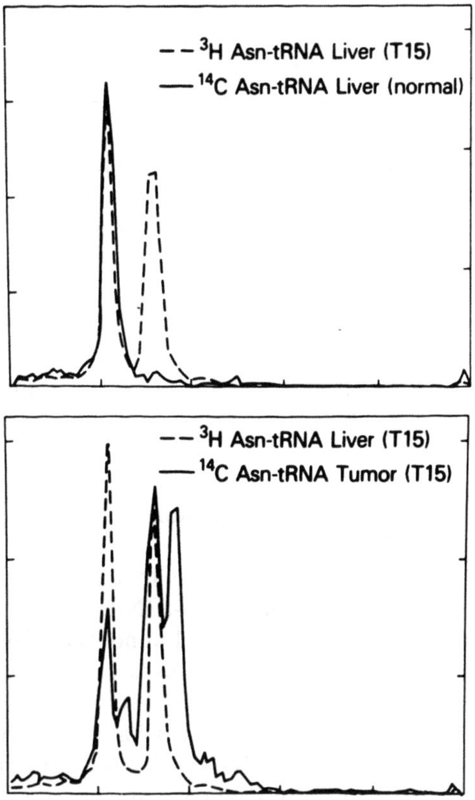

Fig. 6. RPC-5 elution profiles of asparaginyl-tRNA from plasmacytoma TEPC15 [tumor(T15)], normal liver, and liver from mice bearing TEPC15 subcutaneously [liver(T15)]

There are reports that a second phenylalanyl-tRNA gene may be activated in bovine lens development (Ortwerth et al. 1975), but all our studies on tumor-specific phenylalanyl-tRNAs implicate changes in the modified nucleosides as the factors responsible for their appearance. Particularly important in determining RPC-5 elution position for phenylalanine isoacceptors is the highly modified Y base, which appears to be defective in the early-eluting tumor-specific peaks seen in many tumors (Grunberger et al. 1975, and this vol. pp. 133–145; Mushinski and Marini 1979). Extra methylated bases were also reported in tumor phenylalanyl-tRNAs (Kuchino and Borek 1978).

The seryl-tRNA patterns of plasmacytomas and hepatomas seem to consist of varying combinations of the peaks of isoaccepting tRNAs seen in normal liver and the different ones seen in normal brain. At least one cause of differences between liver and brain tRNA has been revealed by RNA sequence determination of two seryl-tRNAs from each organ. The two brain tRNAs lack the 2′-*O*-methylation of guanosine at position 17 which is present in the corresponding tRNAs in liver (Rogg et al. 1977). This *O*-methylation difference resulted in the shift in elution position seen on RPC-5 chromatography. A similar lack of guanosine *O*-methylation was found in a rat hepatoma seryl-tRNA (Randerath et al. 1981). Thus structural differences consisting of hypo- or hypermethylation of tRNAs are likely to be the cause of many of the chromatographic variations presented here for seryl-tRNAs and perhaps other isoacceptors (Randerath et al., this vol. pp. 103–120).

Three of the four Q-base-containing tRNAs, asparaginyl-, histidinyl-, and tyrosinyl-tRNAs, are involved in the plasmacytoma tRNA variations reported here. Differences in Q-base structure due to incomplete post-transcriptional modification or subsequent partial breakdown of this highly modified nucleoside is a prime suspect as explanation for at least some of the pattern differences seen for these isoacceptors. We have reported that plasmacytomas growing subcutaneously cause the appearance of an abnormal peak of asparaginyl-tRNA in the grossly and histologically normal liver of tumor-bearing animals (Marini et al. 1979), as shown in Fig. 6. Although not yet clearly established by analysis of the modified nucleoside content of these tissues, this finding is reminiscent of the results of Katze (1978) and Marshall et al. (1978), which suggest that the Q-base content of tRNAs can be altered by a soluble factor. The Q base is charged, so its presence or absence would certainly affect the RPC-5 elution characteristics of an aa-tRNA. Another chapter in this volume (Katze et al., pp. 146–159) concentrates on Q-base alterations in tumors.

Conclusions and Discussion

Our working hypothesis is that most and possibly all variations in chromatographic profiles of isoaccepting aa-tRNAs result from variation in one or more of the modified nucleosides which abound in normal tRNAs. More sequence determinations need to be done to confirm this in all cases, but the Y base, Q base, and *O*-methylated bases do appear to be significantly involved.

It is still unclear, however, what causes the content of modified nucleosides to vary in some but not all tRNAs and some but not all tumors. No single alteration is found in every tumor, although once an altered chromatographic pattern is formed it seems to remain fixed in the tumor. Characteristic chromatographic profiles remain virtually unchanged in plasmacytoma tumor lines derived from a parent tumor by mutation, adaptation to tissue culture, etc., as demonstrated by cluster analysis and displayed in Figs. 3–5. The question of how this stability is maintained is worthy of further study.

The functional significance of the changes in isoaccepting tRNA patterns is a key question that has yet to be resolved. It has two aspects:

1. Are the modified nucleoside abnormalities that are seen as tRNA alterations primarily directed at tRNA, or are they merely coincidental by-products of enzymatic alterations found in tumors for unrelated reasons?
2. What effect do these variations have on the tRNA function as adaptors in protein synthesis?

In addressing the latter point our studies of Y-base-deficient tumor-specific phenylalanyl-tRNA (Hatfield et al. 1981) have detected no change in codon recognition or ability to function in protein synthesis. In fact the only difference so far documented is a small alteration in rate of aminoacylation and deacylation, but our studies are continuing.

Finally, the relationship of tRNA alterations in modified nucleosides to carcinogenesis or tumor biology remains tantalizing, fascinating, yet obscure. Computer analysis of all the profiles points out a significant difference in aa-tRNA profiles between plasmacytomas and normal tissues, but the effects of these alterations have not yet been delineated. We feel that very subtle changes in rate of protein synthesis, accuracy of codon translation, or other functions that tRNAs might have in cellular physiology and biochemistry could result in alterations in key regulatory molecules. These small alterations might well have profound effects on the control of cell growth and metabolism and may play an important role in some aspect of the cancer process.

Summary

RPC-5 chromatography has been used to analyze the aa-tRNA populations found in normal organs and in various tumors in experimental animals. The most extensively studied animal systems have been mineral-oil-induced mouse plasmacytomas and carcinogen-induced rat hepatomas. Certain aa-tRNA species appear to be tumor-specific, e.g., rat hepatoma phenylalanyl-$tRNA_1$ and plasmacytoma asparaginyl-$tRNAs_{2-4}$. In addition, one of the tumor-specific peaks of asparaginyl-tRNA can be found in normal livers of animals bearing plasmacytomas at a distant site. Many other significant quantitative and qualitative differences among histologically similar plasmacytomas and between normal tissues and plasmacytomas were observed in the chromatographic patterns of isoaccepting aa-tRNAs for 11 of 20 amino acids. Some of the qualitative differences in chromatographic patterns could be correlated with the tumorous nature of the tissue using computer analysis. The program utilized cluster analysis to compare the RPC-5 patterns of aa-tRNAs from 11 plasmacytomas and two normal tissues for each of the 20 amino acids. The variations in these chromatographic profiles are thought to be caused by varying degrees of incomplete synthesis of some of the normally modified nucleosides in tRNAs.

Abbreviations

aa-tRNA, aminoacyl-tRNA; *DI*, dissimilarity index; *IgA(κ)*, immunoglobulin A containing α-type heavy chains and κ-type light chains; *$IgG_{2b}(\kappa)$*, immunoglobulin G_{2b} containing γ_{2b}-type heavy chains and κ-type light chains; *dpm*, disintegrations per minute; *Vκ* and *Vα*, variable regions of the κ and α chains respectively.

References

Borek E, Kerr SJ (1972) Atypical transfer RNA's and their origins in neoplastic cells. Adv Cancer Res 15: 163–190

Gonano F, Chiarugi VP, Pirro G, Marini M (1971) Transfer ribonucleic acids in rat liver and Morris 5123 minimal deviation hepatoma. Biochemistry 10: 900–908

Grunberger D, Weinstein IB, Mushinski JF (1975) Deficiency of the Y base in a hepatoma phenylalanine tRNA. Nature 253: 66–67

Hatfield DL, Rice MJ, Mushinski JF (1981) Comparison of the codon recognition properties and of the utilization of normal and tumor specific Phe-tRNAs in protein synthesis. Cancer Lett 12: 251–258

Katze JR (1978) Q-factor: A serum component required for the appearance of nucleoside Q in tRNA in tissue culture. Biochem Biophys Res Commun 84: 527–535

Kelmers AD, Heatherly DE (1971) Columns for the rapid chromatographic separation of small amounts of tracer-labeled transfer ribonucleic acids. Anal Biochem 44: 486–495

Kuchino Y, Borek E (1978) Tumor specific phenylalanine transfer RNA contains two supernumerary methylated bases. Nature 271: 126–129

Marini MS, Mushinski JF (1979) Transfer ribonucleic acids from eleven immunoglobulin-secreting mouse plasmacytomas – constant and variable chromatographic profiles compared with the myeloma protein sequence. Biochim Biophys Acta 562: 252–270

Marini M, Muldoon WP, Mushinski JF (1979) Biochemical changes induced by tumors at distant sites: altered transfer RNA profiles in livers of mice bearing plasmacytomas. Cancer Lett 8: 177–181

Marshall MV, Adams DL, Griffin AC (1978) Regulation of an aspartyl-tRNA species in BHK cells in culture and in solid tumor form II. The effect of different sera on aspartyl-tRNA in culture. Cancer Lett 4: 147–153

Morris HP, Wagner BP (1968) Induction and transplantation of rat hepatomas with different growth rate including "minimal deviation" hepatomas. Methods Cancer Res 4: 124–139

Mushinski JF (1971) Stability of chromatographic patterns of aminoacyl transfer ribonucleic acid from individual mouse plasmacytomas and variability among different immunoglobulin A producing plasmacytomas and normal organs. Biochemistry 10: 3917–3924

Mushinski JF, Marini MS (1979) Tumor-associated phenylalanyl-transfer RNA found in a wide spectrum of rat and mouse tumors but absent in normal adult, fetal and regenerating tissues. Cancer Res 39: 1253–1258

Mushinski JF, Koziol JA, Marini M (1980) Cluster analysis of aminoacyl-tRNAs from mouse plasmacytomas correlates chromatographic profiles with myeloma protein similarity, clonal origin of tumor lines, and the neoplastic nature of the tissues. J Theor Biol 85: 507–521

Ortwerth BJ, Yonuschot GR, Heidlege JF, Chu-Der OMY, Juarez D, Hedgcoth C (1975) Induction of a new species of phenylalanine transfer RNA during lens cell differentiation. Exp Eye Res 20: 417–426

Potter M (1972) Immunoglobulin-producing tumors and myeloma proteins of mice. Physiol Rev 52: 631–719

Rogg H, Muller P, Keith G, Staehlin M (1977) Chemical basis for brain-specific serine transfer RNAs. Proc Natl Acad Sci USA 74: 4243–4247

Randerath E, Gopalakrishnan AS, Gupta RC, Agrawol HP, Randerath K (1981) Lack of a specific ribomethylation at guanosine 17 in Morris hepatoma 5123D $tRNA^{Ser}_{IGA}$. Cancer Res 41: 2863–2867

Volkers SAS, Taylor MW (1971) Chromatographic comparison of the transfer ribonucleic acids of rat livers and Morris hepatomas. Biochemistry 10: 488–497

Weiss JF, Kelmers AD (1967) A new chromatographic system for increased resolution of transfer ribonucleic acids. Biochemistry 6: 2507–2513

*Alterations in Post-Transcriptional Modification of the Y Base in Phenylalanine tRNA from Tumor Cells**

D. Grunberger[1], R. G. Pergolizzi[1], Y. Kuchino[2], J. F. Mushinski[3], and S. Nishimura[2]

[1] Cancer Center/Institute of Cancer Research, Columbia University College of Physicians & Surgeons, New York, NY 10032, USA; [2] Biology Division, National Cancer Center Research Institute, Chuo-ku, Tokyo, Japan; [3] Laboratory of Cell Biology, National Cancer Institute, Bethesda, MD 20205, USA

Introduction

In the search for a possible role of tRNA in regulatory processes in higher organisms, a number of studies have compared chromatographic profiles of tRNA from different tissues, organs, tumors, and cell cultures (Nishimura 1978). These studies have revealed that tumor cells frequently contain tRNA species which differ in their chromatographic mobility from the corresponding tRNAs present in normal adult tissues. However, in only a few cases have structural studies on these tRNAs been carried out to clarify whether the isoaccepting species are due to a new transcript of a gene or to a different degree of modification (Shindo-Okada et al. 1981; Raba et al. 1979; Roe et al. 1979; Randerath et al. 1981). The primary transcripts of tRNA genes are known to undergo several processing steps prior to their emergence as mature functional tRNA molecules (Altman 1978). In addition to cleavage of the precursor molecules, the formation of modified nucleosides occurs post-transcriptionally (Nishimura 1978).

One of the most consistent differences reported for tumor tRNAs involves phenylalanine tRNA ($tRNA^{Phe}$). Several laboratories have demonstrated by reverse-phase column chromatography (RPC-5) that many types of tumors contain, in addition to the single species of $tRNA^{Phe}$ found in normal tissues, an early-eluting peak not normally present (Gonano et al. 1971; Volkers and Taylor 1971; Mushinski and Marini 1979). It is known that $tRNA^{Phe}$ of eukaryotic cells contains a highly fluorescent and hydrophobic base, called wye (Y), which is located next to the 3′ end of the anticodon (RajBhandary and Chang 1968). The Y compound represents the most highly modified nucleic acid base characterized so far, consisting of a tricyclic imidazo derivative of guanine to which is usually attached a 4-carbon side chain (Blobstein et al. 1973; Kasai et al. 1979) (Fig. 1). Due to the very hydrophobic character of the Y base, $tRNA^{Phe}$ elutes as the latest peak on the RPC-5 column. This base can be selectively excised from $tRNA^{Phe}$ by a mild acid treatment without breaking the polynucleotide chain (Thiebe and Zachau 1968). In this case, the modified tRNA ($tRNA_{-Y}$) appears on the RPC-5 as an early-eluting peak.

* This study was supported partly by Grants CA21111 and CA31696 from the National Cancer Institute, USA, and by the US-Japan Cooperative Cancer Research Program

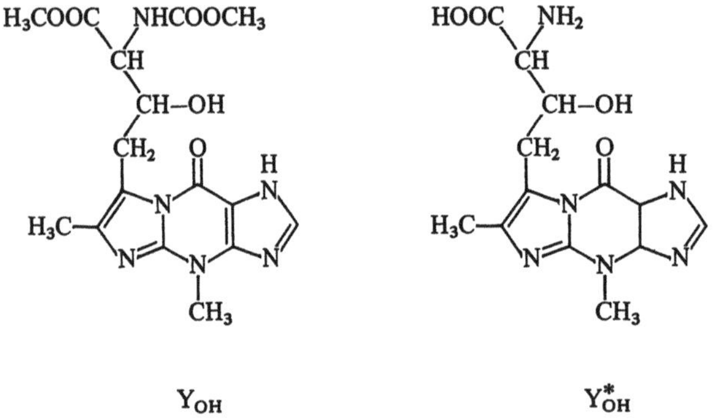

Fig. 1 Structure of Y_{OH} base and Y^{*}_{OH} base

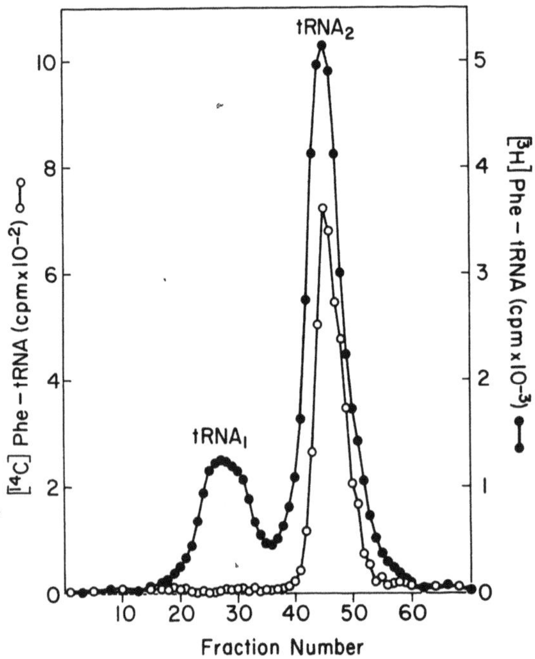

Fig. 2. Elution profiles of liver and hepatoma $tRNA^{Phe}$ from RPC-5 columns. [^{3}H]Phe-tRNA from Morris hepatoma 7777 (●) cochromatographed with [^{14}C]Phe-tRNA from normal rat liver (○). Grunberger et al. (1975)

Phenylalanine tRNA in Hepatoma and Neuroblastoma Tissues

We have shown (Grunberger et al. 1975) that tRNA isolated from rat liver and Morris hepatoma 7777, aminoacylated with [^{14}C]- and [^{3}H]phenylalanine respectively and cochromatographed on the RPC-5, have different chromatographic profiles (Fig. 2). The rat liver contained only one $tRNA^{Phe}$ species and the hepatoma two. The major hepatoma peak eluted at the same position as rat liver $tRNA^{Phe}$. The minor hepatoma peak ($tRNA_1^{Phe}$) eluted earlier at the position where the $tRNA^{Phe}_{-Y}$ appears. In similar studies, Salomon et al. (1976) have shown by affinity chromatography on anti-Y antibody immobilized to Sepharose that about 85% of the $tRNA^{Phe}$ from mouse neuroblasts lacks the Y base.

We have also compared the chromatographic profiles of $tRNA^{Phe}$ isolated from mouse liver and N18/6TG neuroblastoma tissue (Mushinski and Marini 1979). Figure 3

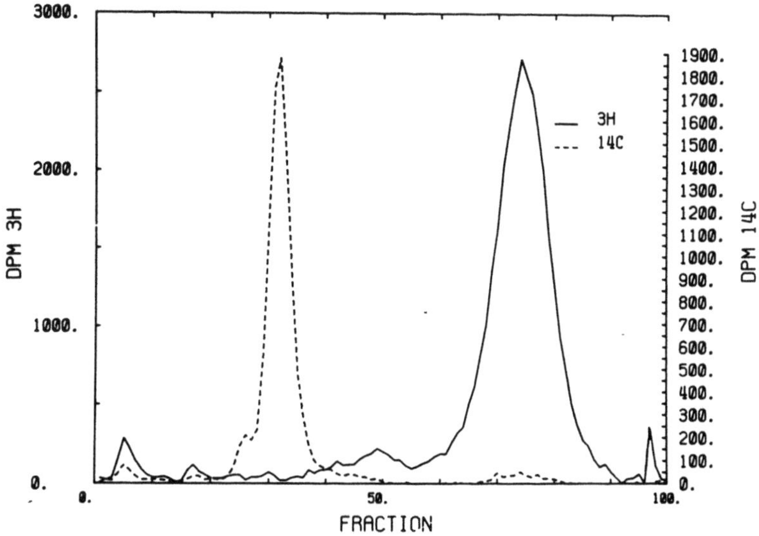

Fig. 3. RPC-5 profiles of [^{3}H]Phe-tRNA (———) from normal Balb/c mouse liver cochromatographed with [^{14}C]Phe-tRNA (— — —) from A/J mouse neuroblastoma. Mushinski and Marini (1979)

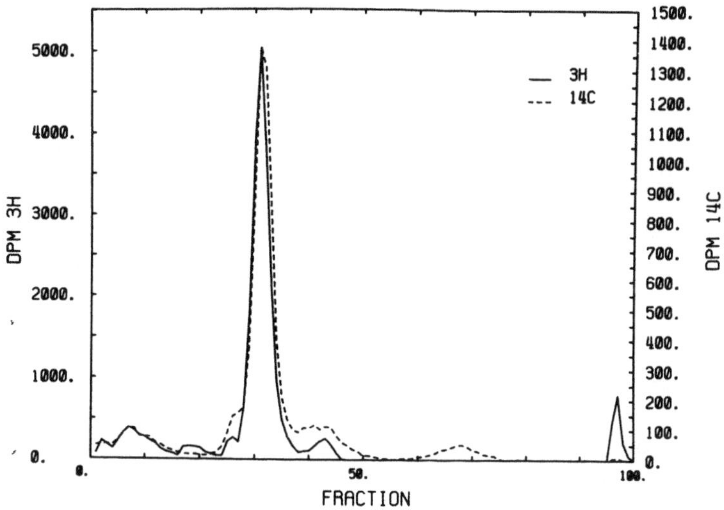

Fig. 4. RPC-5 chromatograms of [^{3}H]Phe-tRNA (———) from normal Balb/c liver which had been incubated with 0,05 *M* sodium citrate pH 2.9 at 37° for 18 h cochromatographed with [^{14}C]Phe-tRNA (- - - -) from A/J neuroblastoma. Mushinski and Marini (1979)

illustrates the RPC-5 of [^{3}H]Phe-tRNA from normal Balb/c mouse liver cochromatographed with [^{14}C]Phe-tRNA from mouse neuroblastoma. It is evident that about 90% of the tRNA^{Phe} from neuroblastoma elutes earlier than the normal tRNA^{Phe}. However, if both tRNAs have been incubated at ph 2.9, which is the condition for Y-base excision, and then cochromatographed there would be no difference in the elution profiles of tRNA^{Phe} from normal and neuroblastoma tRNA^{Phe} (Fig. 4). These experiments clearly indicated that the tumor-specific tRNA^{Phe} lacks the fully modified Y base.

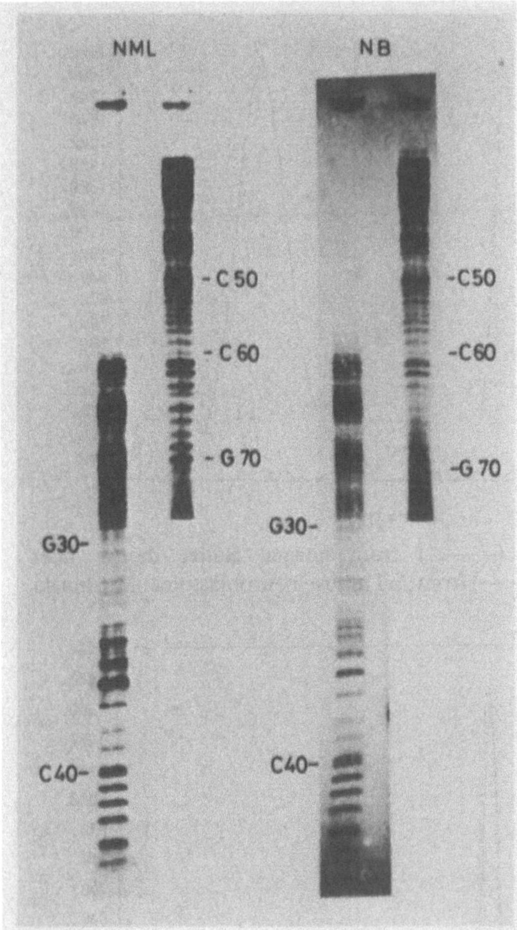

Fig. 5. Autoradiograms of 5′-[^{32}P]oligonucleotides derived from normal mouse liver *(NML)* and neuroblastoma *(NB)* $tRNA_1^{Phe}$ fractionated on 20% polyacrylamide, 7 *M* urea gel

Nucleotide Sequence of Neuroblastoma $tRNA^{Phe}$

From the results with Morris hepatoma and neuroblastoma, it was not possible to decide whether the tumor-specific $tRNA^{Phe}$ species represents the expression of a separate tRNA gene or only an undermodified form of normal $tRNA^{Phe}$ resulting from a failure to complete the synthesis of the Y base from its precursor guanosine molecule (Li et al. 1973). Therefore, we have determined the nucleotide sequence of $tRNA^{Phe}$ from mouse liver and N18/6TG neuroblastoma tissue (Kuchino et al. 1982). Isolation of $tRNA^{Phe}$ was achieved by successive application of RPC-5, BD cellulose, DEAE-Sephadex A-50, and repeated RPC-5 column chromatography. Final purification of $tRNA^{Phe}$ was performed by two-dimensional polyacrylamide gel electrophoresis, as previously described (Kuchino et al. 1979b, 1980). For sequencing of tRNA, the postlabeling procedures were essentially the same as previously reported (Kuchino et al. 1979a, 1980). Figure 5 shows that the pattern of the bands of 5′-[^{32}P]oligonucleotides of neuroblastoma $tRNA^{Phe}$ produced by partial alkaline hydrolysis was similar to that of mouse liver $tRNA^{Phe}$. Analysis of 5′-terminal nucleotides of the oligonucleotides of neuroblastoma $tRNA^{Phe}$ showed that the

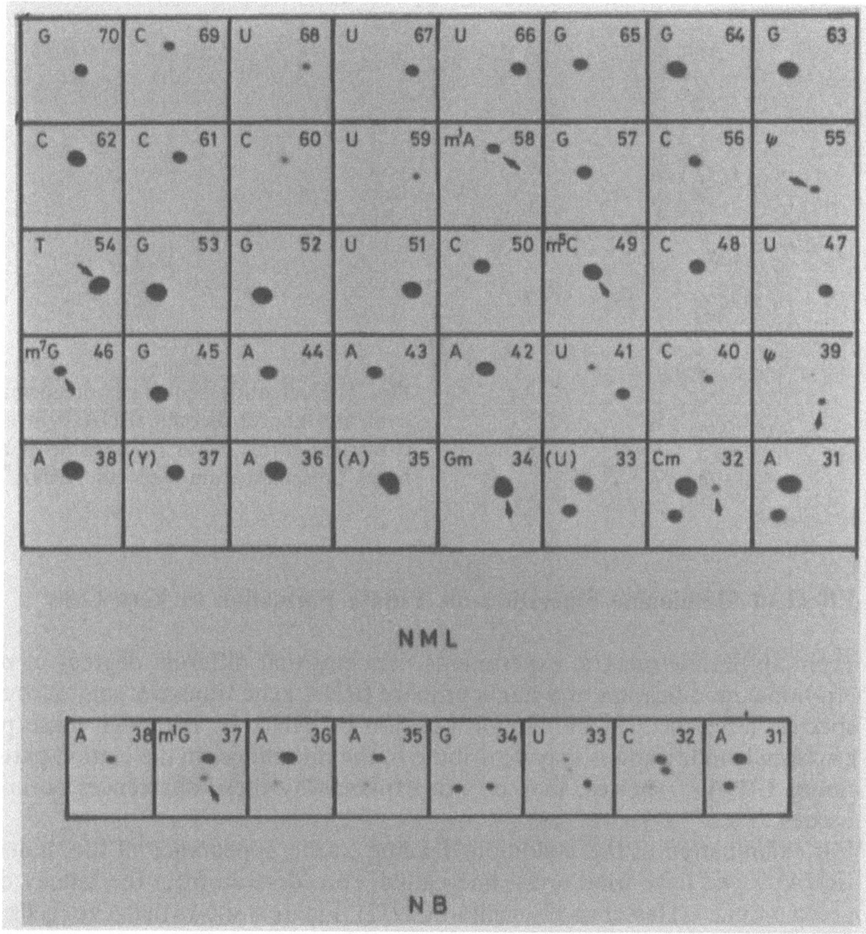

Fig. 6. Autoradiograms of 3′-end labeled tRNA^{Phe} sequenced by chemical degradation. The electrophoresis was carried out on 20% polyacrylamide 7 *M* urea gel for 9 h at 700 V

primary nucleotide sequence from residues 31–70 is the same as that of normal tRNA^{Phe} (Fig. 6). With respect to modification in the anticodon loop, neuroblastoma tRNA^{Phe} contained mostly C_{32}, G_{34}, and m^1G_{37}. Onyl very small amounts of Cm_{32} and Gm_{34} were detected (Fig. 6). It can therefore be concluded that neuroblastoma tRNA^{Phe} consists mostly of m^1G-containing tRNA^{Phe} (75%) with small amounts of undermodified Y^*_{OH}-containing tRNA^{Phe} (25%) (Fig. 1). The presence of the undermodified Y^*_{OH} was confirmed by fluorescent spectra specific for Y^*_{OH} and by high-pressure liquid chromatography. Similar results were obtained with tRNA^{Phe} from Ehrlich ascites cells, the only difference being that these cells contained mostly Y^*_{OH}-containing tRNA^{Phe} (Kuchino et al. 1982).

These results clearly indicate that alteration of modification in tumor-specific tRNA^{Phe} takes place in specific modified nucleosides located in the anticodon loop, but not in all modified nucleosides. The structures of tRNA^{Phe} from mouse liver and neuroblastoma are summarized in a cloverleaf diagram in Fig. 7. The only difference occurs in the anticodon loop: if m^1G is in the position next to the anticodon, there is C_{32} and C_{34} instead of Cm_{32} and Gm_{34}.

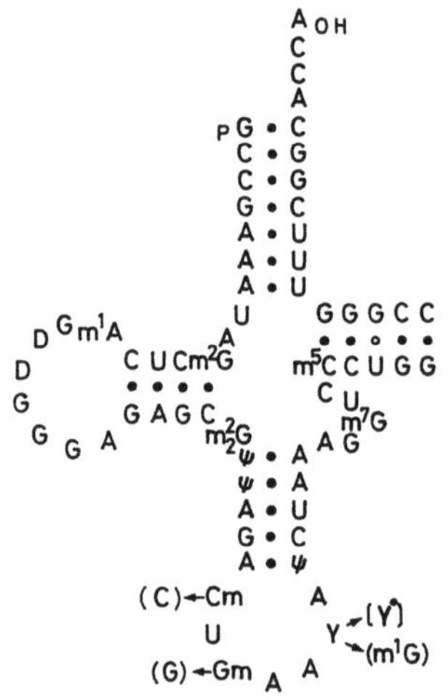

Fig. 7. Nucleotide sequences of normal mouse liver and neuroblastoma $tRNA^{Phe}$ arranged in cloverleaf form. *Bases in parentheses* are altered bases present in tumor-specific $tRNA^{Phe}$

Effect of Methionine Starvation on Y-Base Formation in Vero Cells

From all these structural experiments, it seems that different degrees of post-transcriptional modification of a single primary tRNA gene transcript may account for the species' differences in the elution position of $tRNA^{Phe}$. Although these post-transcriptional modifications may contribute to the differences in the elution pattern of the tumor $tRNA^{Phe}$ species, they do not explain why these differences occur in tumor tissues.

For examination of the conditions leading to the appearance of the undermodified $tRNA_1^{Phe}$, we have used a cell line called Vero derived from the kidney of African green monkey (Hassel and Engelhardt 1977). Figure 8 shows that Vero cells harvested after 2 days growth in Dulbecco's modified Eagle's (DME) medium containing 10% calf serum displayed only one normal $tRNA^{Phe}$ species, $tRNA_2^{Phe}$ (Pergolizzi et al. 1978). However, by the time these cells had been incubated for several days without any change of medium growth had slowed down, and a new early-eluting $tRNA^{Phe}$ species became a prominent feature of the $tRNA^{Phe}$ profile. The shift in position of the $tRNA^{Phe}$ species indicate that the new $tRNA^{Phe}$ lacks the fully modified Y base. Disappearance of the early-eluting $tRNA_1^{Phe}$ is complete by 20 h after replacing the exhausted medium with fresh medium.

To determine which component of the medium was required for elimination of the abnormal $tRNA_1^{Phe}$, amino acid analysis of the exhausted medium was performed. It showed that methionine was completely depleted from the medium. If methionine was added back to the exhausted medium or medium containing methionine was used, $tRNA_1^{Phe}$ disappeared (Fig. 9). These results suggested that $tRNA_1^{Phe}$ could be an undermodified precursor of $tRNA_2^{Phe}$. In order to confirm this, an experiment was performed in which medium containing [methyl-^{3}H]methionine was added to starved cells in the presence of 0.01 mg/ml actinomycin D. Figure 10 shows that ^{3}H counts appear in $tRNA_2^{Phe}$ and that $tRNA_1^{Phe}$ was completely eliminated. Since under these conditions new RNA synthesis was blocked, the radioactivity in $tRNA_2^{Phe}$ could only have come from modification of $tRNA_1^{Phe}$. Thin-layer chromatography of the acid-excised Y base (Blobstein et al. 1973) revealed that ^{3}H counts comigrated with

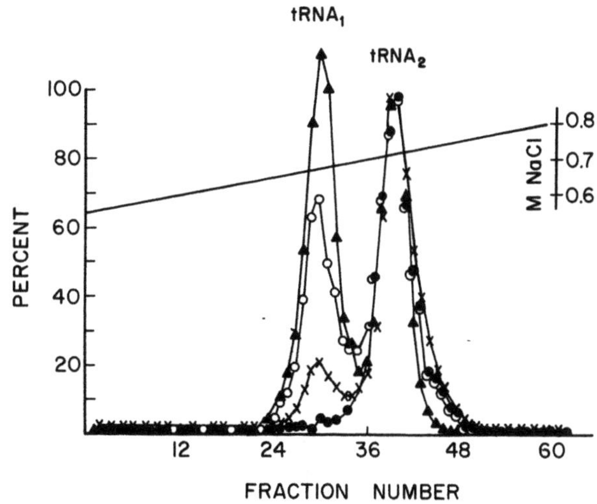

Fig. 8. Patterns of elution of $tRNA^{Phe}$ from RPC-5 columns. tRNA was isolated from Vero cells after 2 days (●–●), 7 days (X–X), 10 days (O–O), or 13 days (▲–▲) in unchanged DME medium. The tRNA was then charged with [^{3}H]- or [^{14}C]Phe. Percent, (counts per min $tRNA_1$/counts per min $tRNA_2$) × 100. This figure is a composite of two double-label experiments. In order to show the relative increase in $tRNA_1^{Phe}$, profiles are plotted with $tRNA_2^{Phe}$ always equal to 100%. Pergolizzi et al. (1978)

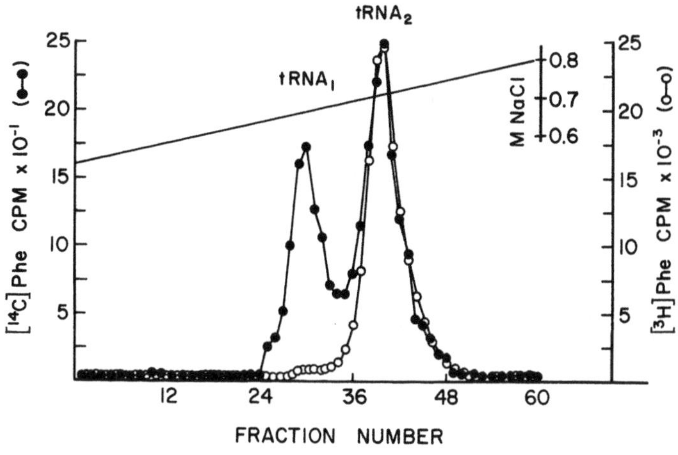

Fig. 9. Effect of methionine in growth medium on RPC-5 profile of $tRNA^{Phe}$ from 10-day-starved cells. Starved cells were harvested 20 h after replacement of medium with complete DME (O–O) or DME medium without methionine (●–●). The tRNAs were charged with [^{3}H]- and [^{14}C]Phe respectively, and analyzed by RPC-5. Pergolizzi et al. (1978)

Y base, suggesting that $tRNA_1^{Phe}$ is an undermodified precursor of $tRNA_2^{Phe}$ and that methionine is required for Y base synthesis. However, from the structure of the Y base it is evident that some other component(s) is also required for the biosynthesis of the Y base from the precursor guanine molecule.

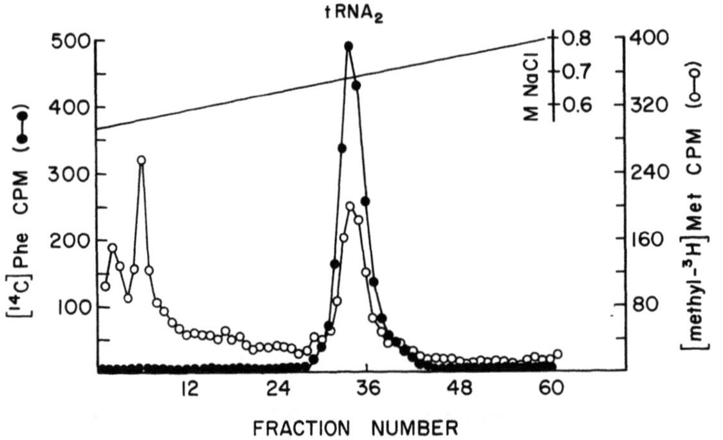

Fig. 10. RPC-5 profile of tRNA from starved cells incubated with [methyl-^{3}H]Met in the presence of actinomycin D. Growth medium was removed from starved cells and replaced by DME without methionine containing 0.01 mg/ml actinomycin D. One hour later, 0.5 mCi/150 mm culture dish of [methyl-^{3}H]Met was added. Cells were incubated for 20 h, and tRNA was harvested and aminoacylated with [^{14}C]Phe. (●–●), [^{14}C]Phe profile; (○–○), [methyl-^{3}H]Met profile. Pergolizzi et al. (1978)

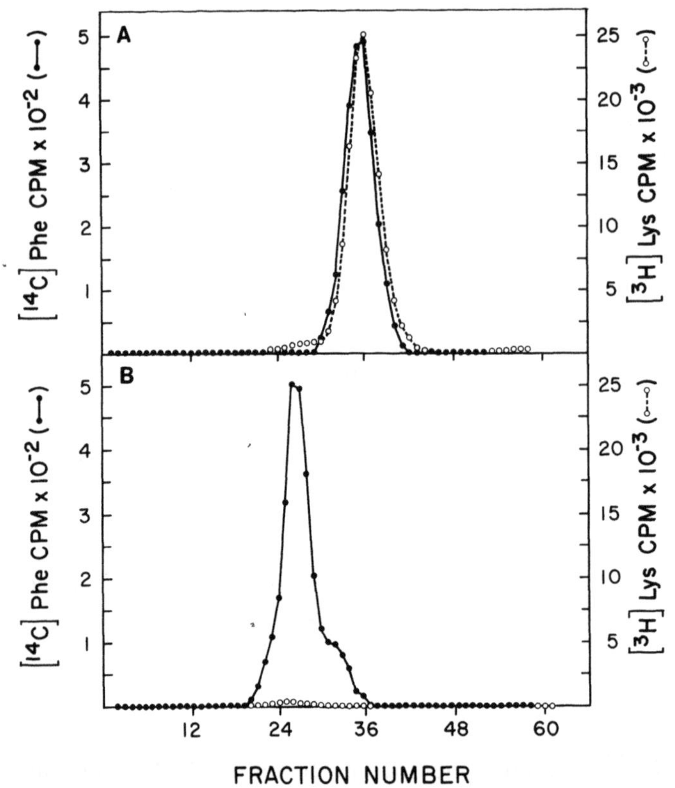

Fig. 11A, B. Elution profiles of Vero tRNAs from RPC-5 columns. **A** [^{14}C]Phe-tRNA from Vero cells incubated with [^{3}H]lysine. **B** [^{14}C]Phe-tRNA from the same cells as **A** after acid excision of the Y-base. (○), [^{3}H]lysine; (●), [^{14}C]phenylalanine. Pergolizzi et al. (1979)

Involvement of Lysine in Biosynthesis of Y Base

To determine whether any of the essential amino acids were direct precursors of Y base, we have adopted an approach similar to that used in the case of methionine. By growing Vero cells in medium in which one of the 14 essential amino acids was replaced by its radioactive counterpart and measuring the extent of labeling of the Y base we could establish that lysine is involved in the biosynthesis of Y base. To do this, Vero cells were grown in medium that was limiting for lysine, and after 8 days incubation were given medium which contained [^{3}H]lysine (Pergolizzi et al. 1979). The isolated tRNA was then separated by RPC-5 to determine whether radioactivity from [^{3}H]lysine comigrated with $tRNA^{Phe}$ aminoacylated with [^{14}C]phenylalanine. Figure 11A shows that under these conditions radioactivity from lysine cochromatographed solely with $tRNA^{Phe}$. Figure 11B shows an RPC-5 profile obtained after excision of the Y base from the tRNA shown in Fig. 11A. The $tRNA^{Phe}$ eluted earlier than in Fig. 11A indicating that the Y base had been excised. Lysine-derived radioactivity no longer cochromatographed with $tRNA^{Phe}$. However, radioactivity from the excised base extracted into ethyl acetate and chromatographed on silical gel comigrated with the standard Y base.

From these results, it is evident that lysine is involved in the biosynthesis of Y base in $tRNA^{Phe}$ of mammalian cells. The structure of lysine is compatible with a proposed biosynthetic pathway which will be discussed later.

Restoration of Y-Base Biosynthesis in Ehrlich Ascites Cells by Exogenous Nutrients

Since in Vero cells deprivation of either methionine or lysine resulted in defects in $tRNA^{Phe}$ modification similar to those in the various tumor cells, the possibility was raised that the appearance of altered $tRNA^{Phe}$ species within a variety of neoplasms is also the result of starvation of tumor cells for some nutritional factors. Since $tRNA^{Phe}$ from Ehrlich ascites cells also contains an undermodified Y base in the anticodon loop (Kuchino and Borek 1978; Kuchino et al. 1982), we have tested the possibility that a similar principle is responsible for the de novo appearance of tumor-specific tRNAs in these cells (Pergolizzi and Grunberger 1980).

Figure 12 shows the cochromatography of [^{3}H]Phe-tRNA from Ehrlich ascites cells with [^{14}C]Phe-tRNA from mouse liver (from the same animals). The $tRNA^{Phe}$ species from these cells were resolved into a broad zone of subspecies, indicating that these are multiple forms of $tRNA_1^{Phe}$ containing various stages of modified Y-base.

To determine whether the tRNA's Phe profile could be altered by the addition of nutrients in vivo, as has been shown in monkey kidney cells in vitro, a group of tumor-bearing mice were given intraperitoneal injections of 1 ml of a solution of essential amino acids and vitamins containing 50 times the concentration in DME-medium. Another group received normal saline. Twenty-four hours later the mice were killed, the tumor cells harvested from both groups, and tRNA prepared. As shown in Fig. 13, the majority of [^{3}H]Phe-tRNA from cells of the group which received additional nutrients now elutes later than [^{14}C]Phe-tRNA from the control group. The results suggest that under these conditions the modification of Y base went to completion. Thus $tRNA^{Phe}$ from tumor cells can be altered by the addition of exogenous factors. This finding supports the contention that some tumor-specific

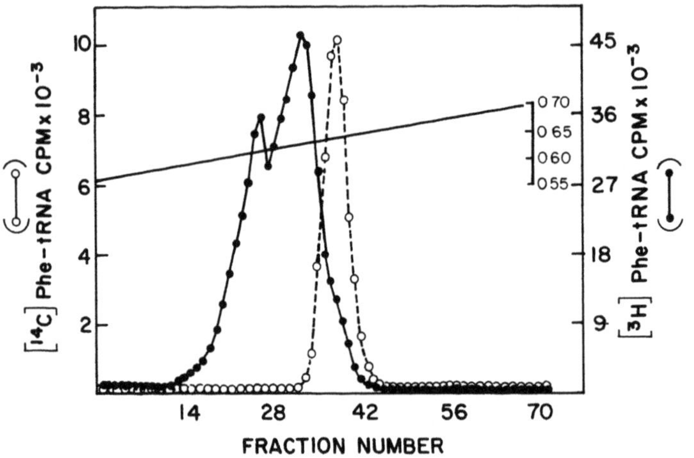

Fig. 12. Elution profiles of Ehrlich ascites cells and mouse liver Phe-tRNAs from RPC-5. [3H]Phe-tRNA (0.5 A_{260}) from Ehrlich ascites cells (●) was cochromatographed with 1.2 A_{260} units of [14C]Phe-tRNA from mouse liver (○). Pergolizzi and Grunberger (1980)

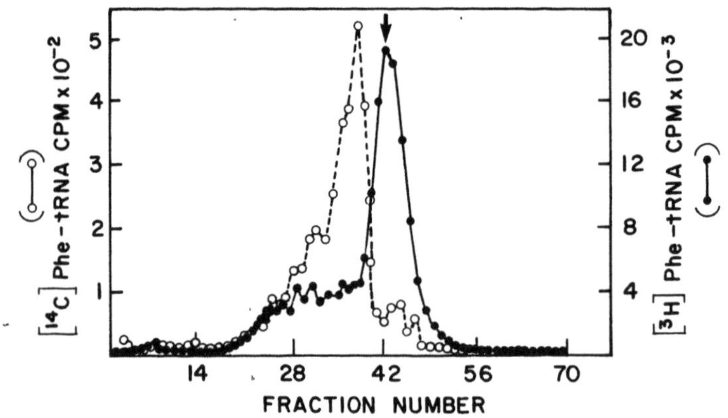

Fig. 13. Cochromatography on RPC-5 of Phe-tRNA from Ehrlich ascites cells of mice injected with saline or a mixture of amino acids and vitamins. The elution position of normal mouse liver Phe-tRNA is marked by an *arrow*. (○), [14C]Phe-tRNA from saline-injected mice; (●), [3H]Phe-tRNA from mice injected with amino acids and vitamins. Pergolizzi and Grunberger (1980)

tRNAs seen in a variety of neoplasms arise from derangements in cellular metabolism and nutrient supply. Their disappearance upon nutritional supplementation and the concomitant appearance of mature tRNA species further suggest a precursor-product relationship similar to that observed in monkey kidney cells, as opposed to the expression of hitherto silent genes. It should be noted, however, that the situation in Ehrlich ascites cells is considerably more complex than that in culture, since the injection of methionine alone had no effect on the $tRNA^{Phe}$ profile.

In accord with our results are the observations that diet also has an effect on the synthesis of the hypermodified nucleoside queuosine (Q) in the family of tRNAs of germ-free mice (Farkas 1980).

Conclusion

Taken together, our results with starved Vero cells and with various tumors suggest that the early-eluting $tRNA_1^{Phe}$ is not the product of a normally repressed gene. Instead, these new species are aberrantly modified transcripts of the same gene product, which would otherwise become normal $tRNA^{Phe}$. The alterations occur mainly in the anticodon loop of the molecule. The Y base present in normal mouse liver is replaced in neuroblastoma $tRNA^{Phe}$ mostly by m^1G, less frequently by undermodified Y base. The m^1G-containing $tRNA^{Phe}$ has C_{32} and G_{34} in the positions of Cm_{32} and Gm_{34} respectively. Otherwise, the primary nucleotide sequences are the same in normal as in tumor-specific $tRNA^{Phe}$. Other new isoaccepting tRNA species found in tumor cells, such as $tRNA^{Ser}$ (Randerath et al. 1981), $tRNA^{Asp}$ (Kuchino et al., to be published), $tRNA^{Val}$ (Shindo-Okada et al. 1981), $tRNA^{Lys}$ (Raba et al. 1979), and $tRNA^{Asn}$ (Roe et al. 1979), have changes only in post-transcriptional modification. No new tRNA species as a transcriptional product of a new gene has been found thus far in tumor cells.

The effect on tRNA function of the presence of m^1G in the position next to anticodon is not yet understood. No significant difference was detected in the codon recognition of neuroblastoma $tRNA^{Phe}$ when it was explored by ribosomal binding of tRNA in the presence of different triplet codons (Hatfield et al. 1981). An interesting observation is that $tRNA^{Phe}$ of *Drosophila* also contains m^1G instead of the Y base (Altweg and Kubli 1979). Further studies are needed to clarify whether these changes have a specific role in these cells.

Structural characterization of tumor-specific $tRNA^{Phe}$ and the methionine and lysine starvation experiments with Vero cells have made it possible to propose a hypothetical pathway for Y-base biosynthesis. According to this scheme the first step is the formation of m^3G, which is suggested as the signal for the synthesis of the Y base. Since lysine residues are incorporated into the Y base and it is established that in liver and kidney α-aminoadipic semialdehyde is a metabolite of lysine (Rothstein and Greenburg 1960), the 2-amino group of guanosine could readily react with the aldehyde to form a Schiff base (Goldschmidt et al. 1968). Closing the third ring and modification of the appropriate positions could complete the biosynthetic pathway of the Y base.

On the other hand, in tumor cells or in methionine-starved cells, at low methionine or *S*-adenosylmethionine concentration, it is proposed that tRNA methylase preferentially methylates the N^1 instead of the N^3 position of G. In such a case, the formation of m^3G is blocked and the Y base synthesis cannot proceed. This mechanism would explain the presence of m^1G instead of Y base in some tumor-specific $tRNA^{Phe}$. Results obtained in vivo with Ehrlich ascites cells, in which the $tRNA^{Phe}$ species lacking the Y-base disappeared after intraperitoneal injection into tumor-bearing mice of a mixture of amino acids and vitamins, strongly support the contention that nutritional factors play the critical role in the appearance of undermodified bases, not only in $tRNA^{Phe}$ but also in other tRNA species of some tumor cells.

Summary

Various tumor cells contain chromatographically distinct isoacceptor tRNA species. To decide whether the tumor-specific species represent an expression of a separate tRNA gene or only an undermodified form of normal $tRNA^{Phe}$, nucleotide sequences of $tRNA^{Phe}$ isolated from neuroblastoma and normal mouse liver were determined by postlabeling techniques. The results showed identical sequences except for the changes of post-transcriptional modifications in the anticodon loop. Normal mouse liver $tRNA^{Phe}$ contained Cm_{32}, Gm_{34}, and the hypermodified Y_{OH} next to the 3′ end of the anticodon. On the contrary, $tRNA^{Phe}$ from neuroblastoma contained C_{32}, G_{34}, and, instead of Y_{OH} base m^1G. A small proportion of $tRNA^{Phe}$ species contained an undermodified Y_{OH} base. For the examination of the conditions leading to the undermodified $tRNA^{Phe}$, Vero cells derived from the kidney of African green monkey in culture were used. In these cells, deprivation of methionine or lysine resulted in changes in $tRNA^{Phe}$ modification similar to those in tumor cells. Ehrlich ascites tumor cells were examined to determine whether the presence of altered $tRNA^{Phe}$ species in various tumors is also the result of starvation of some nutritional factors. Results obtained with these cells showed that $tRNA^{Phe}$ species lacking the Y base disappeared in tumor-bearing mice after intraperitoneal injection with a mixture of amino acids and vitamins. Thus it is concluded that tumor-specific $tRNA^{Phe}$ species are the products of aberrant post-transcriptional modification, not the transcripts of different, normally repressed genes.

References

Altman S (1978) Biosynthesis of tRNA. In: Altman S (ed) Transfer RNA. MIT Press, Cambridge, MA, pp 48–77

Altwegg M, Kubli E (1979) The nucleotide sequence of phenylalanine $tRNA_2$ of *Drosophila melanogaster:* four isoacceptors with one basic sequence. Nucleic Acids Res. 7: 93–105

Blobstein SH, Grunberger D, Weinstein IB, Nakanishi K (1973) Isolation and structure determination of the fluorescent base from bovine liver phenylalanine transfer RNA. Biochemistry 12: 188–193

Farkas WR (1980) Effect of diet on the queuosine family of tRNAs of germ-free mice. J Biol Chem 255: 6832–6835

Goldschmidt BM, Blazej TP, Van Duuren BL (1968) The reaction of guanosine and deoxyguanosine with glycidaldehyde. Tetrahedron Lett 13: 1583–1586

Gonano F, Chiarugi VP, Pirro G, Marini M (1971) Transfer ribonucleic acid in rat liver and Morris 5123 minimal deviation hepatoma. Biochemistry 10: 900–908

Grunberger D, Weinstein IB, Mushinski JF (1975) Deficiency of the Y base in a hepatoma tRNA. Nature 253: 66–67

Hassell J, Engelhardt DL (1977) Factors regulating the multiplication of animal cells in culture. Exp Cell Res 107: 159–167

Hatfield DL, Rice MJ, Mushinski J (1981) Comparison of the codon recognition properties and of the utilization of normal and tumor specific Phe-tRNAs in protein synthesis. Cancer Lett 12: 251–258

Kasai H, Yamaizumi Z, Kuchino Y, Nishimura S (1979) Isolation of hydroxy-Y base from rat liver $tRNA^{Phe}$. Nucleic Acids Res 6: 993–999

Kuchino Y, Borek E (1978) Tumor-specific phenylalanine tRNA contains two supernumerary methylated bases. NAture 271: 126–129

Kuchino Y, Kasai H, Yamaizumi Z, Nishimura S, Borek E (1979a) Under-modified Y base in a $tRNA^{Phe}$ isoacceptor observed in tumor cells. Biochim Biophys Acta 565: 215–218

Kuchino Y, Kato M, Sugisaki H, Nishimura S (1979b) Nucleotide sequence of starfish initiator tRNA. Nucleic Acids Res 6: 3459–3469

Kuchino Y, Watanabe S, Harada F, Nishimura S (1980) Primary structure of AUA-specific isoleucine transfer ribonucleic acid from E. coli. Biochemistry 19: 2085–2089

Kuchino Y, Grunberger D, Borek E, Mushinski JF, Nishimura S (1982) Changes of post-transcriptional modification of wye base in tumor specific $tRNA^{Phe}$. Nucleic Acids Res 10: 6421–6432

Kuchino Y, Shindo-Okada N, Ando N, Watanabe S, Nishimura S (1981) Nucleotide sequences of two aspartic acid tRNAs from rat liver and rat ascites hepatoma. J Biol Chem 256: 9059–9062

Li HJ, Nakanishi K, Grunberger D, Weinstein IB (1973) Biosynthetic studies of the Y base in yeast phenylalanine tRNA. Incorporation of guanosine. Biochem Biophys Res Commun 55: 818–823

Mushinski JF, Marini M (1979) Tumor-associated phenylalanyl transfer RNA found in a wide spectrum of rat and mouse tumors but absent in normal adult, fetal and regenerating tissues. Cancer Res 39: 1253–1258

Nishimura S (1978) Modified nucleosides and isoaccepting tRNA. In: Altman S (ed) Transfer RNA. MIT Press, Cambridge, MA, pp 168–195

Pergolizzi RG, Grunberger D (1980) The effect of exogenous nutrients on the biosynthesis of Y base in $tRNA^{Phe}$ from Ehrlich ascites carcinoma. Cancer Lett 8: 329–333

Pergolizzi RG, Engelhardt DL, Grunberger D (1978) Formation of phenylalanine transfer RNA lacking the wye base in Vero cells during methionine starvation. J Biol Chem 253: 6341–6343

Pergolizzi RG, Engelhardt DL, Grunberger D (1979) Incorporation of lysine into Y base of phenylalanine tRNA in Vero cells. Nucleic Acids Res 6: 2209–2216

Raba M, Limburg K, Burghagen M, Katze JR, Simsek M, Heckman JE, RajBhandary UL, Gross HJ (1979) Nucleotide sequence of three isoaccepting lysine tRNAs from rabbit liver and SV40-transformed mouse fibroblasts. Eur J Biochem 97: 305–318

RajBhandary UL, Chang SH (1968) Yeast phenylalanine tRNA: Partial digestion with ribonuclease T_1 and derivation of the total primary structure. J Biol Chem 243: 598–608

Randerath E, Gopalakrishnan AS, Gupta RC, Agrawal HP, Randerath K (1981) Lack of a specific ribose methylation at guanosine 17 in Morris hepatoma 5123D $tRNA^{Ser\,1}_{IGA}$. Cancer Res 41: 2863–2867

Roe BA, Stankiewicz AF, Ritzi HL, Weisz C, DiLauro MN, Pike D, Chen CY, Chen EY (1979) Comparison of rat liver and Walker 256 carcinosarcoma tRNAs. Nucleic Acids Res 6: 673–688

Rothstein M, Greenburg DM (1960) The metabolism of DL-Pipecolic acid-2-C_1. J Biol Chem 235: 714–718

Salomon R, Giveon D, Kimhi Y, Littauer NZ (1976) Abundance of $tRNA^{Phe}$ lacking the peroxy Y-base in mouse neuroblastoma. Biochemistry 15: 5258–5262

Shindo-Okada N, Kuchino Y, Harada F, Okada N, Nishimura S (1981) Biological and structural differences between $tRNA^{Val}$ species isolated from rat ascites hepatoma cells and normal rat liver. J Biochem 90: 535–544

Thiebe R, Zachau HG (1968) Specific modification next to anticodon of phenylalanine transfer ribonucleic acid. Eur J Biochem 5: 546–555

Volkers AS, Taylor MW, (1971) Chromatographic comparison of the tRNA of rat livers and Morris hepatoma. Biochemistry 10: 488–497

*Why Is Tumor tRNA Hypomodified with Respect to Q Nucleoside?**

J. R. Katze[1], W. T. Beck[2], C. S. Cheng[3], and J. A. McCloskey[3]

[1] Department of Microbiology and Immunology, University of Tennessee Center for the Health Sciences, Memphis, TN, USA; [2] Division of Biochemical and Clinical Pharmacology, St. Jude Children's Research Hospital, Department of Pharmacology, University of Tennessee Center for the Health Sciences, Memphis, TN, USA; [3] Departments of Medicinal Chemistry and Biochemistry, University of Utah, Salt Lake City, UT, USA

Introduction

Nucleoside Q is found exclusively in the first position of the anticodon in $tRNA^{Tyr}$, $tRNA^{His}$, $tRNA^{Asn}$, and $tRNA^{Asp}$ (Kasai et al. 1975b, 1976). Its function is unknown, and long-term Q-deficient, germ-free mice appear normal (Reyniers et al. 1981). However, queuine metabolism is altered in neoplasia. Many tumors exhibit Q-deficient tRNA (Katze 1975; Okada et al. 1978; Roe et al. 1979) and queuine addition to tumor-bearing mice can reverse tumor tRNA Q deficiency (Katze and Beck 1980; Nishimura et al., this volume pp. 401–412) and may inhibit tumor growth (Katze and Beck 1980). It is unlikely that Q-deficient tRNA is necessary for the neoplastic state since the careful study of Marini and Mushinski (1979; Mushinski and Marini, this volume pp. 121–132) shows widely varying, repeatable isoaccepting patterns (largely due to differences in Q content) for the Q family of tRNAs from several Balb/c mouse plasmacytomas with similar growth rates and size at harvest. These large differences among such a similar group of tumors suggest that the alteration in Q metabolism is secondary to the neoplastic process.

The aberrant Q metabolism of tumors, however, may influence the tumor-host relationship. In addition to tumors, the "normal" livers of tumor-bearing mice exhibit Q-deficient tRNA (Marini et al. 1979; Katze and Beck 1980; Mushinski and Marini, this volume pp. 121–132). Therefore, to the extent that normal Q metabolism is required for optimal tissue function, a tumor-induced systemic depletion of Q would favor the tumor in the tumor-host struggle. In this regard, Q-deficient germ-free mice appear normal, however; their immune systems are unstressed. Before addressing the question of why tumor tRNA is hypomodified with respect to Q, we will discuss how [Q+]tRNA is formed normally.

Queuine is a Dietary Factor for Animals

Unlike other tRNA modifications, Q is synthesized first as a base and is then incorporated irreversibly in an exchange reaction in which guanine is removed, into

* This work was supported by grants from the National Institutes of Health, CA-23099 and CA-21765 (W.T.B.), CA-20919 (J.R.K.), GM-29812 (J.A.M.); and ALSAC (W.T.B.). We thank P. Moore for her excellent assistance

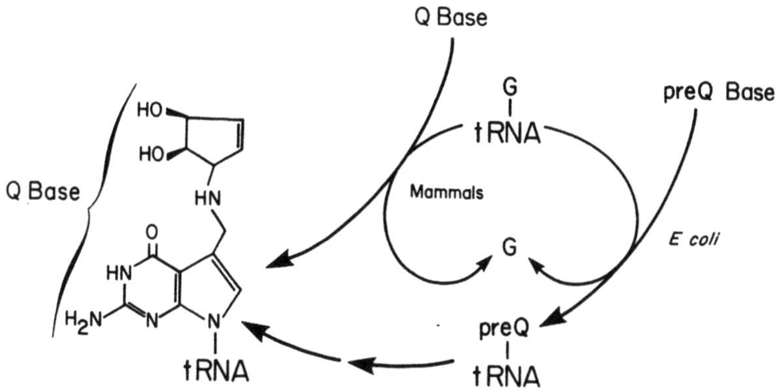

Fig. 1. Comparison of guanine, queuine tRNA transglycosylase catalyzed step in mammals and in *Escherichia coli*. *PreQ base,* 7-(aminomethyl)-7-deazaguanine (Okada et al. 1979). Figure from Katze and Beck 1980

preformed tRNA by the enzyme guanine, queuine tRNA transglycosylase (Fig. 1). Queuine, the base of Q, appears to be the immediate precursor of Q in mammalian tRNA (Katze and Farkas 1979; Shindo-Okada et al. 1980, 1981; Katze and Beck 1980; Reyniers et al. 1981). However, animals apparently cannot synthesize queuine de novo, since germ-free mice on a defined diet do not synthesize [Q+]tRNA unless enabled to do so by loss of germ-free state, consumption of a normal laboratory diet, parenteral injection of queuine, or addition of queuine or [Q+]tRNA to the defined diet (Farkas 1980; Reyniers et al. 1981).

The contribution of diet to the synthesis of [Q+]tRNA is explained at least in part by the recent discovery that free queuine is distributed widely among eukaryotes, with significant levels in plant and animal products common to the diet (Table 1). However, the ability of germ-free mice to use dietary [Q+]tRNA implies a mechanism for the salvage of free queuine from [Q+]tRNA. Therefore, diet must provide queuine both directly and indirectly (after salvage). Indeed, salvage would also explain the contribution of gut flora to Q formation in mice, because rodents practice coprophagy and the digestive tract of rodents contains some microbial flora (Barnard 1969). Salvage may account as well for the high concentration of queuine in bovine sources (Table 1), since salvaged material from the degradation of microbial RNA (from rumen microflora) contributes significantly to tissue nucleic acid synthesis in ruminants (Smith et al. 1974; Rassaque et al. 1981). Finally, the possibilities remain that diet and/or gut flora may contribute a precursor of queuine, e.g., the cyclopentenediol moiety, and that gut flora may contribute free queuine.

Direct queuine synthesis has not yet been observed in any organism, although the high concentration of queuine in some plant sources (Table 1) suggests that plants may do so. *Escherichia coli,* the best studied organism in this regard, does not synthesize queuine directly and no free queuine has been detected in *E. coli* extracts (Okada et al. 1979). Instead, a precursor of queuine is incorporated into tRNA (queuine is not a substrate for this reaction), with further modification occurring to yield queuosine only at the polynucleotide level.

Support for the ability of mice to salvage free queuine from dietary [Q+]tRNA has been obtained as part of a study of queuine excretion in mice. Normal mice were injected with saline, queuine, or queuosine; Ehrlich ascites tumor-bearing mice were

Table 1. Queuine content of natural products. Queuine was estimated from the appearance of [Q+]tRNA^{Asp} in the LM cell line, using authentic queuine as a standard and a m*M* extinction coefficient for queuine of 10.5 at 260 nm in H_2O (S. Nishimura, unpublished work). For multiple samples (number in parentheses) the range of values is given. Katze et al., to be published

Source	Content (ng/g or ng/ml)
Bovine amniotic fluid (3rd trimester) (3)	2300–3600
Drosophila melanogaster (wild type + mutants) (15)	0–1100
Coconut water (ripe) (5)	87– 530
Bovine pineal body	300
Wheat germ	190
Bovine seminal vesicle (adult)	110
Bovine testicle (adult)	58
Bovine serum (fetal) (2)	33– 54
Tomato (fresh, ripe)	21
Bovine milk (whole + skim) (2)	16– 17
Bovine serum (calf)	14
Bovine milk (evaporated skim, canned)	12
Yogurt (commercial + homemade) (2)	4– 6
Goat milk (fresh)	3
Goat milk (evaporated, canned)	1
Human milk	1

Table 2. Queuine recovery from mouse urine. Tumor-bearing mice were inoculated intraperitoneally with 2×10^6 Ehrlich ascites tumor cells on day 0 and test injected on day 7; tumor yield, day 9, was 2–3 ml packed cells. Queuine was assayed by the method of Horton, Farkas, and Katze (unpublished work). Urines, collected from mice in metabolism cages, were adjusted to 1.0 ml with H_2O, then 0.4 ml was mixed with 2 ml 0.05 *M* NH_4HCO_3, pH 7.5, and absorbed to a small column containing 1 g C_{18} reverse phase packing (BondElute, Analytichem International, Inc.) previously washed with 0.05 *M* NH_4HCO_3, pH 7.5. The column was eluted with 3 ml 0.05 *M* NH_4HCO_3, pH 7.5, 3 ml 10% methanol, and 2 ml 1 *M* acetic acid. The acetic acid fraction was lyophilized, taken up in H_2O (75–200 µl), then subjected to HPLC analysis on a C_{18} column (Altex Ultrasphere ODS, 4.6 × 250 mm). Mobile phase: 0.005 *M* heptane sulfonate; 0.02 *M* ammonium acetate, pH 3.20; methanol; tetrahydrofuran (85: 14.5: 0.5, v/v: 0.95 ml/min) at room temperature. Detection was at 254 nm. Quantitation was from peak heights compared to a standard, and values were corrected for a 55% yield of queuine from the BondElute columns. Queuine for injection was isolated from 3rd-trimester bovine amniotic fluid (Katze and Farkas 1979; Crain et al. 1980). Queuosine was from *E. coli* tRNA (Kasai et al. 1975b). Both queuine and queuosine were purified by HPLC (C_{18} column and elution with 0.05 *M* ammonium formate, pH 4.0, 4.5% methanol) prior to use. *NA* signifies not analyzed

Injection	A_{260} Queuine in 24-h urine	
	Normal	Tumor-bearing
Saline	0.03	NA
Queuosine (2 A_{260})	0.11	NA
Queuine (2 A_{260})	0.72	0.48

injected with queuine. The 24-h urine yield of each mouse was then assayed for queuine by high-performance liquid chromatography. The results are shown in Table 2. Controls (normal saline-injected mice) excreted 0.03 A_{260} units queuine/day. After the injection of 2 A_{260} units queuine, normal and tumor-bearing mice excreted 0.72 and 0.43 A_{260} units per day respectively. Similar values have been obtained using the LM-cell assay for queuine determination (data not shown). When queuosine was injected, a small but significant increase in queuine excretion was observed; however, no queuosine was detected (< 0.005 A_{260}) in the urine of either control or queuosine injected mice. These data are consistent with a capacity for the salvage of free queuine from its nucleoside, but the fate of most of the injected queuosine is unknown.

Queuine Catabolism in Animals

Little is known about how queuine, either free or as [Q+]tRNA, is catabolized. It is apparent from Table 2 that much of a large dose of injected queuine is excreted within 24 h in an unchanged form, but the fate of the remaining queuine remains to be determined.

Our ignorance regarding queuine catabolism derives in large part from the difficulty in obtaining radioactively labeled queuine. We have attempted to label queuine by a procedure involving catalytic deuteration or tritiation (Kinoshita et al. 1981), but have been unable to label the molecule without reducing the double bond in the cyclopentenediol moiety. These derivatives, in which the proton at the 8 position of the 7-deazaguanine moiety has been exchanged and the cyclopentene has been reduced, contain 3 mol isotope/mol and are referred to as rQD_3 and rQT_3. Each appears to be faithfully and irreversibly incorporated into tRNA in place of queuine by LM cells, but approximately ten times more derivative than queuine is required for a similar effect (see below).

A large portion of injected rQT_3, like injected queuine, was eliminated unchanged in the urine within 24 h (Table 3). In normal mice, however, only 60% appeared in the urine within 4 days and even less was accounted for in the tumor-bearing mouse. Where is the rest of the material? Urinary catabolic products are unlikely, because HPLC examination of the urine from the normal and the tumor-bearing mice (Fig. 2) shows that more than 95% of the material elutes in the position of rQT_3. The

Table 3. Recovery of rQT_3 from mouse urine. rQT_3 (0.5 A_{260}, 6.3 × 10^6 CPM) was injected, as in Table 2. The recovery is calculated from direct counting of an aliquot of urine. rQT_3 was synthesized (by Amersham) by catalytic reduction and tritiation of queuine, and was purified by HPLC (using the ammonium formate buffer in Table 2) prior to use; details will be published elsewhere. *NA* signifies not analyzed

Days after injection	Recovery (%) in 24-h urine of injected CPM	
	Normal	Tumor-bearing
1	53	39
2	8	2
3	1	NA
4	1	NA

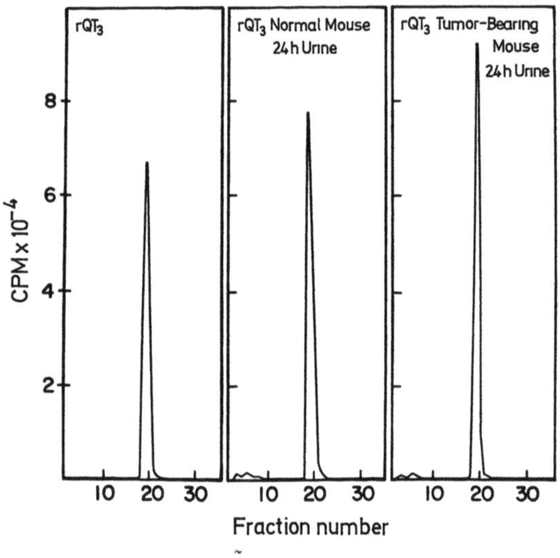

Fig. 2. HPLC analysis of rQT_3 and 24 h urines of rQT_3-injected mice, normal and tumor-bearing. This is an analysis from the experiment described in Table 3. Urines (first 24 h collection) were adjusted to 1.0 ml with H_{20}, 50 µl of this was subjected directly to HPLC analysis (ammonium acetate buffer of Table 2), 1.0 min fractions were collected, and the radioactivity was measured. The rQT_3 HPLC analysis was performed on 1/40 of the dose injected into the mice. Under these conditions queuosine and queuine would be expected to elute near fractions 10 and 15 respectively. No marker is available for rQT_3 nucleoside. Essentially 100% of the radioactivity added to the HPLC column was recovered in the fractions shown

decreased excretion of rQT_3 (Table 3) and queuine (Table 2) by the tumor-bearing mice is consistent with the known uptake of exogenous queuine into [Q−]tRNA in tumors (Katze and Beck 1980; Nishimura et al., this volume pp. 401−412). The fate of the remainder of the injected rQT_3 in both normal and tumor-bearing mice remains to be determined.

Queuine Salvage Occurs in AGMK Primary Cells, but is Absent or Deficient in Several Cell Lines

A factor in serum enables tissue cultured cells to make [Q+]tRNA (Katze 1978a). This factor has been identified as queuine (Katze and Farkas 1979; Crain et al. 1980). Data on the appearance of serum factor-dependent [Q+]tRNA were obtained first with the SV40-transformed mouse fibroblast cell line SVT2 (Katze 1975), and later with the mouse fibroblast cell line LM adapted to serum-free growth (Katze 1978a; Katze and Farkas 1979). LM cells cultured in serum-free medium contain only traces of [Q+]tRNA, but the addition of saturating amounts of queuine to the cultures brings about nearly complete conversion to [Q+]tRNA within 24 h (Fig. 4). In a reverse experiment (Table 4), when LM cells containing [Q+]tRNA are transferred to queuine-free medium, the proportion of $tRNA^{Asp}$ which contains Q declines from 99% to 48% in 24 h. This decline requires RNA synthesis, i.e., it is eliminated by actinomycin D. These data are consistent with irreversible queuine incorporation, and furthermore imply that LM cells do not salvage queuine upon turnover of [Q+]tRNA. Therefore, the decline in the proportion of $[Q+]tRNA^{Asp}$ simply reflects tRNA turnover plus dilution from the net increase in tRNA due to cell division. Similar results were obtained with rQD_3, indicating that it too is irreversibly incorporated into tRNA. In contrast, 8azaG is reversibly incorporated by the transglycosylase into tRNA, since its loss from LM-cell tRNA is not inhibited by actinomycin D. It is known that 8azaG is incorporated into the same position occupied by Q (Shindo-Okada et al.

Fig. 3. Representative reversed-phase (RPC-5) cochromatographic comparison of LM-cell $tRNA^{Asp}$. The *dashed line* depicts [^{14}C]Asp-tRNA from LM cells cultivated serum free, with fresh serum-free medium (25 ml/150 cm^2 flask) replacement 24-h before harvest. The *solid line* depicts [^{3}H]Asp-tRNA from cultures parallel except for a serum-free medium containing 0.2 A_{260} queuine/100 ml replacement 24-h before harvest. Isolation of tRNA, aminoacylation, and reversed-phase chromatography have been described (Katze 1978a). Peaks 1 and 3 are [Q+]$tRNA^{Asp}$; peaks 2 and 4 are [Q−]$tRNA^{Asp}$. The radioactivity present in each peak is used to determine the percentage [Q+]$tRNA^{Asp}$, i.e., the CPM in 1 + 3 divided by the CPM in 1 + 2 + 3 +4. The percentage [Q+]$tRNA^{Asp}$ is 3% and 96% in the serum-free cells and queuine-treated cells respectively

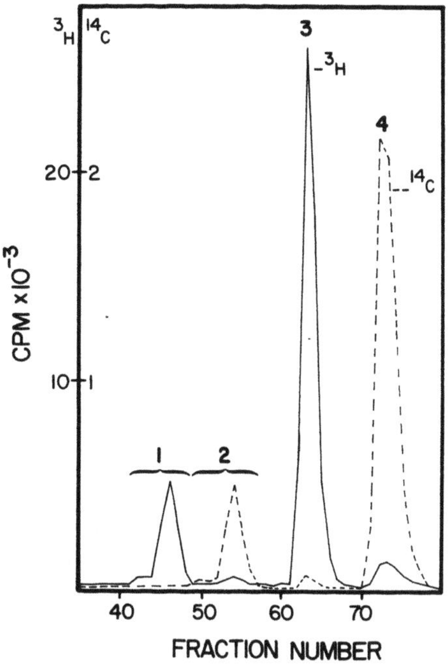

Table 4. Queuine and rQD_3 are incorporated irreversibly into LM-cell tRNA; 8azaG is not. LM cells, cultivated in serum-free medium to nearly confluent monolayers in 150 cm^2 flasks, were subjected to treatment: 25 ml of 50 ml medium to which the designated additions had been made was used to replace the medium in each of two flasks. After 24 h, each flask was subjected to chase: the medium was removed, the cells were rinsed with serum-free medium, then 25 ml of fresh serum-free medium was added. After 24 h (exp. 1) or 16 h (exp. 2), the cells were harvested and the $tRNA^{Asp}$ isoaccepting distribution determined as in Fig. 3. Actinomycin D (4 μg/ml) was present during both treatment and chase in exp. 2. Note that [Q−]$tRNA^{Asp}$ values are presented. rQD_3-containing $tRNA^{Asp}$ coelutes with [Q+]$tRNA^{Asp}$ (peaks 2 and 4, Fig. 3), but 8azaG-containing $tRNA^{Asp}$ elutes later than [Q−]$tRNA^{Asp}$ (peaks 2 and 4, Fig. 3). rQD_3 was synthesized by catalytic reduction and deuteration, in an analogous fashion to rQT_3 synthesis (Table 3). *NA*, signifies not analyzed

Experiment	Treatment	Actinomycin D	[Q−]$tRNA^{Asp}$ (%)	
			After treatment	After chase
1	No addition	−	99	99
	0.1 A_{260} Queuine	−	< 1	42
	1 A_{260} rQD_3	−	1	46
	5 A_{260} 8azaG	−	20	84
2	No addition	+	NA	97
	0.1 A_{260} Queuine	+	14	6
	1 A_{260} rQD_3	+	1	2
	5 A_{260} 8azaG	+	45	97

Table 5. [Q+]tRNA in tissue cultured cells requires queuine in medium. N-18 line (courtesy of H. Herschman, UCLA) basal medium: Dulbecco's modified Eagle's medium (DMEM), buffered with HEPES and Tricine (Katze 1978b). BeWo line cells (from Am. Type Culture Collection) basal medium: DMEM. AGMK primary cells (from Flow Labs.) basal medium: minimal essential Eagle's medium. After continuous culture, or culture for the designated times, and, where noted, a 24-h queuine treatment in the same medium, the cells were harvested and the percentage [Q+]tRNA^{Asp} was determined as in Fig. 3

Cell	Medium	Treatment (24 h)	[Q+]tRNA^{Asp} (%)
Neuroblastoma mouse line Cl1300	10% FBS	None	76
clone N-18	Serum-free (3 days)	None	42
Choriocarcinoma Human line BeWo	15% FBS	None	99
	15% [Q−]FBS (6 days)	None	23
	15% [Q−]FBS (6 days)	0.01 A_{260}/50 ml	81
	15% [Q−]FBS (6 days)	0.05 A_{260}/50 ml	97
	15% [Q−]FBS (4 months)	None	6
Kidney	15% FBS	None	99
AGMK primary	15% [Q−]FBS (11 days)	None	50

1981). These data also indicate that the low efficiency (relative to queuine) of rQD_3 incorporation into LM-cell tRNA cannot be attributed to reversible incorporation. Queuine-dependent [Q+]tRNA formation is not restricted to mouse fibroblasts. Marshal et al. (1978) reported similar results with the baby hamster kidney cell line BHK 21, and the data in Table 5 demonstrate serum factor dependent [Q+]tRNA formation in both the mouse neuroblastoma and human choriocarcinoma cell lines, as well as primary cultures of African green monkey kidney cells. Since animals do not synthesize queuine de novo, a requirement for queuine in the medium for the appearance of [Q+]tRNA in tissue culture cells is not surprising. What is of interest, however, is that different cell types utilize queuine in the growth medium with greatly differing efficiencies.

When the mouse neuroblastoma cell line is placed in serum-free medium, the cells cease dividing but remain viable, so that the attendant decrease in [Q+]tRNA^{Asp} (Table 5) is largely from tRNA turnover. The data, therefore, allow an estimate of the half-life of the [Q+]tRNA^{Asp}: $t_{1/2}$ = 3.5 days. Similarly, when the human choriocarcinoma cell line (BeWo) is placed in medium supplemented with serum treated to remove queuine (Katze 1978), the relative [Q+]tRNA^{Asp} content falls dramatically. Since the BeWo cells continue to divide in the queuine-depleted medium, the decrease in [Q+]tRNA is due to both tRNA turnover and cell growth, and the rate of decline is comparable to that for the LM cells (above). The BeWo cells, like the LM cells, rapidly regain [Q+]tRNA upon addition of queuine to the queuine-depleted medium.

Table 6. Queuosine enables AGMK cells, but not LM cells, to synthesize [Q+]tRNA. Cells were cultivated and the percentage [Q+]tRNA^{Asp} determined as described in Tables 4 and 5 and Fig. 3

Cell	Medium	Treatment (24 h)	[Q+]tRNA^{Asp} (%)
AGMK	5% FBS	–	97
	5% [Q–]FBS 11 days	–	17
	5% [Q–]FBS 11 days	0.01 A_{260} Queuine/50 ml	98
	5% [Q–]FBS 11 days	0.15 A_{260} Queuosine/50 ml	98
	5% [Q–]FBS 11 days	5% FBS	98
LM	Serum-free	–	1
	Serum-free	0.15 A_{260} Queuosine/50 ml	1
	Serum-free	5% FBS	6
	Serum-free	5% [Q–] FBS	1

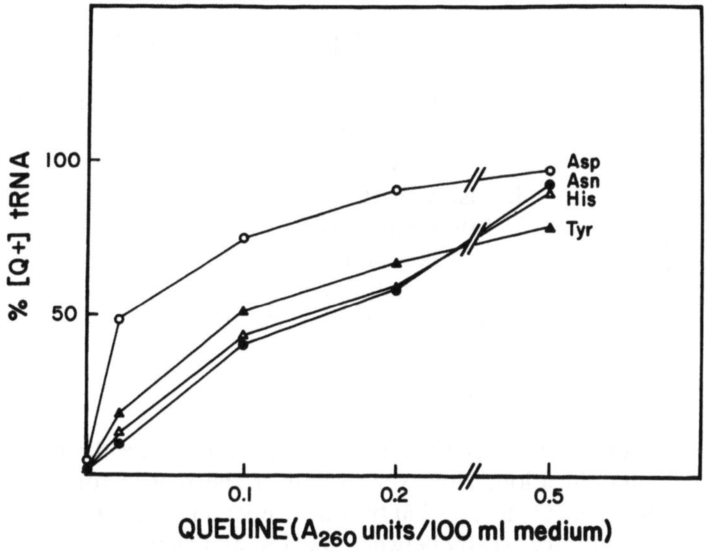

Fig. 4. tRNA^{Asp} is the preferred in vivo substrate for guanine, queuine tRNA transglycosylase. LM cells were grown in serum-free medium and then exposed to increasing concentrations of queuine 24 h before harvest and tRNA isolation, as in Fig. 3. Each of the Q family of tRNAs was then subjected to aminoacylation and chromatographic analysis, essentially as described in Fig. 3 and Katze 1978b

In contrast, African green monkey kidney primary cells (AGMK) lose [Q+]tRNA very slowly. After 11 days in queuine-depleted medium, the relative [Q+]tRNA^{Asp} content had decreased only 50%, even though the cell number had increased more than tenfold. These results (Table 5) were taken as evidence for net queuine synthesis in AGMK cells; however, the data from germ-free mice (above) make this

interpretation unlikely. A second possibility is that AGMK cells can salvage free queuine upon tRNA turnover. In order to test this possibility, queuosine was added to AGMK cells cultivated in queuine-depleted medium. The results (Table 6) show that AGMK cells, but not LM cells, can utilize queuosine to synthesize [Q+]tRNA. We take this as evidence for queuine salvage in AGMK cells. It should be noted that ribothymidine is the only other modified ribonucleoside known to be salvaged in mammalian cells (Nielsen et al. 1974; Lothrop and Uziel 1981). However, the data also indicate that AGMK cells use queuine much more efficiently than do LM cells: in 5% FBS medium LM cells exhibit 6% [Q+]$tRNA^{Asp}$, while AGMK cells exhibit 98% [Q+]$tRNA^{Asp}$. This large difference between the two cell types in ability to use queuine is unlikely to be explained simply by a difference in salvage.
Even if 100% salvage were assumed, it is difficult to envisage how 99% [Q+]$tRNA^{Asp}$ could be diluted tenfold and still be 50% [Q+]$tRNA^{Asp}$. One possible explanation is contained in Fig. 4, which shows that the best tRNA substrate (by a factor of 5) for queuine incorporation is $tRNA^{Asp}$: in the absence of exogenous queuine, assuming salvage upon turnover, $tRNA^{Asp}$ would become enriched relative to and at the expense of the other [Q+]tRNAs.

What is the Cause of the Q Hypomodification in Tumors?

There are several factors of possible significance to the control of [Q+]tRNA expresssion in mammals:

1. Queuine Availability Dietary (free) Dietary (salvaged)
2. Transport rate
3. tRNA synthesis rate
4. Insertion rate
5. Competitor level
6. Catabolic rate
7. tRNA half-life
8. Salvage rate (intracellular)

Queuine Availability

Queuine availability to the host is unlikely to be directly responsible for tumor Q hypomodification. However, whatever the reason for the Q hypomodification, the extent (penetrance) of that trait will depend in part on the availability of queuine. The latter will vary greatly between species, and even within a species, depending on both type of stomach and diet. Thus man (with a simple stomach) appears to have lower systemic queuine levels than the mouse (a coprophage with a cecum), while the bovine (with the large microbial content of the rumen) contains very large amounts of queuine. This dietary factor may be significant during cancer therapy, especially when hyperalimentation or total parenteral nutrition are employed.

Queuine Transport Rate

The transport of queuine into normal or tumor cells has not been studied. The transport of nucleosides and purines in mammalian cells is via facilitated diffusion, and the rate-limiting step in their uptake is not transport, but incorporation (into nucleotides) (Plagemann and Wohlhueter 1980). These observations may be valid for queuine uptake by LM Cells as well, since the queuine concentration that yields 50% [Q+]tRNA^{Asp} (Fig. 4) is about 0.03 A_{260} units/100 ml, or 3×10^{-8} *M*, and the K_m for queuine exchange into yeast tRNA^{Asp} by the rabbit reticulocyte glycosyltransferase is 4.5×10^{-8} *M* (Katze and Farkas, 1979). As noted, AGMK cells utilize queuine much more efficiently than do LM cells, in part because of queuine salvage. An active (concentrative) queuine transport mechanism also may be present in AGMK cells. Alternatively, a more active transglycosylase may be present, but this seems unlikely (see below).

Synthesis Rate of tRNA

Does the tRNA synthesis rate in tumors influence Q metabolism? The rate of tRNA synthesis per se is unlikely to differ between host and tumor cells, though tRNA synthesis in tumors may be relatively greater because of relatively rapid cell growth and/or increased tRNA turnover (see below). It is unlikely that queuine is stored to any extent in the body, because situations in which normal animals are forced to synthesize large amounts of new tissue rapidly (e.g., phenylhydrazine induction of reticulocytosis or partial hepatectomy to induce liver regeneration) result in tRNA hypomodified with respect to Q (Farkas and Chernoff 1976; DuBrul and Farkas 1976; McNamara and Smith 1978; Okada et al. 1978). During rapid tumor growth, therefore, queuine intake may be inadequate to meet demand. The latter cannot explain the entire difference in Q metabolism between normal and tumor cells, however, because the infusion of far greater than physiological amounts of exogenous queuine into Ehrlich ascites tumor-bearing mice partially restored the Q content of the tumor tRNA, but not to normal levels (Katze and Beck 1980).

Insertion Rate

Is the activity of guanine, queuine tRNA transglycosylase lower in tumor cells? Available data do not support this possibility: tumor tissues have been reported to contain adequate levels of guanine, queuine tRNA transglycosylase (Shindo-Okada et al. 1980). The enzyme is probably constitutive, as it is present in LM cells grown in serum-free medium (Katze and Farkas 1979), and in germ-free mice maintained on a defined diet (Reyniers et al. 1981), even though neither source contains more than traces of [Q+]tRNA.

Competitor Level

Do tumors produce a factor that interferes with Q metabolism? Naturally occuring pteridines inhibit queuine incorporation into tRNA both in vivo, using the LM-cell assay, and in vitro, using reticulocyte guanine, queuine tRNA transglycosylase (Jacobson et al. 1981). Furthermore, high levels of pigment pteridines in the skin of fishes of the genus *Xiphophorus* may be responsible for the apparent Q hypomodification in the skin tRNA (H. Kersten, this volume pp. 255–263). These observations, coupled with alterations in pteridine metabolism associated with neoplastic disease

(Wachter et al. 1979; Saleh et al. 1980; Rokos et al. 1980), are suggestive of a tumor-elicited inhibitor of Q metabolism, though none has been identified.

Catabolic Rate

Do tumors inactivate queuine by catabolism or derivatization? As indicated, very little is known about Q catabolism. No catabolites or derivatives of Q have been identified as yet, but it is hoped that any such compounds will be discovered as a result of further studies on the fate of rQT_3 in normal and tumor-bearing animals and in normal and transformed cells in culture.

Half-life of tRNA

Does the half-life of tRNA in tumors influence the Q content? The elevated excretion of tRNA-derived modified nucleosides and bases, which occurs in cancer patients and tumor-bearing animals, has led to the hypothesis that the turnover rate of tRNA in tumors is very high (Borek et al. 1977). The present workshop was convened in part to discuss the diagnostic potential of this elevated excretion, and the data of Borek, Schöch, Björk, Rasmuson, Gehrke, Salvatore, Thomale and Clark in this volume hold promise for the clinical application of the analysis of modified nucleosides in urine or serum. As indicated, even normal animals exhibit Q hypomodified tRNA when required to synthesize large quantities of tRNA rapidly; apparently the result of queuine demand exceeding queuine availability. An analogous situation would result from rapid tumor growth coupled with a high turnover rate for tRNA, especially if queuine salvage were compromised or inefficient (see below).

Whether the increase in tRNA turnover involves the tumor exclusively or some contribution of both tumor and host is not clear. Borek (Borek et al. 1977, and this volume pp. 301–316) favors tumor tRNA turnover exclusively, even though it might require "a 500-fold greater rate of tRNA breakdown" – corresponding to a half-life of less than 30 min – to account for observed urinary excretion of modified nucleosides in patients with tumors. However, since the measured values for tRNA half-lives vary between 22 h and 5 days (Abelson et al. 1974; Schlegel et al. 1978; Kleiman et al. 1980; Smith and Weinberg 1981), and systemic effects of tumors, such as enhanced muscle protein breakdown (Shapot 1979; Karlberg et al. 1981), are common, it would seem more reasonable to postulate a tumor-induced mobilization of tRNA turnover by the host. K. Randerath et al. (this volume pp. 283–297) has diagrammed excellently the sources and fates of "undermodified" tRNA in tumors. In that diagram, increased degradation of undermodified tRNA results from "destabilization" or activation of nucleases. To the extent that the signal which leads to increased degradation of tRNA is a systemic one, aberrant tRNA in a tumor could induce increased tRNA catabolism in other tissues.

Salvage Rate

Is queuine salvage blocked or attenuated in tumors? Evidence for salvage by normal tissues and a salvage deficiency in several tissue culture cell lines has been presented (above). The possibility of a salvage deficiency in tumors remains to be tested, but such a deficiency could contribute to the Q hypomodification of tumor tRNA, especially if salvaged queuine, in contrast to transported extracellular queuine, is more efficiently incorporated into tRNA.

In conclusion, the available data suggest that tumor tRNA is Q-deficient in part because the demand for queuine exceeds the dietary intake, the result of increased tRNA turnover and cell growth, and in part because tumor cells may not salvage queuine efficiently after tRNA turnover. However, it is likely that this simple description is incomplete and other factors have yet to be identified.

Abbreviations

Q or *nucleoside Q* or *queuosine,* 7-(4,5-*cis*-dihydroxy-1-cyclopenten-3-ylaminomethyl)-7-deazaguanosine; *Q base* or *queuine*, the aglycone of queuosine; *[Q+]tRNA,* tRNA containing Q in the first position of the anticodon; *[Q−]tRNA,* the unmodified or precursor form of [Q+]tRNA containing guanosine instead of Q in the first position of the anticodon; rQD_3, the reduced and deuterated derivative of queuine (see text); rQT_3, the reduced and tritiated derivative of queuine (see text); *8azaG,* 8-azaguanine; *FBS,* fetal bovine serum; *[Q−]FBS,* FBS treated with charcoal plus dextran to remove queuine (Katze, 1978b); *HPLC* high-performance liquid chromatography; *HEPES,* *N*-2-hydroxyethylpiperazine-*N′*-2ethane sulfonic acid; *Tricine,* *N*-Tris(hydroxymethyl)methyl glycine; A_{260} *unit,* the amount of material giving an absorbance of 1.0 at 260 nm when dissolved in 1 ml of water and measured in a cell of a 1-cm light path. In this study, Q is used generically to designate Q, and Q* denotes queuosine containing galactose or mannose bound to carbon 4 of the cyclopentenediol substituent.

References

Abelson HT, Johnson LF, Penman S, Green H (1974) Changes in RNA in relation to growth of the fibroblast: II the lifetime of mRNA, rRNA, and tRNA in resting and growing cells. Cell 1: 161–165

Barnard EA (1969) Biological function of pancreatic ribonuclease. Nature 221: 340–344

Borek E, Baliga BS, Gehrke CW, Kuo KW, Belman S, Troll W, Waalkes TP (1977) High turnover rate of transfer RNA in tumor tissue. Cancer Res 37: 3362–3366

Crain PF, Sethi SK, Katze JR, McCloskey JA (1980) Structure of an amniotic fluid component, 7-(4,5-*cis*-dihydroxy-1-cyclopenten-3-ylaminomethyl)-7-deazaguanine (queuine), a substrate for tRNA: guanine transglycosylase. J Biol Chem 255: 8405–8407

DuBrul EF, Farkas WR (1976) Partial purification and properties of the reticulocyte guanylating enzyme. Biochim Biophys Acta 442: 379–390

Farkas WR (1980) Effect of diet on the queuosine family of tRNAs of germ-free mice. J Biol Chem 255: 6832–6835

Farkas WR, Chernoff D (1976) Identification of the minor guanylated tRNAs of rabbit reticulocytes. Nucleic Acids Res 3: 2521–2529

Jacobson KB, Farkas WR, Katze JR (1981) Presence of queuine in *Drosophila melanogaster:* correlation of free pool with queuosine content of tRNA and effect of mutations in pteridine metabolism. Nucleic Acids Res 9: 2351–2366

Karlberg I, Edström S, Ekman L, Johansson S, Scherstén T, Lundholm K (1981) Metabolic host reaction response to the proliferation of nonmalignant cells versus malignant cells in vivo. Cancer Res 41: 4154–4161

Kasai H, Kuchino Y, Nihei K, Nishimura S (1975a) Distribution of the modified nucleoside Q and its derivatives in animal and plant transfer RNA's. Nucleic Acids Res 2: 1931–1939

Kasai H, Ohashi Z, Harada F, Nishimura S, Oppenheimer NJ, Crain PF, Liehr JG, von Minden DL, McCloskey JA (1975b) Structure of the modified nucleoside Q isolated from *Escherichia coli* transfer ribonucleic acid. 7-(4,5-*cis*-dihydroxy-1-cyclopenten-3-ylaminomethyl)-7-deazaguanosine. Biochemistry 14: 4198–4208

Kasai H, Nakanishi K, MacFarlane RD, Torgerson DF, Ohashi Z, McCloskey JA, Gross HJ, Nishimura S (1976) The structure of Q* nucleoside isolated from rabbit liver transfer ribonucleic acid. J Am Chem Soc 98: 5044–5046

Katze JR (1975) Alterations in SVT2 cell transfer RNAs in response to cell density and serum type. Biochim Biophys Acta 383: 131–139

Katze JR (1978a) Q-Factor: A serum component required for the appearance of nucleoside Q in tRNA in tissue culture. Biochem Biophys Res Commun 84: 527–535

Katze JR (1978b) Relation of cell type and cell density in tissue culture to the isoaccepting spectra of the nucleoside Q containing tRNAs: $tRNA^{Tyr}$, $tRNA^{His}$, $tRNA^{Asn}$ and $tRNA^{Asp}$. Nucleic Acids Res 5: 2513–2524

Katze JR, Beck WT (1980) Administration of queuine to mice recieves modified nucleoside queuosine deficiency in Ehrlich ascites tumor tRNA. Biochem Biophys Res Commun 96: 313–319

Katze JR, Farkas WR (1979) A factor in serum and amniotic fluid is a substrate for the tRNA-modifying enzyme tRNA-guanine transferase. Proc Natl Acad Sci USA 76: 3271–3275

Katze JR, Basile B, McCloskey JA (1982) Queuine, a modified base incorporated posttranscriptionally into eukaryotic tRNA: Wide distribution in nature. Science 216: 55–56

Kinoshita T, Schram KH, McCloskey JA (1981) Preparation of deuterium-labelled nucleosides by platinum-catalyzed exchange and reduction. J Label Compound Radiopharm 9: 525–534

Kleiman L, Peters S, Woodward-Jack J, Myers J (1980) Alterations in the metabolism of transfer RNA during erythroid differentiation of the Friend erythroleukemia cell. Exp Cell Res 129: 415–424

Lothrop CD, Uziel M (1981) Salvage of ribothymidine from RNA turnover. Fed Proc 40: 1763

Marini M, Mushinski JF (1979) Transfer ribonucleic acids from eleven immunoglobulin-secreting mouse plasmacytomas: constant and variable chromatographic profiles compared with the myeloma protein sequences. Biochim Biophys Acta 562: 252–270

Marini M, Muldoon WP, Mushinski JF (1979) Biochemical changes induced by tumors at distant sites: altered transfer RNA profiles in livers of mice bearing plasmacytomas. Cancer Lett 8: 177–181

Marshall MV, Adams DL, Griffin AC (1978) Regulation of an aspartyl-tRNA species in BHK cells in culture and in solid tumor form. II The effect of different sera on aspartyl-tRNA in culture. Cancer Lett 4: 147–153

McNamara AL, Smith DWE (1978) The function of the histidine tRNA isoaccepting species in hemoglobin synthesis. J Biol Chem 253: 5964–5970

Nielsen HR, Sjlin K-E, Nyholm K, Baliga BS, Wong R, Borek E (1974) β-Aminoisobutyric acid, a new probe for the metabolism of DNA and RNA in normal and tumorous tissue. Cancer Res 34: 1381–1384

Okada N, Shindo-Okada N, Sato S, Itoh YH, Oda K-I, Nishimura S (1978) Detection of unique tRNA species in tumor tissues by *Escherichia coli* guanine insertion enzyme. Proc Natl Acad Sci USA 75: 4247–4251

Okada N, Noguchi S, Kasai H, Shindo-Okada N, Ohgi T, Goto T, Nishimura S (1979) Novel mechanism of post-transcriptional modification of tRNA, insertion of bases of Q precursors into tRNA by a specific tRNA transglycosylase reaction. J Biol Chem 254: 3067–3073

Plagemann PGW, Wohlhueter RM (1980) Permeation of nucleosides, nucleic acid bases, and nucleotides in animal cells. Curr Top Membr Transp 14: 225–330

Razzaque MA, Topps JH, Kay RNB, Brockway JM (1981) Metabolism of the nucleic acids of rumen bacteria by preruminant and ruminant lambs. Br J Nutr 45: 517–527

Reyniers JP, Pleasants JR, Wostmann BS, Katze JR, Farkas WR (1981) Administration of exogenous queuine is essential for the biosynthesis of the queuosine-containing transfer RNAs in the mouse. J Biol Chem 256: 11591–11594

Roe BA, Stankiewicz AF, Rizi HL, Weisz C, Dilauro MN, Pike D, Chen CY, Chen EY (1979) Comparison of rat liver and Walker 256 carcinosarcoma tRNAs. Nucleic Acids Res 6: 673–688

Rokos H, Rokos K, Fisius H, Kirstaedter H-J (1980) Altered urinary excretion of pteridines in neoplastic disease, determination of biopterin, neopterin, and pterin. Clin Chim Acta 105: 275–286

Saleh AM, Pheasant AE, Blair JA, Allan RN (1980) The effect of malignant disease on the metabolism of pteroylglutamic acid in man. Biochem Soc Trans 8: 566–567

Schlegel RA, Iversen P, Rechsteiner M (1978) The turnover of tRNAs microinjected into animal cells. Nucleic Acids Res 5: 3715–3729

Shapot VS (1979) On the multiform relationships between the tumor and the host. Adv Cancer Res 30: 89–150

Shindo-Okada N, Okada N, Ohgi T, Nishimura S (1980) Transfer ribonucleic acid guanine transglycosylase isolated from rat liver. Biochemistry 19: 395–400

Shindo-Okada N, Terada M, Nishimura S (1981) Changes in amount of hypo-modified tRNA having guanine in place of queuine during erythroid differentiation of murine erythroleukemia cells. Eur J Biochem 115: 423–428

Smith DWE, Weinberg WC (1981) Transfer RNA in reticulocyte maturation. Biochim Biophys Acta 655: 195–198

Smith RC, Moussa NM, Hawkins GE (1974) Utilization of the nucleic acids of *Escherichia coli* and rumen bacteria by sheep. Br J Nutr 32: 529–537

Wachter H, Hausin A, Grassmayr K (1979) Erhöhte Ausscheidung von Neopterin im Harn von Patienten mit malignen Tumoren und mit Viruserkrankungen. Z Physiol Chem 360: 1957–1960

The Effects of Growth Factors on tRNA^{Lys} Modification

B. J. Ortwerth and V. K. Lin*

Departments of Ophthalmology and Biochemistry, University of Missouri,
Columbia, MO 65201, USA

Introduction

One of the more interesting questions in tRNA research is whether the redundancy of tRNA isoaccepting species has any functional meaning. Numerous reports have indicated that the distributions of these isoaccepting tRNA species are altered under different physiological conditions (Sueoka and Kano-Sueoka 1970; Littauer and Inouye 1973). The multiplicity of isoaccepting tRNA species seen in living cells suggests that these species may arise as a result of differences in base modification, which may play a role in regulating tRNA function (Agris and Söll 1977). Several laboratories have shown that RPC-5 chromatography can resolve tRNA^{Lys} into three to nine isoaccepting species (Ortwerth and Liu 1973; Juarez et al. 1974; Katze 1975). All these species, however, share only two code words, AAA and AAG (Ortwerth et al. 1973; Rudloff and Hilse 1975). One of the tRNA^{Lys} isoacceptors, tRNA$_4^{Lys}$, has been proposed as being a requirement for cell division (Ortwerth and Liu 1973). This tRNA is present in all tissues and cultured cells which have the ability to divide, but absent in tissues which have become terminally differentiated. Furthermore, the level of this tRNA correlated exactly with the doubling time of cells in culture (Conlon-Hollingshead and Ortwerth 1980). The levels of this tRNA remained high during log growth in Balb/c 3T3 cells, but decreased sharply just before the cells became confluent. Upon trypsinization and replating, the levels of this tRNA rose immediately and reached log growth levels before the cells began to divide. These alterations in tRNA^{Lys} isoacceptors may be due to the modulation of the activity of certain tRNA modification enzymes brought about by cell density, medium depletion, or serum factors.

It is clear that the serum is the controlling element in mouse 3T3 cell proliferation (Todaro et al. 1966; Holley and Kiernan 1974). Recently, trophic hormones and purified protein factors from serum or tissues have successfully replaced serum in stimulating DNA synthesis and cell proliferation in quiescent mouse 3T3 cells (Gospodarowicz and Moran 1974; Wyche and Noteboom 1977). The experiments

* The authors would like to thank Dr. Orchid Chu-Der for providing the LM-cell tRNA^{Lys} and Mary Harrison for her excellent work on the isolation of purified tRNA^{Lys} species. This work was supported in part by USPHS Grant Ca-26423 and in part by the Eye Research Foundation of Missouri, Inc.

described herein show that purified growth factors cause specific changes in several $tRNA^{Lys}$ species and that these factors appear to act at the level of $tRNA^{Lys}$ modification.

Results

Properties of $tRNA^{Lys}$ Isoacceptors

Lysine-tRNA samples isolated from Balb/c 3T3 cells have been resolved into as many as nine isoacceptors, possibly reflecting alterations in tRNA modification. A composite profile showing these species is presented in Fig. 1, with a rat liver $tRNA^{Lys}$ profile for comparison. The numbering system is that used previously (Chu-Der and Ortwerth 1980). We have isolated $tRNA_2^{Lys}$, $tRNA_4^{Lys}$, $tRNA_5^{Lys}$, and $tRNA_{5A}^{Lys}$ by RPC-5 and BD-cellulose chromatography in a manner similar to that described by Wittig et al. (1973). Each preparation was electrophoresed in a 20% polyacrylamide slab gel (Efstratiadis and Kafatos 1976); this gel is also shown in Fig. 1. $tRNA_2^{Lys}$ from mouse leukemic cells separated into two major bands. This is consistent with the $tRNA_2^{Lys}$ isolated and sequenced by Raba et al. (1979). They have shown that these two tRNAs differ by only one base pair in the anticodon stem. The same bands were seen in $tRNA_4^{Lys}$ isolated from mouse leukemic cells and faintly in $tRNA_{5A}^{Lys}$ peak. The major band in $tRNA_5^{Lys}$ electrophoresed between the two $tRNA_2^{Lys}$ bands and represents a completely different $tRNA^{Lys}$ sequence. No $tRNA_2^{Lys}$-related tRNAs were seen in the $tRNA_5^{Lys}$ from mouse leukemic cells, which is consistent with the fact that no changes have been observed in $tRNA_5^{Lys}$ during the growth of these cells (Ortwerth and Liu 1973). One and possibly two $tRNA_2^{Lys}$-related species are present in rat liver $tRNA^{Lys}$ (data not shown). This correlates with the tRNA changes during liver regeneration (Ortwerth and Liu 1973) and with the presence of an iodine-resistent $tRNA^{Lys}$ in the $tRNA_5^{Lys}$ peak from rat liver (Ortwerth and Carlson 1977). This $tRNA^{Lys}$ is designated $tRNA_{5B}^{Lys}$ in Fig. 1. These data suggest that the two species seen in $tRNA_2^{Lys}$, $tRNA_4^{Lys}$, and $tRNA_{5A}^{Lys}$ in mouse leukemic cells and in $tRNA_{5B}^{Lys}$ in rat liver represent different modified forms of the same transcripts. Surprisingly, Raba et al. (1979) were only able to demonstrate one isoacceptor under the $tRNA_4^{Lys}$ peak from SV40-transformed Balb/c 3T3 cells.

Mouse LM-cell $tRNA^{Lys}$ contains most of the species shown in Fig. 1. These cells were therefore grown in quantity and the tRNA was isolated, aminoacylated with [^{3}H]lysine, and fractionated by RPC-5 chromatography. Each of the peaks was pooled and compared for ability to bind to ribosomes in response to the lysine codons AAA and AAG. These data are shown in Table 1. $tRNA_2^{Lys}$ and $tRNA_4^{Lys}$ bind in response to AAG only, and $tRNA_5^{Lys}$ binds mainly, but not exclusively, with poly(A). These results are identical to ribosomal binding data for these species isolated from several different sources (Ortwerth et al. 1973; Rudloff and Hilse 1975). $tRNA_{5A}^{Lys}$ and $tRNA_6^{Lys}$ two late-eluting tRNAs, show coding properties very similar to those of $tRNA_5^{Lys}$. In fact, the percentage of each of these species bound in response to poly A was almost identical. In general, the ribosomal binding data presented here, along with a similar study from another laboratory (Bjercke and Hedgcoth 1981), show that the early-eluting $tRNA^{Lys}$ species all code for AAG while the late-eluting tRNAs code for AAA.

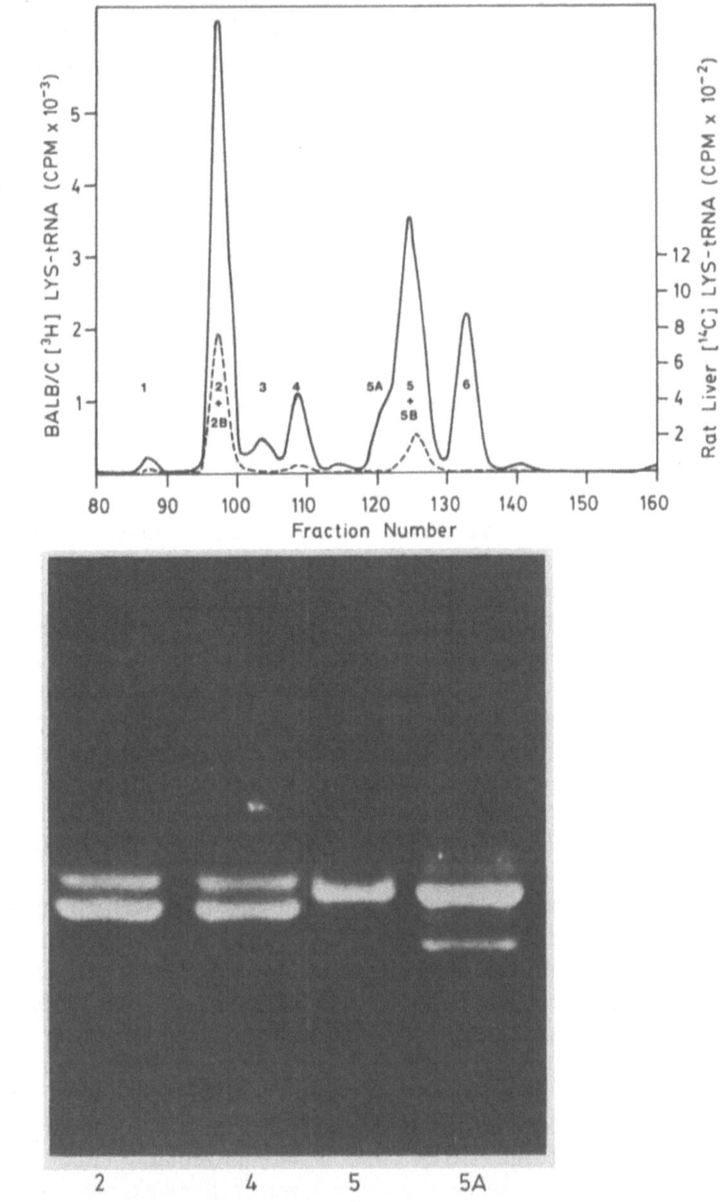

Fig. 1. Composite profile of tRNA^{Lys}. The *solid line* shows a profile of tRNA^{Lys} from Balb/c 3T3 cells which contains all of the species which we have been able to resolve by RPC-5 chromatography. The numbers above each peak represent the numbering system employed in our laboratory. The *dashed line* represents a typical RPC-5 profile of rat liver tRNA^{Lys} which is routinely included in every chromatography as a standard to aid in the identification of the various tRNA^{Lys} species

Previous results from our laboratory showed that tRNA^{Lys} was able to incorporate lysine into protein in a rat liver system. Recently Hatfield et al. (1980) were able to compare the relative utilization of tRNA$_2^{Lys}$ and tRNA$_4^{Lys}$ in globin synthesis. In their system, tRNA$_4^{Lys}$ was utilized only 35% as well as tRNA$_2^{Lys}$. We have compared the

Table 1. Binding of LM-cell lysyl-tRNAs to *Escherichia coli* ribosomes

Input	Codon	cpm bound	Δ cpm bound	Percent bound
$tRNA_2^{lys}$	poly A	7,200	0	0
33,500 cpm	AAG	21,200	13,200	39.4
	–	8,000		
$tRNA_4^{lys}$	poly A	8,000	0	0
34,300 cpm	AAG	12,200	3,100	9.0
	–	9,100		
$tRNA_{5A}^{lys}$	poly A	10,300	3,700	19.0
19,700 cpm	AAG	6,300	0	0
	–	6,600		
$tRNA_5^{lys}$	poly A	27,500	6,800	19.0
34,900 cpm	AAG	22,200	1,500	4.3
	–	20,700		
$tRNA_6^{lys}$	poly A	8,700	5,200	20.0
25,900 cpm	AAG	4,500	1,000	3.9
	–	3,500		

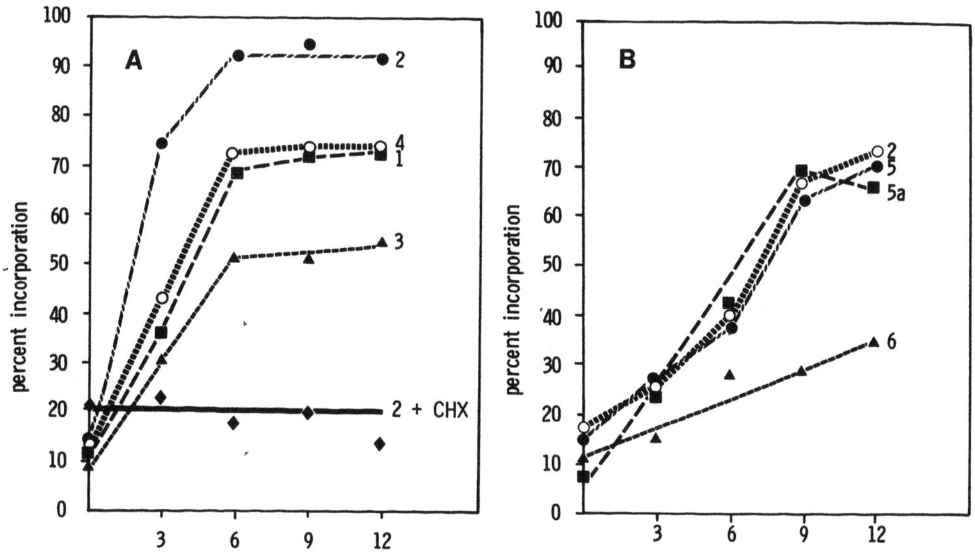

Fig. 2A, B. The relative ability of several tRNA^{Lys} species to incorporate lysine into protein. **A** The incorporation from the early-eluting, AAG-coding tRNA^{Lys} species into protein. *CHX* indicates the incorporation from [^{3}H]Lys-tRNA$_2$ in the presence of 100 μg/ml cycloheximide. **B** The incorporation from the late-eluting, AAA-coding tRNA^{Lys} species with $tRNA_2^{Lys}$ included as a control. *Ordinate values* are percent incorporation, which was determined by comparing hot TCA precipitable counts to cold TCA precipitable counts by the filter-paper disc method of Mans and Novelli (1961): 100% incorporation varied from 3×10^3 to 8×10^3 cpm/aliquot. Precharged tRNA^{Lys} species were obtained from an RPC-5 chromatographic separation of a [^{3}H]Lys-tRNA preparation from mouse LM cells. Incorporation into protein was measured in a reticulocyte lysate (Crystal et al. 1974) supplemented with GTP, a creatine kinase ATP regenerating system, and 0.3 μmol cold lysine to prevent recharging of any released [^{3}H]lysine

incorporation of lysine into globin from a variety of $tRNA^{Lys}$ species. Several time points were taken and the rate of incorporation from each species is shown in Fig. 2. Panel A shows that all the $tRNA^{Lys}$ species from LM cells were able to incorporate lysine into protein. Incorporation was very rapid with $tRNA_2^{Lys}$, with 90% of the input [^{3}H]lysine being transferred into hot TCA precipitable material in 6 min. The protein synthesis inhibitor cycloheximide prevented this incorporation. $tRNA_4^{Lys}$ and $tRNA_1^{Lys}$, both incorporated lysine at a somewhat slower rate than $tRNA_2^{Lys}$, whereas incorporation from $tRNA_3^{Lys}$ was very poor. This experiment was also carried out with the late-eluting $tRNA^{Lys}$ species, and these results are shown in panel B of Fig. 2. Incorporation from $tRNA_5^{Lys}$ and $tRNA_{5A}^{Lys}$ was less rapid, but this reflected the activity of the reticulocyte lysate, since $tRNA_2^{Lys}$ showed similar incorporation kinetics. $tRNA_6^{Lys}$ showed very little ability to transfer lysine into protein. Therefore, those $tRNA^{Lys}$ species which are increased in tissue culture cells are all less efficient in protein synthesis, with the single exception of $tRNA_{5A}^{Lys}$. Raba et al. (1979) have reported that $tRNA_4^{Lys}$ is an undermodified form of $tRNA_2^{Lys}$ and it is possible that perhaps all of these new species arise due to incomplete modification, which would be consistent with their reduced protein synthesis activity. Similar results have also been recently obtained by Bjercke and Hedgcoth (1981).

Growth Factors and $tRNA^{Lys}$ Profiles

Of all the species shown in Fig. 1, only the levels of $tRNA_4^{Lys}$ seem to correlate with cell proliferation (Conlon-Hollingshead and Ortwerth 1980). Whenever cells were treated in a manner which inhibited cell division there was a decrease in $tRNA_4^{Lys}$ occurring prior to the inhibition of proliferation. This decrease in $tRNA_4^{Lys}$ was always accompanied by a quantitative increase in another $tRNA^{Lys}$ species. There was an increase in $tRNA_2^{Lys}$ in mouse leukemic cells (Ortwerth and Liu 1973), in 3T3 cells at confluency, and in Balb/c 3T3 cells in serum-starved medium (Conlon-Hollingshead and Ortwerth 1980). An increase in $tRNA_3^{Lys}$ was seen in confluent LM cells (Chu-Der and Ortwerth 1980), whereas either $tRNA_5^{Lys}$ or $tRNA_6^{Lys}$ increased in confluent Balb/c 3T3 cells and in Balb/c 3T3 cells placed in medium containing calf plasma instead of fetal calf serum (Ortwerth et al. 1982). One interpretation of these data is that each of these tRNAs represents a different intermediate in a given $tRNA^{Lys}$ biosynthetic pathway.

It has long been recognized that serum contains several protein growth factors which are required for cell proliferation. These growth factors are being identified and isolated, and several media have been designed where serum can be completely replaced by purified growth factors and hormones (Wyche and Noteboom 1977; Hutchings and Sato 1978). Recent work has shown that two different types of growth factor are present in serum. These are competence factors, which are believed to move cells from G_0 to G_1 and make them competent to move through the cell cycle (Scher et al. 1979), and progression factors, which are required for cells to progress through G_1 and initiate DNA synthesis (Stiles et al. 1979). We felt that it was possible that these factors could act by controlling different modification reactions necessary for $tRNA_4^{Lys}$ synthesis. This was tested by growing Balb/c 3T3 cells in medium containing 10% plasma in place of 10% fetal calf serum, since plasma has been reported to be deficient in competence factors (Stiles et al. 1979). As predicted, the growth of Balb/c 3T3 cells was inhibited by the plasma-containing medium. The cell number continued to

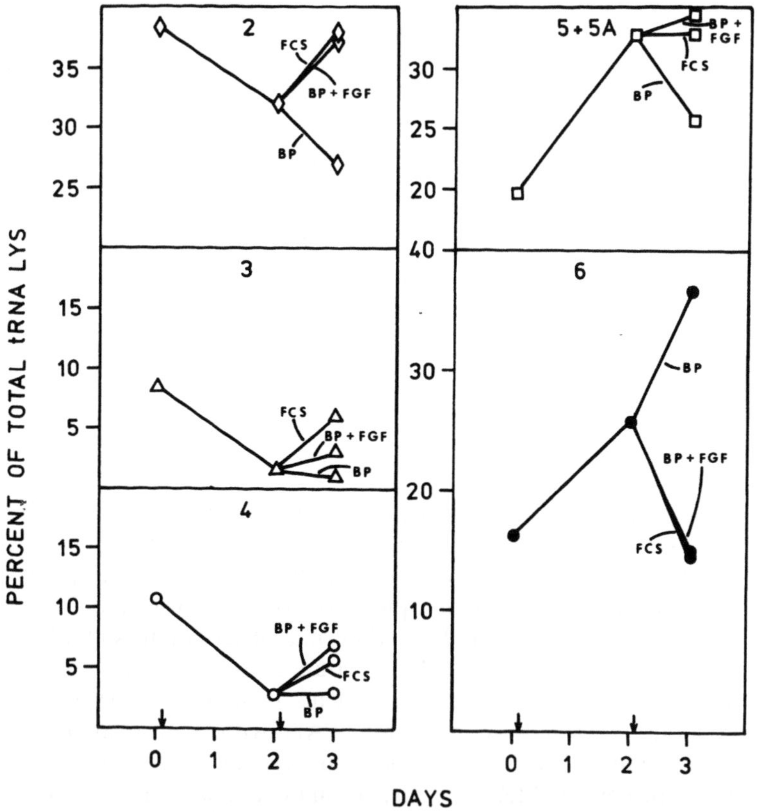

Fig. 3. Changes in the RPC-5 chromatographic profile of [^{3}H]Lys-tRNA isolated from Balb/c 3T3 cells in response to fetal calf serum (FCS), bovine plasma (BP), and BP plus FGF. Cells were plated in Dulbecco's modified Eagle's medium (DME) with 10% FCS and transferred to medium with 10% BP at day 0. After 2 days, the medium was changed to medium containing 10% BP, 10% BP plus 10 µg/ml FGF, or 10% FCS for an additional day. At each point tRNA was isolated, aminoacylated, and fractionated by RPC-5 chromatography as described previously (Conlon-Hollingshead and Ortwerth 1980)

increase for 24 h, but remained relatively constant over the next 3 days, even if new plasma-containing medium was supplied. An increase in cell number did occur, however, if the plasma-containing medium was replaced with medium containing either 10% fetal calf serum or 10% plasma and 10 µg/ml fibroblast growth factor (FGF). No increase was seen at 24 h, but the cells doubled between 24 and 48 h (data not shown). The changes in the tRNA^{Lys} profile during this experiment are shown in Fig. 3. After 48 h in the plasma-containing medium, there was a marked decrease in tRNA$_2^{Lys}$, tRNA$_3^{Lys}$, and tRNA$_4^{Lys}$ and an increase in tRNA$_5^{Lys}$ and tRNA$_6^{Lys}$. These changes continued during the next 24 h, with tRNA$_6^{Lys}$ increasing to 37% of the total tRNA^{Lys} profile. When the cells were placed in medium with either 10% fetal calf serum or 10% bovine plasma with FGF, the tRNA^{Lys} profile returned to normal. tRNA$_6^{Lys}$ decreased sharply, the decrease in tRNA$_5^{Lys}$ was prevented, and tRNA$_2^{Lys}$, tRNA$_3^{Lys}$, and tRNA$_4^{Lys}$ all increased. These data are consistent with an alteration in tRNA^{Lys} modification in which the absence of competence factors causes a block in

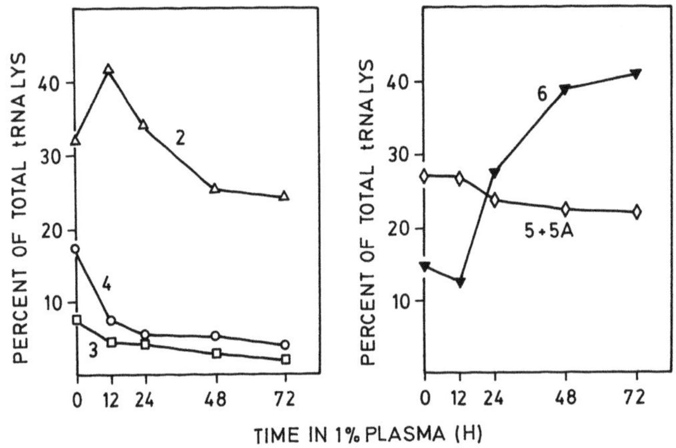

Fig. 4. Time course of tRNA^{Lys} changes in Balb/c 3T3 cells transferred to 1% BP. Cells were grown in DME with 10% FCS and then shifted to DME with 1% BP at day 0. tRNA^{Lys} profiles were determined at several points over the next 72 h

tRNA^{Lys} modification, leading to a build-up of tRNA$_5^{Lys}$ and tRNA$_6^{Lys}$. The addition of FGF appears to release this block, allowing tRNA$_2^{Lys}$, tRNA$_3^{Lys}$, and tRNA$_4^{Lys}$ to be synthesized. While many other interpretations are certainly possible, we were encouraged to believe that a pure growth factor was able to alter the distribution of tRNA^{Lys} species in vivo. Two additional observations should be pointed out: (1) the FGF-induced increase in tRNA$_4^{Lys}$ could be seen at 24 h, before there was an increase in cell numbers; and (2) calf plasma caused an increase in species which we have shown in mouse LM cells to code for AAA with a corresponding decrease in all the AAG-coding species. These data suggest an alteration in the anticodon loop.

The time course of tRNA^{Lys} alteration in bovine plasma medium is shown in Fig. 4. In this experiment, the Balb/c 3T3 cells were transferred from medium with 10% fetal calf serum to medium containing 1% plasma. Two different changes were seen. At 12 h, there was a sharp decrease in tRNA$_4^{Lys}$ with a corresponding increase in tRNA$_2^{Lys}$. Little or no change in the other isoacceptors was seen at this time. With continued incubation in the 1% plasma medium there was a gradual decrease in tRNA$_2^{Lys}$ and an increase in tRNA$_6^{Lys}$. The other species also decreased slightly. In similar experiments there was an early increase in tRNA$_5^{Lys}$, but this increase disappeared later as tRNA$_6^{Lys}$ increased. If tRNA$_6^{Lys}$ was not present in the cells originally, the entire increase occurred in the tRNA$_5^{Lys}$ peak. Despite a considerable number of experiments we have not been able to determine when tRNA$_6^{Lys}$ will be present in a given Balb/c tRNA^{Lys} profile; however, it is routinely observed in HeLa and mouse LM cells.

Cells arrested in calf plasma medium were also stimulated to proliferate by the addition of purified platelet-derived growth factor (PDGF), but insulin and hydrocortisone had little or no effect on either growth rate or tRNA^{Lys} profiles (data not shown). The effects of PDGF on tRNA^{Lys} profiles are shown in Fig. 5. Balb/c 3T3 cells were plated, shifted to 1% calf plasma medium for 48 h, and treated with various levels of PDGF. The cells were maintained for 24 h in the PDGF-containing medium and tRNA^{Lys} profiles were determined. Figure 5 shows tRNA^{Lys} changes similar to those seen previously with FGF. As PDGF levels were increased, tRNA$_6^{Lys}$ levels decreased, with increases in the other tRNA^{Lys} species. Low levels of PDGF caused a 10% decrease in tRNA$_6^{Lys}$ with little change in tRNA$_4^{Lys}$. Higher concentrations of PDGF appeared to be necessary to show an increase in tRNA$_4^{Lys}$. This correlates with the previous data (Fig. 4), which showed that tRNA$_4^{Lys}$ decreased rapidly when the

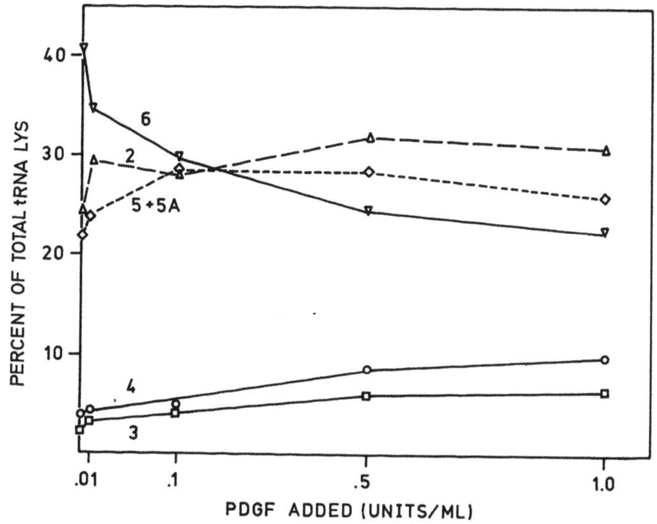

Fig. 5. The effect of increasing concentrations of PDGF on the tRNA^{Lys} profile of Balb/c 3T3 tRNA. Cells were grown in DME with 10% FCS and shifted to DME with 1% BP for 48 h. The medium was then changed to DME with 1% BP containing various levels of PDGF. After 24 h in these media the tRNA was isolated and the tRNA^{Lys} profile was determined

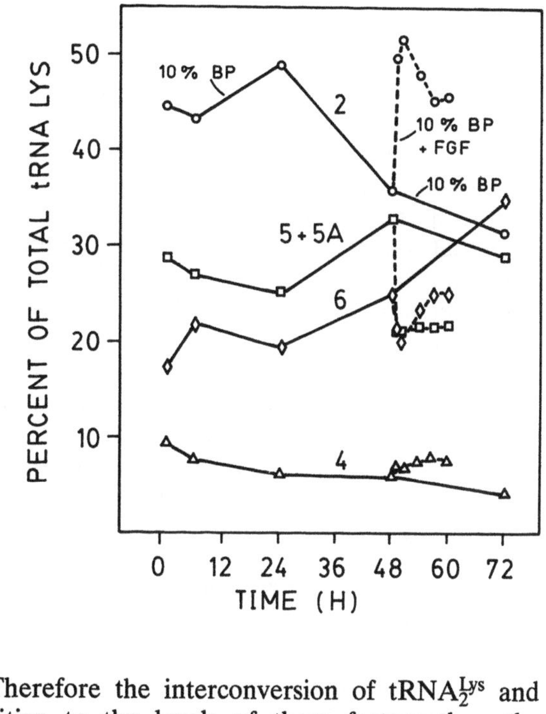

Fig. 6. Time course of the tRNA^{Lys} changes in response to FGF. Balb/c 3T3 cells were grown in DME with 10% FCS and shifted to DME with 10% BP at time zero. tRNA^{Lys} profiles were determined at 0, 6, 24, 48, and 72 h in the BP medium. After 48 h the medium was changed to DME with 10% BP and 20 ng/ml FGF and tRNA^{Lys} profiles were determined at 1, 2, 6, 9, and 12 h. The *solid lines* represent cells in 10% BP only, the *dashed lines* represent cells in 10% BP plus FGF

cells were placed in calf plasma. Therefore the interconversion of tRNA$_2^{Lys}$ and tRNA$_4^{Lys}$ appears to be more sensitive to the levels of these factors than the interconversion of tRNA$_6^{Lys}$ and tRNA$_2^{Lys}$.

The data presented here are consistent with a sequence of tRNA^{Lys} modification reactions which are limiting under certain cell growth conditions and cause certain tRNA^{Lys} species to accumulate. This sequence could be controlled by inhibiting certain modification enzymes or alternatively tRNA^{Lys} synthesis could increase with a constant, limiting amount of modification enzymes. An experiment to distinguish these possibilities is shown in Fig. 6. The design is similar to the previous experiments.

Balb/c 3T3 cells were grown in medium with fetal calf serum and then transferred to medium with 10% plasma. After 48 h in this medium, purified FGF was added to one set of dishes and tRNA was isolated at 1, 2, 6, 9, and 12 h in order to measure the rate at which the $tRNA^{Lys}$ profile became altered. When the cells were shifted to 10% plasma, the same changes occurred as shown in Fig. 4 for cells in 1% plasma; however, the changes did not occur as rapidly. $tRNA_2^{Lys}$, $tRNA_3^{Lys}$, and $tRNA_4^{Lys}$ decreased as $tRNA_5^{Lys}$ increased. $tRNA_6^{Lys}$ did not increase until late in the experiment. The addition of FGF caused an immediate and significant alteration in the $tRNA^{Lys}$ profile. Both $tRNA_5^{Lys}$ and $tRNA_6^{Lys}$ decreased, with a large increase in $tRNA_2^{Lys}$ and a small increase in $tRNA_4^{Lys}$. These data are what one would predict if the FGF was affecting the activity of a specific $tRNA^{Lys}$ modification enzyme. The simplest interpretation of the data is that FGF results in a stimulation of the enzyme which catalyzes the conversion of $tRNA_6^{Lys}$ and a $tRNA^{Lys}$ species in the $tRNA_5^{Lys}$ peak (presumably $tRNA_{5B}^{Lys}$) to $tRNA_2^{Lys}$. Several other mechanisms could give rise to the same results; however, it is unlikely one could generate these data by controlling $tRNA^{Lys}$ transcription rates alone. Therefore it appears likely that FGF can act to modulate the activity of a specific $tRNA^{Lys}$ modification enzyme.

Discussion

Our efforts to describe the events which control $tRNA_4^{Lys}$ levels in tissue culture cells have shown that a variety of $tRNA^{Lys}$ isoacceptors are present in cultured cells which have quantitative and reciprocal relationships with $tRNA_4^{Lys}$. Five different $tRNA^{Lys}$ peaks seem to be involved: $tRNA_2^{Lys}$, $tRNA_3^{Lys}$, $tRNA_4^{Lys}$, $tRNA_{5B}^{Lys}$, and $tRNA_6^{Lys}$. These isoacceptors designate RPC-5 peaks, but each of these peaks appears to contain two or more species. In previous work we have suggested that these tRNA species represent intermediates in a $tRNA^{Lys}$ modification pathway. Confluent Balb/c cells contained increased levels of $tRNA_5^{Lys}$ (presumably $tRNA_{5B}^{Lys}$) and $tRNA_6^{Lys}$ and decreased levels of $tRNA_2^{Lys}$, $tRNA_3^{Lys}$, and $tRNA_4^{Lys}$. Essentially identical results were seen in subconfluent Balb/c 3T3 cultures in plasma-containing medium. Both cultures should represent cells in G_0 phase. The $tRNA^{Lys}$ changes suggest that both cultures are altered in $tRNA^{Lys}$ modification. This conclusion is supported by the rapid loss of $tRNA_5^{Lys}$ and $tRNA_6^{Lys}$ and increase in $tRNA_2^{Lys}$ brought about by the addition of FGF or PDGF to cells in calf plasma. These changes would appear to be much too rapid to represent a stimulation in total $tRNA_2^{Lys}$ transcription with a corresponding loss of $tRNA_5^{Lys}$ by turnover. This could also be explained, however, by activation of a processing enzyme or rapid release of a precursor from the nucleus which overloads a limiting step in $tRNA^{Lys}$ biosynthesis. Proof of the existence of a pathway must await precursor-product studies and tRNA sequence and modified base analyses on the various $tRNA^{Lys}$ species.

It is also premature to consider that the conversion of $tRNA_5^{Lys}$ to $tRNA_2^{Lys}$ in Fig. 6 represents a single reaction. When the FGF was added, all the other medium components and factors were at optimal levels. Therefore, the product of the FGF-stimulated reaction could be rapidly modified to the mature species, $tRNA_2^{Lys}$. The fact that $tRNA_4^{Lys}$ did not reach higher levels may be due to the fact that the cells were 50% confluent at the time the FGF was added. At this cell density, $tRNA_4^{Lys}$ synthesis may be restricted by contact inhibition. It could also be argued that the levels of FGF were insufficient to stimulate $tRNA_4^{Lys}$ levels, since the experiment with PDGF (Fig. 5) showed that high concentrations of growth factor were required to show increases in $tRNA_4^{Lys}$. To resolve the exact reaction(s) stimulated by FGF a cell system will be needed where other serum components are absent or depleted. Cell lines which remain viable in very low serum or in serum-free medium have been tested, but in these cases $tRNA_4^{Lys}$ levels appeared constitutive and remained high under all conditions. The same fact is true for transformed cells. Therefore, the $tRNA^{Lys}$ changes described here may be characteristic for contact-inhibited cells only. Cells which have lowered or no serum requirements appear to have lost the need for serum growth factors, and in these cases the modification enzymes are no longer controllable and $tRNA_4^{Lys}$ becomes a constitutive isoacceptor.

We have shown a rapid alteration in $tRNA^{Lys}$ isoacceptors in response to a pure polypeptide growth factor. A specific tRNA modification enzyme appears to be stimulated but the extent to which this event is linked to FGF binding to the cell is not known. We are encouraged by the fact that this FGF-mediated reaction is capable of controlling the levels of $tRNA_4^{Lys}$. It must be pointed out, however, that as yet there is no evidence that $tRNA_4^{Lys}$ has any direct role in controlling cell proliferation. Such a model, though, would be consistent with the cell hybridization studies of Rao et al. (1977), which led them to conclude that cell division is controlled by a single cytoplasmic molecule, and with recent work by Smith and Stiles (1981) which suggests that competence factors act by stimulating the formation of a stable RNA species.

Summary

The $tRNA^{Lys}$ population from tissue culture cells contains several isoaccepting species which are not present in the $tRNA^{Lys}$ population from tissue sources. These isoacceptors were isolated from mouse LM cells and tested for their coding properties in ribosomal binding assays and their ability to incorporate lysine into protein in a reticulocyte lysate. $tRNA_{5A}^{Lys}$ and $tRNA_6^{Lys}$ eluted in the area of $tRNA_5^{Lys}$. All three species coded preferentially for AAA and bound with equal efficiency. $tRNA_1^{Lys}$, $tRNA_3^{Lys}$, $tRNA_4^{Lys}$, and $tRNA_6^{Lys}$ all transferred lysine into protein at a slower rate than $tRNA_2^{Lys}$ and $tRNA_5^{Lys}$, which are the native species.

Several purified growth factors were tested for their ability to affect the levels of $tRNA_4^{Lys}$, a tRNA possibly associated with cell division. When Balb/c 3T3 cells were grown in medium containing plasma instead of serum, there was a decrease in $tRNA_2^{Lys}$, $tRNA_3^{Lys}$, and $tRNA_4^{Lys}$ and an increase in $tRNA_5^{Lys}$ and $tRNA_6^{Lys}$. The addition of either FGF or PDGF returned the $tRNA^{Lys}$ profile to normal. The extent of the $tRNA^{Lys}$ changes depended upon the concentration of growth factor added. FGF was able to cause a 35% decrease in the $tRNA_5^{Lys}$ peak with a corresponding increase in $tRNA_2^{Lys}$ within 1 h of the addition of the factor. These data suggest that competence factors have the ability to stimulate the modification of specific $tRNA^{Lys}$ isoacceptors.

References

Agris PF, Söll D (1977) The modified nucleosides in transfer RNA. In: Vogel HJ (ed) Nucleic acid-protein recognition. Academic Press, New York London, pp 321–344

Bjercke RJ, Hedgcoth C (1981) Codon binding and translational properties of isoaccepting lysine tRNA peculiar to virus-transformed cells. MGG 183: 528–531

Chu-Der OMY, Ortwerth BJ (1980) Lys-tRNA and cell division. Changes in lys-tRNA during the growth of mouse LM cells. Exp Cell Res 128: 159–170

Conlon-Hollingshead C, Ortwerth BJ (1980) Lys-$tRNA_4$ levels and cell division in mouse 3T3 cells. Exp Cell Res 128: 171–180

Crystal RG, Elson NA, Anderson WF (1974) Initiation of globin synthesis : assays. In: Moldave K, Grossman L (eds) Methods in enzymology, XXX part F. Academic Press, New York London, pp 101–123

Efstratiadis A, Kafatos FC (1976) The chorion of insects. Methods Mol Biol 8: 58–65

Gospodarowicz D, Moran JS (1974) Stimulation of division of sparse and confluent 3T3 cell population by a fibroblast growth factor, dexamethasone and insulin. Proc Natl Acad Sci USA 71: 4584–4588

Hatfield DY, Richer L, Lyon J, Rice M (1980) Relative utilization of mammalian lys-tRNA isoacceptors in protein synthesis. FEBS Lett 113: 249–252

Holley RW, Kiernan JA (1974) Control of the initiation of DNA synthesis in 3T3 cells: serum factors. Proc Natl Acad Sci USA 71: 2908–2911

Hutchings SE, Sato GH (1978) Growth and maintenance of HeLa cells in serum-free medium supplemented with hormones. Proc Natl Acad Sci USA 75: 901–905

Juarez H, Juarez D, Hedgcoth C (1974) Seven lysine isoaccepting tRNA's from polyoma virus-transformed cells. Biochem Biophys Res Commun 61: 110–116

Katze JR (1975) Relation of cell type and cell density to the degree of post-transcriptional modification of $tRNA^{Lys}$ and $tRNA^{phe}$. Biochim Biophys Acta 407: 392–398

Littauer UZ, Inouye H (1973) Regulation of tRNA. Annu Rev Biochem 42: 439–470

Mans RJ, Novelli GD (1961) Measurement of the incorporation of radioactive amino acids into protein by a filter paper disc method. Arch Biochem Biophys 94: 48–57

Ortwerth BJ, Carlson JV (1977) Lysine transfer RNA from liver: A sulfur-containing species that codes for AAG. Arch Biochem Biophys 178: 278–284

Ortwerth BJ, Liu LP (1973) Correlation between a specific isoaccepting lysyl transfer ribonucleic acid and cell division in mammalian tissues. Biochemistry 12: 3978–3984

Ortwerth BJ, Yonuschot GR, Carlson JV (1973) Properties of $tRNA_4^{lys}$ from various tissues. Biochemistry 12: 3985–3991

Ortwerth BJ, Wolters J, Nahlik J, Conlon-Hollingshead C (1982) Cell growth and $tRNA_4^{Lys}$ synthesis in Mouse 3T3 cells. Exp Cell Res 138: 241–250

Raba M, Limburg K, Burghagen M, Katze JR, Simsek M, Heckman JE, Rajbhandary UL, Gross JH (1979) Nucleotide sequence of three isoaccepting lysine-tRNAs from rabbit liver and SV40-transformed mouse fibroblasts. Eur J Biochem 97: 305–318

Rao PN, Sunkara PS, Wilson BA (1977) Regulation of DNA synthesis: Age-dependent cooperation among G_1 cells upon fusion. Proc Natl Acad Sci USA 74: 2869–2873

Rudloff E, Hilse K (1975) Properties of isoaccepting $tRNA^{lys}$, $tRNA^{glu}$ and $tRNA^{gln}$ from rabbit reticulocytes and liver. Multiplicity, codon recognition and inactivation by iodine. Hoppe Seylers Z Physiol Chem 356: 1359–1367

Scher CD, Stone ME, Stiles CD (1979) Platelet-derived growth factor prevents G_0 growth arrest. Nature 281: 390–392

Smith JC, Stiles CD (1981) Cytoplasmic transfer of the mitogenic response to platelet-derived growth factor. Proc Natl Acad Sci USA 78: 4363–4367

Stiles CD, Capone GT, Scher CD, Antonaides HN, Van Wyk JJ, Pledger WJ (1979) Dual control of cell growth by somatomedins and platelet-derived growth factor. Proc Natl Acad Sci USA 76: 1279–1283

Sueoka N, Kano-Sueoka T (1970) Transfer RNA and cell differentiation. Prog Nucleic Acid Res Mol Biol 10: 23–55

Todaro GJ, Lazar GK, Green H (1966) The initiation of cell division in a contact-inhibited mammalian cell line. J Cell Comp Physiol 66: 325–334

Wittig B, Reuter S, Gottschling H (1973) Purification of the four lysine-specific transfer ribonucleic acids from chick embryos. Biochim Biophys Acta 331: 221–230

Wyche JH, Noteboom WD (1977) Requirement of a specific factor for the multiplication of ovarian cells in serum-free medium. Exp Cell Res 110: 135–141

*Perturbation of the Mitochondrial Lysine tRNA Population by Virus-Induced Transformation or Stress of Mammalian Cells: Functional Properties and Nucleotide Sequence of a Mitochondrially Associated Lysine tRNA**

C. Hedgcoth[1] K. Hayenga[1] K. Scheets[1] K. R. Thomas[1]
M. Harrison[2] V. K. Lin[2] and B. J. Ortwerth[2]

[1] Department of Biochemistry, Kansas State University, Manhattan, KS 66506, USA; [2] Departments of Biochemistry and Ophthalmology, University of Missouri, Columbia, MO 65201, USA

Introduction

Depending on the source of mammalian cells and their growth state, 11 isoaccepting tRNAs for lysine can be demonstrated by RPC-5 chromatography or in combination with polyacrylamide gel electrophoresis. A composite profile illustrating these isoacceptors is shown in Fig. 1. The isoacceptors 1, 2, 5a, and 5 are observed in tRNA preparations from most mammalian tissues with insignificant variations from tissue to tissue. In contrast, $tRNA_4^{Lys}$ is present in greater amounts in growing cells than in resting cells (Ortwerth and Liu 1973; Juarez et al. 1975). Variations in amounts of $tRNA_4^{Lys}$ are correlated with the ability of cells to divide, and the isoacceptor was proposed as a requirement for cell division (Ortwerth 1971). It is not detectable in permanently differentiated tissues. The level of $tRNA_4^{Lys}$ is directly related to the doubling time of cells and drops sharply just prior to confluency (Conlon-Hollingshead and Ortwerth 1980; Katze 1975; Ortwerth 1971). Isoacceptors 2b, 3, 4a, 4b, and 5b are not observed routinely, either because of their presence in small amounts and cochromatography with other isoacceptors or because they occur only in certain tissues. $tRNA_{4a}^{Lys}$ is not shown in the profile, but it elutes with $tRNA_4^{Lys}$. $tRNA_6^{Lys}$ occurs in some cell lines transformed by viruses; polyoma-virus-transformed 3T3 and Balb/3T3 (Jacobson et al. 1974), murine sarcoma virus transformed Balb/3T3 (Hedgcoth et al. 1980a, b), and Rous-sarcoma-virus-transformed NRK (C. Hedgcoth, K. Scheets, and S. Allen, unpublished results). This isoacceptor has also been observed in some cell lines not known to be transformed by viruses (Chu-Der and Ortwerth 1980).

The large number of isoaccepting tRNAs for a family of only two codons and the cell sources and variations of some of the species have led to studies of the structures and functional characteristics of the lysine isoacceptors. The sequences of $tRNA_2^{Lys}$, $tRNA_{2b}^{Lys}$, and $tRNA_5^{Lys}$ from rabbit liver and $tRNA_4^{Lys}$ from SV40-transformed Balb/3T3 are known (Raba et al. 1979). We shall present results on functional properties, cellular location, and the nucleotide sequence of $tRNA_6^{Lys}$.

* This work was supported by grants CA12741 (to C.H.) and CA26423 (to B.J.O.) from the National Cancer Institute, HHS, the Eye Research Foundation of Missouri, Inc., and the Kansas Agricultural Experiment Station

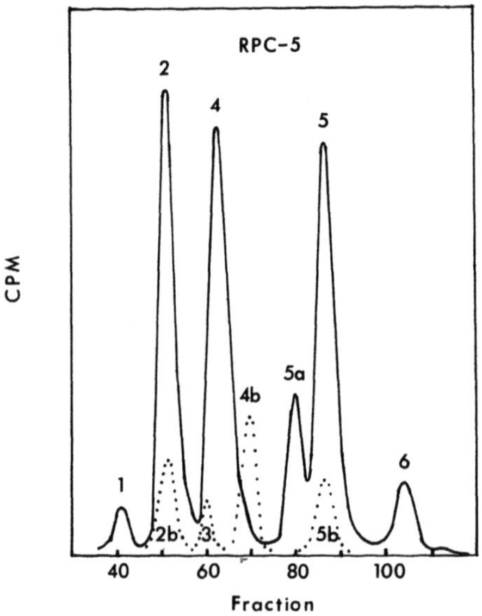

Fig. 1. Composite RPC-5 profiles of isoacceptors of $tRNA^{Lys}$

Codon-Binding and Translational Properties of $tRNA_6^{Lys}$

The codon-binding responses of the six separable isoaccepting lysine tRNAs from PY3T3 cells were studied (Bjercke and Hedgcoth 1981) in a ribosomal binding system prepared with *Escherichia coli* ribosomes (Nirenberg and Leder 1964) and using the trinucleotides AAA and AAG. As reported by others (Ortwerth et al. 1973; Rudloff and Hilse 1971), $tRNA_2^{Lys}$ and $tRNA_4^{Lys}$ are highly specific for AAG and our data include $tRNA_1^{Lys}$ in this group as well (Table 1). $tRNA_5^{Lys}$ and $tRNA_{5a}^{Lys}$ bind preferentially to AAA by a factor of about 2, and $tRNA_6^{Lys}$ appears to have an even stronger preference for AAA. On the other hand, part of the response of species 5a and 5 to AAG may be a result of contamination by $tRNA_{5b}^{Lys}$, which responds to AAG (Ortwerth and Carlson 1977). With respect to relative binding, $tRNA_6^{Lys}$ binds only about 25% as much as the other isoacceptors. The codon-binding response of $tRNA_5^{Lys}$ is in agreement with that reported earlier (Ortwerth et al. 1973).

Functional abilities of the isoacceptors in protein synthesis were compared in a wheat germ translational system with TMV RNA as messenger. Ribosomes and a crude enzyme fraction from wheat germ were prepared (Marcu and Dudock 1974) with additional washing of ribosomes (Marcus 1972) and by passing the supernatant solution from a centrifugation at 150,000 *g* through DEAE cellulose to remove endogenous tRNA (Sharma et al. 1975). The assay was done essentially according to Marcu and Dudock (1976).

The isoacceptors function reasonably well in translation (Table 2) with the exception of $tRNA_6^{Lys}$, which is only 14%–24% as effective as the other isoacceptors (Bjercke and Hedgcoth 1981).

All of the isoaccepting lysine tRNAs, including $tRNA_6^{Lys}$, aminoacylate well in vitro with lysyl-tRNA ligase from either mammalian sources or *E. coli*. The results of the in vitro translation experiments, however, raised the question of the functional ability of $tRNA_6^{Lys}$ in vivo.

Table 1. Binding of lysyl-tRNA to *E. coli* ribosomes

Input $tRNA^{lys}$	Triplet added	Lysyl-tRNA bound (fmol)	Binding ratio AAA/AAG
1	AAA	10.4	1/4.7
	AAG	48.6	
2	AAA	1	1/47.5
	AAG	47.5	
4	AAA	1.36	1/28.5
	AAG	40.0	
5a	AAA	13.1	1.6/1
	AAG	8.37	
5	AAA	36.6	2.4/1
	AAG	15.4	
6	AAA	22.4	3/1
	AAG	7.47	

Assays were performed with [^{3}H]lysyl-tRNA, and data were corrected for binding in the absence of either triplet. The input amount of each isoacceptor was 113 fmol. The total number of determinations varied from three to eight depending on the isoacceptor

Table 2. Utilization in protein synthesis in vitro in a wheat germ system of isoaccepting lysyl-tRNAs in response to TMV RNA

Input $tRNA^{lys}$	[^{3}H]Lysine incorporated (fmol)	Relative utilization (%)
1	20.6	61
2	30.2	90
4	25.5	75
5a	19.2	57
5	33.8	100
6	4.6	14

Data are corrected for incorporation in the absence of TMV RNA. The input amount of each isoacceptor was 113 fmol. The total number of determinations varied from 7 to 13 depending on the isoacceptor used

Aminoacylation In Vivo and In Vitro of Lysine Isoaccepting tRNAs

The level of aminoacylation in vivo of the lysine isoacceptors was determined with KA31 cells in Dulbecco's modified Eagle's minimum essential medium buffered for growth without a CO_2 incubator in 10% calf serum (Hedgcoth et al. 1980a, b). The level of lysine was lowered to that used in Eagle's minimum essential medium and the medium was adjusted to 10 µCi/ml in [^{3}H]lysine (75 Ci/mmol). Experiments were done with cells prior to confluency where rapid growth is occurring and after the transformed cells reached a heavy growth state where growth is tapering off, probably due to high levels of acid in the medium and rapid depletion of essential components. The times for labeling were 0.5, 1, 2, and 3 h. Isolation of tRNA under conditions preserving the aminoacyl linkage and RPC-5 chromatography revealed typical amounts of the isoacceptors 1, 2, 4, 5a, and 5 for the respective growth state. The results for $tRNA_6^{Lys}$ were striking. For labeling periods of 2 h or less $tRNA_6^{Lys}$ was not labeled, regardless of the degree of confluency of the cell monolayer. For each labeling period, a sample of the isolated [^{3}H]lysyl-tRNA was aminoacylated in vitro to serve as a control on the actual presence or absence of $tRNA_6^{Lys}$ in the preparation; it was present in all preparations. When cells were labeled for 3 h, $tRNA_6^{Lys}$ also appeared aminoacylated in vivo, although not to the full extent.

The appearance of [^{3}H]lysine in $tRNA_6^{Lys}$ takes longer than for the other isoacceptors, and endogenous unlabeled lysyl-$tRNA_6^{Lys}$ is not fully exchanged for [^{3}H]lysyl-$tRNA_6^{Lys}$ in labeling periods up to 3 h. Possible explanations for these findings include defective functioning of $tRNA_6^{Lys}$ in vivo with a correspondingly slow turnover of attached lysine or a sequestered or compartmented state of $tRNA_6^{Lys}$.

An additional result from these experiments is the observation that $tRNA_4^{Lys}$ is aminoacylated in vivo to the same extent as when isolated tRNA is aminoacylated: a large proportion of lysyl-$tRNA^{Lys}$ in dividing cells is in the form of lysyl-$tRNA_4^{Lys}$, whereas in slowly dividing or nondividing cells, lysyl-$tRNA_4^{Lys}$, in vivo, is only a small proportion of total lysyl-$tRNA^{Lys}$. This adds support to the importance of $tRNA_4^{Lys}$ in cell division (Ortwerth and Liu 1973) by demonstrating that results from aminoacylating this isoacceptor in vitro accurately reflect the situation in vivo.

Subcellular Location of $tRNA_6^{Lys}$

Differential centrifugation of cell extracts of KA31 provided a 600-*g* pellet, a 15,000-*g* pellet, a 105,000-*g* pellet, and a supernatant from 105,000 *g*, which was passed over a Bio-Rad A5m column to yield a high-molecular-weight complex containing lysyl-tRNA ligase. Each of these fractions was examined for the content of $tRNA^{Lys}$ isoacceptors. $tRNA_6^{Lys}$ was absent from the ligase complex, the 105,000-*g* supernatant applied to the gel filtration column, and the 105,000-*g* pellet. The 15,000-*g* pellet, consisting of mitochondria, lysosomes, and fragments of endoplasmic reticulum, is greatly enriched in $tRNA_6^{Lys}$ (Hedgcoth et al. 1980a, b). Observation of the preferential accumulation of $tRNA_6^{Lys}$ with the 15,000-*g* pellet led to a more detailed study of the possible association of this isoacceptor with mitochondria. Several methods for preparing clean mitochondria were evaluated, and the procedure of Schnaitman and Greenawalt (1968) with some modifications by Malkin (1971) was selected because it involves removal of the outer membrane from mitochondria, thus reducing contamination by lysosomes and membranous fragments. As shown in Fig. 2, mitoplasts prepared by this method have $tRNA_6^{Lys}$ as essentially the sole isoacceptor of lysine when assayed with cytoplasmic ligase (Hedgcoth et al. 1980b). Several attempts at aminoacylating mitochondrial tRNA preparations using ligases prepared from mitochondria failed to aminoacylate a lysine tRNA other than $tRNA_6^{Lys}$.

Nucleotide Sequence of $tRNA_6^{Lys}$

The results of functional studies and the apparent subcellular location of $tRNA_6^{Lys}$ led to questions of whether the origin of this isoacceptor is nuclear or mitochondrial. Because the nucleotide sequences of the genes for the human and bovine

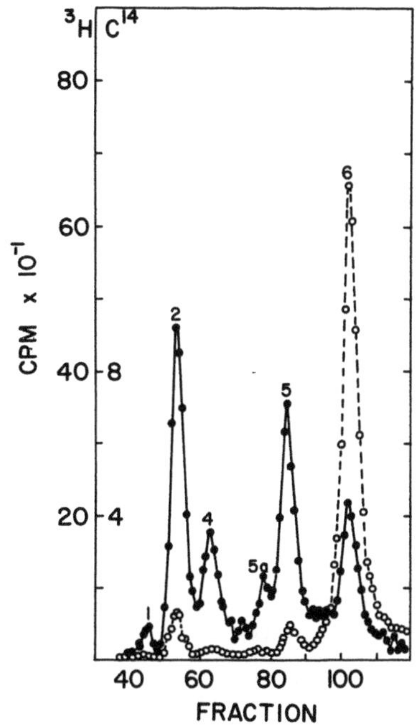

Fig. 2. RPC-5 profile of [^{3}H]lysyl-tRNA from mitoplasts prepared from KA31 cells. Cells were broken in buffer (100 m*M* Tris, pH 7.8, 1 m*M* magnesium acetate, 10 m*M* potassium chloride, 6 m*M* 2-mercaptoethanol, 250 m*M* sucrose, and 0.25% Nonidet P-40) with a Dounce homogenizer. A mitochondrial pellet was obtained by centrifugations of the homogenate for 10 min at 1,200 *g* and for 10 min at 5,000 *g*. Mitochondria were resuspended in buffer with 0.5 mg/ml bovine serum albumin and centrifuged for 15 min at 11,000 *g*. The resuspended pellet was treated for 15 min at 0° C with digitonin (1 mg/100 mg mitochondrial protein) to remove membranous contaminants adhering to mitochondria. After centrifugation for 10 min at 10,000 *g*, the pellet was resuspended and treated for 15 min at 0° C with digitonin (15 mg/100 mg mitochondrial protein) to remove the outer membrane. Mitoplasts were collected by centrifugation for 10 min at 10,000 *g*, centrifuged again for 15 min at 15,000 *g*, and then used to prepare a mitoplast tRNA preparation. ●---●, total [^{14}C]lysyl-tRNA, ○---○, mitoplast [^{3}H]lysyl-tRNA

mitochondrial lysine tRNAs are available (Barrell et al. 1979; Young and Anderson 1980) and because of the poor performance of $tRNA_6^{Lys}$ in translation in vitro, we determined the nucleotide sequence of $tRNA_6^{Lys}$ in order to provide the most definitive information about this isoacceptor. Purification, through the BD-cellulose chromatography step, was done in Dr. Ortwerth's laboratory by following a purification scheme similar to that of Wittig et al. (1973). tRNA containing $tRNA_6^{Lys}$ was obtained from Balb/3T3 cells after stressing the cultures by lowering the serum level to 1% calf serum. After chromatography on RPC-5, pooled fractions containing $tRNA_6^{Lys}$ were rechromatographed on RPC-5, and $tRNA_6^{Lys}$ was recovered, acylated with [^{14}C]lysine, and chromatographed on DEAE cellulose. The recovered [^{14}C]lysyl-$tRNA_6^{Lys}$ was converted into the naphthoxyacetyl derivative. The reaction probably gave naphthoxyacetyl moieties on both the alpha and epsilon amino groups of lysyl-tRNA, as subsequent elution from a column of BD cellulose required 30% ethanol in 1 *M* NaCl for elution of the tRNA. A sample of $tRNA_6^{Lys}$, which had not been discharged, was electrophoresed in a 10% polyacrylamide gel with 7 *M* urea and located by staining with methylene blue. A discharged sample was labeled on the 3′ end with [5-^{32}P]pCp using RNA ligase (Peattie 1979), electrophoresed, and located by autoradiography. $tRNA_6^{Lys}$ located in the polyacrylamide gel by either method gave a single major band and some faint bands (Fig. 3). The major band was eluted and used in sequencing procedures immediately after recovery.

Limited hydrolysis in foramide and subsequent labeling of the newly formed 5′ ends of fragments using polynucleotide kinase and [γ-^{32}P]ATP (Stanley and Vassilenko 1978) were done to produce sequencing ladders in 12% and 20% polyacrylamide gels (Fig. 4). Each band was cut from the gel, and the individual oligonucleotide fragments were eluted and precipitated with ethanol along with 10 μg carrier tRNA. The

Fig. 3. Autoradiogram of $tRNA^{Lys}_{6}$ after purification by electrophoresis in a polyacrylamide gel. [^{32}P]$tRNA^{Lys}_{6}$, prepared by labeling the 3′ end with [5′-^{32}P]pCp (Peattie 1979), was adjusted to 7 *M* urea, applied to a 10% polyacrylamide gel (30 cm × 0.4 mm) containing 7 *M* urea and electrophoresed with a buffer of 90 m*M* Tris-borate, pH 8.3, 1 m*M* EDTA. Autoradiography was for 1.5 min with a Dupont Lighting-plus intensifying screen. $tRNA^{Lys}_{6}$ was eluted from the major band in 300 µl 50 m*M* Tris-HCl, pH 7.5, 0.4 *M* NaCl, and 0.5% SDS for 2 h at 37° C. After addition of 10 µg carrier tRNA, $tRNA^{Lys}_{6}$ was recovered by ethanol precipitation. This preparation was employed for sequencing using nucleases for specific cleavages

[5′-^{32}P]nucleoside-3′,5′-diphosphate was released from the 5′ end of each fragment by digestion with RNase T_2.

Each residue was identified by thin-layer chromatography on PEI cellulose in two chromatographic solvents (Gupta and Randerath 1979). Chromatograms fro nucleotides in positions 30–55 of the tRNA are shown in Fig. 5. A problem with RNase T_2 produced the vague results for positions 33–37, which includes the anticodon. These nucleotides and the nucleotide in position 46 were identified by treating the respective oligonucleotides with nuclease P_1 to yield nucleoside 5′-phosphates and chromatographing the products on cellulose thin layers in two dimensions (Silberklang et al. 1979). The result of this procedure for the nucleotide in position 46, pm^{7}G, is shown in Fig. 6. This approach to sequencing yielded information sufficient to assign all positions in the sequence of $tRNA^{Lys}_{6}$ except for the 3′-terminal A, which could not be identified because the derivatized lysine was not removed before sequencing. While the structure of the nucleotide in position 34 is not known, it has the chromatographic properties of U*, which is found in the anticodons of some mitochondrial tRNAs (Sibler et al. 1980; K. Randerath, personal communication).

There are indirect data supporting the probability that U* is a thiolated derivative of uridine. $tRNA^{Lys}_{5}$ from rabbit liver has a thiolated nucleoside, s^{2}mcm^{5}U, in the first position of the anticodon (Raba et al. 1979); its acceptor capacity is reversibly inactivated by I_2 oxidation (Carbon et al. 1965). $tRNA^{Lys}_{5}$ from rat liver (Liu and Ortwerth 1972) and $tRNA^{Lys}_{5}$, $tRNA^{Lys}_{5a}$, and $tRNA^{Lys}_{6}$ from mouse LM cells (B. J. Ortwerth, unpublished results) are sensitive to I_2 oxidation. Similarly, $tRNA^{Lys}_{5a}$, $tRNA^{Lys}_{5}$, and $tRNA^{Lys}_{6}$ from Py3T3 cells are inactivated by I_2 treatment (Bjercke and Hedgcoth 1981). The only qualitative differences in nucleoside composition of

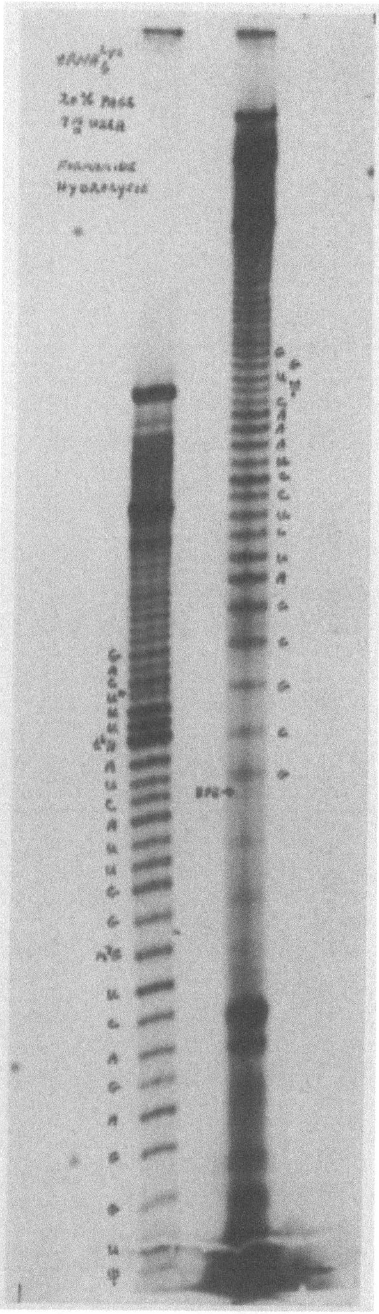

Fig. 4. Autoradiogram of a sequencing ladder of tRNA$_6^{Lys}$. For purification of unlabeled tRNA$_6^{Lys}$, 0.05 A_{260} unit in 80% formamide was heated for 3 min at 37° C and applied to a polyacrylamide gel as in Fig. 3. The gel was stained for 2 min with 0.2% methylene blue. tRNA was eluted in 200 µl buffer for 2 h at 37° C. After recovery by ethanol precipitation, tRNA$_6^{Lys}$ was heated for 4 min at 95° C in 100% formamide to produce limited hydrolysis products, which were recovered by precipitation and labeled with ^{32}P (Stanley and Vassilenko 1978). Labeled fragments were precipitated, dissolved in 80% formamide, heated for 3 min at 55° C, and electrophoresed on 12% and 20% polyacrylamide gels (40 cm × 0.4 mm) containing 7 *M* urea. A second addition to the gel was made after xylene cyanole of the first addition had traveled 23 cm. Bands of the sequencing ladder were located by autoradiography for 1.5 h at −70° C with an intensifying screen. Each band was excised and the oligonucleotide fragment was eluted in 300 µl buffer for 6 h at 37° C. Fragments with 10 µg carrier tRNA were precipitated with ethanol and dissolved in 10 µl 10 m*M* ammonium acetate, pH 4.9, containing 0.05 unit RNase T_2. After 5 h at 37° C, the mixture was taken to dryness in vacuo. The residue was dissolved in 4 µl deionized water

tRNA$_2^{Lys}$, tRNA$_4^{Lys}$, and tRNA$_5^{Lys}$ (Raba et al. 1979) are the presence of t^6A in tRNA$_2^{Lys}$, an unknown derivative of adenosine in tRNA$_4^{Lys}$, and s^2mcm^5U and ms^2t^6A in tRNA$_5^{Lys}$. We have data indicating that tRNA$_{5a}^{Lys}$ contains t^6A and not ms^2t^6A, and the sequence of tRNA$_6^{Lys}$ reported here has no unusual nucleotides, other than U*, which are not present in the other lysine isoacceptors. It is likely, then, that U* is a thiolated uridine derivative involved in the I_2 inactivation of tRNA$_6^{Lys}$.

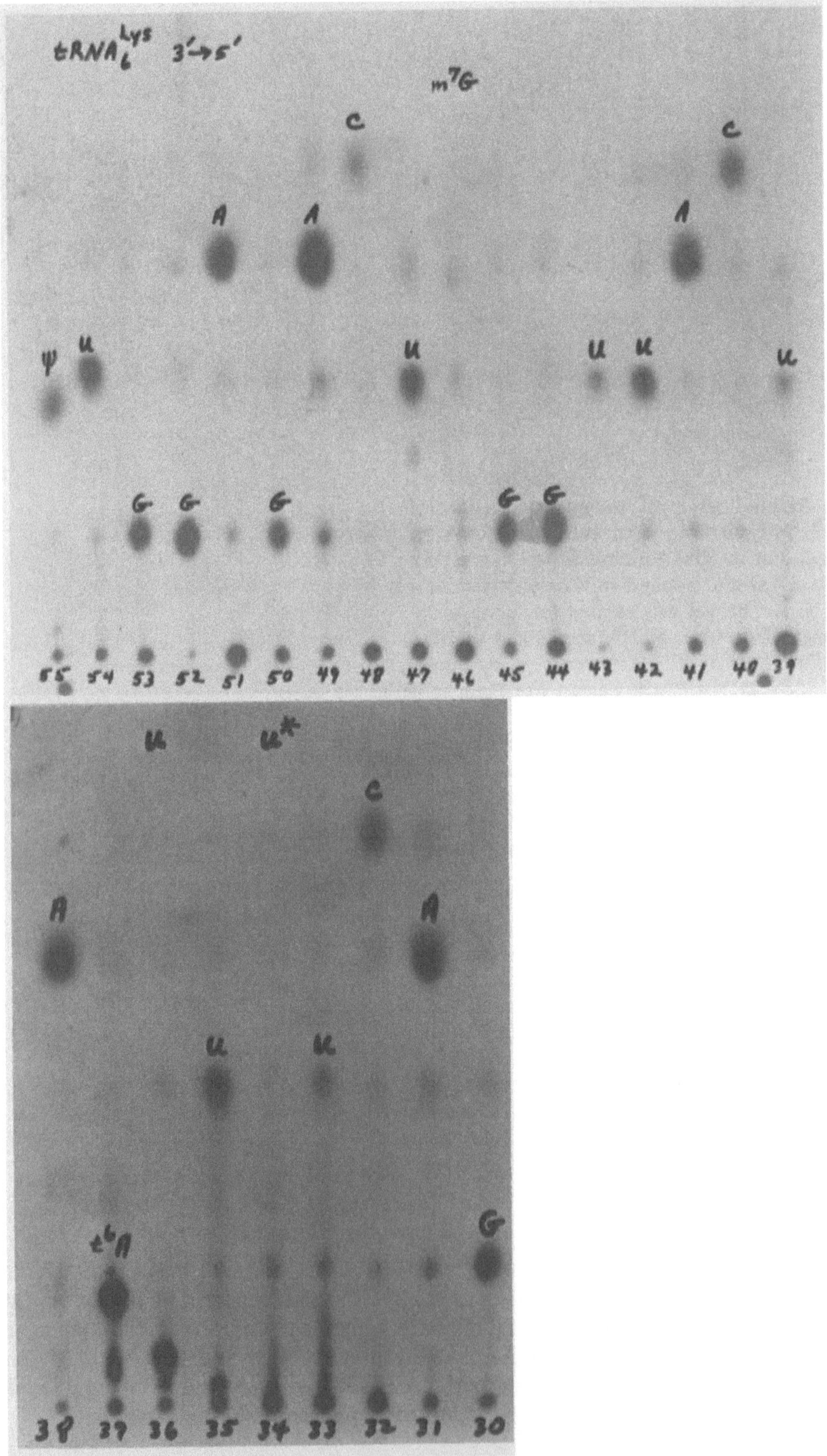
tRNA$_6^{Lys}$ 3'→5'
m^{7}G
t^{6}A
55 54 53 52 51 50 49 48 47 46 45 44 43 42 41 40 39
38 37 36 35 34 33 32 31 30

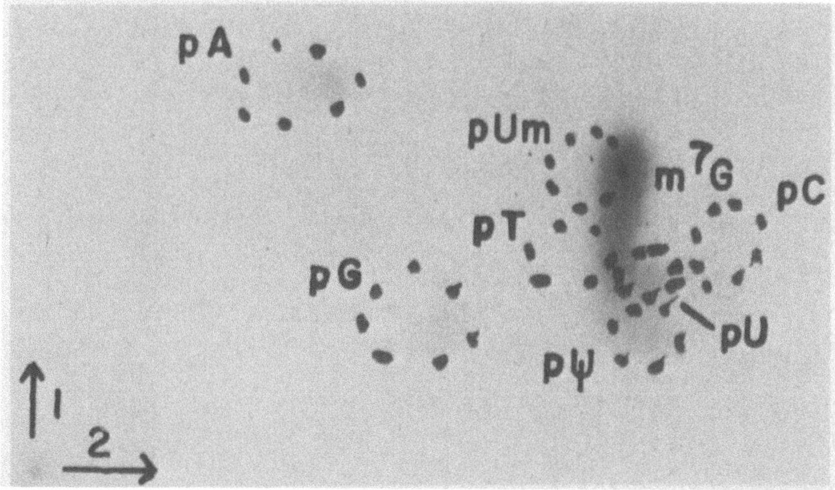

Fig. 6. Autoradiogram of a bidimensional-cellulose chromatogram of the nucleotide from position 46 of $tRNA_6^{Lys}$. A sample (2 μl) of the [5′-^{32}P]-nucleoside 3′,5′-diphosphate from the band corresponding to position 46 of $tRNA_6^{Lys}$ was mixed with 2 μl nuclease P_1 (1 μg) in 50 m*M* Tris-HCl, pH 7.5, and incubated overnight at 37° C. A sample (1 μl) was chromatographed in the bidimensional system of Silberklang et al. (1979). First dimension: isobutyric acid/NH_4OH/HOH (66/1/33); second dimension: 0.1 *M* sodium phosphate, pH 6.8/ammonium sulfate/n-propanol (100/60/2, v/w/v). Autoradiography was for 3 days with an intensifying screen

The positions of major nucleotides were confirmed by a modified method of partial nuclease digestion (Donis-Keller et al. 1977) with limited digestions with RNases T_1 (G-specific), U_2 (A-specific), Phy M (U- and A-specific), a RNase from *Bacillus cereus* (U- and C-specific), and including the cytosine-specific RNase Cl_3 from chicken liver (Levy and Karpetsky 1980).

Discussion of $tRNA_6^{Lys}$ Structure and Mitochondrial Association

The nucleotide sequence of $tRNA_6^{Lys}$ is shown in Fig. 7. This structure differs from all of the lysine tRNAs of known structure, whether of mammalian, yeast, or bacterial origin (Gauss and Sprinzl 1981). It has the U*UU anticodon for recognition of the AAA codon, with U* probably restricting interaction in favor of AAA over AAG. The structure has invariant and semi-invariant nucleotides common to tRNAs and the

◀

Fig. 5. Autoradiograms of PEI-cellulose chromatograms of nucleotide diphosphates 30–55 of $tRNA_6^{Lys}$. [5′-^{32}P]Nucleoside 3′,5′-diphosphates, prepared as in Fig. 4, were chromatographed on thin layers of PEI cellulose in each of two solvent systems (Gupta and Randerath 1979): 1.75 *M* ammonium formate, pH 3.5, and 0.55 *M* ammonium sulfate. Results for nucleotides 30–55 of $tRNA_6^{Lys}$ in the ammonium formate system are shown. Autoradiography was for 18 h with an intensifying screen

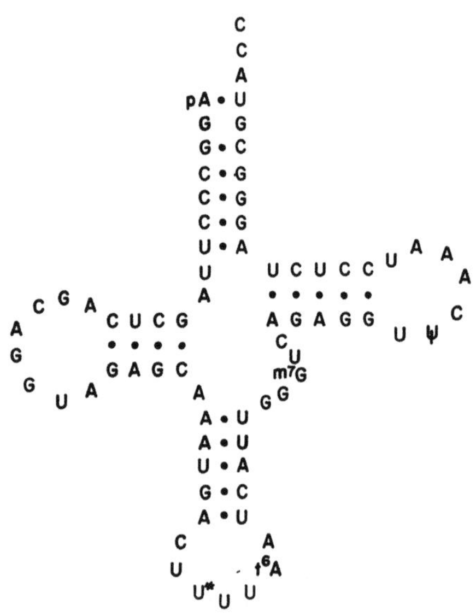

Fig. 7. Nucleotide sequence of tRNA$_6^{Lys}$ in cloverleaf form

sequence GUΨC instead of the fully modified GTΨC. There is an unusual G-G pair in the acceptor stem.

Comparison of the structure with the genes for tRNA^{Lys} from human (Barrell et al. 1979) and bovine (Young and Anderson 1980) mitochondria eliminates the possibility that tRNA$_6^{Lys}$ is encoded in mitochondrial DNA. Furthermore, the structure of tRNA^{Lys} from rat liver mitochondria also differs significantly from tRNA$_6^{Lys}$ (K. Randerath, personal communication). Nucleotide sequences of cytoplasmic isoacceptors of tRNA^{Lys} (Raba et al. 1979) indicated that there were three distinct nuclear genes for lysine tRNAs. Our data suggest that there are at least four different classes of tRNA^{Lys} genes in the nucleus.

Thus we propose that tRNA$_6^{Lys}$ is a nuclear product that associates with mitochondria. It may be the product of a gene that is transcribed to a very limited extent or not at all unless the cell is stressed, for example by viral transformation. There is precedent for importation of lysine tRNA into mitochondria (Martin et al. 1979): in *Saccharomyces cerevisiae* one of the two cytoplasmic lysine tRNAs is associated with mitochondria. Because yeast mitochondria contain a mitochondrially encoded tRNA^{Lys}, which responds to both lysine codons, and because the imported lysine tRNA is not acylated by the mitochondrial aminoacyl-tRNA ligase preparation, Martin et al. proposed a regulatory role of the imported species. Perhaps tRNA$_6^{Lys}$ has a similar role in mammalian cells in mediating nuclear and mitochondrial interactions.

Summary

Eleven isoaccepting lysine tRNAs from mammalian sources are demonstrable by RPC-5 chromatography and polyacrylamide gel electrophoresis. The appearance and amounts of these isoacceptors varies with the source and growth state of cells. One isoacceptor, tRNA$_6^{Lys}$, observed in preparations of tRNA from some virus-transformed cells in culture, has been characterized by determining functional properties, cellular

location, and its nucleotide sequence. $tRNA_6^{Lys}$ responds primarily to the lysine codon AAA, but it is not used efficiently in a wheat germ translational system in vitro. Compared with lysine isoacceptors 1, 2, 4, 5a, and 5, [^{3}H]lysine appears in vivo in $tRNA_6^{Lys}$ with a delay of about 3 h. This delay may in part be a result of a less functional tRNA, but a compartmented state of $tRNA_6^{Lys}$ also appears to be important. $tRNA_6^{Lys}$ is associated with mitoplasts prepared from KA31 fibroblasts.
The nucleotide sequence of $tRNA_6^{Lys}$ was determined by rapid postlabeling procedures involving limited hydrolysis in formamide, ^{32}P-labeling of 5′ ends of fragments with polynucleotide kinase, separation of the nested set of fragments in polyacrylamide denaturing gels, release of 5′-labeled nucleotides with RNase T_2, and identification of the released nucleotides by chromatography on PEI cellulose. Confirmation of the positions of major nucleotides was done by using limited digestions by RNases of $tRNA_6^{Lys}$ labeled with ^{32}P on the 3′ terminus in a gel readout procedure. The nucleotide sequence of $tRNA_6^{Lys}$ differs from that of cytoplasmic lysine tRNAs and mammalian mitochondrial lysine tRNAs. It contains U*, an unidentified modified uridine occurring in the anticodon of some mitochondrial tRNAs. $tRNA_6^{Lys}$ appears to occur in very limited amounts, or not at all, in most cells unless stressed, but when present it is associated with mitochondria, although it is probably coded in the nucleus.

Abbreviations

Py3T3, polyoma-virus-transformed 3T3 mouse fibroblasts; *TMV,* tobacco mosaic virus; *KA31,* murine-sarcoma-virus-transformed Balb/3T3 mouse fibroblasts; *BD cellulose,* benzoylated DEAE cellulose; *pm^{7}G,* *N*-7-methylguanosine 5′-phosphate; *pUm,* 2′-*O*-methyluridine 5′-phosphate (and other nucleoside 5′-phosphates are indicated similarly as *pN*); *s^{2}mcm^{5}U,* 2-thio-5-methylcarboxymethyluridine; *t^{6}A,* *N*-[9-(β-D-ribofuranosylpurin-6-yl)carbamoyl] threonine; *ms^{2}t^{6}A,* the 2-methylthio derivative of *t^{6}A*; *A_{260} unit,* the amount of tRNA in 1 ml aqueous solution that gives an absorbance of 1 for a 1-cm light path and is about 40 μg tRNA when measured in water; *SDS,* sodium dodecylsulfate; *PEI cellulose,* polyethyleneimine-impregnated cellulose.

References

Barrell BG, Bankier AT, Drouin J (1979) A different genetic code in human mitochondria. Nature 282: 189–194
Bjercke RJ, Hedgcoth C (1981) Codon binding and translational properties of an isoaccepting lysine tRNA peculiar to virus-transformed cells. MGG 183: 528–531
Carbon JA, Hung L, Jones DS (1965) A reversible oxidative inactivation of specific transfer RNA species. Proc Natl Acad Sci USA 53: 979–986
Chu-Der OMY, Ortwerth BJ (1980) Lys-$tRNA_4$ and cell division. Changes in lys-tRNA during the growth of mouse LM cells. Exp Cell Res 128: 159–170
Conlon-Hollingshead C, Ortwerth BJ (1980) Lys-$tRNA_4$ levels and cell division in mouse 3T3 cells. Exp Cell Res 128: 171–180
Donis-Keller H, Maxam AM, Gilbert W (1977) Mapping adenines, guanines, and pyrimidines in RNA. Nucleic Acids Res 8: 2527–2538
Gauss DH, Sprinzl M (1981) Compilation of tRNA sequences. Nucleic Acids Res 9: r1–r22
Gupta RC, Randerath K (1979) Rapid print-readout technique for sequencing RNAs containing modified nucleotides. Nucleic Acids Res 6: 3443–3458

Hedgcoth C, Thomas K, Scheets K, Allen S (1980a) Differences in aminoacylation in vivo and in vitro of lysine isoaccepting tRNAs from virus-transformed cells. Biochem Biophys Res Commun 95: 880–886

Hedgcoth C, Thomas K, Allen S, Scheets K (1980b) Differences in mitochondrial lysine tRNAs from normal and virus-transformed cells. Fed Proc 39: 2024

Jacobson EL, Juarez H, Hedgcoth C, Consigli RA (1974) An extra species of lysine transfer ribonucleic acid in polyoma virus-transformed cells in tissue culture. Arch Biochem Biophys 163: 666–670

Juarez H, Juarez D, Hedgcoth C, Ortwerth BJ (1975) Amounts of isoaccepting lysine tRNAs change with the proliferative state of cells. Nature 254: 359–360

Katze JR (1975) Relation of cell type and cell density to the degree of post-transcriptional modification of $tRNA^{Lys}$ and $tRNA^{Phe}$. Biochim Biophys Acta 407: 392–398

Levy CC, Karpetsky TP (1980) The purification and properties of chicken liver RNase. An enzyme which is useful in distinguishing between cytidylic and uridylic acid residues. J Biol Chem 255: 2153–2159

Liu LP, Ortwerth BJ (1972) Specificity of rat liver lysine transfer ribonucleic acid for codon recognition. Biochemistry 11: 12–17

Malkin LI (1971) Minor species of ribonucleic acid associated with rat liver mitochondria. Biochemistry 10: 4752–4756

Marcu K, Dudock B (1974) Characterization of a highly efficient protein synthesizing system derived from commercial wheat germ. Nucleic Acids Res 1: 1385–1397

Marcu K, Dudock B (1976) Effect of ribothymidine in specific eukaryotic tRNAs on their efficiency in in vitro protein synthesis. Nature 261: 159–162

Marcus A (1972) Protein synthesis in extracts of wheat embryo. In: Last JA, Laskin AL (eds) Protein biosynthesis in nonbacterial systems. Dekker, New York, pp 127–145

Martin RP, Schneller J-M, Stahl AJC, Dirheimer G (1979) Import of nuclear deoxyribonucleic acid coded lysine-accepting transfer ribonucleic acid (anticodon C-U-U) into yeast mitochondria. Biochemistry 18: 4600–4605

Nirenberg M, Leder P (1964) RNA code words and protein synthesis. Science 145: 1399–1407

Ortwerth BJ (1971) Isoaccepting transfer-ribonucleic acid in specialized mammalian tissue. Biochemistry 10: 4190–4197

Ortwerth BJ, Liu (1973) Correlation between a specific isoaccepting lysyltransfer ribonucleic acid and cell division in mammalian tissue. Biochemistry 12: 3978–3984

Ortwerth BJ, Carlson JV (1977) Lysine transfer RNA from liver: A sulfur-containing species that codes for AAG. Arch Biochem Biophys 178: 278–284

Ortwerth BJ, Yonuschot GR, Carlson JV (1973) Properties of $tRNA_4^{Lys}$ from various tissues. Biochemistry 12: 3985–3991

Peattie DA (1979) Sequencing RNA by a chemical method. Proc Natl Acad Sci USA 76: 1760–1764

Raba M, Limburg K, Burghagen M, Katze JR, Simsek M, Heckman J, RajBhandary UL, Gross HJ (1979) Nucleotide sequence of three isoaccepting lysine tRNAs from rabbit liver and SV40-transformed mouse fibroblasts. Eur J Biochem 97: 305–318

Rudloff E, Hilse K (1971) Properties of isoaccepting species of lysine tRNA from rabbit reticulocytes in codon recognition and in haemoglobin biosynthesis in vitro. Eur J Biochem 24: 313–320

Schnaitman C, Greenawalt JW (1968) Enzymatic properties of the inner and outer membranes of rat liver mitochondria. J Cell Biol 38: 150–175

Sharma OK, Roberts WK, Beezley DN, Borek E (1975) A transfer RNA-dependent protein synthesizing system from Ehrlich ascites extracts. Biochim Biophys Acta 390: 327–331

Sibler A-P, Bordonne R, Dirheimer G, Martin R (1980) Structure primaire d'un tryptophane-tRNA de mitochondrie de Levure capable de traduire le codon de terminaison U-G-A. C R Acad Sci [D] (Paris) 290: 695–698

Silberklang M, Gillum AM, RajBhandary UL (1979) Use of in vitro ^{32}P labeling in the sequence analysis of nonradioactive tRNAs. Methods Enzymol 59: 58–109

Stanley J, Vassilenko S (1978) A different approach to RNA sequencing. Nature 274: 87–89

Wittig B, Reuter S, Gottschling H (1973) Purification of the four lysine-specific transfer ribonucleic acids from chick embryos. Biochim Biophys Acta 331: 221–230

Young IG, Anderson S (1980) The genetic code in bovine mitochondria: sequence of genes for the cytochrome oxidase subunit II and two tRNAs. Gene 12: 257–265

Involvement of tRNA in Retrovirus Expression: Biological Implications of Reverse Transcriptase-Primer tRNA Interactions

S. Litvak[1] L. Sarih[1] M. Fournier[1] F. von der Haar[2]
B. Labouesse[1] and A. Araya[1]

[1] Institut de Biochimie Cellulaire et Neurochimie du C.N.R.S., 1 rue Camille Saint Saëns, 33000 Bordeaux, France; [2] Max-Planck-Institut für Experimentelle Medizin, Abteilung Chemie, Göttingen, FRG

Introduction

The RNA genome of retrovirus is reverse transcribed by the virus-coded and virion-encapsidated RNA-dependent DNA polymerase (reverse transcriptase) (Bishop 1978; Coffin 1979). The product of reverse transcription, a double-stranded circular DNA, is integrated in the nuclear genome of the transformed cell by a still unknown mechanism (Gilboa et al. 1979).

Reverse transcriptase initiates cDNA synthesis at the 3′ OH of a tRNA partially base paired near the 5′ end of the viral RNA genome. The base pairing between the primer tRNA and the viral genome involves about 16 bases of the 3′ end of tRNA (Panet et al. 1975).

How does tRNA become associated with retrovirus RNA? We have tried to answer this question, assuming that reverse transcriptase may play a role in the annealing of primer and template. It has been shown that pure avian reverse transcriptase will form a specific complex with $tRNA^{Trp}$, the in vivo primer of avian retrovirus reverse transcriptase; in the case of total chicken tRNA the polymerase will bind selectively to $tRNA^{Trp}$ (Haseltine et al. 1977).

In our laboratory we have studied the topography and functional implications of this recognition and shown that the $tRNA^{Trp}$ regions best recognized by avian myeloblastosis reverse transcriptase are the anticodon region and the 3′ end of primer $tRNA^{Trp}$. Both subunits of AMV reverse transcriptase are found cross-linked to $tRNA^{Trp}$ after ultraviolet irradiation of the enzyme-tRNA complex (Araya and Litvak 1979; Araya et al. 1980a). Moreover, the CCA end of tRNA is found covalently bound to the α subunit of AMV reverse transcriptase after affinity labeling of the enzyme to periodate-oxidized $tRNA^{Trp}$ (Araya et al. 1980b). Besides, we have several pieces of evidence indicating that the viral polymerase is able to mediate the binding of primer tRNA to the viral genome through the partial unwinding of the 3′ end of primer tRNA (Araya et al. 1979).

* The authors are indebted to Dr. J. W. Beard for donating the AMV and AMV reverse transcriptase and to Dr. J. E. Dahlberg for a sample of chicken $tRNA^{Trp}$ modified with acrylonitrile. This work was supported by the D.G.R.S.T. and the University of Bordeaux II

We present here our findings that reverse transcriptase is able to deacylate Trp-tRNA^{Trp} under conditions different to those in which the tRNA stripping by tryptophanyl-tRNA synthetase occurs. Also reported are findings on the primer activity of tRNA^{Trp} modified with acrylonitrile on the ψ residues, as well as with primer tRNA carrying adenosine analogs.

Materials and Methods

Avian myeloblastosis virus and reverse transcriptase were from Life Sciences Inc., Florida, USA. Isotopes were purchased from New England Nuclear (Europe). Other reagents were of the highest purity commercially available.

AMV 35-S RNA Purification. The phenol method described previously (Araya et al. 1979) was used for isolating viral RNA devoided of endogenous primer.

Purification of Beef Pancreas Tryptophanyl-tRNA Synthetase. The method used for preparing homogeneous synthetase has been published (Merault et al. 1978).

Purification of Beef Liver tRNA^{Trp}. The tRNA^{Trp} was purified as described previously (Fournier et al. 1976). The accepting capacity of the purified tRNA^{Trp} was higher than 1600 pmol/OD$^{260\ nm}$.

Modification of tRNA with Acrylonitrile. We used the method described by Ofengand (1971) for the cyanoethylation of beef liver tRNA^{Trp}.

Incorporation of ATP Analogs into tRNA. Yeast tRNA nucleotidyltransferase was used for the incorporation of ATP analogs into tRNA previously digested with venom phosphodiesterase (Sprinzl et al. 1977).

Aminoacylation Assay of tRNA^{Trp}. In a final volume of 0.1 ml the incubation mixture contained 100 m*M* Tris-HCl pH 8, 0.1 m*M* EDTA, 10 m*M* magnesium acetate, 1 m*M* dithiothreitol, 10 m*M* ATP, 50 μ*M* [^{14}C]Trp (specific activity = 56 mCi/mmol), 0.1 OD^{260} beef tRNA^{Trp}, and TRS to a final concentration of about 10 n*M*. Radioactivity was determined after incubation at 25° C using the paper disk method.

Deacylation of Trp-tRNA^{Trp}. The deacylation of aminoacyl tRNA was assayed following the system optimized by Peyrie and Labouesse (unpublished results). In a final volume of 0.2 ml the incubation mixture contained 0.1 *M* Tris-HCl pH 8, 0.1 m*M* EDTA, 1 m*M* dithiothreitol, 1 m*M* magnesium acetate, 5 μ*M* [^{14}C]Trp-tRNA^{Trp} (specific activity = 1500–1700 pmol/OD), and 230 n*M* TRS or 230 n*M* reverse transcriptase. Incubation was carried out at 25° C or 37° C for various lengths of time. Radioactivity was determined as described above.

Assay of cDNA Synthesis with AMV Reverse Transcriptase. The final volume was 0.050 ml and the incubation mixture contained 50 m*M* Tris-HCl pH 8.3, 40 m*M* KCl, 6 m*M* $MgCl_2$, 0.1 m*M* each of dCTP, dATP, and dGTP, 5 μM [^{32}P]dGTP (specific activity = 2000 cpm/pmol), 2 m*M* dithiothreitol, 10 μg bovine serum albumine, 0.1 OD^{260} 35-S RNA, 0.1 OD^{260} tRNA^{Trp}, and 10–20 units reverse transcriptase.

Incubation was carried out at 37° C for the indicated times. Radioactivity was determined after trichloroacetic acid precipitation and filtration on nitrocellulose membranes. The annealing between viral RNA and normal or modified $tRNA^{Trp}$ at 75° C was performed as described previously (Araya et al. 1979).

Results and Discussion

Effect of Reverse Transcriptase on the Deacylation of Trp-tRNA^{Trp}

It is an accepted fact that most total tRNA is aminoacylated in the cell. If this is the case it is foreseeable that primer tRNA will serve as initiator for cDNA synthesis only if the terminal adenosine is not aminoacylated. We have investigated the possibility that reverse transcriptase is involved in the hydrolysis of Trp-$tRNA^{Trp}$. As seen in Fig. 1, the charged tRNA is rapidly deacylated by TRS; under the same conditions, reverse transcriptase activity for the deacylation of primer tRNA is very poor. However, as seen in Fig. 2, the viral polymerase can release Trp from charged tRNA if the 35-S viral RNA is present in the reaction mixture. The enzyme alone, the enzyme plus dNTPs, and the spontaneous hydrolysis of Trp-$tRNA^{Trp}$ showed low deacylation. We have observed that reverse transcriptase can use charged $tRNA^{Trp}$, but when the kinetics of cDNA synthesis is compared in the presence of charged or deacylated primer tRNA, a lag time is observed with Trp-$tRNA^{Trp}$ (not shown). This difference can be attributed to the time necessary for the hydrolysis of the aminoacyl-tRNA. The effect of 35-S RNA recalls the situation we described previously (Araya et al. 1979), where viral RNA enhances the protection of the 3′ end against nuclease digestion of primer tRNA by reverse transcriptase. The partial base pairing between tRNA and viral RNA can modify the exposure of the aminoacylated terminus of tRNA, thus allowing hydrolysis of the ester bond by the polymerase.

Modification of Primer tRNA with Acrylonitrile

Some residues of tRNA can be cyanoethylated by acrylonitrile, as described by Ofengand (1971). In the case of beef $tRNA^{Trp}$, the only target of cyanoethylation is ψ. It has already been shown that cyanoethylation at 40° C will not affect the GTψC loop, while at 60° C all ψ residues will be modified. As seen in Table 1A, the modification at 40° C led to a 25% inhibition of aminoacylation. Control was done with propionitrile, a nonalkylating analog of acrylonitrile. However, if the modification with acrylonitrile is performed at 60° C, the cyanoethylated primer tRNA is not acylated at all by the beef synthetase. A similar experiment was performed with reverse transcriptase and modified $tRNA^{Trp}$. In Table 1B it can be seen that no effect on the primer activity of $tRNA^{Trp}$ (modified at 40° C or 60° C) is obtained if the annealing between primer and template is done at 75° C, while a marked decrease in the ability of tRNA to serve as initiator of DNA synthesis is observed when the annealing is performed at 37° C. We have described previously the capacity of reverse transcriptase to partially unwind $tRNA^{Trp}$, as well as to anneal primer and template at 37° C. Our results suggest that extensive cyanoethylation would lead to the inhibition of the ability of the viral polymerase to open the acceptor stem of primer tRNA. Moreover, we have followed the formation of a complex between cyanoethylated $tRNA^{Trp}$ and AMV reverse

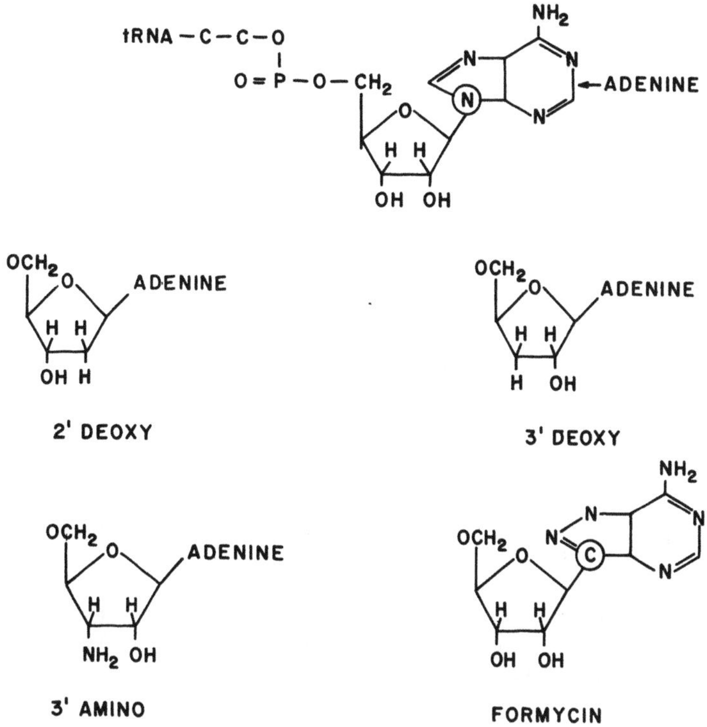

Fig. 1. ATP analogs incorporated into the 3′ end of tRNA^{Trp}. The analogs were incorporated by yeast tRNA nucleotidyltransferase as described by Sprinzl et al. (1977)

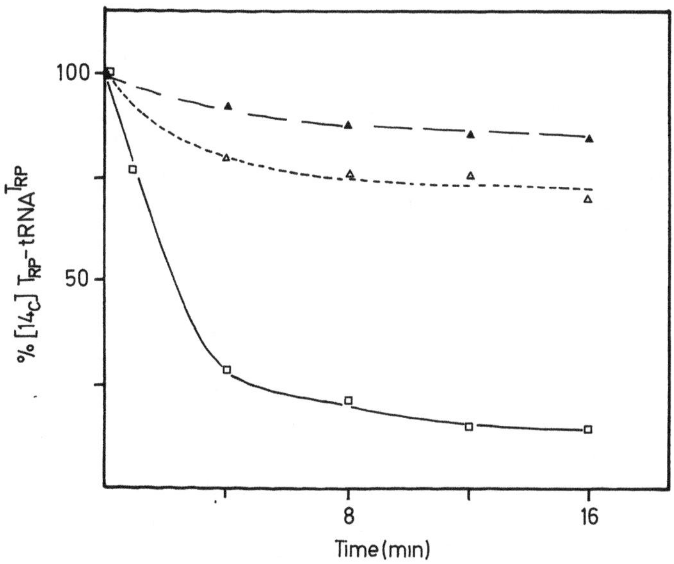

Fig. 2. Deacylation of Trp-tRNA^{Trp} under different conditions: ▲, spontaneous hydrolysis; △, plus reverse transcriptase; □, plus TRS. The incubation conditions are described in Material and Methods

Table 1A, B. Effect of cyanoethylation on the aminoacylation and priming activities of $tRNA^{Trp}$. **A** Aminoacylation of beef $tRNA^{Trp}$ modified with acrylonitrile. Incubation with TRS was carried out as described in Materials and Methods for 30 min at 25° C. **B** Reverse transcription with $tRNA^{Trp}$ modified with acrylonitrile. The assay conditions are described in the text. DNA synthesis was carried out for 60 min at 37° C

A	tRNA	Temperature of modification	[^{14}C] Trp (cpm)
	$tRNA^{Trp}$	40° C	10942
	$tRNA^{Trp}$ (propionitrile)	40° C	10571
	$tRNA^{Trp}$ (acrylonitrile)	40° C	7455
	$tRNA^{Trp}$	60° C	8662
	$tRNA^{Trp}$ (propionitrile)	60° C	7987
	$tRNA^{Trp}$ (acrylonitrile)	60° C	341

B	tRNA	Temperature of modification	Annealing at 37° C (cpm)	Annealing at 75° C (cpm)
	$tRNA^{Trp}$	40° C	46404	28334
	$tRNA^{Trp}$ (propionitrile)	40° C	41750	25365
	$tRNA^{Trp}$ (acrylonitrile)	40° C	36704	28599
	$tRNA^{Trp}$	60° C	40485	31110
	$tRNA^{Trp}$ (propionitrile)	60° C	35518	26167
	$tRNA^{Trp}$ (acrylonitrile)	60° C	0	24230

transcriptase on a Sephadex G-100 column under the same conditions described previously for the complex with normal $tRNA^{Trp}$ (Araya et al. 1980a, b). No complex was detected in the conditions in which propionitrile-modified $tRNA^{Trp}$ or normal tRNA did form a stable complex (not shown).

Primer Activity of $tRNA^{Trp}$ with Different Analogs of Adenosine at the 3′ End

The terminal adenosine of $tRNA^{Trp}$ was substituted with the following analogs: 2′dA, 3′dA, 3′NH_2-3′dA, and formycin (Fig. 3). All these analogs can be incorporated into tRNA by the yeast tRNA nucleotidyltransferase (Sprinzl et al. 1977).

As shown for other aminoacyl-tRNA synthetases, TRS can recognize formycin-modified tRNA very efficiently, while other tRNAs are charged at very low extents (Table 2). The low but significant incorporation of Trp into 2′dA- or 3′dA-modified $tRNA^{Trp}$ is in good agreement with previous reports on other eukaryotic tRNAs (Fraser et al. 1979). The situation with reverse transcriptase is quite different, since besides normal tRNA, only the 2′dA $tRNA^{Trp}$ can serve as primer for cDNA synthesis with the AMV polymerase (Table 3). The inability of reverse transcriptase to initiate with a formycin-modified $tRNA^{Trp}$ is very interesting, since it has been shown that this adenine analog can base-pair to U and T in a way similar to that in which A base-pairs with them. However, a polyformycin-poly U duplex has a lower Tm than poly A-poly U (Ward et al. 1969). Formycin incorporated in the terminal position of tRNA can be placed in such a way as to avoid interaction with the polymerase site involved in the formation of the phosphodiester group. Whether the lack of primer activity of formycin-modified $tRNA^{Trp}$ is related to the antitumor activity of this analog (Ward et al. 1969) remains to be established.

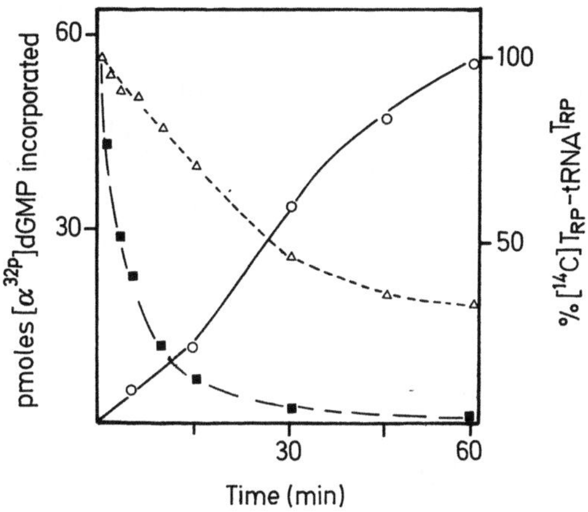

Fig. 3. Deacylation of Trp-tRNA^{Trp} and DNA synthesis catalyzed by reverse transcriptase: ○, dGMP incorporation into DNA; △, deacylation in the absence of enzyme, plus reverse transcriptase, or plus reverse transcriptase and dNTPs; ■, deacylation in the presence of reverse transcriptase and 35-S RNA. See experimental conditions under Material and Methods

Table 2. Aminoacylation of tRNA^{Trp} with adenosine analogs incorporated at the 3′ end of tRNA. The incorporation of Trp into beef tRNA^{Trp} by TRS was performed as described in Materials and Methods. Incubation was carried out for 30 min at 25° C

tRNA	[^{14}C]Trp (cpm)
tRNA^{Trp}	10182
tRNA^{Trp}-2′dA	776
tRNA^{Trp}-3′dA	647
tRNA^{Trp}-3′NH_2-3′dA	0
tRNA^{Trp}-formycin	10343

Table 3. Reverse transcription of 35-S RNA using tRNA^{Trp} with adenosine analogs at the 3′ end. The incorporation of dGMP into DNA was followed as detailed in Materials and Methods. Incubation was for 60 min at 37° C

tRNA	dGMP incorporated (cpm)	
	Annealing at 37° C	Annealing at 75° C
tRNA^{Trp}	66582	36544
tRNA^{Trp}-2′dA	53653	25689
tRNA^{Trp}-3′dA	546	5923
tRNA^{Trp}-3′NH_2-3′dA	732	6647
tRNA^{Trp}-formycin	08	4851

Summary

We have previously studied the topographical and functional implications of the recognition of primer tRNA^{Trp} by avian retrovirus reverse transcriptase. Here we have presented evidence that the enzyme is able to deacylate beef liver Trp-tRNA^{Trp}, provided that 35-S viral RNA is present in the incubation mixture. No effect of dNTPs on this activity was observed.

The extensive modification of $tRNA^{Trp}$ with acrylonitrile led to a marked loss of priming activity by $tRNA^{Trp}$ if the annealing between primer and template was performed at 37° C, while the annealing of cyanoethylated tRNA with the viral genome at 75° C gave almost normal levels of cDNA synthesis. We have also studied the priming behaviour of $tRNA^{Trp}$, modified by incorporation of various analogs of adenosine. Only $tRNA^{Trp}$-2′dA was active in cDNA initiation; 3′dA, $3'NH_2$-3′dA, and primer tRNA with formycin in the 3′ end showed low or nonexistent priming activity.

Abbreviations

Trp, tryptophan; *TRS,* tryptophanyl-tRNA synthetase; *Trp-tRNA^{Trp},* tryptophanyl-$tRNA^{Trp}$; *AMV,* avian myeloblastosis virus; *2′dA,* 2′deoxyadenosine; *3′dA,* 3′deoxyadenosine; *$3'NH_2$-3′dA,* 3′amino-3′deoxyadenosine; *ψ*, pseudouridine.

References

Araya A, Litvak S (1979) Study of the interaction of $tRNA^{Trp}$ with AMV reverse transcriptase. Cold Spring Harbor Symp Quant Biol 43: 631–637

Araya A, Sarih L, Litvak S (1979) Reverse transcriptase mediated binding of primer tRNA to the viral genome. Nucleic Acids Res 6: 3831–3844

Araya A, Keith G, Fournier M, Gandar JC, Labouesse J, Litvak S (1980a) Photocrosslinking studies of the interaction between AMV reverse transcriptase with primer $tRNA^{Trp}$. Arch Biochem Biophys 205: 437–448

Araya A, Hevia E, Litvak S (1980b) Study of the interactions between AMV reverse transcriptase and primer tRNA. Affinity labeling and inactivation of the enzyme by periodate treated $tRNA^{Trp}$. Nucleic Acids Res 8: 4009–4020

Bishop JM (1978) Retrovirus Annu Rev Biochem 47: 35–88

Coffin JM (1979) Structure, replication and recombination of retrovirus genomes. Some unifying hypotheses. J Gen Virol 42: 1–26

Fournier M, Dorizzi M, Sarger C, Labouesse J (1976) Purification of $tRNA^{Trp}$, $tRNA^{Val}$ and partial purification of $tRNA^{Ileu}$ and $tRNA^{Met}$ from beef liver. Biochimie 58: 1159–1165

Fraser TH, Julius DJ, Rich A (1979) Determination of aminoacylation specificity using tRNA terminating in $3'$-NH_2-3′ dA and $2'$-NH_2-2′ dA. Methods Enzymol 59: 272–282

Gilboa E, Mitra SW, Goff S, Baltimore D (1979) A detailed model of reverse transcription and tests of crucial aspects. Cell 18: 93–100

Haseltine WA, Panet A, Smoler D, Baltimore D, Peters G, Harada F, Dahlberg JE (1977) Interactions of $tRNA^{Trp}$ and AMV reverse transcriptase. Further characterization of the binding reaction. Biochemistry 16: 3625–3632

Merault G, Graves PV, Labouesse B, Labouesse J (1978) Influence of magnesium on the steady state derived order of substrate addition and product release in $tRNA^{Trp}$ aminoacylation by beef pancreas tryptophanyl tRNA synthetase. Eur J Biochem 87: 541–550

Panet A, Haseltine WA, Baltimore D, Peters G, Harada F, Dahlberg JE (1975) Specific binding of $tRNA^{Trp}$ to AMV reverse transcriptase. Proc Natl Acad Sci USA 72: 2535–2539

Ofengand J (1971) Cyanoethylation of nucleotides and tRNA by acrylonitrile. Methods Enzymol 20: 150–168

Sprinzl M, Sternbach H, von der Haar F, Cramer F (1977) Enzymatic incorporation of ATP and CTP analogues into the 3′ end of tRNA. Eur J Biochem 81: 579–589

Ward DC, Cerami A, Reich E, Acs G, Altwerger L (1969) Biochemical studies of the analogue formycin. J Biol Chem 244: 3243–3250

Session II

Biosynthesis and Degradation of Modified Nucleosides in Cancer Cells

DNA-Specific Enzymes

Enzymatic Methylation of Chicken Erythrocyte DNA Modified by Two Carcinogens, 2-(N-Acetoxyacetylamino) Fluorene and Methylnitrosourea

A. Pfohl-Leszkowicz, R. P. P. Fuchs, G. Keith, and G. Dirheimer

Institut de Biologie Moléculaire et Cellulaire du CNRS et Faculté de Pharmacie, Université Louis Pasteur, 15 rue Descartes, 67084 Strasbourg, France

Introduction

2-(*N*-acetoxyacetylamino)fluorene (AcO-AAF), a model of ultimate carcinogen of 2-(acetylamino)fluorene (AAF), reacts with DNA to give essentially *N*-(deoxyguanosine-8-yl)AAF (for a review, see Grunberger and Weinstein 1979). This substitution induces a conformational change in the vicinity of the adduct, leading to a local denaturation of the double helix (Daune and Fuchs 1976).

N-methyl-*N*-nitrosourea (MNU), a potent carcinogen in mammals, induces tumors in a variety of tissues, e.g., gastrointestinal tract, skin, and kidney. MNU does not require metabolic activation, but directly alkylates DNA (for a review, see Leaver et al. 1969, and IARC 1978).

We have investigated whether the enzymatic methylation of DNA by a *S*-adenosyl DNA cytosine 5-methyltransferase (DNA methylase) is affected by these modifications.

Materials and Methods

Chicken erythrocyte DNA was a gift from Professor Daune and was prepared as described elsewhere (Kay et al. 1952). *S*-Adenosyl-L[methyl-^{3}H]methionine (SAM) was from New England Nuclear (NEN), [^{14}C]SAM was from Commissariat à l'Energie Atomique (CEA), nonradioactive SAM was from Boehringer-Mannheim, proteinase K was from Merck, Unisolv was from Koch Light, DEAE cellulose (DE52) was from Whatman, and Dyematrex columns were from Amicon.

AcO-AAF was synthesized as described elsewhere (Lotlikar et al. 1966). Reaction of DNA with AcO-AAF and subsequent purification of modified DNA have been described (Miller et al. 1966; Fuchs and Daune 1972).

N[methyl-^{14}C]nitrosourea (MNU) was from NEN and nonradioactive MNU was a gift from Professor Kleihues. Reaction of DNA with MNU was carried out as follows: the reaction mixture, 600 μg DNA in sodium citrate pH 7, 1.6 m*M* and MNU (0.15 m*M* up to 15 m*M*), was stirred for 24 h at 37° C. DNA was then precipitated with 2 volumes cold ethanol.

Recent Results in Cancer Research. Vol 84

Enzymatic Methylation Assay and DNA Recovery

The methylation assay was as described previously (Pfohl-Leszkowicz et al. 1981). For kinetic studies of DNA methylation, the methylated DNA must be recovered quantitatively. We elaborated a new method because neither the classical methods (Kalousek and Morris 1968) nor phenol extraction gave satisfactory recovery of the labeled DNA. In these methods large amounts of DNA (60%) are eliminated by coextraction with the proteins during the enzyme elimination step. In our method only 12% of the DNA was lost during enzyme elimination (Pfohl-Leszkowicz and Dirheimer 1982). Normally 20 μl proteinase K solution (1 mg/ml Tris-HCl 10 m*M* pH 7.8, 10 m*M* NaCl, 0.5% SDS) was added to 200 μl reaction mixture (50 m*M* Tris-HCl pH 7.6, 0.5 m*M* dithiothreitol (DTT), 10 μg chicken erythrocyte DNA, 0.35 μg pancreatic RNase, 9 nmol [^{3}H]- or [^{14}C]SAM, 50 μg partially purified rat brain DNA methylase) and the mixture was incubated for 30 min at 60° C. After cooling, 500 μl carrier DNA (1 mg/ml) and 70 μl 2 *M* sodium acetate buffer pH 5 were added, then 2 volumes cold (−20° C) ethanol. After 30 min at −20° C the DNA pellet was recovered by centrifugation, dissolved in 0.5 ml 0.5 *M* NaOH, and incubated for 10 min at 60° C. Finally it was recovered by precipitation at 0° C with 2 ml cold 15% trichloroacetic acid, filtered on GFC filters, washed, and counted in 4 ml Unisolv.

Column Chromatography Procedures

Chromatography on DEAE cellulose (15 mm × 150 mm) was with a linear gradient of NaCl 20–750 m*M* in Tris-HCl pH 7.6 10 m*M* and dithioerythritol (DTE) 0.5 m*M*. Purification on standard blue A, orange A, and green A Dyematrex columns (9 mm × 32 mm) was as follows. The columns were prewashed with 12 ml Tris-HCl 5 m*M* pH 7.6, DTE 0.5 m*M*. The enzyme sample (3 mg in 0.5 ml) was applied and allowed to fix to the ligand. The nonfixed proteins were washed out after 30 min with the buffer described above. Finally the methylase was eluted with NaCl 1 *M* in the same buffer.

Results

Preparation of Rat Brain DNA Methylase

The DNA methylase was prepared from 7-day-old Wistar rat brain cortex nuclei because this organ displays high methylase levels during early postnatal development (Salas and Selinger 1978). The DNA methylase was liberated from nuclei and prepared according to Pogo et al. (1966) by Triton X100 (0.5% solution) treatment. After centrifugation the DNA methylase in the supernatant was precipitated with ammonium sulfate (80% saturation) and dialyzed overnight against 10 m*M* Tris-HCl pH 7.6. Further purification was by DEAE cellulose (DE52) column chromatography, for the DNA-AAF methylation experiments, or by orange A and green A Dyematrex affinity column chromatography, for the methylase used in MNU-DNA alkylated methylation experiments. The latter procedure gave much better yields (60% recovery) than the DEAE cellulose column (10% recovery) and was therefore prefered for further experiments.

Table 1. Purification of DNA methylase on Dyematrex columns

Enzyme fraction	Total ammonium sulfate protein applied on the column (mg)	Eluted proteins (mg)	Specific activity (units/mg[a])	Total activity (units recovered)	Puri-fication (-fold)	Yield (%)
Ammonium sulfate	–	–	157	470[b]	1	100
Dyematrex blue A	3	0.79	710	560	4.5	119
Dyematrex green A	3	0.65	446	290	2.8	62
Dyematrex orange A	3	0.40	1334	535	8.5	113
Dyematrex green A methylase fraction applied on Dyematrex orange A	0.65	0.12	1953	254	12.5	54

[a] One unit equals 1 pmol CH_3 incorporated into DNA in 60 min
[b] In 3 mg proteins

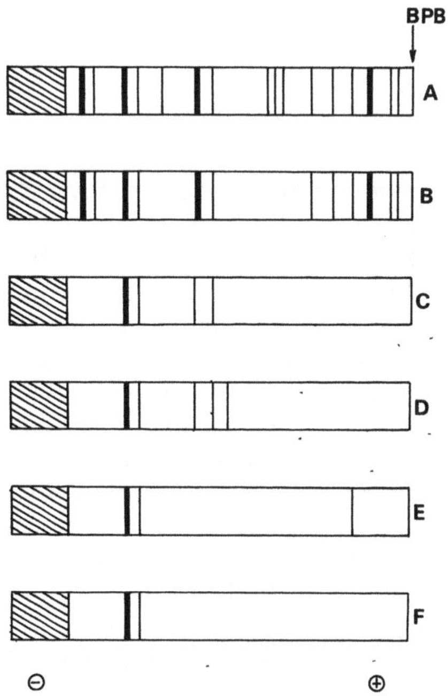

Fig. 1A–F. Polyacrylamide gel electrophoresis on DNA methylase containing protein fractions. **A** total proteins from nuclei; **B** ammonium sulfate precipitate; **C** Dyematrex green A; **D** Dyematrex blue A; **E** Dyematrex orange A; **F** Dyematrex green A and orange A successive columns

Table 1 shows the results of a typical purification experiment using the different Dyematrex affinity columns. It shows that the combination of the green A and orange A columns gives a 12-fold purification over the ammonium sulfate precipitation fraction. This combination results in a major and a minor band on polyacrylamide gel (Fig. 1). We do not yet know which of these two bands contains DNA methylase.

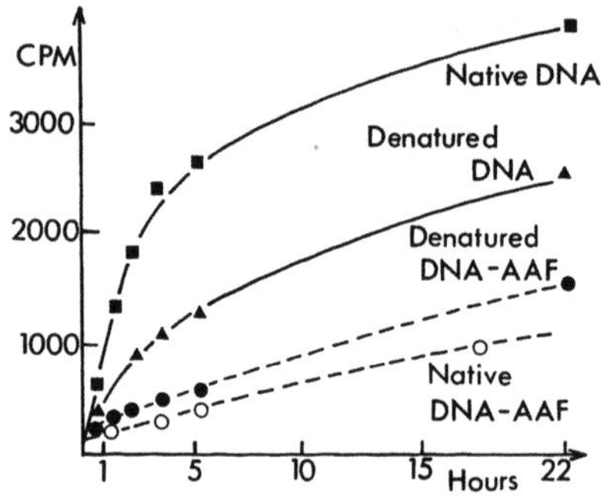

Fig. 2. Methylation of double- and single-stranded DNAs substituted or not with AAF (4.6% of substituted bases)

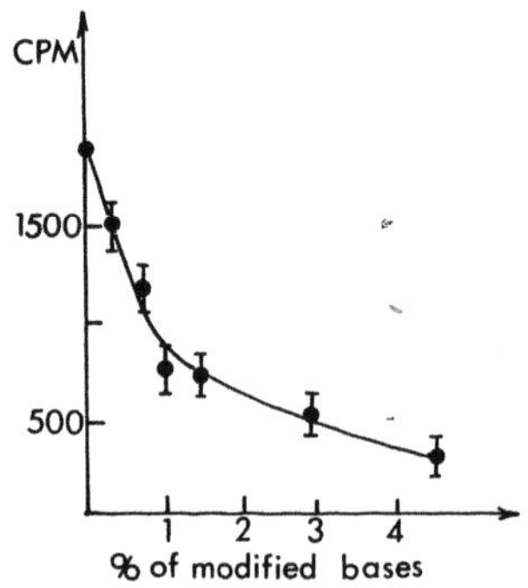

Fig. 3. Methylation of DNA substituted with various amounts of AAF. Methylation for 45 min

Enzymatic Methylation of DNA-AAF

Figure 2 shows the results obtained when double- or single-stranded DNA, AAF-substituted or not, was enzymatically methylated. In the AAF-substituted DNA samples, both the initial velocity of methylation and the overall methylation plateau were lower than in the nonmodified DNA samples.

Figure 3 shows that an inverse relation can be established between the degree of DNA modification and its methyl acceptor capacity. Moreover, the substituted DNA is not only less methylated, but added simultaneously with native DNA it inhibits the methylation of the native DNA (Fig. 4). It appears that about 1 μg DNA-AAF inhibits to about 50% the rate of methylation of 20 μg nonmodified DNA.

The initial methylation velocities of variable amounts of nonmodified DNA were measured in both the presence and absence of DNA-AAF modified to variable extents. Plotting of the reciprocals (1/v versus 1/S) shows a mixed type of inhibition (Fig. 5). The K_m for nonmodified DNA expressed in phosphate residues is 250 μ*M*. The K_i can also be calculated from the curves obtained (Segal 1975); it is 37 μ*M* for a DNA with 1.4% modified bases. Thus the affinity of the enzyme for the substituted DNA is higher than for native DNA.

This higher affinity could be due to the AAF-induced local denaturation regions in the substituted DNA (insertion-denaturation model) (Fuchs and Daune 1972). This was not the case, however, since the Lineweaver and Burk plot of the affinity of the enzyme for heat-denatured DNA showed that the affinity of the single-stranded DNA was 62.5% that of the native double-stranded DNA (K_m 400 μ*M*).

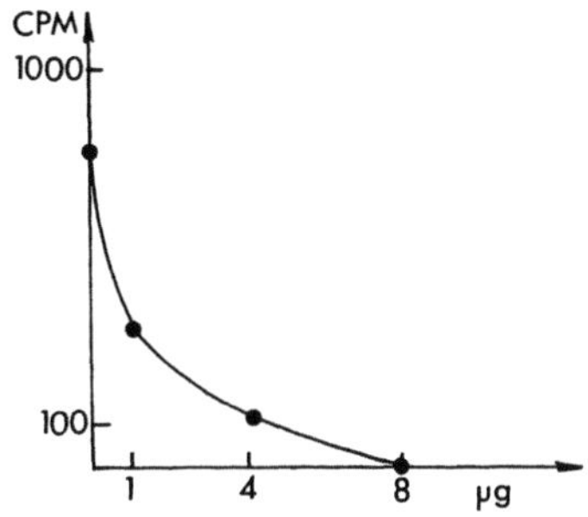

Fig. 4. Inhibition of native DNA (20 µg) methylation by various amounts of DNA-AAF (4.6% of substituted bases). The CPM due to the methylation of DNA-AAF were subtracted. Methylation for 120 min

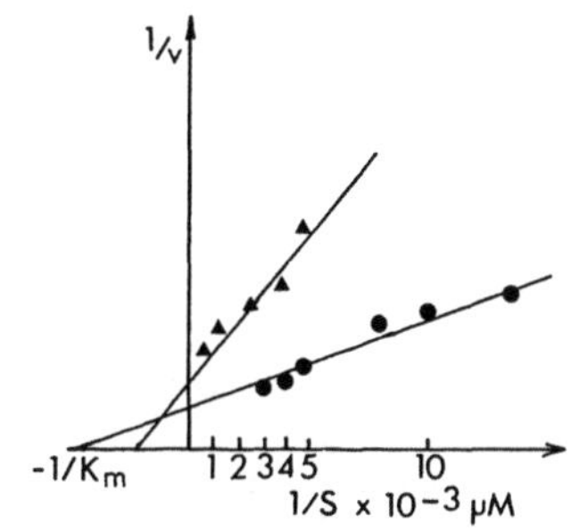

Fig. 5. Lineweaver and Burk plot of inhibition of native DNA methylation by DNA-AAF

Additional experiments were performed in which instead of mixing DNA and DNA-AAF simultaneously before adding the enzyme, either the DNA or the DNA-AAF was mixed with the enzyme prior to addition of the other substrate. When 4 µg DNA-AAF (1.8% of modified bases) is incubated with SAM and limited amounts of DNA methyltransferase for 5 min followed by addition of 30 µg native DNA, the methylation does not increase and remains the same as in the control where only DNA-AAF was present. Thus native DNA does not displace the enzyme from DNA-AAF and the binding of the enzyme to DNA-AAF is irreversible.
On the other hand, if one preincubates native DNA with the enzyme and adds DNA-AAF afterwards, one finds that the inhibition of methylation starts only after a lag.

MNU Methylation of DNA and Enzymatic Methylation of the Alkylated DNA

Chemical Methylation. Methylation with MNU is described in Materials and Methods. Figure 6 shows the kinetics of methylation using different amounts of MNU. The modification ranged from 4/100 to 1/1500 of the deoxynucleotides. Figure 7 shows a two-dimensional cellulose TLC separation of modified DNA constituants. The major modified deoxynucleotide (71%) was found to be 7-methyldeoxyguanosine and a minor one (15%) corresponds to 3-methyldeoxyadenosine. Another radioactive spot found in the deoxyguanosine spot could be accounted for by O^6-methyldeoxyguanosine. Triesters could also exist, and indeed, acid hydrolysis of modified DNA yields a spot (10% of total radioactivity) which migrates with the solvent front and could be accounted for by methylated triesters.

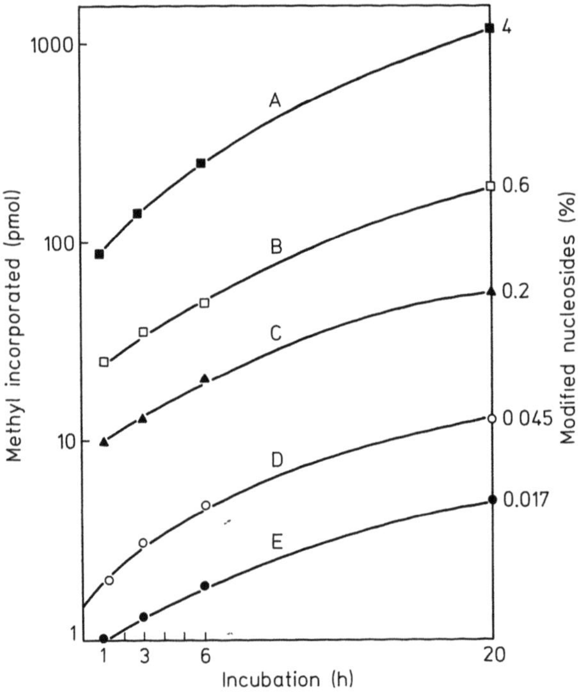

Fig. 6. MNU methylation of DNA. The reaction was as described in Material and Methods. The methyl groups incorporated into DNA (100 μg) were determined using [^{14}C]MNU. After incubation the reaction mixture was applied to Whatman 3MM disks and the DNA was precipitated into the filters by 10% trichloroacetic acid, washed twice in the same solution and twice in cold 95° ethanol, dried, and counted by liquid scintillation

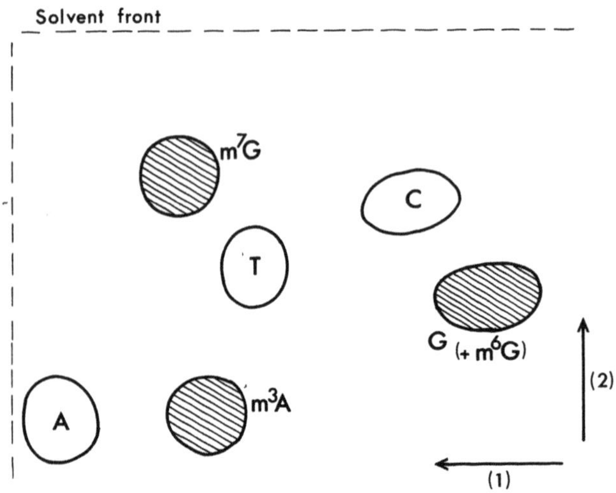

Fig. 7. Two-dimensional separation of MNU-methylated DNA hydrolysate. The deoxynucleosides were separated on cellulose-coated aluminium foil in the first dimension by descending chromatography developed with *n*-butanol, isobutyric acid, conc. ammonium hydroxide, and water (150 : 75 : 5 : 50 by vol) and in the second dimension by ascending chromatography using saturated ammonium sulfate, 0.1 *M* sodium acetate pH 6, and isopropanol (79 : 19 : 2 by vol) (Rogg et al. 1976). The chemically modified DNA (500 μg) (see Fig. 6) was hydrolyzed for 2 h at 37° C in $MgCl_2$ 10 m*M* pH 6.5 containing 50 units pancreatic DNase (Worthington) followed by further incubation for 12 h at 37° in Tris-HCl 0.05 *M* pH 8 (final concentration) in the presence of 1 unit venom phosphodiesterase (Worthington) and 1 unit bacterial alkaline phosphatase (Worthington). *Hatched spots* correspond to ^{14}C-labeled deoxynucleosides

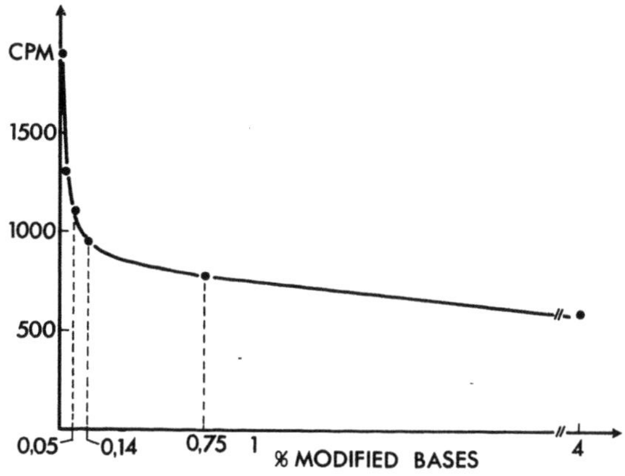

Fig. 8. Enzymatic methylation of MNU-methylated DNA. Chicken erythrocyte DNA modified by various amounts of MNU was incubated with [^{3}H]SAM and rat brain DNA methylase as described under Material and Methods for 90 min at 37° C

Enzymatic Methylation of MNU-modified DNA. The results in Fig. 8 show an inverse proportion between the level of DNA modification and its methylacceptor capacity. Alkylation of 0.15% of the bases inhibits 50% of the enzymatic methylation. However, a residual methylation is still seen even with highly alkylated DNA (4% of the nucleotides).

As the DNA-AAF has an inhibitory effect on native DNA methylation, we wondered whether the MNU-modified DNA could have the same effect. In fact, after incubation of 20 μg native DNA with amounts of MNU-alkylated DNA (4% of alkylated nucleotides) ranging from 2 μg to 20 μg the amount of methylation of the native DNA was not inhibited.

Discussion

The lesser methylation of DNA-AAF compared to the native DNA can be explained if we consider the model proposed for the methylation reaction (Kalousek and Morris 1969; Drahovsky and Morris 1971b), which assumes that the enzyme "walks" along the DNA strand to methylate several cytosine residues before leaving the nucleic acid. We may therefore expect the AAF-guanine residues to hinder the movement of the enzyme along the helix. Once stopped at the AAF-substituted site, the enzyme stays there irreversibly.

The lesser degree of methylation of double-stranded DNA-AAF than of single-stranded DNA-AAF (Fig. 2) can be tentatively explained by the presence of AAF in the guanine residues opposite potential cytosine methylation sites preventing the methylation of these cytosines. This mechanism would occur only in double-stranded DNA.

The MNU-methylated DNA, like DNA-AAF, is less enzymatically methylated than the native DNA. However, the inhibition of enzymatic methylation of chemically modified DNA is much greater for MNU-alkylated DNA than for DNA-AAF: 50% inhibition is reached with only 0.15% of modified bases for the MNU-methylated DNA, compared with 0.9% for the DNA-AAF.

Alkylated DNA therefore seems to behave differently in enzymatic methylation than DNA-AAF. The probable explanation is that in MNU-methylated DNA, the DNA methylase has a much lower affinity for the modified DNA than for the native DNA, in contrast to DNA-AAF, where the enzyme has a greater affinity for DNA-AAF than for the native DNA. This is consistent with preliminary results which show that MNU-methylated DNA inhibits the enzymatic methylation of native DNA much less than DNA-AAF does, or at all. This could be explained by the fact that MNU-methylated DNA has its electrostatic charge highly disturbed by the presence of the cationic charges of 7-methylguanines; the enzyme is bound to the DNA strands in two steps, the first one being an electrostatic fixation on the double helix. (Drahovsky and Morris 1971a).

Methylation of cytosine is the only postreplicational modification so far detected in DNA of higher eukaryotes and has thus been made the basis of several proposed mechanisms of gene activity, cellular differentiation, and oncogenesis (for reviews see Razin et al. 1980, 1981; Drahovsky and Boehm 1980; Ehrlich and Wang 1981). The hypomethylation of DNA caused by its substitution could have an importance in these biological mechanisms.

Summary

Both DNA-AAF and MNU-alkylated DNA are methylated less than nonmodified DNA by rat brain nuclei cytosine 5-methyltransferase purified either by chromatography on DEAE cellulose or by Dyematrex. The inhibition of methylation is proportional to the modification of the DNA, and DNA having a given percentage of bases modified with MNU is less methylated than DNA modified to the same extent with AAF. Moreover, DNA-AAF irreversibly inhibits the methylation of native DNA, whereas MNU-alkylated DNA does not inhibit the methylation of native DNA.

The AAF-substituted DNA has a higher affinity for the enzyme than native DNA. However, this is probably not due to the AAF-induced local destabilization of the DNA helix, since heat-denatured DNA shows a lower affinity for the enzyme than double-stranded DNA.

Addition of DNA-AAF to the enzyme preincubated with native DNA inhibits methylation, but only after a lag period. This agrees with the model in which the methylase walks along the strand to methylate cytosine residues before being detached from the DNA. AAF bound to guanine residues may block the movement of the enzyme along the helix. The in vitro hypomethylation of DNA, caused by carcinogens, could explain the in vivo observations made by several authors and could have significance in gene activity, cellular differentiation, and oncogenesis.

References

Beranek DT, Weiss CC, Swenson DH (1980) A comprehensive quantitative analysis of methylated and ethylated DNA using high pressure liquid chromatography. Carcinogenesis 1: 595–606

Daune MP, Fuchs RPP (1976) Structural modification of DNA after covalent binding of a carcinogen. In: Mécanismes d'altérations et de réparation du DNA, relation avec la mutagénèse et la cancérogénèse chimique. CNRS (ed.) pp 83–102

Drahovsky D, Boehm TLJ (1980) Enzymatic DNA methylation in higher eukaryotes. Int J Biochem 12: 523–528

Drahovsky D, Morris NR (1971a) Mechanism of action of rat liver DNA methylase. I: Interaction with double-stranded methyl-acceptor DNA. J Mol Biol 57: 475–489

Drahovsky D, Morris NR (1971b) Mechanism of action of rat liver DNA methylase. II: Interaction with single-stranded methyl-acceptor DNA. J Mol Biol 61: 343–356

Ehrlich M, Wang RYH (1981) 5-Methylcytosine in eukaryotic DNA. Science 212: 1350–1357

Fuchs R, Daune M (1972) Physical studies on deoxyribonucleic acid after covalent binding of a carcinogen. Biochemistry 11: 2659–2666

Grunberger D, Weinstein IB (1979) Conformational changes in nucleic acids modified by chemical carcinogens. In: Grower P (ed) Chemical carcinogens and DNA, vol 2. CRC Press, Boca Raton, pp 59–94

IARC (1978) Monographs on the evaluation of the carcinogenic risk of chemicals to humans n° 17. Some N-nitroso compounds. International Agency for Research on Cancer, Lyon, pp 125–134 and pp 227–236

Kalousek F, Morris NR (1968) Deoxyribonucleic acid methylase activity in rat spleen. J Biol Chem 243: 2440–2442

Kalousek F, Morris NR (1969) The purification and properties of deoxyribonucleic acid methylase from rat spleen. J Biol Chem 244: 1157–1193

Kay FRM, Simmons NS, Dounce AL (1952) An improved preparation of sodium desoxyribonucleate. J Am Chem Soc 74: 1724–1726

Leaver DP, Swann PF, Magee PN (1969) The induction of tumours in the rat by a single oral dose of N-nitroso-methylurea. Br J Cancer 23: 177–187

Lotlikar PD, Scribner JD, Miller JA, Miller EC (1966) Reaction of esters of aromatic N-hydroxy amines and amides with methionine in vitro: A model for in vivo binding of amine carcinogens to protein. Life Sci 5: 1263–1269

Miller EC, Juhl U, Miller JA (1966) Nucleic acid guanosine: reaction with the carcinogen N-acetoxy-2-acetylaminofluorene. Science 153: 1125–1127

Pfohl-Leszkowicz A, Dirheimer G (1982) Comparison of different methods of recovering DNA from a methylation assay. Biochimie 64: 293–296

Pfohl-Leszkowicz A, Salas CE, Fuchs RPP, Dirheimer G (1981) Mechanism of inhibition of enzymatic deoxyribonucleic acid methylation by 2-(acetylamino)fluorene bound to deoxyribonucleic acid. Biochemistry 20: 3020–3024

Pogo AO, Allfrey UG, Mirsky A (1966) Evidence for increased DNA template activity in regenerating liver nuclei. Proc Natl Acad Sci USA 56: 550–557

Razin A, Friedman F (1981) DNA methylation and its possible biological roles. Prog Nucleic Acids Res Mol Biol 25: 33–51

Razin A, Riggs AD (1980) DNA methylation and gene function. Science 210: 604–610

Rogg H, Brambilla R, Keith G, Staehelin M (1976) An improved method for the separation and quantitation of the modified nucleosides of transfer RNA. Nucleic Acids Res 3: 285–295

Salas CE, Selinger OZ (1978) Methylation of *E.coli* transfer ribonucleic acids by tRNA adenine 1-methyltransferase from rat brain cortex and bulk isolated neurons. J Neurochem 31: 85–91

Segal IH (1975) Enzyme kinetics. John Wiley Interscience Press, New York, pp 183–184

*Inhibition of DNA Methylation by 5-Azacytidine**

P. A. Jones, S. M. Taylor, and V. L. Wilson

Division of Hematology-Oncology, Childrens Hospital of Los Angeles and Departments of Pediatrics and Biochemistry, University of Southern California School of Medicine, Los Angeles, CA 900 27, USA

DNA Methylation and Cellular Differentiation

The process by which eukaryotic cells control the expression of their genes constitutes one of the key unanswered questions in biology. While it is clear that post-transcriptional controls are involved in the fine tuning of gene expression it also seems clear that the primary level of control is exhibited at the transcriptional level. Considerable evidence accumulated over the past few years strongly suggests that the methylation of specific cytosine residues within and around genes may exert such transcriptional control (Razin and Riggs 1980).

Human (van der Ploeg and Flavell 1980), rabbit (Waalwijk and Flavell 1978), and chicken (McGhee and Ginder 1979) globin genes contain sequences within and around the genes which are undermethylated in cells active in the expression of those genes, whereas the same sequences tend to be more methylated in cells not active in globin synthesis. Viral sequences such as herpes (Desroisiers et al. 1979), adenovirus (Sutter and Doerfler 1980), and mouse mammary tumor virus (Cohen 1980) are more extensively methylated in nonproducer cells, whereas the same sequences are unmethylated in cells active in viral expression. It should be noted that methylation sites exist in three states: (1) sites which are never methylated, (2) those which are always methylated irrespective of the differentiated state of the cell, and (3) those which demonstrate tissue-specific variability in the degree of methylation (Mandel and Chambon 1979). The relationship between DNA modification and gene expression is therefore not an all-or-none situation, and van der Ploeg and Flavell (1980) have suggested that low methylation levels may be a necessary but not a sufficient condition for gene expression.

Inheritance of Methylation Patterns

The tissue-specific DNA methylation patterns present in the cells of vertebrates suggest that they must be copied during cell division. Vertebrate DNAs contain 5-methylcytosine (5mC) as a minor base and the modification is introduced specifically

* This work was supported by grants GM25739 and T32-CA09320 from the National Institutes of Health

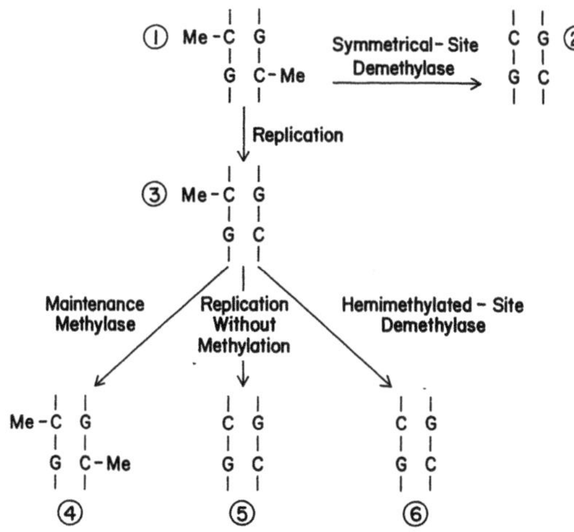

Fig. 1. Possible pathways for the generation of symmetrically demethylated CG doublets

into the progeny strand following DNA replication (Bird 1978; Jones and Taylor 1980, 1981) predominantly, but not exclusively, in the sequence CpG (Doskocil and Sorm 1962). The elegant studies by Bird (1978) showed that in the sequence −C−G−/−G−C either both cytosines are methylated or neither is methylated, and hemimethylated sites do not occur in eukaryotic DNA. Studies with cellular DNA (Bird 1978) and with cells infected with DNA sequences containing modifications introduced into specific sequences (Pollack et al. 1980; Wigler et al. 1981), have shown that a methylation pattern can be semiconservatively copied after replication so that it is passed to the daughter cells after division. The heritability of the methylation pattern is of fundamental importance, since it immediately suggests how differentiated cells breed true.

Mechanisms to explain the heritability of the pattern have been proposed by Holliday and Pugh (1975) and Riggs (1975). Central to these hypotheses were the suggestions that cells contain "maintenance methylases" which would only be capable of the modification of a cytosine residue which occurred opposite to a methylated CpG doublet (Fig. 1 ③→④). The substrate for this enzyme would therefore be hemimethylated DNA arising in cells immediately after DNA replication in which one DNA strand was modified and the other not. The maintenance enzyme would be incapable of the modification of completely unmethylated sites, and thus its action would ensure the heritability of the methylation patterns. The existence of such enzymes is suggested by the existence of specific modification patterns (see above) and by our recent demonstration that hemimethylated duplex DNA is a good substrate for a crude DNA methylase extracted from mouse spleen (Jones and Taylor 1981).

Changes in Methylation Patterns

The action of maintenance DNA methylases would ensure the heritability of methylation patterns, and thus ensure that differentiated cells bred true following DNA synthesis. However, coordinate changes in these patterns, which may be responsible for changes in gene expression, are likely to be of singular importance during cell differentiation. While we know that the pattern can be inherited (Pollack et al. 1980; Wigler et al. 1981), and also that specific sequences become demethylated during differentiation (Razin and Riggs 1980), the processes controlling the loss of methyl groups are totally unknown.

The hypomethylation associated with gene expression might be achieved by the action of sequence-specific symmetrical-site demethylase enzymes (Fig. 1, ①→②). However, there is no evidence for the presence or action of such enzymes in eukaryotic cells (Razin and Riggs 1980).

The failure to apply methyl groups during critical cell cycles is a more likely mechanism for cells to achieve the hypomethylation of DNA sequences observed in differentiated cells. Hemimethylated CG sites (Fig. 1, ③) are normally converted to symmetrically modified sites immediately after DNA synthesis (Fig. 1, ③→④), but if cell division occurred before such a site had been modified, an unmethylated sequence would be generated (Fig. 1, ③→⑤). This might occur if chromosomal proteins or RNA masked the site before the action of the methylase, and the model would predict that two cell divisions were required for differentiation. Since cell division is often required for cell differentiation (Dientsman and Holtzer 1975; Groudine and Weintraub 1981), the failure to methylate during certain specific S phases may represent the quantal cell cycles of Dientsman and Holtzer (1975). It is also possible that hemimethylated-site demethylases might operate within cells to remove the methyl groups from half-modified sequences and thus generate unmodified sites after one cell division (Fig. 1, ③→⑥).

I will present experiments in which we have utilized analogs of cytidine modified in the 5 position to perturb DNA methylation patterns and induce changes in the differentiated state of cells.

Effects of 5-Azacytidine on Cell Differentiation

The nucleoside analog 5-azacytidine (z^5C) has profound effects on the differentiated state of cultured cells (Constantinides et al. 1977, 1978; Taylor and Jones 1979). Thus, cells of the $10T^1/_2$ or 3T3 lines of mouse embryo cells are converted into fully functional and biochemically differentiated muscle cells, adipocytes, or chondrocytes several days or weeks after exposure to this analog (Fig. 2). The ability of z^5C to induce changes in the differentiated state of cells is not due to a selection of cells with a predisposition to differentiate. The maximal rate of conversion of synchronized cells was seen in cells treated in the early part of the S phase of the cell cycle (Constantinides et al. 1978).

The induction of new phenotypes in z^5C-treated cultures is dependent upon cell division, and more than two divisions are required after z^5C treatment for the expression of the muscle phenotype in $10T^1/_2$ cultures (Taylor and Jones 1982). The maximum number of myotubes was seen in cultures which had undergone 11 divisions before reaching confluence.

These results have been confirmed in several other laboratories, and z^5C has been used to induce the expression of a human gene located on an inactive X chromosome in a mouse/human hybrid (Mohandas et al. 1981), the differentiation of human HL60 cells (Mendelsohn et al. 1981), the expression of endogenous chicken viral genes (Groudine et al. 1981), and metalothienin inducibility (Compere and Palmiter 1981).

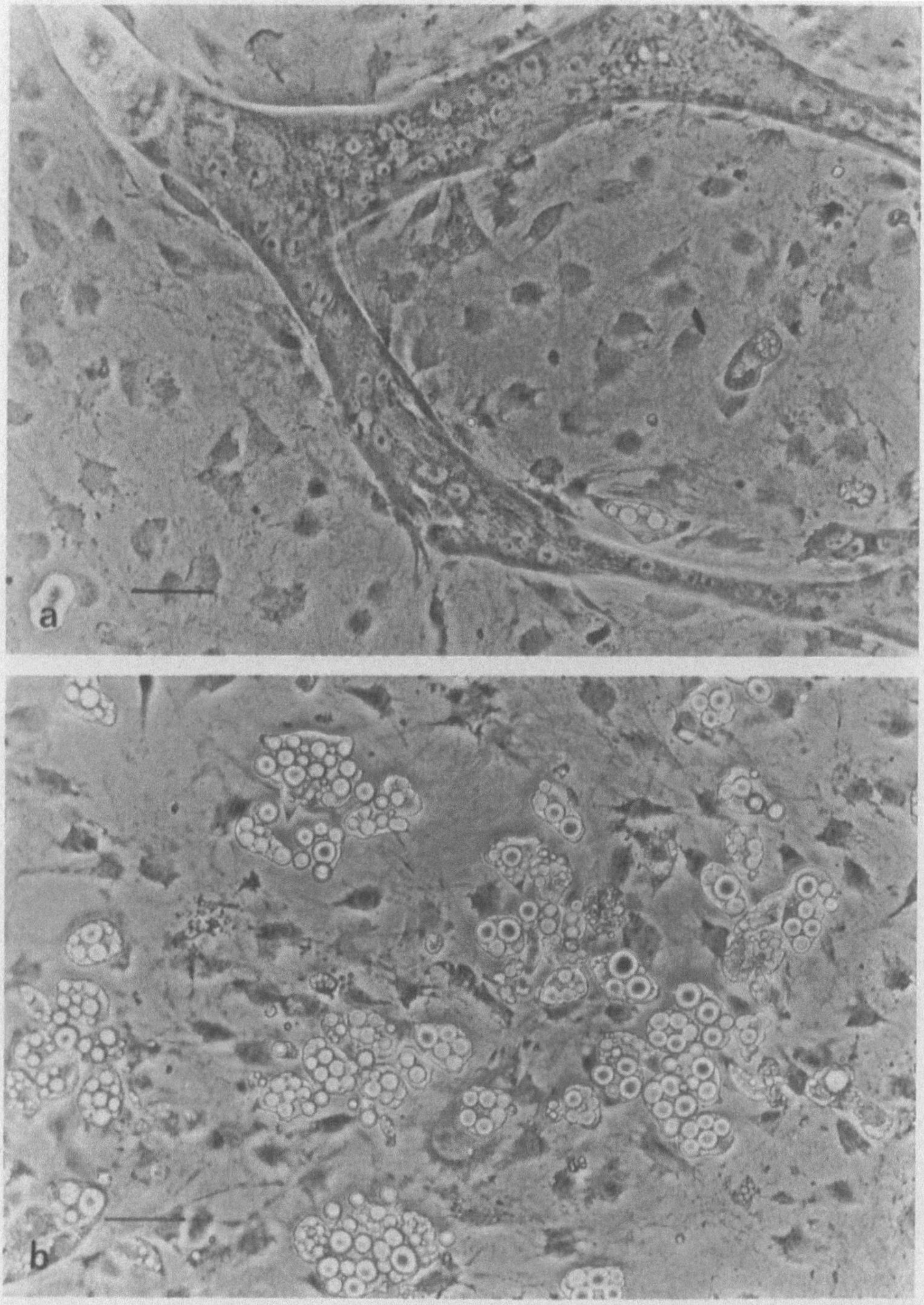

Fig. 2a–c. New phenotypes induced in C3H $10T^{1}/_{2}$ C18 cells treated with 5-azacytidine. **a** myotubes; **b** adipocytes

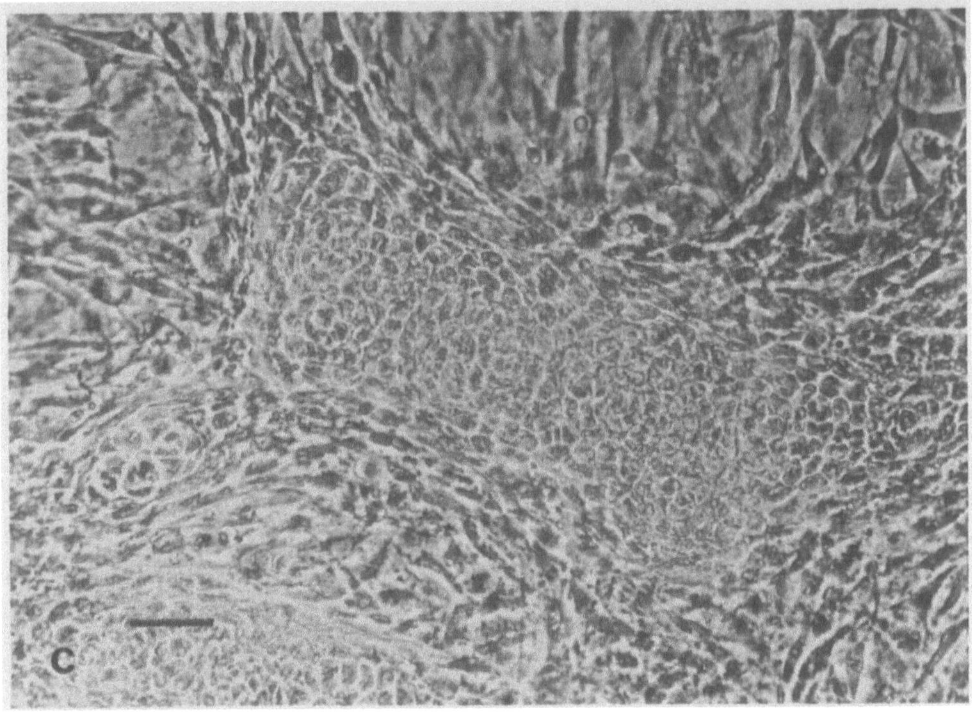

Fig. 2c. Chondrocytes. The *bar* represents 50 μm

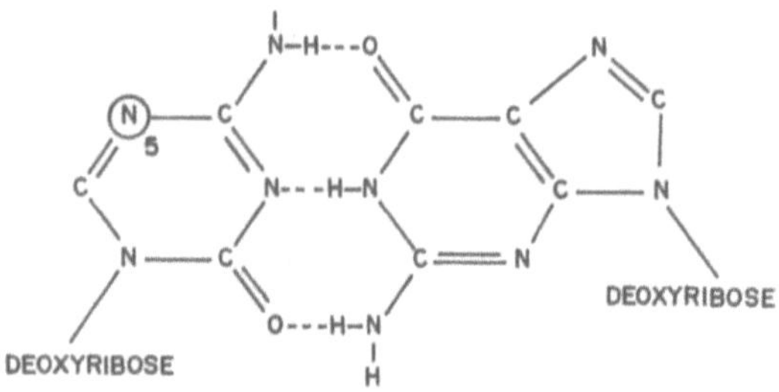

Fig. 3. 5-Azacytosine-guanine base pair

Inhibition of DNA Methylation by 5-Azacytidine

The facts that 5-aza-2′-deoxycytidine was more active than 5-aza-cytidine in inducing muscle formation and that maximal induction occurred in cells treated in early S phase suggested a DNA-linked mechanism of action for z^5C (Constantinides et al. 1978). However, the 5 position of cytosine is not involved in hydrogen bonding, so that 5-azacytosine would be expected to base pair with guanine in the normal manner (Fig. 3).

We therefore discounted a mutagenic mechanism of action for the analog and have recently demonstrated directly that z^5C is, at best, a very weak mutagen in $10T^1/_2$ cells (Landolph and Jones 1982). On the other hand, the occurrence of the nitrogen atom in the 5 position would be expected to render the ring refractory to enzymic methylation following incorporation into DNA.

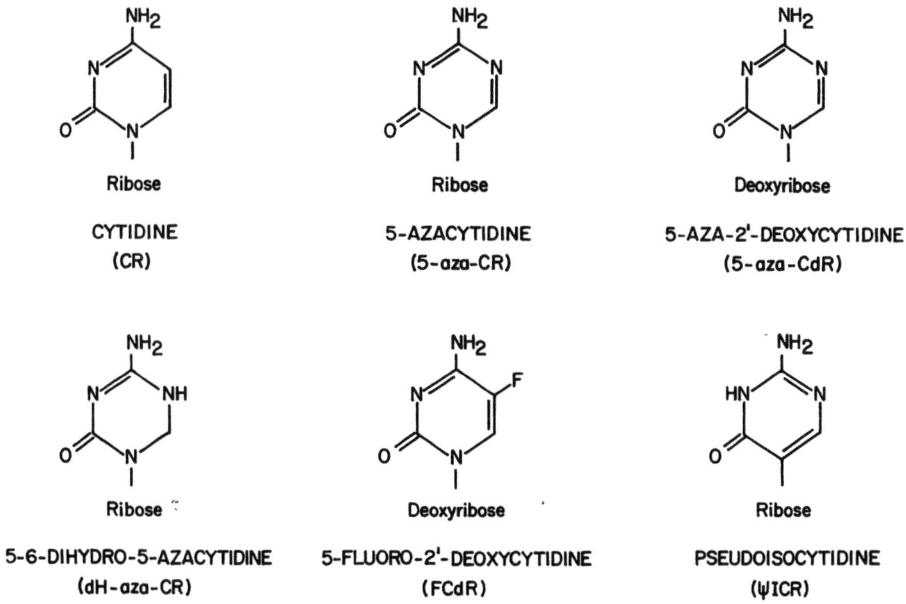

Fig. 4. Chemical structures of cytidine analogs

Table 1. Induction of myotubes and inhibition of DNA methylation by cytosine nucleosides

Treatment	Nuclei in myotubes/dish	Cytosine methylation in newly synthesized DNA (% of control)
3 μ*M* Cytidine	0	100
3 μ*M* z^5C	22411	33
0.3 μ*M* z^5dC	28190	55
30 μ*M* ψ-iso-C	5920	40
10 μ*M* 5FdC	1168	63
30 μ*M* hz^5C	0	104
10 μ*M* z^6C	0	106
0.3 μ*M* Ara-C	0	127

10T½ cells were treated with the indicated agents for 24 h and stained and scored for muscle cells 10–12 days later. Cultures were exposed to the analogs in the presence of ^3H-methionine and ^{14}C-dT to determine the inhibition of DNA methylation. The DNA was hydrolysed and the bases separated by TLC. The ^3H radioactivity present in m^5C was compared to the ^{14}C radioactivity in thymine to correct for the extent of DNA synthesis during the treatment period. *Ara-C*, cytosine arabinoside; *z^6C*, 6-azacytidine; *hz^5C*, 5,6-dihydro-5-azacytidine; *5FdC*, 5-fluoro-2′-deoxycytidine; *ψ-iso-C*, pseudoisocytidine; *z^5dC*, 5-azadeoxycytidine; *z^5C*, 5-azacytidine; *m^5C*, 5-methyl-cytosine

If the mechanism action of z^5C was linked to the alteration in the 5 position, and therefore its ability to inhibit DNA methylation, one might anticipate that other analogs of cytidine (Fig. 4) would also inhibit DNA methylation and change the differentiated state of cells. Indeed, all the analogs which inhibited DNA methylation induced the formation of muscle cells in treated cultures (Table 1).

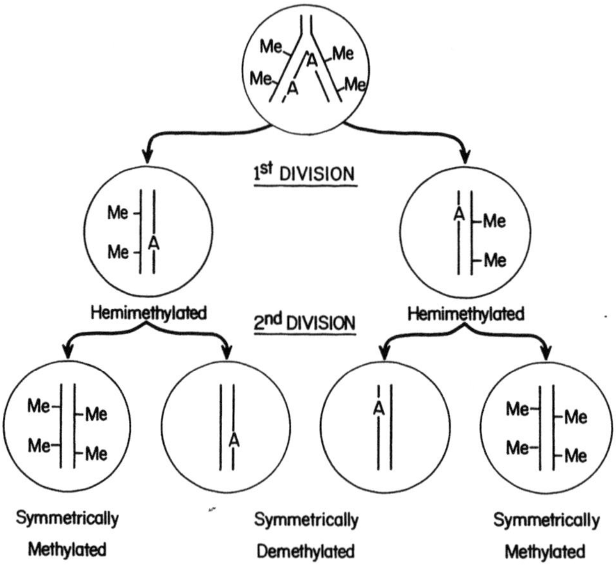

Fig. 5. Proposed mechanism of action of 5-aza-CR. The replication of DNA containing 5-methylcytosine (*Me*) in the S phase is shown at the top of the diagram. If 5-azacytosine (*A*) was incorporated into the newly synthesized DNA and inhibited DNA methylation, the daughter cells of the first division would contain hemimethylated DNA in the sequence controlling gene expression. Symmetrically demethylated DNA in this sequence would result after the second division following treatment, because of the specificity of the DNA methyltransferase (see text)

Since the only chemical similarity of the active analogs is the modification in the 5 position, these results provide strong evidence for a controlling role for this position in cellular differentiation.

Mechanism of Action of 5-Azacytidine

The mechanism by which z^5C induces heritable changes in DNA methylation patterns is summarized in the model presented in Fig. 5. The incorporation of 5-azacytosine into DNA would inhibit the action of the DNA methylase, leading to the formation of hemimethylated DNA in the daughter cells of the subsequent mitosis. Evidence that the DNA is hemimethylated has been obtained by direct measurement (Jones and Taylor 1981). Symmetrically demethylated DNA would result in the second division following z^5C treatment. This would result if the maintenance methylase only applied methyl groups to hemimethylated newly synthesized duplex DNA as proposed by Holliday and Pugh (1975) and Riggs (1975). The existence of such maintenance methylases is implied by the heritability of methylation patterns (Pollack et al. 1980; Wigler et al. 1981) and by our recent demonstration that hemimethylated duplex DNA is a much better substrate for mouse spleen methylase than unmethylated duplex DNA (Jones and Taylor 1981). Note that once symmetrically demethylated sites have been generated in the DNA of treated cells, this condition would be heritable and would ultimately lead to the expression of new genes.

Table 2. Inhibition of DNA methyltransferase activity by chemical carcinogens[a]

Agent	Dose (γb)[b]	Inhibition of DNA methylation (%)
MNNG	17.7	58.9
ENU	100.0	55.1
BCNU	24.0	81.1
HN2	0.2	53.2
BPDE	2.0	49.7

MNNG, *N*-methyl-*N*-nitroso-*N'*-nitroguanidine; *ENU*, ethylnitrosourea; *BCNU*, 1,3-bis(2-chloroethyl)-1-nitrosourea; *HN2*, nitrogen mustard; *BPDE*, (anti)-r-7t-8-dihydroxy-t-9,10-oxy-7,8,9,10-tetrahydrobenzo(a)pyrene

[a] Hemimethylated DNA was incubated with carcinogen, or in buffer alone, for 2 h at 37° C. Aliquots of treated DNA were assayed for their methyl-accepting abilities in the presence of mouse spleen methyltransferase and ^{3}H-S-adenosylmethionine

[b] The molar ratio of the agent to DNA base pairs in the reaction mixture

Inhibition of DNA Maintenance Methylation by Chemical Carcinogens

We have recently taken advantage of the ability of z^{5}C to inhibit DNA methylation to prepare milligram quantities of hemimethylated DNA (Fig. 5). This DNA is a good acceptor of methyl groups from ^{3}H-*S*-adenosylmethionine incubated in the presence of a crude mouse spleen methyltransferase (Jones and Taylor 1981). The methyl groups are transferred specifically to cytosine residues located in the hypomethylated strand of the hemimethylated duplex DNA. The in vitro reaction therefore satisfies several of the criteria for maintenance DNA methylation (see Fig. 1).

Preliminary data has shown that the abilities of these hemimethylated DNA substrates to act as methyl acceptors is markedly impaired if they are pretreated with a variety of ultimate chemical carcinogens (Table 2). We have not yet determined the extent of adduct formation by the different carcinogens, but the data suggests that chemical carcinogens may also be capable of inhibiting DNA methylation. Therefore if DNA methylation has a major role in controlling gene expression, certain carcinogens may perturb cellular phenotypes directly, by changing pre-existing methylation patterns in a heritable manner.

Summary

The nucleoside analog z^{5}C induced marked changes in the differentiated state of mouse embryo cells and inhibited the methylation of newly synthesized DNA. Other analogs of cytidine containing modifications in the 5 position (5-aza-2'-deoxycytidine, 5-fluoro-2'-deoxycytidine, and pseudoisocytidine) also induced the formation of striated muscle cells in treated cultures and inhibited DNA methylation. Together the data suggests a causative role for the methylation of specific cytosine residues in the control of gene expression. Hemimethylated duplex DNA was extracted from cultures treated with z^{5}C and was an efficient acceptor of methyl groups from *S*-adenosylmethionine in the presence of a mouse spleen methyltransferase. The ability of this hemimethylated DNA to accept methyl groups was markedly impaired if it was pretreated with several different ultimate chemical carcinogens.

References

Bird AP (1978) Use of restriction enzymes to study eukaryotic DNA methylation: The symmetry of methylated sites supports semi-conservative copying of the methylation pattern. J Mol Biol 118: 49–60

Cohen JC (1980) Methylation of milk-borne and genetically transmitted mouse mammary tumor virus proviral DNA. Cell 19: 653–662

Compere SJ, Palmiter RD (1981) DNA methylation controls the inducibility of the mouse metallothionein-l gene in lymphoid cells. Cell 25: 233–240

Constantinides PG, Jones PA, Gevers W (1977) Functional striated muscle cells from non-myoblast precursors following 5-azacytidine treatment. Nature 267: 364–366

Constantinides PG, Taylor SM, Jones PA (1978) Phenotypic conversion of cultured mouse embryo cells by aza pyrimidine nucleosides. Dev Biol 66: 57–71

Desrosiers RC, Mulder C, Fleckenstein B (1979) Methylation of herpesvirus samiri DNA in lymphoid tumor cell lines. Proc Natl Acad Sci USA 76: 3839–3843

Dientsman SR, Holtzer H (1975) Myogenesis: A cell lineage interpretation. In: Reinert J, Holtzer H (eds) Results and problems in cell differentiation. Springer, Berlin Heidelberg New York, pp 1–25

Doskocil J, Sorm F (1962) Distribution of 5-methylcytosine in pyrimidine sequences of deoxyribonucleic acids. Biochim Biophys Acta 55: 953–959

Groudine M, Weintraub H (1981) Activation of globin genes during chicken development. Cell 24: 393–401

Groudine M, Eisenman R, Weintraub H (1981) Chromatin structure of endogenous retroviral genes and activation by an inhibitor of DNA methylation. Nature 292: 311–317

Holliday R, Pugh JE (1975) DNA modification mechanisms and gene activity during development. Science 187: 226–232

Jones PA, Taylor SM (1980) Cellular differentiation, cytidine analogs and DNA methylation. Cell 20: 85–93

Jones PA, Taylor SM (1981) Hemimethylated duplex DNAs prepared from 5-azacytidine treated cells, Nucleic Acids Res 9: 2933–2947

Landolph JR, Jones PA (1982) Mutagenicity of 5-azacytidine and related nucleosides in C3H/10T$^1/_2$CL8 and V79 cells. Cancer Res 42: 817–823

Mandel JL, Chambon P (1979) DNA methylation: Organ specific variations in the methylation pattern within and around ovalbumin and other chicken genes. Nucleic Acids Res 7: 2081–2103

McGhee JD, Ginder GD (1979) Specific DNA methylation sites in the vicinity of the chicken β-globin genes. Nature 280: 419–420

Mendelsohn N, Herzog D, Christman JK (1981) 5-Azacytidine (5-aza-CR) as an inducer of differentiation in human leukemia cells (HL-60). Proc Am Assoc Cancer Res 22: 190

Mohandas T, Sparkes RS, Shapiro LJ (1981) Reactivation of an inactive human X chromosome: Evidence for X inactivation by DNA methylation. Science 211: 393–396

Pollack Y, Stein R, Razin A, Cedar H (1980) Methylation of foreign DNA sequences in eukaryotic cells. Proc Natl Acad Sci USA 77: 6463–6467

Razin A, Riggs AD (1980) DNA methylation and gene function. Science 210: 604–610

Riggs AD (1975) X-inactivation, differentiation and DNA methylation. Cytogenet Cell Genet 14: 9–25

Sutter D, Doerfler W (1980) Methylation of integrated adenovirus type 12 DNA sequences in transformed cells is inversely correlated with viral gene expression. Proc Natl Acad Sci USA 77: 253–256

Taylor SM, Jones PA (1979) Multiple new phenotypes induced in $10T^{1}/_{2}$ and 3T3 cells treated with 5-azacytidine. Cell 17: 771–779

Taylor SM, Jones PA (1982) Changes in phenotypic expression in embryonic and adult cells treated with 5-azacytidine. J Cell Physiol 111: 187–194

van der Ploeg LHT, Flavell RA (1980) DNA methylation in the human $\gamma\delta\beta$-globin locus in erythroid and nonerythroid tissue. Cell 19: 947–958

Waalwijk C, Flavell RA (1978) DNA methylation at a CCGG sequence in the large intron of the rabbit β-globin gene: tissue specific variations. Nucleic Acids Res 5: 4631–4641

Wigler M, Levy D, Perucho M (1981) The somatic replication of DNA methylation. Cell 24: 3340

Alteration of Enzymatic DNA Methylation by Chemical Carcinogens

T. L. J. Boehm and D. Drahovsky

Zentrum der Biologischen Chemie, Universität Frankfurt, Theodor-Stern-Kai 7, D-6000 Frankfurt a. M. 70, FRG

Enzymatic Methylation of Eukaryotic DNA

Experiments analyzing the methylation patterns in the vicinity of various eukaryotic genes in gamete DNA and in DNA of various differentiated cells of one organism have shown that during development, the fully methylated zygote DNA becomes devoid of 5-methylcytosines at certain sequences (McGhee and Ginder 1979; Kuo et al. 1979; Mandel and Chambon 1979; Shen and Maniatis 1980; van der Ploeg and Flavell 1980; Weintraub et al. 1981; Groudine and Weintraub 1981). Although there are no gross changes of enzymatic DNA methylation during development and cellular differentiation (Baur et al. 1979; Fabricant et al. 1979; Pollock et al. 1978; Singer et al. 1979; Lapeyre et al. 1980), it was shown that such a hypomethylation correlates with the expression of these particular genes (McGhee and Ginder 1979; Kuo et al. 1979; Mandel and Chambon 1979; Shen and Maniatis 1980; van der Ploeg and Flavell 1980; Weintraub et al. 1981; Groudine and Weintraub 1981; Boehm and Drahovsky 1981a; Chistman et al. 1977; Christman et al. 1980; Boehm and Drahovsky 1981).

These findings raised the question of how the enzymatic methylation of DNA in developing organisms is regulated, i.e., what mechanism(s) govern(s) the maintenance of the methylation pattern in the differentiated cells and what directs the demethylation and remethylation processes during cellular differentiation. The experimental evidence for two different kinds of DNA methylating activities suggests that the maintenance activity of DNA methylases produces an identical methylation pattern in the progeny DNA strand via a semiconservative copying mechanism directed by the 5-methylcytosine residue of the parental strand (Bird 1978; Pollack et al. 1980; Wigler et al. 1981). The initiation of methylation at sites previously not methylated was first shown in in vitro experiments with DNA-methylating enzymes isolated from various tissues using methyl-accepting DNA polymers essentially free of 5-methylcytosines (Drahovsky and Morris 1971a,b, 1972; Roy and Weissbach 1975; Simon et al. 1978; Salas et al. 1979; Adams et al. 1979; Sneider et al. 1975). The finding that integrated viral DNA became methylated in eukaryotic cells (Desrosiers et al. 1979; Sutter and Doerfler 1981) and the observation of hypermethylated DNA in somatic cells hybrids (Drahovsky et al. 1980, 1981) are compatible with the existence of an initiation methylation process in vivo. Figure 1 schematically describes the maintenance demethylation, and remethylation processes in eukaryotic DNA.

Recent Results in Cancer Research. Vol 84

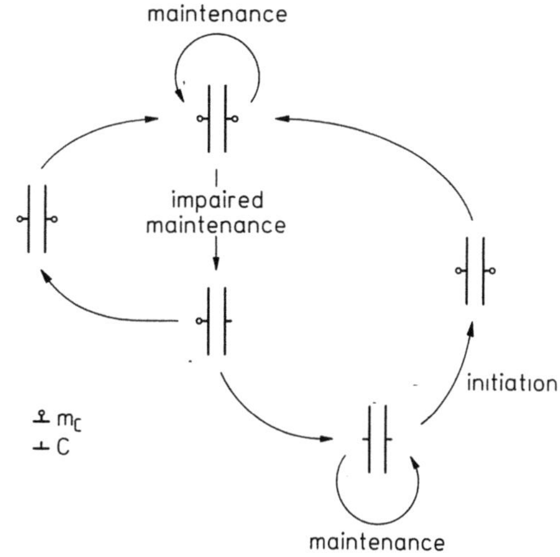

Fig. 1. Maintaining methylation, demethylation, and initiation of methylation in eukaryotic DNA. The maintenance activity ensures the copying of the parental methylation pattern in the progeny cells, since the methylation of the parental strand determines the methylation in the progeny strand. Demethylation at a specific site probably occurs via a hemimethylated intermediate, which, after an additional round of replication, becomes fully devoid of 5-methylcytosine. Although no information has been obtained regarding the factor(s) regulating this process under physiological conditions, evidence presented here favors such a mechanism, and the possibility of demethylation during a single step of replication of DNA thus seems unlikely. The information regarding the initiation of methylation is also sparse; it is likely, however, that this occurs through a symmetrical methylation on both DNA strands at a potentially methylatable site. A certain degree of sequence specificity can be anticipated. *^{m}C*, 5-methylcytosine at methylation site; *C*, cytosine at methylation site

Since the lack of methylation at certain DNA sequences can be correlated to the transcription of these DNA segments, one may expect that compounds interfering with the enzymatic methylation of DNA may lead to a pertubed program of gene expression. In this chapter we present evidence showing that the carcinogenic substances *N*-methyl-*N*-nitrosourea (MNU), *N*-methyl-*N*-nitro-*N*-nitrosoguanidine (MNNG), and L-ethionine are capable of altering the pattern of enzymatic DNA methylation in treated cells. We also found that carcinogen-induced hypomethylation of DNA is accompanied by an increased nucleotide sequence complexity in the nRNA of treated cells. This suggests the initiation of transcription at sites previously inactive in this respect. Since the carcinogen-induced changes in the process of enzymatic DNA methylation are clonally inherited, i.e., passed through progeny cell generations, they may initiate the sequence of biochemical changes ultimately leading to a malignant phenotype.

The Effect of Some Chemical Carcinogens on the Enzymatic Methylation of Mammalian DNA

In order to study the effects of carcinogens on the process of enzymatic DNA methylation, we have concentrated on MNU, which interacts directly with DNA to

Table 1. Sequence specificities of restriction enzymes pertinent to this study

Enzymes	5′ → 3′ Sequence	
	Cleaved	Not cleaved
*Hpa*II	CCGG, MCGG	MMGG, CMGG
*Msp*I	CCGG, CMGG	MCGG, MMGG
*Hha*I	GCGC	CMGC
*Hae*II	PuGCGCPy	PuGMGCPy
*Ava*I	CpyCGPuG	CPyMGPuG
*Hind*III	AAGCTT	?
*Hae*III	GGCC, GGCM	GGMC

Recognition sequences have been compiled from Bird and Southern (1978), Bird et al. (1979), Mann and Smith (1977), Roberts (1978), Sneider (1980), van der Ploeg and Flavell (1980), and Waalwijk and Flavell (1978)

form covalent adducts, and on L-ethionine, which, probably via activation into *S*-adenosyl-L-ethionine, is either transferred into nucleic acids or in this form inhibits the action of these methylating enzymes. MNNG, which both alkylates DNA and inhibits enzyme activities responsible for methylation of newly replicated DNA, will also be discussed.

In the studies described here, we have employed three different methods to analyze the process of enzymatic DNA methylation:

1. The overall extent of methylation of newly replicated DNA has been measured by estimating the conversion of labeled incorporated cytosine into 5-methylcytosine, a method which will be referred to as the absolute extent of enzymatic DNA methylation (Kappler 1970).
2. In certain cases, this method gives insufficient sensitivity, especially if portions of the cellular DNA are to be analyzed. We have then used a simultaneous labeling of the cells under study with both (a) labeled deoxycytidine or thymine (in order to assess the replication of DNA), and (b) labeled L-methionine (the labeled methyl group of which becomes incorporated into 5-methylcytosine). This method will be referred to as the relative extent of enzymatic DNA methylation (Craddock 1970; Drahovsky et al. 1976).
3. In addition to measuring the total amount of 5-methylcytosine formed in the DNA during replication, we have used bacterial restriction enzymes to probe the extent of methylation at specific DNA sequences determined by the recognition specificity of these endonucleases. Table 1 gives a representative sample of CpG enzymes, so called because their recognition sequence involves a CpG dinucleotide; they are sensitive to 5-methylcytosine present at these sites (compare the structure of sequences cleaved and those not cleaved by the particular enzyme).

Each of the methods described above has its advantages, but also certain limitations. For example, the absolute and relative extents of DNA methylation can only be measured in cell systems in which DNA replication takes place; furthermore, they measure total methylation and do not differentiate between methylations at particular nucleotide sequence specific sites. The latter is the great advantage of restriction enzyme analysis of eukaryotic DNA methylation. However, with this method one measures only a small fraction, approximately 5%–15%, of the total DNA methylation.

As will become apparent below, it is of great value to combine these methods when analyzing the modification of DNA methylation patterns in cells treated with carcinogens and other compounds. For instance, pulse labeling of cells treated with a carcinogen allows estimation of the methylation of newly replicated DNA in every cell cycle, whereas analysis by use of restriction enzymes only gives valid results if one can be certain that symmetrical methylation sites (i.e., fully demethylated or methylated) occur in the DNA under study. For example, if the action of a carcinogenic compound induces an impaired maintenance methylation, a hemimethylated site may appear in the DNA of the progeny cell. This situation will only be detected by parallel labeling experiments, since restriction enzymes cleave only if both strands are devoid of 5-methylcytosine.[1]

Clonal Inheritance of Carcinogen-Induced Hypomethylation of DNA

When Raji cells were cultured in the presence of MNU, we observed a dose-dependent decrease of enzymatic methylation in the newly replicated DNA (Boehm and Drahovsky 1981b) which was not detected with restriction enzyme analysis after the first round of replication. However, when cells were grown further in the absence of the carcinogen, we found an increased digestibility of DNA isolated from treated cells while the absolute extent of enzymatic methylation was still decreased (Fig. 2b). These results suggested that MNU-induced hypomethylation of DNA occurred via hemimethylation at certain methylation sites, which appear as fully demethylated sites only after an additional round of replication.

The same experimental system, using a similar experimental approach, has been used to test MNNG, and the results have been found to be qualitatively similar (Boehm and Drahovsky 1981d). One interesting observation in these experiments is worth mentioning. In contrast to the effects of MNU, found only with *Hpa*II, not with *Msp*I, suggesting the hypomethylation of internal cytosines at 5′-CCGG-3′ sequences only, MNNG caused a decrease in the methylation of both internal and external cytosines at 5′-CCGG-3′ sites, albeit to a different extent (Fig. 3). The reason for the observed differential inhibition of enzymatic DNA methylation at different sites is not clear at present. MNNG (Drahovsky and Wacker 1975), but not MNU (Cox 1980) inhibits DNA methylation in an in vitro system, and thus alkylation of DNA (caused by both MNU and MNNG) and inhibition of DNA methylases (exerted only by MNNG) may both contribute to the effects of MNNG on the enzymatic DNA methylation in these cells. Alternatively, since the actual degree of DNA alkylation by MNNG was not determined and compared to that caused by the MNU treatment, one can speculate that if there are different methylating enzymes, each with a different specificity in selection of the methylation sites, a differential sensitivity to inhibition by MNNG might explain the observed effects. Such an explanation is even more likely in

1 Recently, it was shown that there are several enzymes which, under appropriate experimental conditions, will cleave hemimethylated DNA also (Gruenbaum et al. 1981). However, this does not apply to the enzymes used in this study, since their cleavage properties have the characteristics described in the text

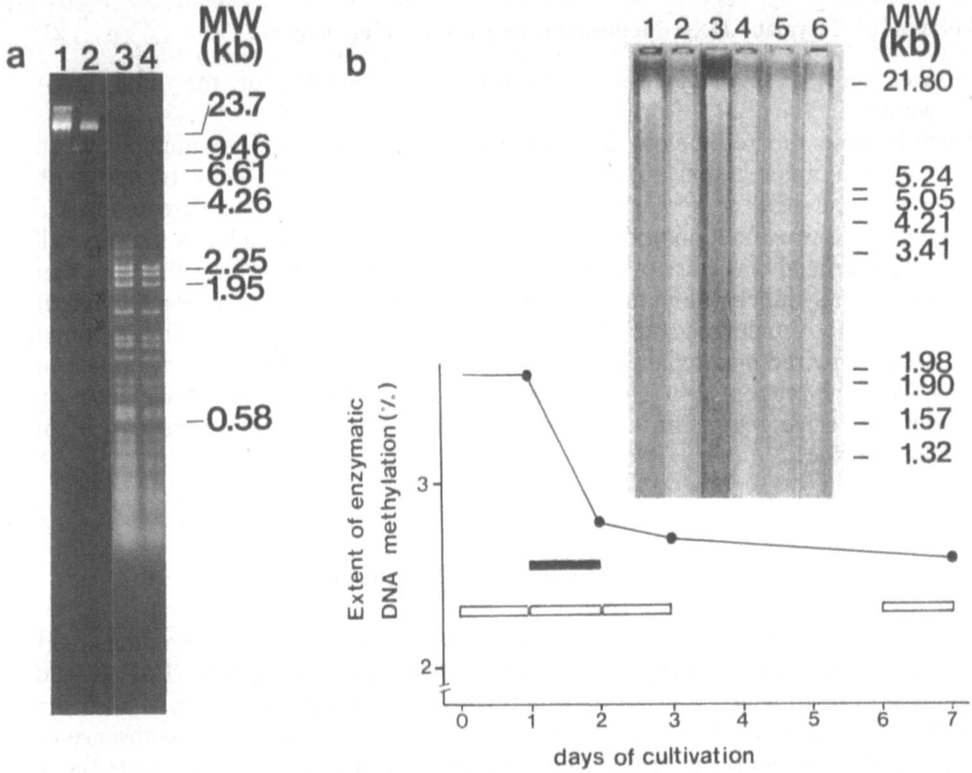

Fig. 2. a Ability of restriction enzymes to cleave DNA substrates treated in vitro with MNU (Boehm and Drahovsky 1980b). The restriction enzymes *Hpa*II, *Msp*I, *Hha*I, *Hae*III, *Hin*dIII, *Eco*RI, and *Bam*HI were all inhibited, suggesting that the sequence-specific restriction enzymes are unable either to recognize carcinogen-modified sequences or to insert endonucleolytic cuts at such sites in a modified substrate. The example here is of such an experiment with phage lambda DNA as a substrate and *Hpa*II as the restriction enzyme. Mock-modified DNA was added in lanes 2 and 4. Lanes 1 and 2 contain uncut DNA, lanes 3 and 4 contain DNA digested with *Hpa*II. The molecular weight standards are from a *Hin*dIII digest of lambda DNA subjected to electrophoresis on the same gel. The appearance of additional bands *(arrows)* reflects impaired restriction and is proportional to the degree of chemical modification of the substrate DNA. MNNG was also positive in this test (T.L.J. Boehm and D. Drahovsky, unpublished work). **b** Extent of enzymatic DNA methylation (percent of total cytosines methylated in newly replicated DNA) in Raji cells cultured in presence of 20 µg/ml initial concentration of MNU and restriction endonuclease digests of Raji cell DNA (inserts). At day 1 the medium was supplemented with MNU and the cells were treated for 24 h *(solid bar)*. Cells were also labeled for 24-h periods with [^{14}C]deoxycytidine in parallel cultures at various intervals *(open bars)*. The extent of enzymatic DNA methylation was analyzed after hydrolysis of the DNA by thin layer chromatography. After termination of the MNU treatment, the lower level of enzymatic DNA methylation of newly synthesized DNA still persists. The insert shows the gel patterns of DNAs treated with the restriction enzymes *Hpa*II and *Msp*I. Control DNA was added in lanes 1 and 2, DNA from cells after 24 h treatment with MNU in lanes 3 and 4, and DNA from cells 5 days after termination of MNU treatment in lanes 5 and 6. *Hpa*II digests are in lanes 1, 3, and 5, *Msp*I digests are in lanes 2, 4, and 6. Note the presence of low-molecular-weight DNA in lane 5, not found in lanes 1 and 3. The patterns of restriction with *Msp*I remain unchanged. This suggests that there is no significant chemical modification of DNA by MNU which would interfere with the restriction endonuclease assay of total DNA (cf. Fig. 2a). This does not exclude the possibility of chemical modification of these DNAs, however, since a level of about 5% of modified recognition sequences in the DNA would not be detected in this assay. The increase in the digestibility of DNAs with *Hpa*II therefore reflects a lower extent of enzymatic methylation at internal cytosines of 5′-CCGG-3′ sequences. The molecular weight standards are from a *Hin*dIII-*Eco*RI double digest of lambda DNA and are given in kilobases

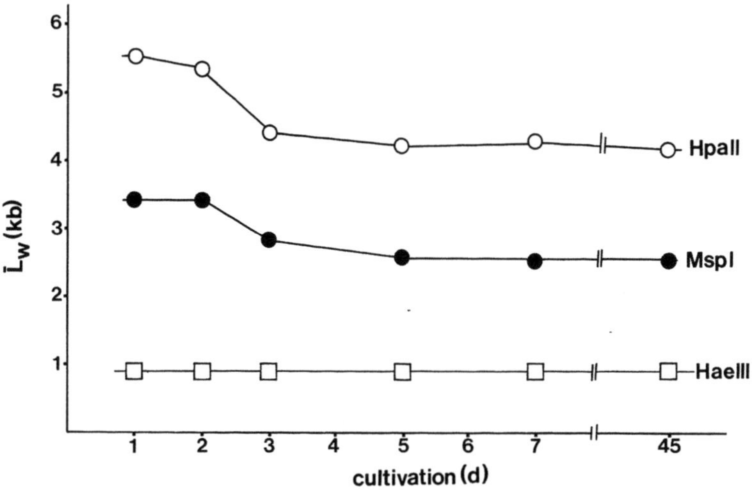

Fig. 3. Weight average lengths ($\bar{L}_w$) of DNA of Raji cells digested with the restriction endonucleases *Hpa*II, *Msp*I, and *Hae*III. The values (average of two independent determinations) were obtained by densitometry of the gels as described in Boehm and Drahovsky (1981d). The period of MNNG treatment was from day 2 to day 3 (3 μg/ml initial concentration). At the indicated time points, cells were taken out of the cultures and the DNA was isolated from the purified nuclei and digested with the restriction endonucleases. The number of cuts made by *Hae*III into DNA of Raji cells is invariant when control DNA and DNAs from MNNG-treated cells are compared. Since no methylation at 5′-GGCC-3′ sequences in Raji cell DNA is likely to occur, this digest serves as an internal control for possible effects of the MNNG modification of DNA (cf. legend to Fig. 2a)

view of the results obtained with L-ethionine (see below), which have demonstrated that methylation is inhibited to different extents at different methylation sites.

The results allow us to propose a model of clonal inheritance of carcinogen-induced aberrant methylation patterns of DNA (Fig. 4). In DNA replicated in the presence of the carcinogen, certain sites in the newly replicated progeny strand are not methylated (impaired maintenance methylation). This lack of methylation was shown by measuring the conversion of labeled cytosine into 5-methylcytosine. The appearance of hemimethylated sites is suggested by the finding that restriction endonucleases do not detect this difference. After the next round of replication fully demethylated sites arise in a subpopulation of the DNA molecules, because the signal for the maintenance activity (i.e., the 5-methylcytosine residue in the opposite strand) is missing. Such sites are now cleaved by restriction enzymes and the lower level of maintenance activity is reflected by the still decreased extent of enzymatic cytosine conversion. The demethylated sites do not become remethylated in the following cell cycles. Thus if a DNA molecule becomes chemically modified prior to replication and the chemical modification still allows a correct DNA synthesis[1], then after the replication the hybrid molecule containing a carcinogen-modified parental strand is insufficiently methylated. This impaired maintenance activity causes the appearance of hemimethylated sites

1 This is not an unrealistic assumption. Abanobi et al. (1980) have shown that certain chemical modifications in DNA molecules do not inhibit a subsequent complete round of DNA replication

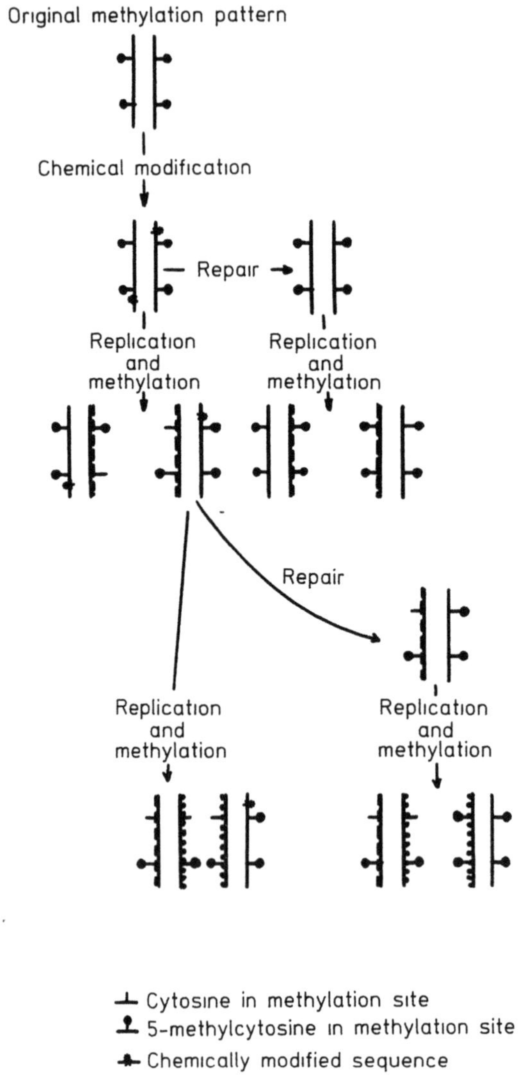

Fig. 4. Putative model for carcinogen-induced hypomethylation of DNA. As detailed in the text, a chemically modified sequence impairs the ability of methylating enzymes to methylate the progeny DNA strand, leading to a clonally inherited aberrant DNA methylation pattern

which become fully demethylated in the next round of replication whether the originally chemically modified site is repaired or not. Note that the repair of such lesions prior to DNA replication does not cause aberrant DNA methylation patterns. It is also apparent from Fig. 4 that there is no need for a continued presence of the carcinogen in the cell cycles following the initial treatment.

Relationship of DNA Methylation to Gene Expression

The results reported in the previous section have shown that MNU and MNNG are capable of inducing clonally inherited aberrant DNA methylation patterns. In this section we will deal with the effects of L-ethionine on enzymatic DNA methylation,

Table 2. Sequence composition of transcribed and nontranscribed regions of the P815 genome

Component	Sequence composition in DNA (% of total DNA)	
	Bound to immobilized heterogeneous nRNA	Not bound to immobilized heterogeneous nRNA
Unique and intermediate repetitive sequences	8.20	62.40
Ordinary highly repetitive sequences	0.90	26.17
Inverted repetitive sequences	0.43	1.90

The sequence composition of the DNA fractions was determined as described previously (Boehm and Drahovsky 1979a, 1980a). Two observations are particularly interesting. First, transcribed DNA contains a higher proportion of inverted repeats than the transcriptionally inactive fraction of the genome. Second, highly repetitive sequences, which comprise mainly of satellite DNA (Drahovsky et al. 1979), are concentrated in nontranscribed regions of the P815 genome

since this carcinogen has been studied in considerable detail respecting a correlation of aberrant DNA methylation and disturbed gene expression.

In previous experiments in our laboratory, we have been interested to study the overall extent of enzymatic methylation of DNA in transcribed genomic regions as compared to transcriptionally inactive sections. Special attention was paid to inverted repetitive sequences, which are generally found to be methylated to a higher extent than other sequence classes in the genome of mammalian cells (Drahovsky et al. 1979; Boehm and Drahovsky 1979b). After denaturation, the inverted repeats form double-stranded structures within a single polynucleotide chain in unimolecular reactions and represent about 3%–5% of mammalian genomes. These sequences were found to be interspersed with sequences of other degrees of repetitiveness and were also found in the vicinity of coding regions. It was therefore suggested that they might have a regulatory role in mammalian DNA (Jelinek 1977; Wallace and Kass 1976; Boehm and Drahovsky 1979a; Jelinek et al. 1980). In P815 mouse mastocytoma cells, we have looked at the extent of methylation in inverted repeats of transcribed and nontranscribed regions of the genome. For the purpose of this study, we separated the DNA molecules of an approximate length of 5000 nucleotides on immobilized heterogeneous nRNA of P815 cells. The fractions complementary to the RNA as well as the DNA which failed to bind to the immobilized RNA were analyzed by reassociation kinetics (Table 2) and by base analysis (Table 3) in order to determine the amount of 5-methylcytosine residues in each kinetic component of the two genomic fractions. With respect to methylation in these DNA portions, the only significant difference was found in inverted repetitive sequences, where the transcribed regions contained only about 40% as much 5-methylcytosine as inverted repeats from nontranscribed DNA. A quantitative estimation shows that this difference represents only about 0.1%–0.5% of the total 5-methylcytosine content in total DNA.

These data suggested that the enzymatic methylation of DNA in inverted repeats correlates inversely with the transcriptional activity in the particular genomic regions.

Table 3. Enzymatic methylation in DNA sequences from transcribed and nontranscribed regions

Component	Relative extent of enzymatic DNA methylation[a]		
	Total DNA	Transcribed DNA	Nontranscribed DNA
Native DNA	1.00		
Nonrepetitive sequences	0.71	0.71 (0.65–0.75)	0.72 (0.70–0.74)
Nonrepetitive and intermediate repetitive sequences	0.91	0.93 (0.83–1.01)	0.95 (0.83–1.06)
Ordinary highly repetitive sequences	2.21	2.16 (1.98–2.34)	2.19 (1.96–2.40)
Inverted repetitive sequences	3.29	1.58 (1.29–1.84)	3.49 (3.33–3.62)

[a] The average and the range of at least three independent experiments (i.e., different preparations of heterogeneous nuclear RNA and DNA) are given

On the basis of these results we have proposed that the extent of methylation in inverted repeats covalently linked to coding sequences negatively controls the transcription of such regions: if they are methylated to an extent comparable to other DNA sequences (an average of one 5-methylcytosine residue per 100 nucleotides) then transcription can proceed in this region. However, if inverted repeats are additionally methylated (to a level of about 2.5 5-methylcytosines per 100 nucleotides), the transcription in this region is inhibited. In a given state of differentiation, with a distinct pattern of methylation in inverted repeats characteristic for this particular cell type, the maintenance methylase activity ensures that the elevated level of methylation will be transferred faithfully to the progeny cells, as will sites of low methylation.

L-Ethionine-Induced DNA Hypomethylation Correlates with Increased Sequence Complexity of nRNA

If the model presented above is correct, one may expect that a lower methylation of inverted repeats will be accompanied by initiation of transcription at sites previously silent, and vice versa. L-Ethionine, an ethyl analog of the essential amino acid L-methionine, is capable of inducing morphological changes in the liver and other organs (Stekol 1963; Farber 1963; Popper et al. 1953). It has also been shown to induce or modulate differentiation in various cell systems and to initiate the expression of certain genes (Christman et al. 1977, 1980; Fitzgerald and Alvizouri 1952; Hancock et al. 1976; Mendelsohn et al. 1980; Sharma and Borek 1977). The mechanism(s) of action has not yet been clarified, even though a possible relationship between the induced phenotypic changes and the effects of L-ethionine on the enzymatic DNA methylation is strongly indicated. To analyze the DNA methylation pattern in P815 cells grown in presence of L-ethionine for a number of cell cycles, we have digested such DNA with different restriction endonucleases. The results shown in Table 4 indicate that the methylation at 5′-CCGG-3′, 5′-GCGC-3′, and 5′-PuGCGCPy-3′ sequences decreased, whereas at 5′-CpyCGPuyG-3′ sequences no such change was

Table 4. Enzymatic methylation at different sequences in P815 DNA

Restriction endonuclease	$\bar{L}_w$ (kb)[a]		No. of cuts		
	Control	+ L-Ethionine (1 m*M*)	Control	+ L-Ethionine (1 m*M*)	Change (%)
*Hpa*II	5.0	3.7	19.0	26.0	37
*Msp*I	2.8	2.6	34.7	37.5	32
*Hha*I	4.7	3.5	20.3	27.0	36
*Hae*II	3.7	2.8	26.0	34.7	34
*Ava*I	3.7	3.7	26.0	26.0	0
*Hin*dIII	3.0	3.0	32.3	32.2	0
*Hae*III	1.2	1.2	82.3	82.3	0

Values of an individual experiment are given; triplicate determinations with different DNA preparations gave similar results and the deviation from the mean did not exceed 5%
[a] Uncut DNA had a weight average length ($\bar{L}_w$) of about 50 kb

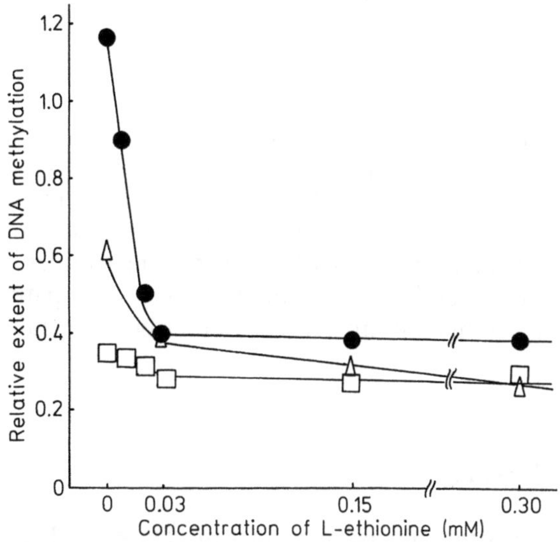

Fig. 5. Enzymatic DNA methylation in P815 cells grown in the presence of different concentrations of L-ethionine. The DNA was isolated and processed through various denaturation and reassociation steps in order to prepare sequence classes of different degrees of repetitiveness (Boehm and Drahovsky 1979a). (–●–), Inverted repetitive sequences; (–△–) ordinary highly repetitive sequences; (–□–), intermediate repetitive and nonrepetitive sequences

observed. These experiments have been done with total cellular DNA and the unmethylated sequences have not been further localized. By analyzing the inhibitory effect of L-ethionine on the enzymatic methylation of DNA of different sequence classes, a more detailed picture was obtained. At a concentration as low as 0.01 m*M* the methylation of inverted repeats was significantly decreased, whereas the methylation in other sequences was virtually unaffected. At higher concentrations, a lower level of methylation appeared in all sequence classes (Fig. 5).

In order to determine whether the L-ethionine-induced lower methylation of DNA is accompanied by a higher nucleotide sequence complexity of nRNA, tracer amounts of radioactively labeled nonrepetitive DNA sequences were hybridized to an excess of nRNA of both control and treated cells. The formation of RNA-DNA hybrids was measured and the results are presented in Table 5. In the control cells, about 6.2% of

Table 5. Nucleotide sequence complexity of nRNA in L-ethionine-treated P815 cells

Source of nRNA	$[^3H]$DNA in RNA-DNA hybrids (%)		Complexity (10^{-6} nucleotides)	No. of nRNA molecules (10^{-3})[b]
	Observed	Corrected for reactability[a]		
Control	6.2 ± 0.2	7.7 ± 0.3	258 ± 8	103
Cells grown in presence of L-ethionine (1 m*M*)	8.8 ± 0.5	11.0 ± 0.6	368 ± 20	147

Values are expressed as mean ± SD

[a] Reactability of nonrepetitive sequences in hybridization reactions is less than 100%. It was found to be in the range of about 80%, and therefore the observed values have to be corrected by a factor of 1.25

[b] Calculated by dividing the complexity of nRNA by the average length of nRNA molecules (about 2500 nucleotides)

the nonrepetitive DNA is complementary to the nRNA, whereas in cells treated with L-ethionine about 8.8% of the DNA is in RNA-DNA hybrids. The estimated sequence complexity is then 2.6×10^8 nucleotides for controls and 3.7×10^8 nucleotides for L-ethionine-treated cells. This corresponds to 103000 vs 147000 nRNA molecules, with an average size of about 2500 nucleotides. The initiation of transcription of DNA sequences previously not expressed is compatible with the activation of certain genes in L-ethionine-treated cells described by Hancock et al. (1976).

Summary

It is generally accepted that the DNA methylation pattern in a particular cell type is stable over the cell generations and is clonally inherited by a semiconservative mechanism in which the methylation of the progeny strand is determined by the 5-methylcytosine residue present in the parental strand. In our experiments, we have been able to show that the chemical carcinogens MNU, MNNG, and L-ethionine affect the methylation process either by modification of the DNA substrate or by interference at the cofactor level. The changes introduced into the cellular methylation pattern persist and are inherited in the progeny cells regardless of whether the carcinogens or their adducts in the DNA persist in the cell or not. The carcinogen-induced hypomethylation correlates with the increased transcriptional complexity of the nRNA of treated cells, indicating the initiation of transcription at sites previously inactive. This means that chemical carcinogens can cause, by interference with the process of DNA methylation, stable changes in the program of genetic expression; the possibility that such changes are related to the process of initiation of carcinogenesis should not be overlooked.

References

Abanobi SE, Columbano A, Mulivor, RA, Rajalakshuni S, Sama DSR (1980) In vivo replication of hepatic deoxyribonucleic acid of rats treated with dimethylnitrosamine: presence of dimethylnitrosamine-induced O^6-methylguanine, N^7-methylguanine, and N^3-methyladenine in the replicated hybrid deoxyribonucleic acid. Biochemistry 19: 1382–1387

Adams RLP, McKay EL, Craig LM, Burdon RH (1979) Mouse DNA methylase:methylation of native DNA. Biochim Biophys Acta 561: 345–347

Baur R, Wohlert H, Kröger H (1979) Methylation of DNA in developing embryos of the sea urchin *Psammechinus miliaris*. Hoppe Seylers Z Physiol Chem 360: 1263–1269

Bird AP (1978) Use of restriction enzymes to study eukaryotic DNA methylation. II. The symmetry of methylated sites supports semi-conservative copying of the methylation pattern. J Mol Biol 118: 49–60

Bird AP, Southern EM (1978) Use of restriction enzymes to study eukaryotic DNA methylation. I. The methylation pattern in ribosomal DNA from *Xenopus laevis*. J Mol Biol 118: 27–47

Bird AP, Taggart MH, Smith BA (1979) Methylated and unmethylated DNA compartments in the sea urchin genome. Cell 17: 889–901

Boehm TLJ, Drahovsky D (1979a) Effect of carcinogen ethionine on enzymatic methylation of DNA sequences with various degrees of repetitiveness. Eur J Cancer 15: 1167–1173

Boehm TLJ, Drahovsky D (1979b) Distribution and enzymatic hypermethylation of inverted DNA repeats in different murine and human cells. Z Naturforsch 34[c]: 558–564

Boehm TLJ, Drahovsky D (1980a) Arrangement of inverted repetitive and unique DNA sequences in genome of mouse P815 mastocytoma cells. Int J Biochem 11: 251–258

Boehm TLJ, Drahovsky D (1980b) Impaired restriction endonuclease cleavage of DNA modified with N-methyl-N-nitrosourea. Carcinogenesis 1: 729–731

Boehm TLJ, Drahovsky D (1981a) Enzymatic hypomethylation of inverted repeats in transcribed DNA regions of mouse P815 mastocytoma cells. Int J Biochem 13: 153–156

Boehm TLJ, Drahovsky D (1981b) Hypomethylation of DNA in Raji cells after treatment with N-methyl-N-nitrosourea. Carcinogenesis 2: 39–42

Boehm TLJ, Drahovsky D (1981c) Elevated transcriptional complexity and decrease in enzymatic DNA methylation in cells treated with L-ethionine. Cancer Res 41: 4101–4106

Boehm TLJ, Drahovsky D (1981d) Inhibition of enzymatic DNA methylation by N-methyl-N-nitro-N-nitrosoguanidine in human Raji lymphoblast-like cells. Int J Biochem 13: 1225–1232

Christman JK, Price P, Pedrinan L, Acs G (1977) Correlation between hypomethylation of DNA and expression of globin genes in Friend erythroleukemia cells. Eur J Biochem 81: 53–61

Christman JK, Weich N, Schoenbrun B, Schneiderman N, Acs G (1980) Hypomethylation of DNA during differentiation of Friend erythroleukemia cells. J Cell Biol 86: 366–370

Cox R (1980) DNA methylase inhibition in vitro by N-methyl-N-nitro-N-nitrosoguanidine. Cancer Res 40: 61–63

Craddock VM (1970) Methylation of DNA in the intact animal and effect of carcinogens dimethylnitrosamine and ethionine. Biochim Biophys Acta 240: 376–383

Desrosiers RC, Mulder C, Fleckenstein B (1979) Methylation of *Herpesvirus saimiri* DNA in lymphoid tumor cell lines. Proc Natl Acad Sci USA 76: 3839–3843

Drahovsky D, Morris RN (1971a) Mechanism of action of rat liver DNA methylase. I. Interaction with double-stranded methyl-acceptor DNA. J Mol Biol 57: 475–489

Drahovsky D, Morris RN (1971b) Mechanism of action of rat liver DNA methylase. II. Interaction with single-stranded methylacceptor DNA. J Mol Biol 61: 343–356

Drahovsky D, Morris RN (1972) The mechanism of action of rat liver DNA methylase. III. Nucleotide requirements for binding and methylation. Biochim Biophys Acta 277: 245–250

Drahovsky D, Wacker A (1975) Inactivation of mammalian DNA methylase activities by N-methyl-N-nitro-N-nitrosoguanidine. Eur J Cancer 11: 517–519

Drahovsky D, Lacko I, Wacker A (1976) Enzymatic DNA methylation during repair synthesis in non-proliferating human peripheral lymphocytes. Biochim Biophys Acta 447: 139–143

Drahovsky D, Boehm TLJ, Kreis W (1979) Distribution pattern and enzymic hypermethylation of inverted repetitive DNA sequences in P815 mastocytoma cells. Biochim Biophys Acta 563: 28–35

Drahovsky D, Kaul S, Boehm TLJ, Wacker A (1980) Enzymatic hypermethylation of DNA in mouse-mouse somatic cell hybrids. Biochim Biophys Acta 607: 201–205

Drahovsky D, Boehm TLJ, Kaul S, Wacker A (1981) The persistence of chromosomes in somatic cell hybrids correlates with the enzymatic hypomethylation of their DNA. Int J Biochem 13: 565–570

Fabricant JD, Wagner EF, Auer B, Schweiger M (1979) 5-Methylcytosine content of DNA during differentiation in mouse teratocarcinoma cells. Exp Cell Res 124: 25–29

Farber E (1963) Ethionine carcinogenesis. Adv Cancer Res 7: 383–418

Fitzgerald PJ, Alvizouri M (1952) Rapid restitution of the rat pancreas following acinar cell necrosis subsequent to ethionine. Nature 170: 929–930

Groudine M, Weintraub H (1981) Activation of globin genes during chicken development. Cell 24: 393–401

Gruenbaum Y, Cedar H, Razin A (1981) Restriction enzyme digestion of hemimethylated DNA. Nucleic Acids Res 9: 2509–2515

Hancock RL, Forrester FL, Lorscheider PC, Lai PCW, Hay DM (1976) Ethionine-induced activation of embryonic genes. In: Fishman WH, Selt S (eds) Oncodevelopmental gene expression. Academic Press, New York, pp 247–251

Jelinek WR (1977) Specific nucleotide sequences in HeLa cell inverted repeated DNA: enrichment for sequences found in double-stranded regions of heterogeneous nuclear RNA. J Mol Biol 115: 591–601

Jelinek WR, Toomey TP, Leinwand L, Duncan CH, Biro PA, Chondary PV, Weissman SM, Rubin CM, Houck CM, Deininger PL, Schmid CW (1980) Ubiquitous, interspersed repeated sequences in mammalian genomes. Proc Natl Acad Sci USA 77: 1398–1402

Kappler JW (1970) The kinetics of DNA methylation in cultures of a mouse adrenal cell line. J cell Physiol 75: 21–32

Kuo MT, Mandel JL, Chambon P (1979) DNA methylation: correlation with DNaseI sensitivity of chicken ovalbumin and conalbumin chromatin. Nucleic Acids Res 7: 2105–2113

Lapeyre JN, Maizel AL, Becker FF (1980) DNA methylation of liver and HTC cells during corticosteroid induction. Biochem Biophys Res Commun 95: 630–637

Mandel JL, Chambon P (1979) DNA methylation: organ specific variations in the methylation pattern within and around ovalbumin and other chicken genes. Nucleic Acids Res 7: 2081–2103

Mann MB, Smith HO (1977) Specificity of DNA methylases from *Haemophilus sp.* Nucleic Acids Res 4: 4211–4222

McGhee JD, Ginder GD (1979) Specific DNA methylation sites in the vicinity of the chicken β-globin gene. Nature 280: 419–420

Mendelsohn N, Michl J, Gilbert HS, Acs G, Christman JK (1980) L-ethionine as an inducer of differentiation in human promyelotic leukemia cells (HL-60). Cancer Res 40: 3206–3210

Pollack Y, Stein R, Razin A, Cedar H (1980) Methylation of foreign DNA in eukaryotic cells. Proc Natl Acad Sci USA 77: 6463–6467

Pollock JM, Swihart M, Taylor JH (1978) Methylation of DNA in early development: 5-methylcytosine content of DNA in sea urchin sperm and embryos. Nucleic Acids Res 5: 4855–4863

Pooper H, delaHuerge J, Yesimiek C (1953) Hepatic tumors due to prolonged ethionine feeding. Science 118: 80–82

Roberts RJ (1978) Restriction and modification enzymes and their recognition sequences. Gene 4: 183–193

Roy PH, Weissbach A (1975) DNA methylase from HeLa cell nuclei. Nucleic Acids Res 2: 4855–4863

Salas CE, Pfohl-Leszkowicz A, Lang MC, Dirheimer G (1979) Effect of modification by N-acetoxy-N-2-acetylaminofluorene on the level of DNA methylation. Nature 278: 71–72

Sharma OK, Borek E (1977) The carcinogen ethionine elevates progesterone levels. Nature 265: 748–749

Shen CKJ, Maniatis T (1980) Tissue-specific DNA methylation in a cluster of rabbit β-like globin genes. Proc Natl Acad Sci USA 77: 6634–6638

Simon D, Grunert F, Vacken U, Döring HP, Kröger H (1978) DNA-methylase from regenerating rat liver: purification and characterization. Nucleic Acids Res 5: 2153–2167

Singer J, Robert-Ems J, Luthardt FW, Riggs AD (1979) Methylation of DNA in mouse early embryos, teratocarcinoma cells and adult tissues of mouse and rabbit. Nucleic Acids Res 7: 2369–2385

Sneider TW (1980) The 5′-cytosine in CCGG is methylated in two eukaryotic DNAs and MspI is sensitive to methylation at this site. Nucleic Acids Res 8: 3829–3840

Sneider TW, Teague WM, Rogachevsky LM (1975) S-adenosylmethionine: DNA-cytosine 5-methyltransferase from a Novikoff rat hepatoma cell line. Nucleic Acids Res 2: 1685–1700

Stekol JA (1963) Biochemical basis for ethionine effects on tissues. Adv Enzymol 25: 369–393

Sutter D, Doerfler W (1981) Methylation of integrated viral DNA sequences in hamster cells transformed by adenovirus 12. Cold Spring Harbor Symp Quant Biol 44: 565–568

van der Ploeg LHT, Flavell RA (1980) DNA methylation in the human $\gamma\delta\beta$-globin locus in erythroid and non-erythroid tissues. Cell 19: 947–958

Waalwijk C, Flavell RA (1978) DNA methylation at a CCGG sequence in the large intron of the rabbit β-globin gene: tissue-specific variations. Nucleic Acids Res 5: 4631–4641

Wallace B, Kass TL (1976) On inverted repeat sequences in chromosomal DNA. Genetics 82: 139–140

Weintraub H, Larsen A, Groudine M (1981) α-globin gene switching during the development of chicken embryos: expression and chromosome structure. Cell 24: 333–344

Wigler M, Levy D, Perucho M (1981) The somatic replication of DNA methylation. Cell 24: 33–40

tRNA-Specific Enzymes

Ethionine-Induced Alterations of tRNA Metabolism*

S. J. Kerr

Department of Biochemistry, Biophysics, and Genetics, University of Colorado, Health Sciences Center, 4200 E. Ninth Avenue, Denver, CO 80262, USA

Introduction

Ethionine, the ethyl analog of methionine, is a hepatocarcinogen when administered chronically in the diet to rats (Farber 1963). Studies with radioactive ethionine revealed that tRNA was the most extensively labeled nucleic acid species after ethionine administration (Farber et al. 1967). Further studies in recent years have led to extremely interesting findings concerning the effect of ethionine on tRNA metabolism.

In the liver of treated animals ethionine is converted enzymatically to SAE, which can accumulate to such an extent as to cause an ATP deficiency severe enough to curtail RNA synthesis (Shull et al. 1966). The latter phenomenon can be prevented by simultaneous administration of adenine (Farber et al. 1974). SAE can serve as an alkyl donor in a variety of enzymatic reactions (Stekol 1965), but it is an extremely poor substrate for tRNA methyltransferases (Rodeh et al. 1967; Moore and Smith 1969; Pegg 1972). Conversely, it is a relatively good inhibitor of tRNA methyltransferases (Moore and Smith 1969; Pegg 1971). The inhibitory effect might be expected to be evidenced in vivo, since SAE can accumulate in the livers of treated animals to levels more than 50-fold greater than SAM levels (Hoffman 1975), and the elevated levels persist for extended periods of time (Ortwerth and Novelli 1969). That inhibition of tRNA methyltransferase activity does occur in vivo was demonstrated by Rajalakshmi (1973), who showed that tRNA isolated from the livers of ethionine-treated rats could serve as a substrate in vitro for homologous tRNA methyltransferases. These observations made it possible for the first time to prepare methyl-deficient tRNA from a mammalian source in order to study its interactions with homologous enzymes (Kerr 1975). Wainfan and Maschio (1975) extended this observation to *Escherichia coli*. Cells grown in the presence of 0.5% DL-ethionine synthesized tRNA which could serve as a substrate for the enzymes from *E. coli*. The tRNA was deficient in 5-methyluracil. The mechanism of action of ethionine on *E. coli* is puzzling. The bacterial adenosyltransferase enzyme responsible for the synthesis of SAM does not accept ethionine as a substrate (Lombardini et al. 1970). Thus SAE does not accumulate in bacterial cells. Also, previous in vitro studies had shown that the uracil methyltransferase of *E. coli* was relatively resistant to inhibition by SAE (Moore 1970), which

* Supported in part by NIH grant CA 12742

is further evidence that SAE is probably not involved in the induction of 5-methyluracil-deficient tRNA in ethionine-treated *E. coli.* Wainfan et al. (1975) reported evidence for the accumulation of inhibitors of tRNA methyltransferases other than SAE in the livers of ethionine-treated rats.

Another interesting effect of ethionine administration is on the level of tRNA methyltransferase activity. Hancock (1968) first observed that the tRNA methyltransferase activity in mice fed an ethionine-supplemented diet was highly elevated before any pathological evidence of tumor was apparent. This was confirmed by Moore and Smith (1969) using rats. The phenomenon of increased tRNA methyltransferase activity at early stages following carcinogen administration has also been observed with other carcinogens (Wilkinson and Pillinger 1971; Stewart and Pegg 1972).

Wainfan et al. (1977) studied the time course of the changes in tRNA methyltransferase activity in rat liver following exposure to ethionine. They found that the specific activity of the enzymes diminished during the first 2 days of treatment and then began to rise steadily for the duration of the experiment, which was 14 days. The tRNA isolated from the livers of animals at the same time points showed a peak of in vitro methyl acceptance at 3 days and declined steadily thereafter.

The finding of a peak in vitro methyl acceptance of tRNA from livers of ethionine-treated rats after 72 h exposure has been confirmed by Friedman (1977). However, another puzzle has been raised by his observations. The minor base content of tRNA can be estimated directly by the method of Randerath et al. (1972), which involves the enzymatic digestion of tRNA to the nucleoside level and oxidation of the ribose moiety with periodate, followed by reduction to the dialcohol with tritiated borohydride of high specific activity. The labeled derivatives are then separated by two-dimensional thin-layer chromatography. Lu et al. (1976) performed analyses of this type on tRNA from livers of ethionine-treated mice. They found a general reduction in all the methylated bases in the tRNA of treated animals, but the individual methylated components were affected to different extents. Their data, however, were at variance with the results of in vitro experiments performed by Kerr (1975). The pattern and extent of bases methylated in vitro by rat liver enzymes was quite different from that which might be expected from the in vivo pattern of methyl deficiency. Furthermore, the data of Lu et al. (1976) suggested that the methyl-deficient tRNA might be expected to accept as much as 1 mol total methyl group/mol tRNA, while in vitro experiments yielded only 10%–15% of that amount (Kerr 1975).

Friedman (1977) studied this phenomenon in detail, combining analysis of tRNA by the method of Randerath et al. (1972) with in vitro enzyme studies during the induction of methyl-deficient tRNA by exposure to ethionine. By direct analysis, tRNA from treated animals had the same degree of methyl deficiency at 4 weeks as at 67 h. Methylation in vitro by rat liver enzymes gave a different pattern, however. Methyl deficiency could be detected in vitro as early as 19 h after ethionine administration. The in vitro methyl acceptance reached a peak 67 h after treatment and then declined to a plateau level of approximately 40% of the peak value, which was maintained for up to 4 weeks. At the peak of methyl acceptance, 67 h, the tRNA accepted only 18% of the theoretically possible maximum amount of methyl groups indicated by the direct analysis, and this acceptance had declined to 7% by 4 weeks. When tRNA from treated animals was methylated in vitro with enzymes from *E. coli,* a different pattern emerged. The methyl acceptance of tRNA reached a peak after

67 h treatment, but this level was maintained for 4 weeks. The enzymes from rat liver synthesized seven or more specific methylated derivatives, while the enzyme from *E. coli* synthesized principally 5-methyluracil. Thus while the other base-specific sites decreased in accessibility during the course of the experiment, the 5-methyluracil site retained its availability.

The conclusion is that not all the methyl-deficient sites induced in mammalian tRNA by ethionine treatment are available for in vitro methylation by extracts of liver and that even those which are accessible initially decline in availability as exposure to ethionine is prolonged. The reasons behind these experimental findings are unclear. The actual substrates for many of the methylation sites may be precursor molecules, or some sort of conformational change or denaturation of the tRNA may occur in the treated animals which makes it a poor substrate; and, as always, the question of the biological similitude of the in vitro reaction conditions arises. The optimum conditions are not the same for different base-specific enzymes (Leboy and Glick 1976; Friedman 1977), and unknown requirements may exist for enzymes specific for sites which are not methylated in vitro.

Studies concerning the interaction of ethionine-induced methyl-deficient tRNA with the aminoacyl synthetases and its participation in protein synthesis have revealed further functional deficiencies of the hypomethylated tRNA. In vitro charging assays with ethionine-induced methyl-deficient tRNA revealed few differences when compared to control tRNA (Harris and Randerath 1978; Ginzburg et al. 1979). However, when the methyl-deficient tRNA was injected into oocytes there was a severe impairment of the aminoacylation capacity of the tRNA (Ginzburg et al. 1979). The effect was not uniform for all species of tRNA; some aminoacyl-specific tRNAs showed no change, while some reactions, such as methionine aminoacylation, revealed very complex patterns of acylation and deacylation. The methyl-deficient tRNA also showed an impaired ability to participate in protein synthesis whether tested in a cell-free system or when injected into oocytes (Ginzburg et al. 1979).

Whether the changes in tRNA structure and activity of the methyltransferases are involved in ethionine carcinogenesis is not known. Ethionine causes at least 100-fold greater ethylation in tRNA than in DNA. It is a unique carcinogen in that it appears to react through an enzymatic mechanism rather than a direct chemical ethylation of nucleic acid or protein. Ortwerth and Novelli (1969; see also Pegg 1972) have suggested that a metabolite of ethionine other than SAE can act as an alkylating agent. Their hypothesis is based on the observations that large quantities of methionine do not prevent the ethylation of tRNA and that the administration of large quantities of actinomycin D to prevent RNA synthesis also does not block ethylation of tRNA, indicating that pre-existing tRNA might be alkylated aberrantly. Ethionine treatment causes alkylation in DNA of 1 of 230000 guanine residues to 7-ethylguanine (Swann et al. 1971). No enzyme with this specificity has been found, and 7-methylguanine does not occur naturally in DNA, suggesting that ethylation of DNA may occur by a nonenzymatic mechanism. The observation by Leopold et al. (1979) that the vinyl analog of ethionine is much more toxic to rodents and is also mutagenic to bacteria may indicate that metabolites of ethionine may be involved in ethionine carcinogenesis as well. However, they found no evidence for the production of vinthionine from ethionine by Aroclor 1254-induced rat liver microsomes.

The specificity of the reaction with tRNA points to an enzymatic reaction, however. Ethylated analogs of all the naturally occurring methylated components of tRNA were detected after ethionine administration (Pegg 1972). Chemical ethylating agents such as diethylnitrosamine do not yield such a broad spectrum of products (Swann and Magee 1971). In fact, different tRNA species from ethionine-treated rats are not equally susceptible to ethylation.

Ortwerth and Novelli (1969) obtained preliminary evidence for this from reversed-phase chromatography of in vivo-labeled tRNA, and Kuchino et al. (1978) isolated from the liver of ethionine-treated rats the major ethylated tRNA species, which is an isoaccepting species of lysyl-tRNA. The results, revealing nonuniform effects on in vivo aminoacylation of tRNA from ethionine-treated rats, provide further evidence for specificity of the interaction of ethionine with tRNA.

Some of the effects of ethionine on RNA metabolism are as follows:

1. Inhibition of RNA synthesis
   ATP depletion (Shull et al. 1966)
   Inhibition or inactivation of RNA polymerase (Smuckler and Koplitz 1969)
2. Disaggregation of polysomes (Stewart and Farber 1967)
3. Inhibition of rRNA maturation (Swann et al. 1975)
4. Ethylation of tRNA (Farber et al. 1967)
   Nonrandom distribution of ethyl groups (Ortwerth and Novelli 1969)
   Specificity for lysine tRNA (Kuchino et al. 1978)
5. Elevation of tRNA methyltransferase activity (Hancock 1968)
6. Inhibition of tRNA methyltransferase by SAE (Moore and Smith 1969; Pegg 1971)
7. Hypomethylation of tRNA (Rajalakshmi 1973)
8. Functional impairment of tRNA
   Interaction with aminoacyl synthetases (Harris and Randerath 1978; Ginsberg et al. 1979)
   Participation in protein synthesis (Ginsburg et al. 1979).

Ethionine has other physiological effects. Ethionine administration can cause a rise in blood progesterone levels. Thus hormonal effects must also be considered in ethionine carcinogenesis. It appears that ethionine, as well as alkylating tRNA, induces a chronic hypomethylated state in the tRNA of the treated animal (Friedman 1977), even though the level of methylating enzymes becomes highly elevated (Wainfan et al. 1977). These are among the earliest effects noted, and they persist throughout the course of the regimen leading to tumor induction. How all these factors interact in the carcinogenic process remains to be shown.

We have undertaken the study of a number of other enzymes involved in methyl metabolism during the course of ethionine carcinogenesis.

A key enzyme in the regulation of cellular levels of SAM is the synthetic enzyme ATP:L-methionine adenosyltransferase, which carries out the direct enzymatic adenosylation of methionine at the expense of ATP. As mentioned earlier, ethionine is also a substrate for this reaction. It has been noted that adenosyltransferase levels are low in fetal tissues and in some tumors (Lombardini and Talalay 1970). The highest levels of the enzyme are found in adult liver, kidney, and pancreas. Two isozyme forms of the enzyme in liver have been identified, one of which disappears in Novikoff ascites tumor (Liau et al. 1979). The isozymes differ in their K_m for methionine. The major form in the liver is a high-K_m (1 m*M*) enzyme, while the low-K_m (0.02 m*M*) enzyme is a minor component. It is the low-K_m form of the enzyme which is found in Novikoff ascites.

SAH hydrolase, which hydrolytically cleaves SAH to adenosine and homocysteine, plays a pivotal role in regulating cellular levels of SAH. The ratio of the levels of SAH

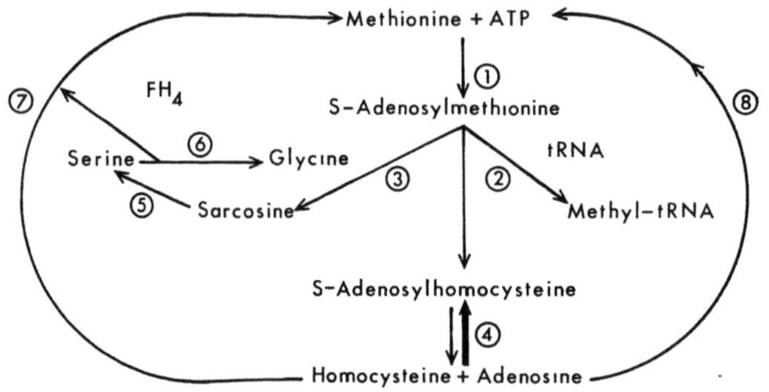

Fig. 1. Synthesis and metabolism of *S*-adenosylmethionine. Enzymes: *1,* ATP:L-methionine adenosyltransferase; *2,* tRNA methyltransferases; *3,* glycine *N*-methyltransferase; *4,* SAH hydrolase; *5,* sarcosine dehydrogenase; *6,* serine hydroxymethyltransferase; *7,* 5-methyltetrahydrofolate-homocysteine methyltransferase; *8,* adenosine kinase

and SAM appears to be the key to the control of a variety of methyltransferases. We have previously noted that the activity of the enzyme is lower in a number of hepatomas than in normal liver (Kerr and Heady 1974).

A third enzyme of interest to our laboratory is glycine methyltransferase, which *N*-methylates glycine to yield sarcosine, and is found in high levels in normal adult liver, kidney, and pancreas (Kerr 1972). In crude extracts this enzyme can inhibit the tRNA methyltransferases, both by competing for SAM and by generating SAH. The glycine methyltransferase is much less sensitive to product inhibition by SAH than are the tRNA methyltransferases. The glycine methyltransferase is absent in fetal liver and either absent or highly diminished in a number of hepatomas (Kerr 1972), a pattern which parallels that of the adenosyltransferase.

Figure 1 indicates the interaction of these enzymes in cellular methylation reactions. The effect of the glycine methyltransferase on the tRNA methyltransferases would appear to be part of a larger system involved in the regulation of cellular levels of SAM and SAH with the consequent effect of the latter compound on a number of methyltransferases.

We report now on perturbations of this system during the course of ethionine carcinogenesis.

Results and Discussion

Holtzmann rats (100–150 g) were placed on a low-protein diet, supplemented with 0.25% DL-ethionine, for experimental induction of hepatocarcinogenesis. tRNA methyltransferase, glycine methyltransferase, SAM synthetase, and SAH hydrolase were assayed in the livers and kidneys of control and treated animals at various times following the start of the carcinogenic regimen.

The tRNA methyltransferase and glycine methyltransferase activity in the livers of control and treated animals and in an ethionine-induced tumor are presented in Table 1. It can be seen that within 3 days of starting ethionine feeding elevations are observed in tRNA-methyl-transferase-specific activity and capacity, while the glycine methyltransferase activity drops by over 50%. These changes persist throughout the course of

Table 1. Alterations in tRNA methyltransferase and glycine methyltransferase activity in rat liver during ethionine carcinogenesis

Regimen	tRNA methyltransferase		Glycine methyltransferase
	Sp. act. (pm/mg prot/min)	Capacity (pm/μg tRNA)	Sp. act. (nm/mg prot/min)
Control	6.58	4.06	2.43
Ethionine			
3 days	9.23	7.16	1.16
6 days	11.05	8.22	1.67
9 days	11.95	7.68	0.79
12 days	16.95	11.31	0.65
21 days	15.42	9.18	1.05
28 days	10.55	8.0	0.80
2 months	10.43	14.02	1.20
3 months	10.05	12.31	1.35
4 months	16.25	15.00	0.72
Tumor	7.07	10.06	0.16

Enzymes were assayed by the methods of Heady and Kerr (1975). *Sp. act.*, specific activity; *prot*, protein

the carcinogenic regime, while in a frank ethionine-induced tumor tRNA methyltransferase capacity is elevated and the glycine methyltransferase is even further reduced by 95%.

Because ethionine is a specific hepatocarcinogen, it was of interest to determine whether the early enzyme changes observed in the target organ, liver, would also occur in nontarget tissues. For this reason, tRNA methyltransferase and glycine methyltransferase activities were also assayed in the kidneys of control and ethionine-treated animals. These results are presented in Table 2. It is evident that while there are some fluctuations in enzyme activities, they are not consistent and are not of the magnitude observed in the liver.

The specificity of D- vs L-ethionine in inducing elevated tRNA methyltransferases in the liver was also examined. As can be seen in Table 3, both were equally effective. This is not too surprising, as Brada et al. (1975) demonstrated that the levels of SAE found in rat liver were equivalent after the administration of D- or L-ethionine. This is probably due to deamination of D-ethionine and reamination to the L form.

It has been reported that female rats are more susceptible than male rats to the acute toxic effects of ethionine, although both sexes do develop tumors after prolonged feeding of ethionine (Farber 1963). Other workers have not noted a sex difference in toxicity of ethionine (Ward et al. 1979). We examined the tRNA methyltransferases in the livers of male and female rats maintained on an ethionine diet. It can be seen in Table 4 that in both males and females the enzymes are elevated both in specific activity and capacity after either 1 week or 2 months of ethionine feeding.

The SAM synthetic enzyme activity was also examined during the course of ethionine feeding. As mentioned earlier, there are at least two isozyme forms of the enzyme in liver, one of which disappears in Novikoff ascites (Liau et al. 1979). Table 5 shows that the high-K_m form of the enzyme is diminished by about 60% after 1 week of ethionine exposure, while the low-K_m enzyme is relatively unaffected. The lowered activity of

Table 2. Transfer RNA methyltransferase and glycine methyltransferase activity in rat kidney during ethionine carcinogenesis

Regimen	tRNA methyltransferase		Glycine methyltransferase
	Sp. act. (pm/mg prot/min)	Capacity (pm/μg tRNA)	Sp. act. (nm/mg prot/min)
Control	1.41	1.75	0.67
Ethionine			
3 days	1.38	3.81	0.70
6 days	1.43	2.12	0.34
9 days	1.34	2.76	0.32
12 days	1.32	2.18	0.39
21 days	1.33	1.88	0.57
28 days	2.01	0.96	0.93
2 months	1.49	2.33	0.77
5 months	1.0	3.22	0.68

Assays performed as in Table 1

Table 3. Comparison of effects of D- and L-ethionine on rat liver tRNA methyltransferase

	Sp. act. (pm/mg prot/min)	Capacity (pm/μg tRNA)
Control	6.04	7.52
Ethionine		
6 days (L)	22.88	17.00
(D)	21.09	16.00
12 days (L)	14.21	14.34
(D)	16.00	15.18

Female Holtzmann rats were injected daily with 1 mmol/kg body wt of either D- or L-ethionine and 0.5 mmol/kg body wt adenine. Assays were performed at the times indicated by Heady and Kerr (1975)

Table 4. Effect of ethionine on tRNA methyltransferase in male and female rats

	Sex	Sp. act. (pm/mg prot/min)	Capacity (pm/μg tRNA)
Control	Female	7.17	6.07
	Male	5.70	7.15
Ethionine			
1 week	Female	30.50	11.4
	Male	23.76	10.9
2 months	Female	10.43	14.02
	Male	11.64	12.71

Male and female Holtzmann rats were fed on ethionine chow and assays were performed at the times indicated by Heady and Kerr (1975)

Table 5. Methionine: adenosyltransferase activity after ethionine exposure

	Sp. act. (pm/mg prot/min)	
	Low K_m	High K_m
Control	3.93	29.47
Ethionine		
2 weeks	2.58	11.79
2 months	3.41	10.22
Tumor	4.47	34.95

Assays were performed on high-speed supernatant extracts of liver according to Liau et al. (1979), except that the product was quantitated by high-pressure liquid chromotography

Table 6. SAH hydrolase activity after ethionine exposure

	Sp. act. (nm/mg prot/min)
Control	8.50
Ethionine	
6 days	11.03
3 months	8.09
Tumor	1.62

Assays were performed on high-speed supernatant extracts of livers from control and ethionine-fed rats according to the method of Trewyn and Kerr (1981)

the high-K_m enzyme persists for at least 2 months. However, in an ethionine-induced tumor the two activities appeared to be present at relatively normal levels. It has been reported that the enzyme level is not altered in minimal deviation hepatomas (Sheid and Bilik 1968) and this particular ethionine-induced tumor may fall into that category. Additional ethionine-induced tumors will have to be examined to determine isozyme patterns following ethionine hepatocarcinogenesis.

SAH hydrolase, the enzyme necessary for preventing the accumulation of the methyltransferase inhibitor SAH, was also determined during the course of ethionine carcinogenesis. As is evident in Table 6, no changes in SAH hydrolase were observed for up to 3 months of ethionine exposure. The ethionine-induced tumor, however, did evidence a reduced activity of about 20% that of control liver. This is in accord with our previous findings on a number of chemically-induced hepatomas (Kerr and Heady 1974).

We also examined the induction of methyl-deficient tRNA during ethionine carcinogenesis, and the results are shown in Table 7. Methyl acceptance reached peak between 24 and 48 h and then declined to a steady-state level which lasted for the duration of the experiment. Ethionine-induced tumor tRNA was not examined for methyl acceptance, but reports have appeared which indicate that some tumor tRNAs are undermodified (Randerath et al. 1974).

Another enzyme of RNA metabolism which we studied in ethionine-exposed rats was ribonuclease. Table 8 shows clearly that after a week of ethionine exposure, alkaline RNase (pH 7.8) activity has diminished by almost 50% in the livers of treated rats, while acid RNase activity has increased. These differences persist and are still evident

Table 7. Induction of methyl-deficient tRNA (pm CH_3/μg tRNA) during ethionine carcinogenesis

Control	Not detected
Ethionine	
24 h	6.79
48 h	7.01
72 h	3.56
1 week	1.20
1 month	1.32
2 months	1.78

The tRNA was isolated from the livers of control and ethionine-treated rats and assayed for methyl acceptance using the homologous tRNA methyltransferases of normal rat liver as described by Kerr (1975)

Table 8. RNase activity in rat liver after ethionine exposure

	ΔOD_{260}/mg protein/min	
	pH 7.8	pH 5.8
Control	0.315	0.484
Ethionine, 7 days	0.170	0.670
Control	0.451	0.474
Ethionine, 3 months	0.209	0.839

High-speed supernatant extracts of control and ethionine-exposed rat livers were assayed for alkaline and acid RNase activity by the method of Roth (1967)

after 3 months ethionine feeding. These results are similar to those found using other carcinogens (Roth 1967). Elevations in acid RNase have also been reported for some hepatomas (Roth 1967).

The data presented here indicate that there are coordinate changes in certain of the enzymes involved in tRNA metabolism and overall methyl metabolism during the course of ethionine carcinogenesis. tRNA methyltransferase activity is elevated very early after ethionine exposure, while glycine methyltransferase is diminished as is the predominant adult differentiated liver isozyme form of methionine:adenosyltransferase.

These changes may indicate an impaired ability of the cell to metabolize and use the methyl group of methionine for one-carbon transfer reactions. SAH hydrolase activity is not altered early in carcinogenesis but its level is diminished in tumor tissue. Control of the expression of SAH hydrolase activity may then be affected at a much later stage during carcinogenesis than the other enzymes examined.

Changes in RNase activity exhibit an interesting pattern during ethionine carcinogenesis. Alkaline RNase activity is diminished early, while conversely, acid RNase activity is increased. The exact function of these RNases is not clear, so how changes in their activity might impinge on the carcinogenic process remains to be explored. The alterations in activity do reflect the derangement of normal cellular control mechanisms which occur very early in carcinogenesis and are not only expressed in the eventual tumor.

Abbreviations

SAM, *S*-adenosylmethionine; *SAH*, *S*-adenosylhomocysteine; *SAE*, *S*-adenosylethionine.

References

Brada Z, Bulba S, Cohen J (1975) The metabolism of ethionine in rats. Cancer Res 35: 2674–2683

Farber E (1963) Ethionine carcinogenesis. Adv Cancer Res 7: 383–474

Farber E, McConomy J, Franzen B, Marroquin F, Stewart GA, Magee PN (1967) Interaction between ethionine and rat liver ribonucleic acid and protein in vivo. Cancer Res 27: 1761–1772

Farber JL, Shinozuka H, Seronni A, Farmar R (1974) Reversal of the ethionine-induced inhibition of rat liver ribonucleic acid polymerases in vivo by adenine. Lab Invest 31: 465–472

Friedman S (1977) Alterations of tRNA modification in mammalian systems: the effect of ethionine. Nucleic Acids Res 4: 1853–1871

Ginzburg I, Cornelis P, Giveon D, Littauer UZ (1979) Functionally impaired tRNA from ethionine treated rats as detected in injected Xenopus oocytes. Nucleic Acids Res 6: 657–672

Hancock RL (1968) Ethionine induced sRNA neomethylase activity. Biochem Biophys Res Commun 31: 77–81

Harris JS, Randerath K (1978) Aminoacylation of undermethylated mammalian transfer RNA. Biochim Biophys Acta 521: 566–575

Heady JE, Kerr SJ (1975) Alteration of glycine N-methyltransferase activity in fetal, adult, and tumor tissues. Cancer Res 35: 640–643

Hoffman J (1975) A rapid liquid chromatographic determination of S-adenosylmethionine and S-adenosylhomocysteine in subgram amounts of tissue. Anal Biochem 68: 522–530

Hyde CL, Ward JM, Wenk ML, Poirier LA (1979) Comparative hepatotoxicity of subchronic doses of ethionine in mice, rats and hamsters. (Abstr) Proc Am Assoc Cancer Res 20: 128

Kerr SJ (1972) Competing methyltransferase systems. J Biol Chem 247: 4248–4252

Kerr SJ (1975) Interaction of mammalian tRNA methyltransferases with heterologous and homologous tRNA. Adv Enzyme Regul 13: 379–390

Kerr SJ, Heady JE (1974) Modulation of tRNA Methyltransferase activity by competing enzyme systems. Adv Enzyme Regul 12: 103–117

Kuchino Y, Sharma OK, Borek E (1978) Mechanisms of ethionine carcinogenesis. Adv Enzyme Regul 16: 391–405

Leboy P, Glick JM (1976) tRNA methyltransferases from rat liver. Differences in response of partially purified enzymes to polyamines and inorganic salts. Biochim Biophys Acta 435: 30–38

Leopold WR, Miller JA, Miller EC (1979) S-vinyl homocysteine (vinthionine): a highly mutagenic analog of ethionine. (Abstr) Proc Am Assoc Cancer Res 20: 28

Liau MC, Chang CF, Belanger L, Grenier A (1979) Correlation of isozyme patterns of S-adenosylmethionine synthetase with fetal stages and pathological states of the liver. Cancer Res 39: 162–169

Lombardini JB, Coulter AW, Talalay P (1970) Analogues of methionine as substrates and inhibitors of the methionine adenosyltransferase reaction. Deductions concerning the conformation of methionine. Mol Pharmacol 6: 481–499

Lu L, Chiang GH, Randerath K (1976) Effects of DL-ethionine on mouse liver tRNA base composition. Nucleic Acids Res 3: 2243–2253

Moore BG (1970) Differential inhibition of bacterial tRNA methylases by S-adenosylethionine and other adenine derivates. Can J Biochem 48: 702–705

Moore BG, Smith RC (1969) S-adenosylethionine as an inhibitor of tRNA methylation. Can J Biochem 47: 561–565
Ortwerth BJ, Novelli CD (1969) Studies on the incorporation of L-ethionine-ethyl-1-^{14}C into the transfer RNA of rat liver. Cancer Res 29: 380–390
Pegg AE (1971) Studies on inhibitors of mammalian tRNA methylases. FEBS Lett 16: 13–16
Pegg AE (1972) Studies of the ethylation of rat liver transfer ribonucleic acid after administration of L-ethionine. Biochem J 128: 59–68
Rajalakshmi S (1973) A liver tRNA for the assay of rat liver methylase in vitro. (Abstr) Proc Am Assoc Cancer Res 14: 39
Randerath E, Yu CT, Randerath K (1972) Base analysis of ribopolynucleotides by chemical tritium labeling: a methodological study with model nucleosides and purified tRNA species. Anal Biochem 48: 172–198
Randerath E, Chia LSY, Morris HP, Randerath K (1974) Transfer RNA base composition studies in Morris hepatomas and rat liver. Cancer Res 34: 643–653
Reid E (1962) Significant biochemical effects of hepatocarcinogens in the rat: a review. Cancer Res 22: 398–430
Rodeh R, Feldman M, Littauer UZ (1967) Properties of soluble ribonucleic acid methylases from rat liver. Biochemistry 6: 451–460
Roth JS (1967) Some observations on the assay and properties of ribonucleases in normal and tumor tissues. Methods Cancer Res 3: 153–242
Sheid B, Bilik E (1968) S-adenosylmethionine synthetase activity in some normal rat tissues and transplantable hepatomas. Cancer Res 28: 2512–2515
Shull KH, McConomy J, Vogt M, Castillo A, Farber E (1966) On the mechanism of induction of hepatic adenosine triphosphate deficiency by ethionine. J Biol Chem 241: 5060–5070
Smuckler EA, Koplitz M (1969) The effects of carbon tetrachloride and ethionine on RNA synthesis in vivo and in isolated rat liver nuclei. Arch Biochem Biophys 132: 62–79
Stekol JA (1965) Formation and metabolism of S-adenosyl derivatives of S-alkylhomocysteines in the rat and mouse. In: Shapiro SK, Schlenk F (eds) Transmethylation and methionine biosynthesis. University of Chicago Press, Chicago Ill, pp. 231–252
Stewart BW, Pegg AE (1972) Changes in tRNA methylase activity of rat kidney following administration of the carcinogen dimethylnitrosamine. Biochim Biophys Acta 281: 416–424
Stewart GA, Farber EM (1967) Reformation of functional liver polyribosomes from ribosome monomers in the absence of RNA synthesis. Science 157: 67–69
Swann PF, Magee PN (1971) Nitrosamine-induced carcinogenesis. The alkylation of N-7 of guanine of nucleic acids of the rat by diethylnitrosamine, N-ethyl-N-nitrosourea and ethyl methanesulphonate. Biochem J 125: 841–847
Swann PF, Pegg AE, Hawks A, Farber E, Magee PN (1971) Evidence of ethylation of rat liver deoxyribonucleic acid after administration of ethionine. Biochem J 123: 175–181
Swann PF, Peacock AC, Bunting S (1975) Carcinogenesis and cellular injury. The effect of ethionine on ribonucleic acid synthesis in rat liver. Biochem J 150: 335–344
Trewyn RW, Kerr SJ (1981) An improved rapid assay for S-adenosyl-L-homocysteine hydrolase. J Biochem Biophys Methods 4: 299–307
Wainfan E, Maschio FA (1975) Inhibition of methylated nucleoside synthesis in vivo: accumulation of incompletely methylated transfer RNA in ethionine-treated cells of Escherichia coli B. Ann NY Acad Sci 255: 567–575
Wainfan E, Moller ML, Maschio FA, Balis ME (1975) Ethionine-induced changes in rat liver Transfer RNA Methylation. Cancer Res 35; 2830–2835
Wainfan E, Tscherne JS, Maschio FA, Balis ME (1977) Time dependence of ethionine-induced changes in rat liver Transfer RNA Methylation. Cancer Res 37: 865–869
Wilkinson R, Pillinger DJ (1971) Effect of the carcinogen N-nitrosomethylurea on the tRNA methylase activity of cells cultured in vitro. Int J Cancer 8: 401–409

Processing of tRNA Is Accomplished by a High-Molecular-Weight Enzyme Complex

P. F. Agris, T. Playl, L. Goldman, E. Horton, D. Woolverton, D. Setzer, and C. Rodi

Division of Biological Sciences, University of Missouri, Columbia, MO 65211, USA

Introduction

A complex of functionally related enzymes is in essence a highly concentrated manufacturing unit completing various steps simultaneously or sequentially on the same or related substrates. The substrates are efficiently available to all enzymes. Enzymes of the complex could influence each other's activities through their physical association or their prior action on the substrate. Such influence affects regulation of metabolic processes. Regulation, or the lack of it, is of primary interest to the elucidation of molecular oncology.

Reviews (Ginsberg and Stadtman 1970; Reed 1974; Reed and Cox 1970) have been written about naturally occurring multiple enzyme aggregates, excluding discussions of enzyme complexes being possibly associated with the protein biosynthetic process and their possible relation with metabolic changes in neoplasia. Components of the protein biosynthetic machinery, such as the aminoacyl-tRNA synthetases, have been thought to exist freely in the cytoplasm, yet as knowledge of protein biosynthesis accumulates, it appears that in mammalian cells there is a more extensive structural organization beyond that of ribosomes and polyribosomes. High-molecular-weight complexes of aminoacyl-tRNA synthetases, reported as early as 1971 (Bandyopadhyay and Deutscher 1971), have been found in rat and mouse liver (Bandyopadhyay and Deutscher 1971; Tscherne et al. 1973; Dang and Yang 1978; Berg 1975), Chinese hamster ovary cells (Hampel and Enger 1973), rabbit reticulocytes (Som and Hardesty 1975), and mouse and chicken embryos (Ussery et al. 1977).

It is an intriguing hypothesis that the processing of tRNA for protein synthesis (Fig. 1) may involve the cytoplasmic ribonucleases and modifying enzymes organized in a specific subcellular fraction. In addition, this enzyme complex may or may not be associated with aminoacyl-tRNA synthetases existing differently in normal and neoplastic cells. This hypothesis is supported by our results.

Modification of tRNA nucleosides has been shown to be important in the regulation of protein synthesis (Agris and Soll 1977; Agris et al. 1973; Agris 1980). Knowledge of how such tRNA modifications are produced and their production regulated through enzyme complexes is important to our understanding of the regulatory functions of tRNA in protein synthesis in normal and neoplastic cells. The hypermodification, especially hypermethylation, of tRNA and the higher activity of modification enzymes in cancer cells than in normal cells has been investigated for many years. The approach

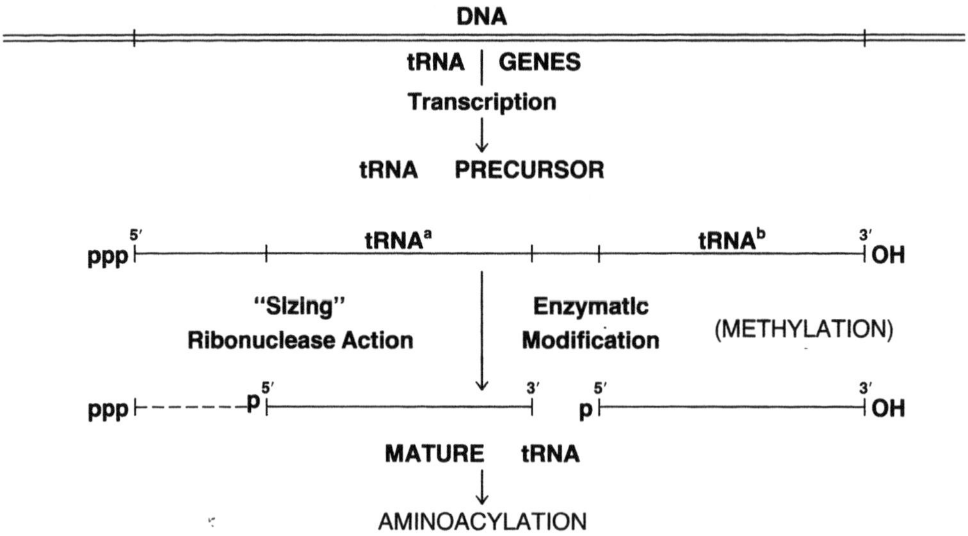

Fig. 1. Maturation of tRNA from transcription to mature size, modified, and functional tRNA

discussed herein has never before been utilized; nor has any other research implicated a direct coupling of tRNA maturation and aminoacylation. Mammalian cell aminoacyl-tRNA synthetases have been shown to occur in high-molecular-weight enzyme complexes. These synthetases may be associated with enzyme complexes for the modification of tRNA nucleosides and the trimming of precursor tRNA (Agris et al. 1976, 1977). Differences in the enzyme's activities have already been shown to exist between normal and leukemic cells (Agris et al. 1976).

Isolation, Purification, and Characterization of the Enzyme Complex

Activities of tRNA methyltransferases and aminoacyl-tRNA synthetases were investigated in subcellular fractions obtained from a Friend's murine-virus-induced leukemic cell (FLC) line (GM86) and from human normal and leukemic cell lines (RPMI 1788 and RPMI 6410 respectively). Suspension cultures were grown to a concentration of 2×10^6 cells/ml. Cells were collected at 4° by centrifugation at 750 *g* for 10 min. The resulting cell pellet was resuspended in physiological saline solution and resuspended cells were collected again by centrifugation. Cells were carefully broken in the presence of 0.05 *M* Tris-HCl, pH 7.5, with brief homogenization in a Potter-Elvehjem homogenizer. Cellular fractions were obtained according to a procedure adapted from that described in detail by Hampel and Enger (1973). This procedure results in the separation of cellular constituents into three fractions: nuclei and membrane debris, microsomal substances having sedimentation rates (svedberg units) between those of nuclei and the 40-S ribosomal subunit, and postribosomal materials having sedimentation rates smaller than 8 S (Fig. 2). Pellets were resuspended in a buffer consisting of 50 m*M* Tris-HCl (pH 7.5), 10 m*M* $MgCl_2$, and 1 m*M* 2-mercaptoethanol (Buffer A). tRNA was isolated from *Escherichia coli* C6 *met-cys-rel* grown either under methionine starvation for use in methyltransferase

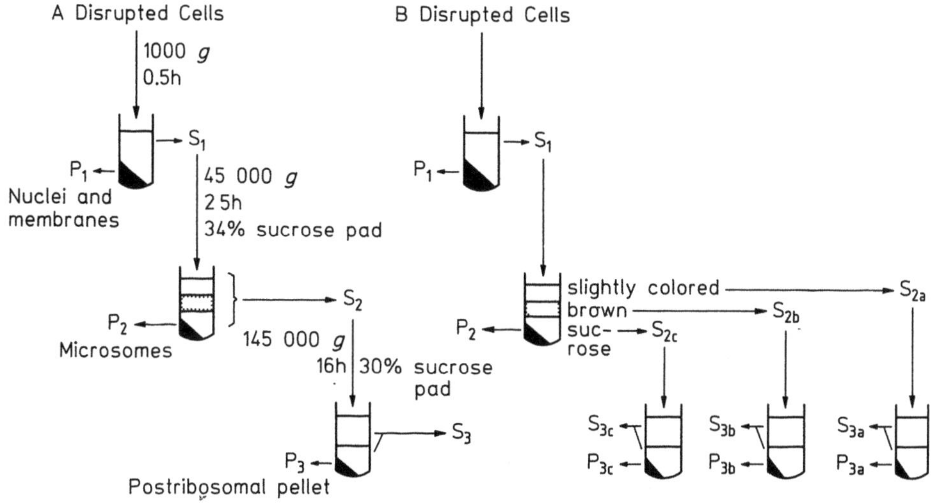

Fig. 2. Diagrammatic representation of enzyme complex preparation. Cell extracts were fractionated by either (**A**) a previously reported method (Agris et al. 1976), or (**B**) a variation resulting in three different postribosomal pellets (Agris et al. 1977)

assays or under cysteine starvation for use in sulfurtransferase assays. tRNA was isolated from each of the cultured mammalian cells for aminoacylation assay.

The highest tRNA methyltransferase activity of FLC(GM86) was found to reside in the postribosomal fraction, P_3. Optimal conditions of tRNA methyltransferase activity for this fraction were obtained by testing five parameters: the concentrations of protein (Fig. 3), tRNA (Fig. 4), and *S*-adenosyl-L-methionine (Fig. 5); the pH; and the cation concentration of reaction mixtures (Fig. 6). There was a distinctly linear response of activity to protein concentrations between 0.02 and 0.1 mg of postribosomal protein per reaction mixture (Fig. 3). Assays, whether with the postribosomal fraction of FLC or with fractions from other cell lines, were carried out under conditions in which the activities responded linearly to protein concentration. An apparent lack of change in enzyme activity with pH (between pH 7.2 and 8.0) was probably due to the assay's measurement of a number of methyltransferase activities, each with a different pH optimum. Decreasing activity above pH 8.0 was due to the alkaline instability of *S*-adenosylmethionine. Activities of the postribosomal fraction of the three cell lines demonstrated optima in the presence of 0.2 *M* NaCl, as has been found for both highly purified, specific methyltransferase activities and crude, unfractionated methyltransferase activities (Agris et al. 1974; Agris 1975).

Purification of the postribosomal enzyme complex was taken a step further by fractionation of the pellet P_3 according to procedure B in Fig. 2. This fractionation more than doubled the specific activity of the methyltransferase (Table 1). Increases in specific activity were accomplished by Sephadex G200 column chromatography (Fig. 7) and sucrose density gradient centrifugation (Fig. 8). Methyltransferase activities eluted from Sephadex G200 at a point corresponding to a molecular weight of approximately 5.5×10^5 daltons. Results obtained from sucrose density gradient centrifugation indicated the presence of complexes of three molecular weights. Peaks of activity were seen at molecular weights of approximately 3×10^5, 6×10^5, and 9×10^5 daltons as shown in Fig. 8. The relative amounts of the three species varied

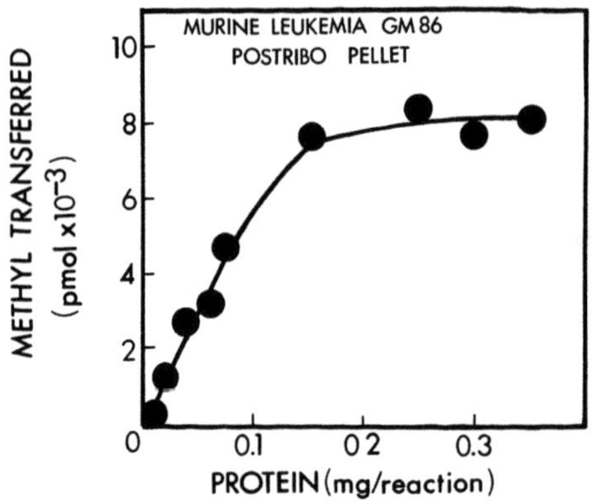

Fig. 3. Methyltransferase activity of FLC postribosomal enzyme complex. Reaction mixtures were prepared to contain the following components in 1 ml final volume buffered with 0.05 *M* Tris-HCl (pH 7.8): 25 μg *E. coli* methyl-deficient tRNA; 40 pmol *S*-adenosyl-L[methyl-^{14}C]methionine; 0.2 mmol NaCl; and varying amounts of the particular subcellular fraction

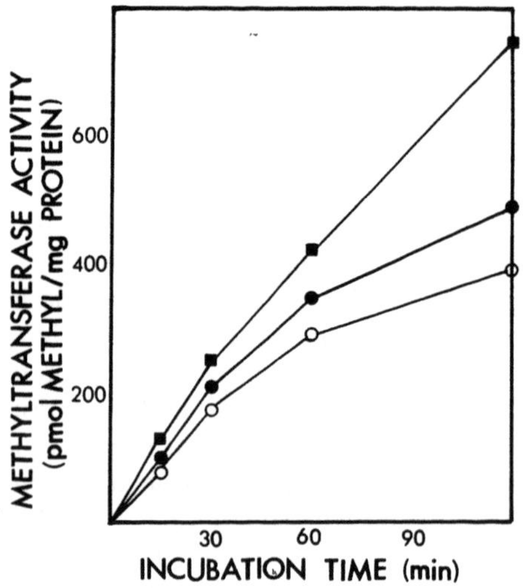

Fig. 4. Methyltransferase activity of FLC high-molecular-weight complex: tRNA dependence. Methyltransferase activity was assayed and the concentration of tRNA in the reaction mixture was varied to test substrate dependence: 16 μ*M* (○); 32 μ*M* (●);, and 62 μ*M* (■). The tRNA is deficient in methyl groups and is obtained from a methionine auxotroph of *E. coli*

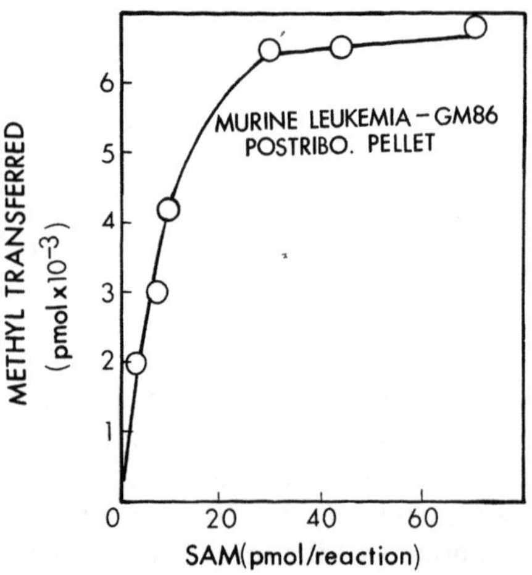

Fig. 5. Methyltransferase activity of FLC enzyme complex: *S*-adenosyl-L-methionine dependence. Methyltransferase activity was assayed and the concentration of *S*-adenosyl-L-methionine in the reaction mixture was varied to test substrate dependence

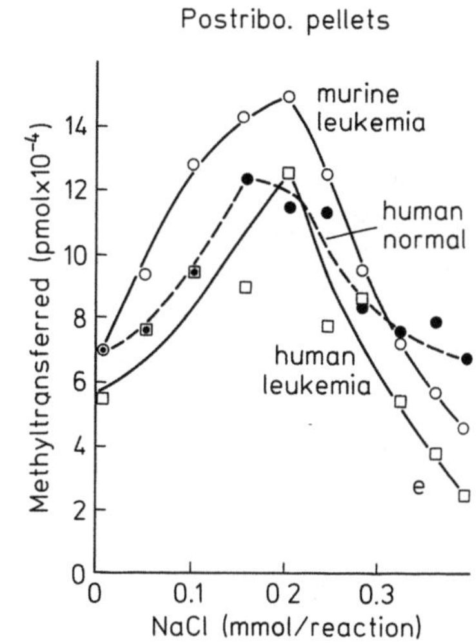

Fig. 6. Methylation of tRNA as a function of NaCl concentration. Reaction mixtures were prepared as described for Fig. 3 except that the amount of NaCl was varied. Postribosomal fraction from FLC GM86 cells (○), RPMI 1788 cells (●), and RPMI 6410 (□) were used to catalyze the transfer of methyl groups. The transfer was plotted as pmol($\times 10^{-3}$) methyl transferred/mg tRNA/mg protein/h

Table 1. Methyltransferase activities of enzyme complex during fractionation

Fraktion[a]	Specific activity (nmol methyl transferred/ mg protein/mg PNA/h)	Percent total activity[c]
P_1	2[b]	15
P_2	3[b]	17
P_3	34[b]	67
P_{3a}	28[b]	14
P_{3b}	74[b]	42
P_{3c}	19[b]	11
Sephadex G200		
Fractions 10–14	128	Not determined
Sucrose ≠ Gradient		
Fractions 8–9	156	Not determined

[a] P_{3a}, P_{3b}, and P_{3c} are subfractions of P_3 (Fig. 2)
[b] Mean value from nine experiments (Fig. 2)
[c] Percent total activity of all cell fractions including those of the supernatant fluids (not shown)

from one preparation to the next, suggesting that the two lower-molecular-weight species were derived from the larger.

Physical characterization of the enzyme complex has been accomplished through electron microscopy with phosphotungstate staining. Photomicrographs of the enzyme complex purified by sucrose density gradient centrifugation showed a complex of three subunits for the highest-molecular-weight (900000 daltons) material, as seen in Fig. 9. However, electron micrographs have also shown complexes of two units and single units (Fig. 9). The latter two would correspond to the 600000- and 300000-dalton units sedimenting in the sucrose gradient. The diameter of the three-subunit complex is approximately 200Å.

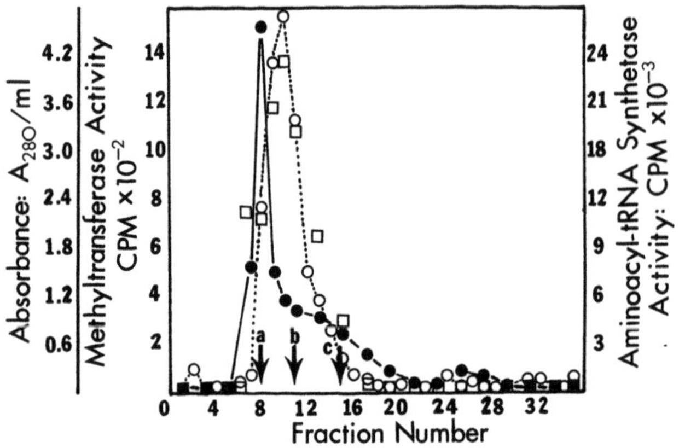

Fig. 7. Sephadex G200 chromatography of semipurified FLC enzyme complex. Enzyme complex was subjected to chromatography on Sephadex G200 (Agris et al. 1977). Protein elution was recorded through absorption at 280 nm (●——●). Column fractions were assayed for both methyltransferase (○---○) and aminoacyl-tRNA synthetase (□---□) activities. *Arrows* indicate the elution position of **a** Blue Dextran; **b** catalase, 232000 daltons; and **c** bovine serum albumin, 67000 daltons

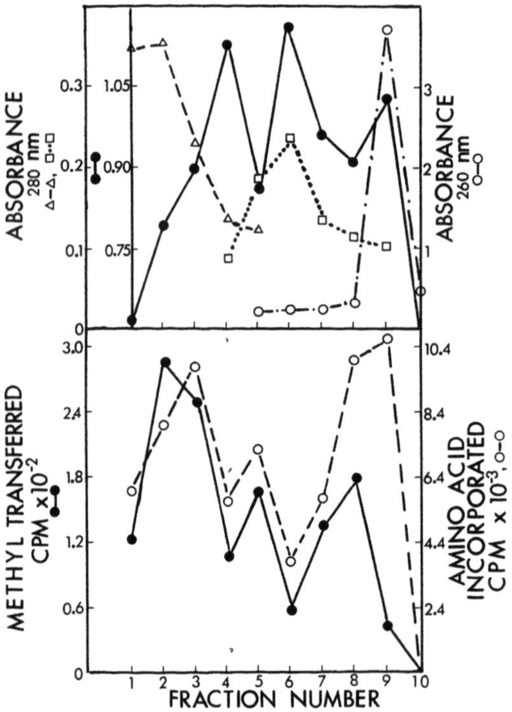

Fig. 8. Sucrose density gradient centrifugation of semipurified FLC enzyme complex. Enzyme complex was subjected to sucrose density gradient centrifugation (Agris et al. 1977). The *upper panel* depicts the migration of complex protein, absorbance at 280 nm (●——●), and molecular weight standards: catalase, 232000 daltons (△---△); thyroglobulin, 669000 daltons (□·····□); and 30-S ribosomal subunit, 1×10^6 daltons (○-·-○). The lower panel shows the comigration of methyltransferase (●——●) and aminoacyl-tRNA synthetase (○---○) activities in three molecular weight species

We have investigated the polypeptide, fatty acid, and sugar composition of the enzyme complex. The fraction having the highest specific activity, P_{3b}, and the complex from the Sephadex chromatography contained some 16 discrete polypeptides ranging in molecular weight from 25000 to 90000 daltons. The microsomal fraction P_2 contained numerous prominent low-molecular-weight peptides, 10000 to 40000 daltons, that

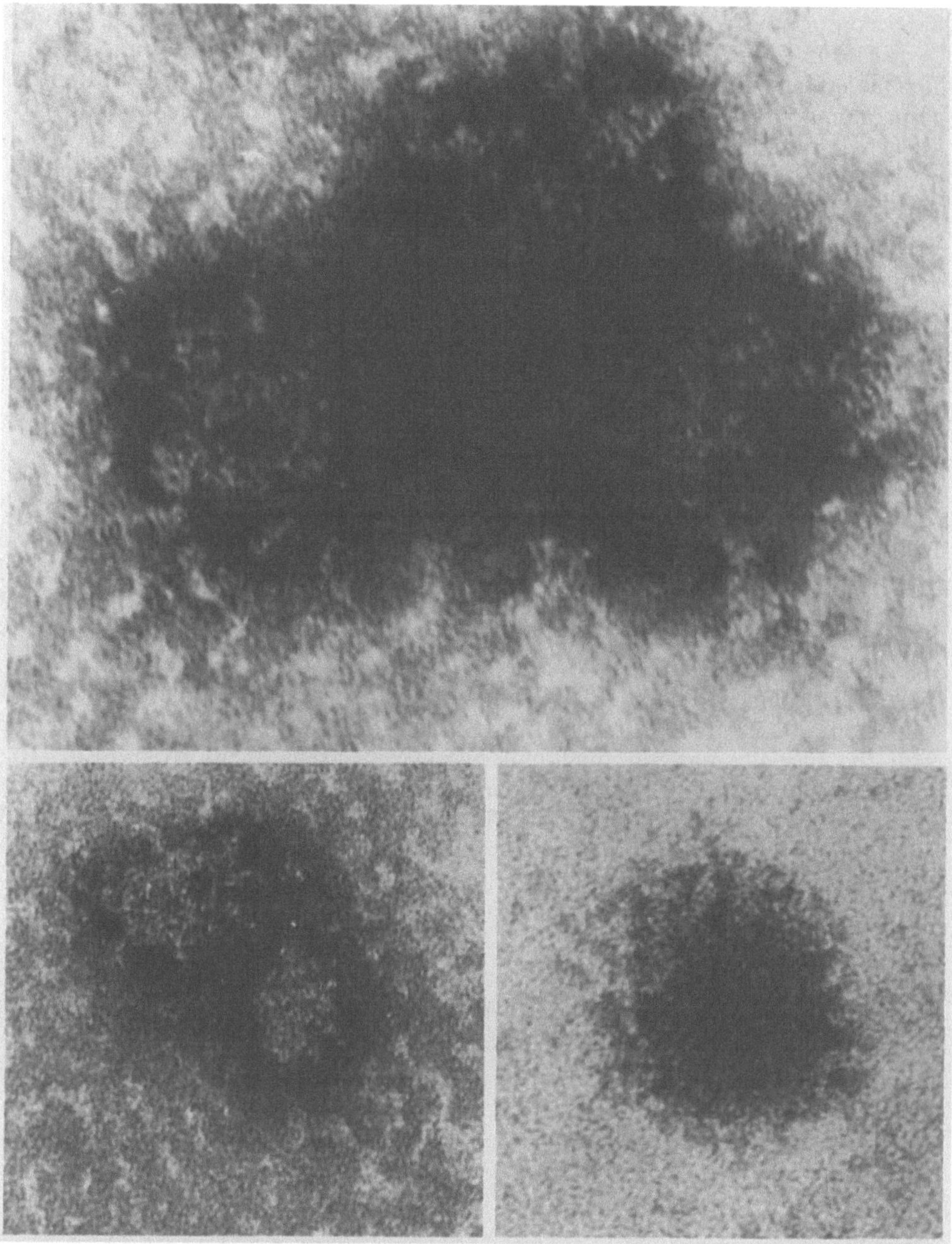

Fig. 9. Transmission electron microscopy of purified FLC enzyme complex. Enzyme complex purified by sucrose gradient centrifugation was prepared for electron microscopy by phosphotungstic acid negative staining. *Top,* the three-subunit complex with the largest dimension approximately 200 Å. One-third of all material in the micrographs was found to be of the three-subunit structure; the other structures found, two subunits and one unit, are shown in the *lower* micrographs

were conspicuously absent from the enzyme complexes. Bandyopadhyay and Deutscher (1973) reported the presence of cholesterol esters in association with a high-molecular-weight complex of aminoacyl-tRNA synthetases. We analyzed various preparations of the methyltransferase/synthetase complex for the presence of lipids by use of high-resolution gas-liquid chromatography of the fatty acids after saponification of lipids. In our preparations of the enzyme complex we found the lowest level of fatty acid content in those preparations exhibiting the highest specific activities. It thus seems likely that only a small quantity of lipid (0.63%) is present in the partially purified complex. The enzyme preparation with highest methyltransferase specific activity and minimal lipid content had a very low amount of sugar, which was detected almost exclusively as glucose.

Methylated Nucleosides Formed by the Enzyme Complex

If a specific methyltransferase were present only in soluble form and not in a high-molecular-weight complex, one might expect to find certain methylated nucleosides in the methylated tRNA resulting from incubation with unfractionated cell extract (S_1) but not in the tRNA resulting from incubation with the resuspended postribosomal pellet (P_3). An examination of the data in Table 2 indicates that a very significant difference in the two cases occurred for the methylated nucleoside T. Whereas T comprised about 10% of the total methylated nucleosides in the tRNA incubated with the crude extract, it was less than 1% of those in the tRNA incubated with the partially purified, high-molecular-weight complex P_3 from FLC. This suggested the absence in the postribosomal pellet of the methyltransferase responsible for the methylation of uracil to riboTp. The enzyme responsible for production of m_bA was the only other methyltransferase having a conspicuously lower activity in the high-molecular-weight fraction than in the unfractionated cell extract.

Table 2. Products of in vitro tRNA methyltransferase activity

Methylated nucleoside	S_1 enzyme fraction		P_3 enzyme fraction	
	Mean[a]	SE	Mean[a]	SE
m^1A	26.7	3.4	30.7	1.6
m^6A	1.7	0.1	0.3	0.1
m^5C	10.7	3.1	17.2	2.5
m^1G	10.9	2.8	6.3	2.3
m^2G	11.1	2.4	7.6	0.9
m^7G	10.9	1.5	15.6	2.3
G_p^mN	3.3	1.0	6.8	2.2
N_p^mN[b]	10.1	1.8	8.4	0.8
T	10.0	2.6	0.6	0.4

[a] Mean relative amounts of nucleosides in tRNA from three separate determinations
[b] Amount of N_p^mN represents the sum of different ribose methylated dinucleoside-phosphates

Comparison of Murine and Human Leukemic and Human Normal Methyltransferase Complexes

Transfer RNA methyltransferase activities of the four subcellular fractions from each of the three cell lines are compared in Fig. 10. The postribosomal fraction from leukemic leukocytes had a methyltransferase specific activity higher than that of the microsomal fraction, while the same two fractions of normal leukocytes had approximately equal activities (Table 3). Seventy-five percent or more of the total methyltransferase activity was found to reside in the combined microsomal and postribosomal fractions of each of the three cell lines (Table 3). Distribution of the enzyme activity between these two subcellular fractions is interesting with respect to the murine or human origin of the cell. The postribosomal fraction from the murine-derived FLC cells contained 67% of those cells' total methyltransferase activity, whereas the microsomal fractions of the two human cell lines, RPMI 1788 and 6410, contained 54% and 50% of their respective total enzyme activities.

Association of Methyltransferase Enzyme Complex with Amimoacyl-tRNA Synthetase Complex

Aminoacyl-tRNA synthetase activity cosediments with tRNA methyltransferase activity in the postribosomal-pellet (P_3) disrupted FLC GM86 cells and the two human leukocyte cell lines (Fig. 8). Microsomal and postribosomal fractions from the three cell lines contained both the highest specific activities and greatest total synthetase

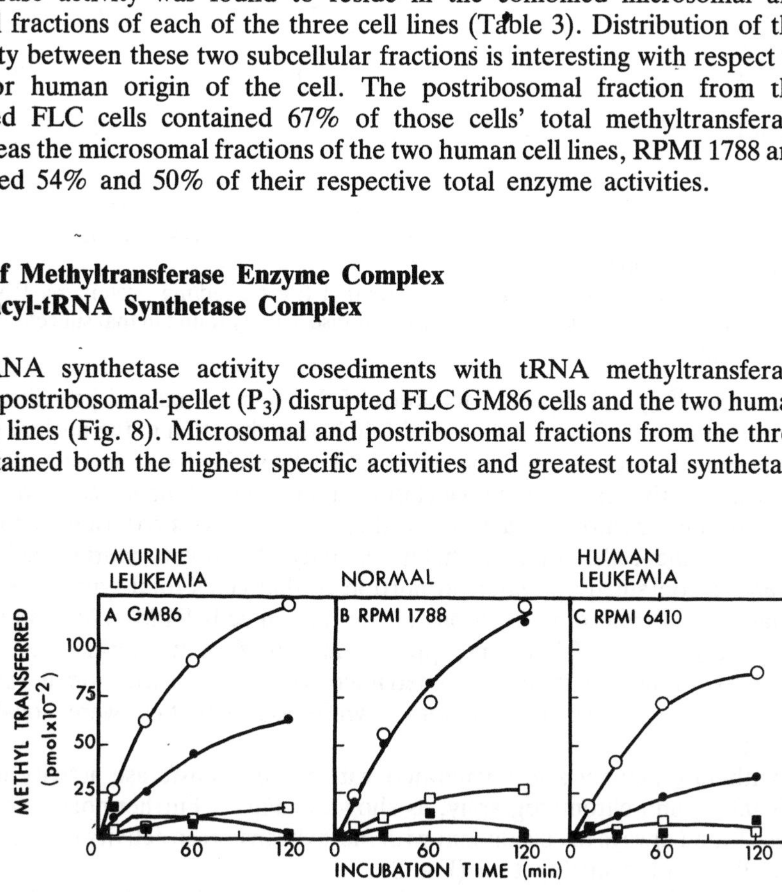

Fig. 10. Comparison of methyltransferase activities for different subcellular fractions from murine leukemic, human normal, and human leukemic cell lines. Reaction mixtures were prepared as described for Fig. 3. The amount of protein was initially tested to insure a linear response of activity with respect to protein concentration. Subcellular fractions were obtained from cultures of the three cell lines. Aliquots were removed from the incubation mixtures at the indicated times and applied to Whatman 3MM filter discs. The discs were then washed at 4° for 10 min each wash, three times in 5% trichloroacetic acid, once in ethanol/ethyl ether (1 : 1, vol/vol), and finally in ethyl ether. The filters were allowed to dry at room temperature and their radioactivities were determined by liquid scintillation counting. Each datum has been corrected for the incorporation of radioactivity into trichloroacetic-acid-precipitable material in the absence of tRNA. Enzymatic activity is plotted as pmol (× 10^{-2}) of methyl transferred/mg of protein from the four subcellular fractions: nuclear and membrane (□), microsomal (●), postribosomal (○), and supernatant (■)

Table 3. Transfer RNA methyltransferase activity of subcellular fractions

Cell line	Fraction							
	Nuclear and membrane (P_1)		Microsomal (P_2)		Postribosomal (P_3)		Supernatant (S_3)	
	Specific activity[a]	%[b]	Specific activity[a]	%[b]	Specific activity[a]	%[b]	Specific activity[a]	%[b]
FLC GM86	1	15	4	17	34	67	0	1
RPMI 1788	2	10	8	54	7	35	ND	ND
RPMI 6410	1	23	2	50	16	26	ND	ND

Comparison of the specific and total methyltransferase activities in subcellular fractions from cultures of three cell lines. Enzyme activities were measured as described in the legend to Fig. 1. *ND*, not determined

[a] Specific activity measured in nmol methyl transferred/mg protein/mg RNA/h

[b] Percent of total subcellular methyltransferase activity found in that subcellular fraction of the cell line

activities (Fig. 11). Specific activities of the microsomal and postribosomal fractions were found to be between 6- and 17-fold higher than that of the nuclear membrane and supernatant fractions. Murine cell (FLC) subcellular fractions had, in general, higher specific activities of aminoacylation than their human cell components. The microsomal fraction of each of the three cell lines was consistently found to contain 40% of the cells' total synthetase activity. However, murine cell postribosomal fraction contained a greater proportion of that cell's total synthetase activity (52%) than the postribosomal fractions of the human cells RPMI 1788 and 6410 (34% and 36% respectively). Therefore, approximately 94% of the murine cells' total synthetase activity was present in the combined microsomal and postribosomal fractions, whereas some 75% of the human cells' synthetase activities were localized in these fractions.

Synthetase activity also comigrated with methyltransferase activity upon Sephadex G200 column chromatography, as shown in Fig. 7. Furthermore, synthetase activity was found always to cosediment with methyltransferase activity during sucrose density gradient ultracentrifugation (Fig. 8).

Aminoacyl-tRNA synthetase activity has previously been shown to be associated with ribosomal and postribosomal subcellular fractions. This activity seems to be altered during the cell cycle, and of the three complexes only the one with the lowest molecular weight is found to exist in a mutant cell line with a temperature-sensitive leucyl-tRNA synthetase. We have compared the activities of the postribosomal and ribosomal fractions from FLC for 17 individual aminoacyl-tRNA synthetases. None of the enzymes are exclusively present in the postribosomal enzyme complex, as shown in Table 4. However, the majority of enzyme activities for Ala, Arg, Gly, His, Lys, Ser, Thr, and Val were found associated with the postribosomal fraction. The majority of enzyme activities for Asp, Cys, Leu, Phe, and Pro were found associated with the ribosomal fraction. Postribosomal total aminoacyl-tRNA synthetase activity was found to be 50% greater than that of the ribosomal fraction.

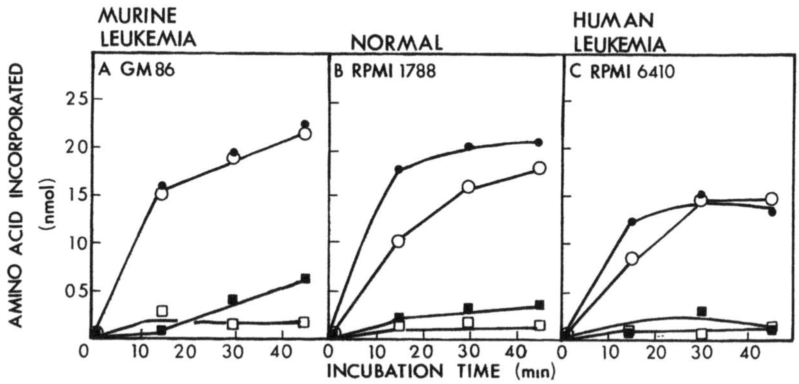

Fig. 11. Comparison of aminoacyl-tRNA synthetase activities for different subcellular fractions from murine leukemic, human normal and leukemic cell lines. Reaction mixtures were prepared as described (Agris et al. 1976). Four subcellular fractions, nuclear and membrane (□), Microsomal (●), postribosomal (○), and supernatant (■), were obtained from cultures of each of the three cell lines and were used to catalyze the aminoacylation of tRNA from the homologous cell line. Aliquots were removed from the incubation mixtures at the indicated times and applied to Whatman 3MM filter discs, which were then washed as described in the legend to Fig. 10. Each datum has been corrected for the incorporation of radioactivity into trichloroacetic-acid-precipitable material in the absence of tRNA. Enzymatic activity is plotted as nmol amino acid incorporated/mg of tRNA/mg protein. This activity was calculated from the average specific activity of the 15 ^{14}C-labeled amino acids (243 mCi/mmol) in the reaction mixture

Table 4. Quantitative comparison of synthetase activity between ribosomal and postribosomal cellular fractions

	Fraction (pmol/A_{260} tRNA/mg protein/min)	
Synthetase	Ribosomal	Postribosomal
Ala	5	39
Arg	25	95
Asp	10	7
Cys	63	13
Glu	27	22
Gly	8	39
His	18	35
Ile	30	25
Leu	90	55
Lys	90	150
Met	32	31
Phe	382	210
Pro	16	1
Ser	42	98
Thr	105	165
Tyr	15	17
Val	56	110

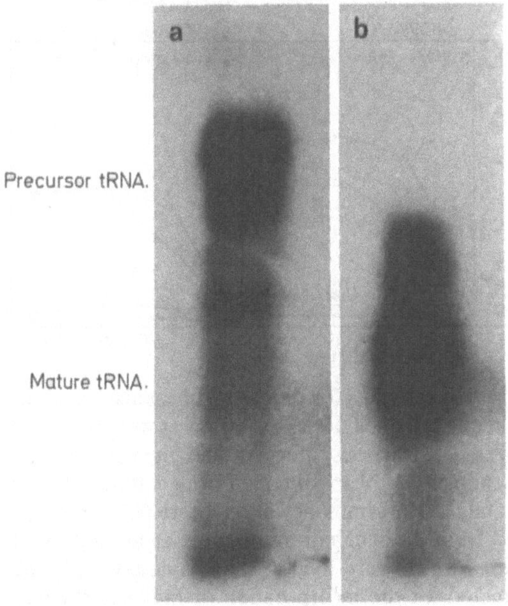

Fig. 12a, b. Autoradiograph of electrophoretically separated precursor tRNA and mature tRNA product of RNase action. *E. coli* A49, a temperature-sensitive mutant of RNase P, was grown at 42° C and radioactive phosphate was added, resulting in an in vivo accumulation of ^{32}P-labeled precursor tRNA. Nucleic acids were extracted and were subjected to electrophoresis on a denaturing polyacrylamide gel. The autoradiograph shows in lane **a** the location of the precursor tRNA and in lane **b** the location of the mature tRNA bands resulting from enzyme action

Analysis for Specific Ribonuclease in the Enzyme Complex

High-molecular-weight enzyme complexes that were found to contain tRNA methyltransferases and aminoacyl-tRNA synthetases were further investigated to determine if specific ribonuclease activity was also present in the complex. The correct substrate for specific ribonuclease processing of tRNA would be the FLC precursor tRNAs. In lieu of isolating these precursors, the more easily isolated and more fully understood precursor tRNAs from *E. coli* A49 were used in the experiments (*E. coli* A49 kindly provided by S. Altman, Yale University). Strain 49 contains a temperature-sensitive RNase P, allowing isolation of precursor tRNA that has not been "sized" by this enzyme. Precursor tRNA and mature-size tRNA, both highly radiolabeled with ^{32}P-phosphate, were isolated from *E. coli* A49 by a procedure similar, but not identical, to that described by Altman (1971) and tested as substrates for the FLC enzyme complex.

The FLC enzyme complex was added to each of the precursor tRNA and mature tRNA solutions, producing incubation mixtures that contained 0.1 *M* NH_4Cl; 5 m*M* $MgCl_2$; 0.1 m*M* EDTA; 0.1 m*M* 2-mercaptoethanol; 30 m*M* Tris-HCl, pH 8; 190000 cpm in ^{32}P-labeled mature or precursor tRNA; and 1.6 mg enzyme complex. The mixtures were incubated at 37° C. Reactions were stopped by heating at 100 degrees for 2 min. The aliquots were subjected to electrophoresis on a denaturing polyacrylamide gel followed by autoradiography. Regions of the gel containing unreacted precursor tRNA and mature tRNA product were then removed from the rest of the gel and the amount of radioactivity was determined for each. An autoradiograph of a gel showing the pre-tRNA substrate and the mature tRNA product is shown in Fig. 12.

In order to ascertain the time course of RNase activity, precursor tRNA was incubated with FLC enzyme complex; the reaction was stopped after 5, 10, 20, 60, and 120 min

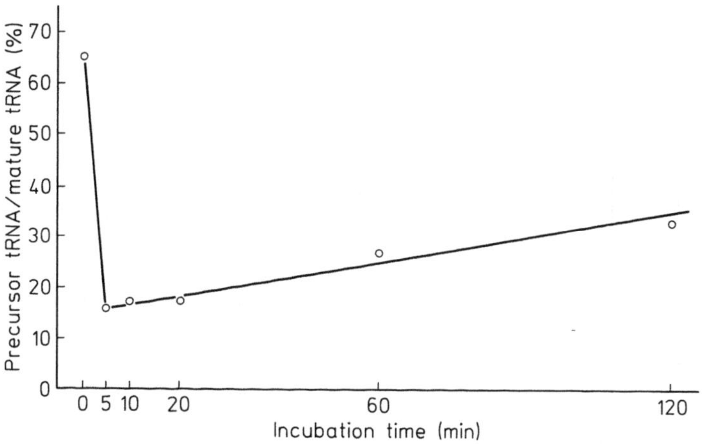

Fig. 13. Ribonuclease activity of postribosomal enzyme complex. FLC enzyme complex was added to incubation mixtures containing either ^{32}P-labeled, precursor tRNA or mature tRNA as a control. Reaction mixtures were incubated at 37° C with aliquots taken at regular intervals. The aliquots were then subjected to electrophoresis and RNase activity quantitated. Radioactivity (cpm of the precursor tRNA bands) was measured by scintillation counting and compared to that of the mature tRNA bands which had been produced from the sizing of precursor. The graph shows the percent of precursor tRNA divided by mature tRNA against the incubation time

and the mixture subjected to electrophoresis on a denaturing polyacrylamide gel. The control for determining the specificity of FLC enzyme for precursor tRNA was to analyze, analogously, the enzyme complex's action on mature-size tRNA. In order to quantitatively analyze the ribonuclease activity over the incubation time course, the radioactivity (cPM) of substrate, precursor tRNA, relative to that of product, mature tRNA, was determined at each time point. As shown in Figure 13, a decrease of precursor tRNA, accompanied by an increase of mature-size tRNA, occurred in the first 5 min incubation time. The rest of the graph is composed of a slightly upward sloping line, due to the small amount of nonspecific ribonuclease activity.

Analysis of Sulfurtransferase Activity in the Enzyme Complex

A cysteine sulfurtransferase activity in rat liver has been described (Harris et al. 1977). The majority (70%) of this enzyme activity was shown to be located in a high-molecular-weight protein complex. We have determined that the FLC enzyme complex has a cysteine to tRNA sulfurtransferase activity.

Enzyme complex sulfurtransferase activity was detected and characterized under various assay conditions. Sulfur-deficient tRNA from *E. coli met-cys-rel* starved of a sulfur source was used as substrate. Figure 14 describes the protein dependency of the activity. Even with high concentrations of enzyme complex the reaction was not complete in 60 min. Modification enzymes of tRNA are known to have slow reactions, even at optimal conditions. Only with low concentrations of tRNA and longer times

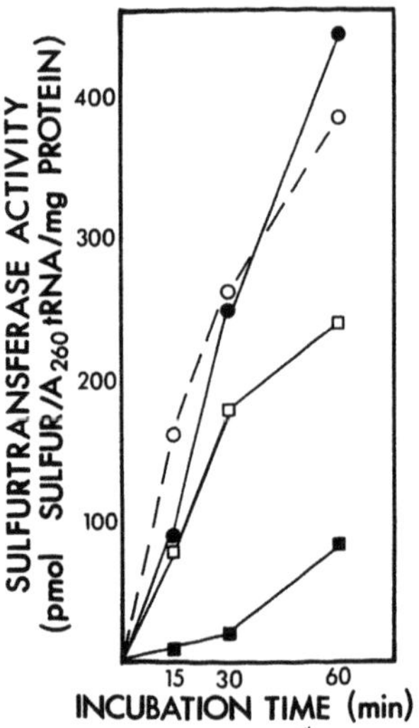

Fig. 14. The optimum conditions for sulfurtransferase activity by the enzyme complex were determined in filter assays similar to that for methyltransferase in which one component was varied while the rest were held constant. The optimum sulfurtransferase conditions were found to be: 50 m*M* Tris-HCl (pH 7.8), 250 m*M* NaCl, 0.2 m*M* 2-mercaptoethanol, 16 μ*M* tRNA, 0.04 μ*M* cysteine, and 0.12 mg/ml enzyme protein. Control assays for sulfurtransferase experiments included incubation mixtures containing all components except tRNA, all components except enzyme, and all components except enzyme and tRNA. All reported results have these three backgrounds (nonspecific sticking of radioactivity to tRNA, enzyme, and filter) subtracted except as noted and are the average of three determinations. This figure demonstrates enzyme dependence of the reaction. The enzyme concentrations were: 0.024 mg/ml (■); 0.036 mg/ml (□); 0.12 mg/ml (○); and 0.24 mg/ml (●)

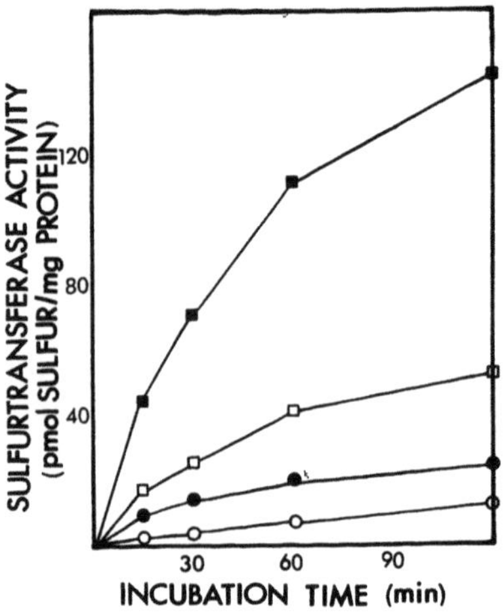

Fig. 15. Transfer RNA dependence of sulfur transfer by the enzyme complex. The figure demonstrates the tRNA substrate dependence of the enzyme complex: 4 μ*M* (○); 8 μ*M* (●), 16 μ*M* (□), and 64 μ*M* (■). The tRNA is deficient in thio groups and is obtained from a cysteine auxotroph of *E. coli.* Note that tRNA has fewer thiolation sites than methylation sites and therefore is more readily saturated with thio groups

were reactions completed as seen in Fig. 15. Reaction dependency on the concentration of the other substrate is seen in Fig. 16. The continual increase in activity with increasing cysteine seen in this figure is an artifact caused by an increasing background of nonspecific sticking of cysteine to the filter in the presence of tRNA and absence of enzyme. When appropriately corrected, the optimum cysteine concentration is 0.04 μ*M*. An optimum NaCl concentration is demonstrated in Fig. 17. Sulfurtransferase activity exhibited an optimum in the presence of 0.25 *M* NaCl, the identical requirement to that of methyltransferases. Thus optimal conditions for this activity (listed in Fig. 14 legend) were determined to be quite similar to those for methyltransferase activity. Analysis of the thiolated tRNA revealed that only s^2U derivatives were produced.

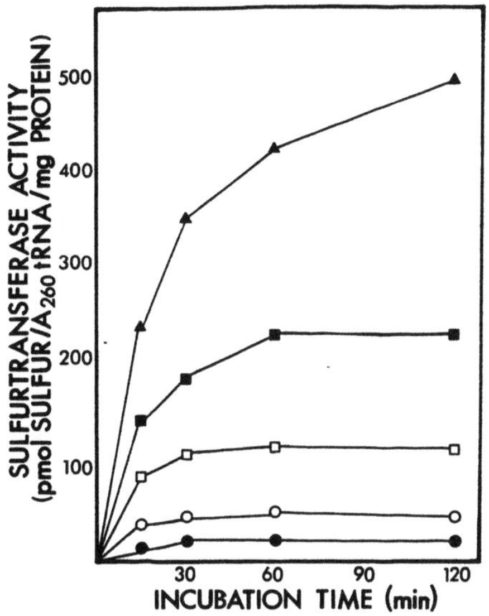

Fig. 16. Cysteine dependence of sulfurtransferase of enzyme complex. Cysteine concentration was varied in the incubation mixtures: 0.008 μ*M* (●), 0.024 μ*M* (○), 0.04 μ*M* (□), 0.08 μ*M* (■), and 0.24 μ*M* (▲). Results of these reactions are plotted in the figure without the subtraction of one of the backgrounds, that due to nonspecific sticking of radioactivity to tRNA. Note the continual increase in acid-precipitable material associated with the assay filters with increasing cysteine yet constant tRNA. When the background due to nonspecific association of ^{35}S-cysteine with tRNA (assay excluding enzyme) is subtracted the optimum concentration is found to be 0.04 μ*M*

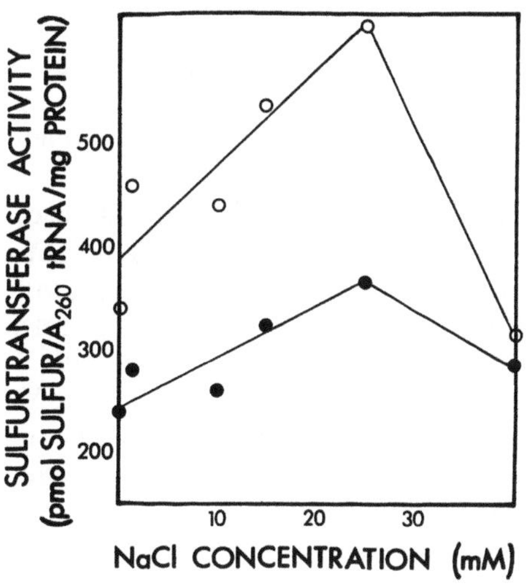

Fig. 17. Optimization of NaCl concentration. Methyltransferases have been shown to be stimulated by monovalent cations with an optimal activity exhibited at 0.25 *M* NaCl. This stimulation may be caused by an affect on tRNA structure. Sulfurtransferase activity exhibited a similar stimulation, as shown in this figure for incubation times of 1 h (●) and 2 h (○)

Conclusion

Knowledge of the separated and purified enzymatic activities of normal and neoplastic cell methyltransferases and other tRNA modifying enzymes has added to our understanding of protein-nucleic acid recognition (Spremulli et al. 1974) in normal and neoplastic cells. But we still have little understanding of (a) the enzymes' involvement in the sequential processing of tRNA molecules in normal cells vs cancer cells, (b) the biochemical interaction of the tRNA-processing enzymes (modification enzymes and RNases) with each other and enzymes involved in the utilization of tRNA for protein synthesis, or (c) the possible regulation and misregulation of protein synthesis by enzymes involved in the maturation of tRNA.

Purification of individual tRNA methyltransferase activities from mammalian cells has been shown to destabilize these activities with respect to that of the crude extract (Agris et al. 1974; Spremulli et al. 1974). Initial steps in the purification entailed ion-exchange chromatography that yielded various active fractions, each with different proportions of all the methyltransferase activities but with essentially no separation of individual activities (Agris et al. 1974). These results are indicative of the ionic disruption of multienzyme complexes into smaller, less stable units. Our analysis of the subcellular distribution of the methyltransferases (Agris et al. 1976), in an analogous manner to that for investigation of aminoacyl-tRNA synthetases, has shown that most of the cells' methyltransferase and sulfurtransferase activity was present in a high-molecular-weight postribosomal pellet. Study of the tRNA modifying activities as present in the high-molecular-weight enzyme complex provides information on the maturation of a set of nucleic acids by a naturally occurring, multifunctional catalytic unit.

The specific methyltransferase activity of the postribosomal fraction of each of the cell lines we studied was found to be either considerably higher than that of all other fractions, or high and comparable to that of the microsomal fraction. Differences were found in the distribution of methyltransferase activities among the subcellular fractions of the three cell lines studied. Leukemia-cell postribosomal methyltransferase had a specific activity significantly higher than that of any other cell fraction; whereas normal-cell postribosomal methyltransferase had a specific activity comparable to that of the microsomal fraction. Specific methyltransferase activities may reside in the various subcellular fractions, but most of the activities are present in the high-molecular-weight enzyme complex of the postribosomal pellet. A notable exception to this is the almost complete lack of m^5U (riboT) methyltransferase activity in the postribosomal pellet.

Methyltransferase, sulfurtransferase, and aminoacyl-tRNA synthetase activities comigrated in high-molecular-weight complexes during sucrose gradient centrifugation and column chromatography, indicating a possible association of these activities. Preliminary investigations of the rat liver high-molecular-weight enzyme complexes were begun in collaboration with Dr. David Yang, Department of Chemistry, Georgetown University (Dang and Yang 1979; Johnson et al. 1980). Sucrose density gradient experiments have shown the presence of high-molecular-weight methyltransferase activity as well as the already-reported rat liver aminoacyl-tRNA synthetase complex.

We have been able to show the presence of other tRNA maturation enzymes in erythroleukemia cells, such as cysteine-tRNA sulfurtransferase, and a possible specific RNase, in high-molecular-weight complexes. The cysteine-tRNA sulfurtransferase comigrates with the tRNA methyltransferases on sucrose density gradient centrifugation. The sulfurtransferase is responsible for the production of such nucleosides as 2-thiouridine in the anticodon of tRNA. Regulation or misregulation of the production of this nucleoside could result in miscoding at the ribosome.

Modification enzyme activity and the modified nucleosides of tRNA change during such phenomena as neoplasia, viral transformation, and differentiation. We have already shown that the modification of nucleosides in tRNA and the tRNA species from FLC cells differs from that in the tRNA of the same cells after erythroid-like differentiation to normablasts has been completed (Agris 1975; Lin and Agris 1980). Detailed analyses of the maturation enzymes' activities and the resulting tRNA nucleoside modification of this cell culture system undergoing differentiation are part of our investigations of modified nucleoside function in translation.

It is with regard to understanding these functions that investigations of tRNA modification enzyme complexes should take note of the presently available eukaryotic mutants. Of particular interest are the aminoacyl-tRNA synthetase mutants of mammalian cell lines. The temperature-sensitive leucyl-tRNA synthetase of a mutant strain of Chinese hamster ovary cells has been shown to be present as the free, unassociated enzyme not in complex with other synthetases, whereas the leucyl-tRNA synthetase of the parent cell is associated with the synthetase complex (Hampel et al. 1978). This and other mutant cell strains should be studied in regard to the modification enzyme complex. Finally, tRNA modification enzyme complexes should be investigated in the lower eukaryotes such as yeast and *Drosophila* in which genetic manipulation has already yielded modification-deficient strains.

Summary

An enzyme complex is a multifunctional catalytic unit that efficiently associates substrates with functionally related enzymes. The enzyme complex provides for the cellular regulation of enzymatic activities by physical interaction of the proteins with each other and by prior alteration of one enzyme's substrate by a related enzyme. Such regulatory abilities may go awry in neoplasia. Components of the protein biosynthetic machinery, such as aminoacyl-tRNA synthetases, have been thought to exist freely in the cytoplasm. However, high-molecular-weight enzyme complexes with aminoacyl-tRNA synthetase activities have been found in mammalian cells. We have been the first to report that the mammalian cell enzymes responsible for modification of tRNA occur in enzyme complexes (molecular weight 900000 daltons) associated with aminoacyl-tRNA synthetases and that the activities of these enzymes differ in normal and leukemic cells. Thus the enzymes responsible for the methylation of tRNA occur in enzyme complexes that provide efficient maturation of tRNA and possible regulation of protein synthesis. In FLC cells a unique enzyme complex composed of tRNA-methyltransferase and aminoacyl-tRNA synthetase activities has also been shown to contain a specific ribonuclease activity and a cysteine-tRNA sulfurtransferase activity. Sulfurtransferase activity has been characterized and optimized for its tRNA and cysteine substrates and mercaptoethanol and cation cofactors. Abnormal activity of this enzyme during neoplasia could result in improper acylation of tRNA and/or infidelity of coding by tRNA. Specific RNase is important in the sizing of percursor tRNA into mature tRNA. Results showed that this sizing was dependent upon the presence of the enzyme complex and the length of the incubation time. Many of the 20 aminoacyl-tRNA synthetases are also found in the complex. Electron microscopy has verified the subunit nature of the complex, seen previously by density gradient centrifugation and gel filtration. Three subunits, each of 300000 daltons, comprise a complex approximately 200 Å in diameter.

References

Agris PF (1975) Alteration of transfer RNA during erythroid differentiation of murine virus-induced leukemia cells. Arch Biochem Biophys 170: 114–123

Agris PF (1980) The modified nucleosides of transfer RNA. Liss, New York

Agris PF, Söll D (1977) The modified nucleosides in transfer RNA. In: Vogel H (ed) Nucleic acid-protein recognition. Academic Press, New York, pp 321–344

Agris PF, Söll D, Seno T (1973) Biological function of 2-thiouridine in *Escherichia coli* glutamic acid transfer ribonucleic acid. Biochemistry 12: 4331–4337

Agris PF, Spremulli LL, Brown GM (1974) tRNA methylases from Hela cells: Purification and properties of an adenine-1-methylase and a guanine-N^2-methylase. Arch Biochem Biophys 162: 38–47

Agris PF, Woolverton DK, Setzer D (1976) Subcellular localization of S-adenosyl-L-methionine: tRNA methyltransferases with aminoacyl-tRNA synthetases in human and mouse: Normal and leukemic leukocytes. Proc Natl Acad Sci USA 73: 3857–3861

Agris PF, Setzer D, Gehrke CW (1977) Characterization of a unique enzyme complex composed of S-adenosyl-L-methionine-tRNA methyltransferase and aminoacyl-tRNA synthetase activities. Nucleic Acids Res 4: 3803–3819

Altman S (1971) Isolation of tyrosine tRNA precursor molecules. Nature 229: 19–21

Bandyopadhyay AK, Deutscher MP (1971) Complex of aminoacyl-transfer RNA synthetases. J Mol Biol 60: 113–222

Bandyopadhyay AK, Deutscher MP (1973) Lipids associated with the aminoacyl-transfer RNA synthetase complex. J Mol Biol 74: 257–261

Berg BH (1975) I. A study of the stages in the quantitative isolation of aminoacyl-tRNA synthetase activities from mouse liver. Biochim Biophys Acta 395: 164–172

Dang CV, Yang DCH (1978) Affinity chromatography of rat liver aminoacyl-tRNA synthetase complex. Biochem Biophys Res Commun 80: 709–714

Dang C, Yang DCH (1979) Disassembly and gross structure of particulate aminoacyl-tRNA synthetases from rat liver. J Biol Chem 254: 5350–5356

Ginsburg A, Stadtman ER (1970) Multienzyme systems. Annu Rev Biochem 39: 429–472

Hampel AE, Enger MD (1973) Subcellular distribution of aminoacyl-transfer RNA synthetases in Chinese hamster ovary cell culture. J Mol Biol 79: 285–293

Hampel AE, Ritter PO, Enger MD (1978) A physically altered leucyl-tRNA synthetase complex in a CHO cell mutant. Nature 276: 844–845

Harris CL, Marin K, Stewart D (1977) tRNA sulfurtransferase: A member of the aminoacyl-tRNA synthetase complex in rat liver. Biochem Biophys Res Commun 79: 657–661

Johnson DL, Dang CV, Yang DCH (1980) Purification and characterization of lysyl-tRNA synthetase after dissociation of the particular aminoacyl-tRNA synthetase from rat liver. J Biol Chem 255: 4362–4366

Lin VK, Agris PF (1980) Alterations in tRNA isoaccepting species during erythroid differentiation of the Friend leukemia cell. Nucleic Acids Res 8: 3467–3480

Reed LJ (1974) Multienzyme complexes. Acc Chem Res 7: 40–46

Reed LJ, Cox DJ (1970) Multienzyme Complexes. In: Boyer PD (ed) The enzymes. Academic Press, New York, pp 213–240

Som K, Hardesty B (1975) Isolation and partial characterization of an aminoacyl-tRNA synthetase complex from rabbit reticulocytes. Arch Biochem Biophys 66: 507–517

Spremulli LL, Agris PF, Brown GM, RajBhandary UL (1974) *Escherichia coli* formylmethionine tRNA: Methylation of specific guanine and adenine residues catalyzed by Hela cell tRNA methylases and the effect of these methylations on biological properties. Arch Biochem Biophys 162: 22–37

Tscherne JS, Weinstein IB, Lanks KW, Gersten NB, Cantor CR (1973) Phenylalanyl transfer ribonucleic acid synthetase activity associated with rat liver ribosomes and microsomes. Biochemistry 12: 3859–3865

Ussery MA, Tanaka WK, Hardesty B (1977) Subcellular distribution of aminoacyl-tRNA synthetases in various eukaryotic cells. Eur J Biochem 72: 491–500

*Alteration of tRNA Modification in Eukaryotes: Causes and Consequences**

H. Kersten

Institut für Physiologische Chemie, Universität Erlangen-Nürnberg,
Fahrstrasse 17, 8520 Erlangen, FRG

Introduction

In eubacteria the patterns of modified nucleosides of tRNA and their biosynthetic pathways show taxa-specific differences. In general, tRNAs in growing microorganisms are fully modified, but alterations of tRNA modifications can be caused by mutations, unbalanced growth conditions, and inhibitors of post-transcriptional modification, and during sporulation (for summarizing references see Kersten 1981).

Common sequences and modifications have been conserved during the evolution of tRNAs, but the number of modified nucleosides has increased. The patterns of tRNA modifications in eukaryotes are almost the same, but they differ in one species depending on cell type or tissue and show alterations during differentiation, morphogenesis, ageing, or neoplastic transformation (for summarizing references see Nishimura 1979; Nishimura and Kuchino 1979). From these observations the following questions arise:

What are the causes of alterations in tRNA modification?
What are the consequences?
Are the patterns of tRNA modifications characteristic or even specific for cells undergoing morphogenesis, differentiation, ageing, or neoplastic transformation?

The prerequisites for answering these questions are: (a) improved methods allowing complete aminoacylation and separation of tRNA isoacceptors, (b) knowledge of cell- or tissue-specific modification patterns, and (c) a better understanding of the role of modified nucleosides in tRNA function.

I should like to discuss experimental approaches to solving these problems in respect to two modified nucleosides that are highly conserved during evolution and are present in eubacterial as well as in eukaryotic tRNAs, namely T and Q.

* This work was supported by Deutsche Forschungsgemeinschaft Grant KE 98/16 and SFB 118. The author thanks Dr. B. Emmerich, München, and Dr. A. Ogilvie, Erlangen, for their cooperation on the work with mouse tumors, Ulrike Lösel and Herbert Brönner for skilful technical assistance, and Sonja Noeth for help with the manuscript

Alteration of Modification of U54 to T

All tRNAs participating in ribosome-dependent peptide elongation contain a modified sequence in the ribosomal binding region which is invariant in gram-positive and gram-negative microorganisms and at positions 54, 55, and 56 comprises T, ψ, and C respectively. Eukaryotic tRNAs have been divided into different classes with respect to this sequence: one major class of elongator tRNAs with TψC, and minor classes with TmψC, UψC, $\psi\psi$C, $N^+\psi$C, or N^+UC (Roe and Tsen 1977). Archaebacteria, the possible ancestors of eukaryotes, have been found to comprise UψCm, $\psi\psi$Cm or ψUCm (Fig. 1a,b).

In contrast to the tRNA of eubacteria, in which U54 is usually fully modified, tRNAs of the major class can occur in eukaryotes with incomplete methylation at this position. Since the number of genes for a specific tRNA is severalfold higher in eukaryotes than in prokaryotes, the amount of tRNA (uridine-5)methyltransferase might become limiting in particular metabolic conditions. As has been shown by Roe and Tsen (1977), the T content in mammalian $tRNA^{Phe}$ can be correlated with efficiency of function in vitro in poly(U)-directed synthesis of poly(Phe).

In the course of our investigations we have studied the role of T54 in prokaryotic tRNA. The absence of T in *Escherichia coli* $tRNA_f^{Met}$ decreases the stability of the tertiary structure (Davanloo et al. 1979). The absence of T reduces the binding of the

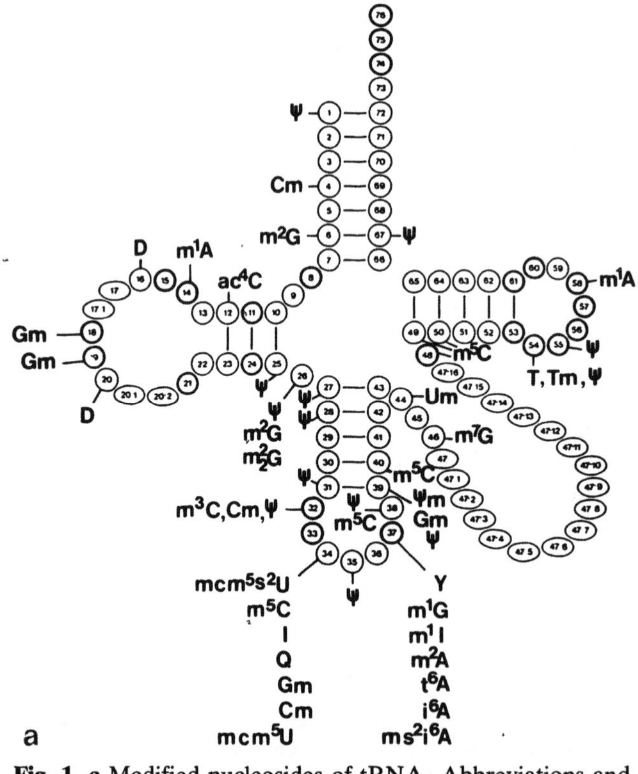

a

Fig. 1. a Modified nucleosides of tRNA. Abbreviations and positions in the two-dimensional cloverleaf according to Sprinzl et al. (1980). **b** Three-dimensional structure of tRNA with modified sequences at the ribosomal binding region and anticodons of $tRNA^{Asn}$, $tRNA^{Asp}$, $tRNA^{Tyr}$, and $tRNA^{His}$ comprising guanosine or queuosine

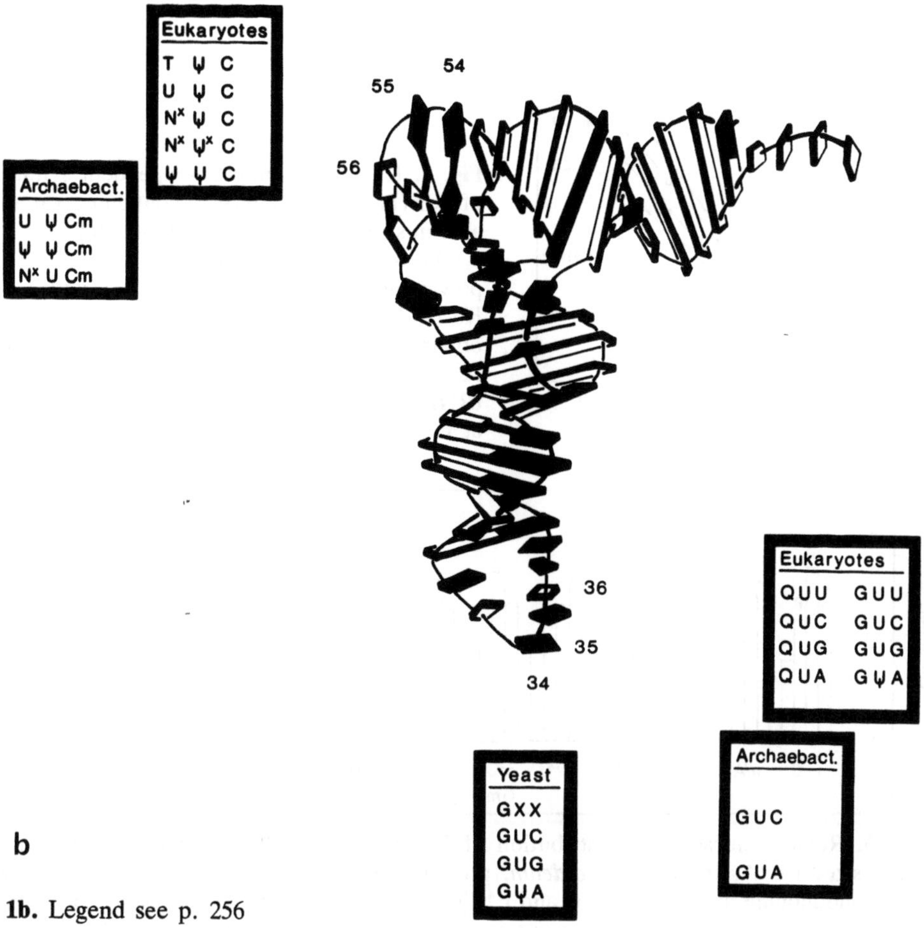

Fig. 1b. Legend see p. 256

elongator tRNA, Lys-$tRNA^{Lys}$, to the ribosomal A-site. No difference was found in poly(U)-dependent poly(Phe) synthesis between the T-comprising and T-lacking $tRNAs^{Phe}$ in peptide elongation using the conventional *E. coli* in vitro system (Kersten et al. 1981). However, in conditions adapted to those in vivo (Jelenc and Kurland 1979), the rate of poly(Phe) formation decreases progressively on successive replacement of *E. coli* $tRNA^{Phe}$ T54 by $tRNA^{Phe}$ U54 (Fig. 2). Correspondingly, at a constant concentration of ribosomes, the saturation level was found to be higher for the T-lacking tRNA. Furthermore, $tRNA_4^{Leu}$ (U54), comprising the anticodon XAA, misreads UUU in this system with significantly higher frequency than the T-comprising counterpart (Praisler et al. 1981). It is therefore possible that the presence of T in elongator tRNAs might be involved in the fine tuning of the translational machinery. In addition, the replacement of T54 by a U residue might disturb other regulatory mechanisms. The T-forming enzyme of *E. coli* – unlike other tRNA methyltransferases – is under stringent control (Ny et al. 1980).

To elucidate the role of T54 in eukaryotic tRNA function we have used *Dictyostelium discoideum* as a model system. This organism grows vegetatively as single amoebae. Upon starvation the cells start a well-defined developmental cycle, resulting in two

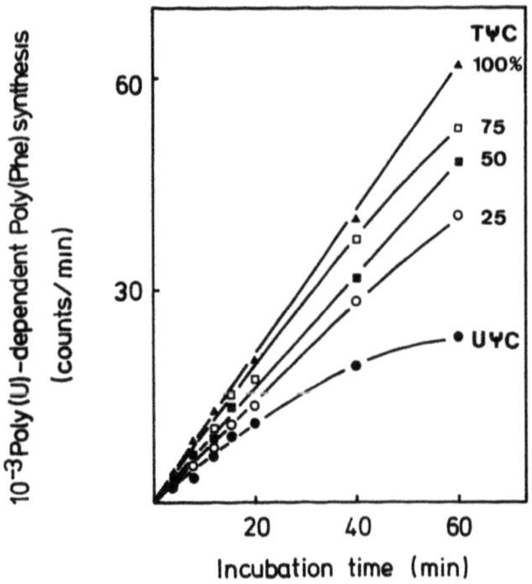

Fig. 2. Kinetics of poly(U)-dependent synthesis of poly(Phe) with $tRNAs^{Phe}$ containing variable amounts of TψC and UψC. Homopeptide synthesis was measured in the polyamine-dependent system (Jelenc and Kurland 1979). tRNAs, lacking T, were obtained from the mutant strain of *E. coli* Trm A^- and were mixed with *E. coli* wild-type tRNA to give the final composition as indicated at the corresponding curves

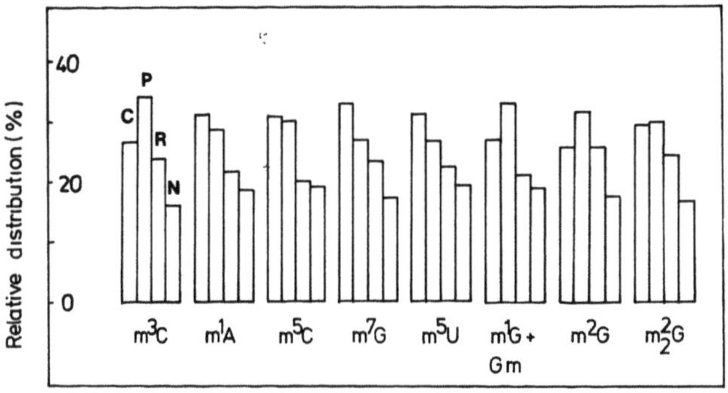

Fig. 3. Relative intracellular distribution of T and other methylated nucleosides in newly synthesized tRNAs from *D. discoideum,* preaggregation stage. The cells were labeled with [^{3}H]-1-methionine as methyl donor and [^{14}C]guanine as tRNA precursor, between 6 and 9 h after the onset of development (suspension culture). The cells were harvested and the cell extract fractionated (Cocucci and Sussman 1970). The tRNAs from the cytosol *(C),* polysomes *(P)* from monoribosomes *(R),* and nuclei *(N)* were isolated, purified, and digested to nucleosides. The methylated nucleosides in newly synthesized tRNA were analysed by high-pressure liquid chromatography (Gehrke and Kuo 1980) and the relative distribution was calculated for different cell fractions (Results from F. Pistel, Dissertation, Erlangen, 1982)

types, spores and stalk cells. tRNAs are newly synthesized during early development, but at successively lower rates as development proceeds. Isolation and analysis of tRNAs from different cell fractions show that fully processed tRNA (4 S) that is less methylated with respect to T accumulates in the nucleus during preaggregation (Fig. 3). Also, the methylation of G to m^7G and to m^2_2G is significantly reduced at this stage. Since the T-comprising species of the major-class tRNAs are utilized preferentially in protein synthesis during growth and development (Dingermann et al. 1980), we suggested that tRNAs of the major class that are completely methylated at U54 become rate limiting in the elongation of peptide chains. That T in this class of tRNAs enhances tRNA-EF-1-directed ribosomal A-site binding in eukaryotes is now well established (Ma et al. 1981). The question of whether the incomplete modification of U to T in the major class of tRNAs is involved in the regulation of the overall rate of translation, as suggested by Roe and Tsen (1977), or whether the nuclear methyl-deficient tRNAs function in regulatory mechanisms at the transcriptional level is currently being investigated in our laboratory.

Alterations of Modification of G34 to the Q base

During Development of D. discoideum

Alterations in tRNA modification during differentiation and neoplastic transformation concern especially the modified nucleoside Q present in $tRNA^{Asn}$, $tRNA^{Asp}$, $tRNA^{His}$, and $tRNA^{Tyr}$ (Okada et al. 1978; Shindo-Okada et al. 1981; Jacobson et al. 1981). tRNA species having G in place of Q34 can be detected by the exchange of G34 with radioactively labeled G, catalyzed by the transglycosylase from *E. coli* (Okada et al. 1978). We have used this reaction to evaluate variations in the amount of G34 in the corresponding tRNAs throughout the developmental cycle of *D. discoideum.* Vegetatively growing amoebae contain considerable amounts of guanylatable tRNAs (mainly tRNAs specific for asparagine and aspartic acid). During aggregation and the pseudoplasmodial stage the amount of tRNAs that are substrates for the transglycosylase reaction increases. However, spores contain only very small amounts of guanylatable tRNA (Fig. 4), suggesting that the amount of Q-containing species increases.

Since development can be induced only by amino acid starvation and unacylated tRNAs might be used as signals in control mechanisms of translation or gene expression (Bergmann and Lodish 1979; Barnes 1978), we have analyzed the level of aminoacylation for several tRNA species during the preaggregation stage of *D. discoideum.* As early as 2 min after the onset of development the aminoacylation of $tRNA^{Asn}$ specifically was reduced to about 30%. One of the two major $tRNA^{Asn}$ isoacceptors, the G34-containing species, was found to be completely uncharged (Dingermann et al. 1981).

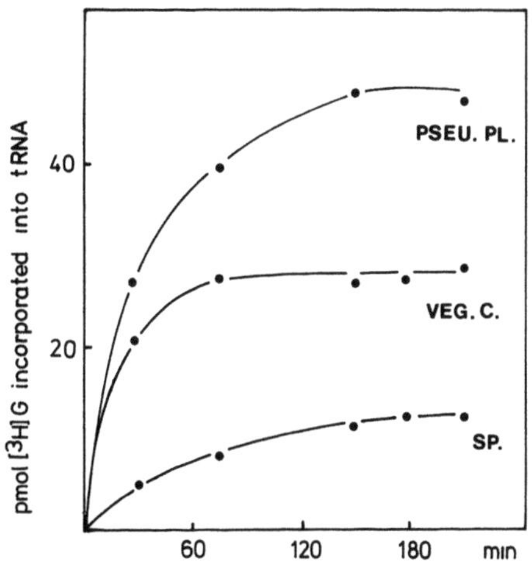

Fig. 4. Alterations in G34 modification of tRNAs during the life cycle of *D. discoideum:* vegetative cells *(VEG. C.)*, pseudoplasmodium *(PSEU. PL.)* and spores *(SP.)*. The purified *E. coli* transglycosylase from Dr. Nishimura was used in these experiments to detect specifically G34 in corresponding tRNAs; pmol [^{3}H]guanine incorporation was referred to the specific activity of the enzyme, set at 110.7 pmol/A_{260} yeast tRNA as substrate. (Okada et al. 1978)

In Heritable Melanomas of the Topminnow Xiphophorus

Another genetically well characterized system suitable for investigation of alterations in the modification of G34 to Q34 in tRNA in relation to differentiation and neoplastic transformation is the pigment system of the skin of the topminnow *Xiphophorus*. The pigment system consists of pterinophores, purinophores, and melanophores, derived from the neural crest. Offsprings of hybrids of two genotypes, *Xiphophorus helleri* and *Xiphophorus maculatus,* can develop heritable melanomas, due to a specific gene, *Tu,* localized at the X chromosome. In 25% of the offspring the melanomas are benign, because the transformed TI melanoblasts differentiate into nondividing T melanophores. In another 25% the melanomas are malignant; the T melanocytes do not differentiate but keep on dividing. These fishes were found to lack a regulatory gene, R_{Diff}, the product of which is necessary for final differentiation (for details see Anders et al. 1980 and references therein). Analyses of tRNAs from skin, liver, and benign and malignant melanomas showed an increase in the amount of guanylatable species in the tRNA from malignant melanomas. Surprisingly, tRNA from the skin of healthy offspring was also found to have a relatively high content of G34 (G. Dess, A. Anders, S. Nishimura, and H. Kersten, unpublished results). The skin of *Xiphophorus* contains pteridines within the pterinophores (Rempters et al. 1981). As shown by Jacobson et al. (1981), pteridines interfere with the formation of Q in eukaryotes. Whether the high content of pteridines in the skin of *Xiphophorus* promotes the formation of malignant melanomas and the mechanism by which Q base is involved in differentiation and/or neoplastic transformation is under current investigation.

In Plasmacytomas of Balb Mice

In higher organisms, the extent to which G34 is modified to Q in specific tRNAs seems to depend on the physiological conditions of cells and tissues and, as shown for mice (Reyniers et al. 1981), on the nutritional environment.

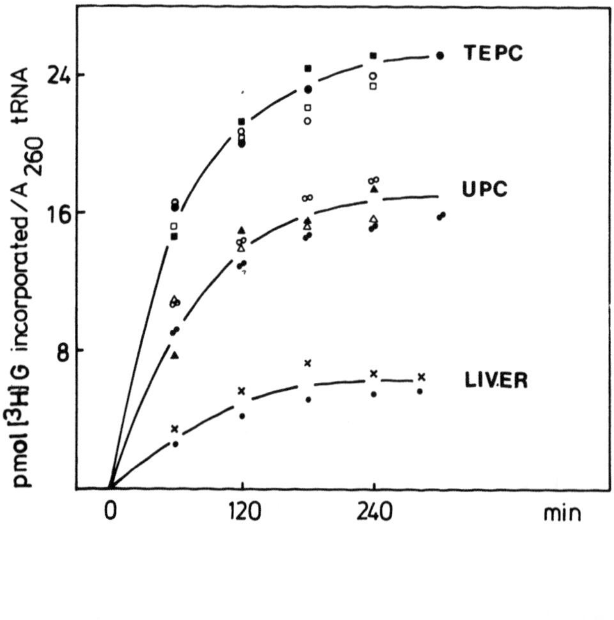

Fig. 5. Differences in G34 modification of tRNAs of two different plasmacytomas of Balb mice: *TEPC,* fast growth; *UPC,* slow growth. A partially purified *E. coli* transglycosylase was used in these experiments. (Results from W. Mühlhofer, Dissertation, Erlangen, 1982)

The occurrence of specific tRNAs with G34 in place of Q is especially high in tumor tissues, but does not seem to be correlated to the growth rate of the tumor (Shindo-Okada et al. 1981). We have isolated tRNAs from the liver and from two solid plasmacytomas of Balb mice, differing in growth rate about twofold. The guanine acceptance was determined with partly purified transglycosylase preparation from *E. coli*. The results of these experiments (Fig. 5) show a positive correlation between the growth rates of the plasmacytomas and the guanine acceptance of the corresponding tumor tRNAs. Another correlation was observed in Ehrlich ascites tumor cells of NMRI mice, between 4 and 8 days after inoculation. In repeated experiments, the tRNAs from fast-growing Ehrlich ascites cells (4 days after inoculation) showed higher guanine acceptance than the tRNAs obtained from the tumor cells 8 days after inoculation when the growth of the tumor had almost ceased. It is possible that the age or the density of the tumor cells, rather than the proliferative stage, is correlated to these changes of tRNA modification.

Concluding Remarks

From the results presented here and those of our colleagues working in this field, some conclusions can be drawn and suggestions made. Alterations in tRNA modification are characteristic in cells and tissues of various organisms – ranging from bacteria to mammals – that undergo metabolic changes during growth, development, or differentiation. Several lines of experimental evidence now support Borek's assertion that the modified nucleosides of tRNA play an important role in these processes (Borek 1977 and references therein).

The enhanced binding to the ribosomal A-site caused by the presence of T in the major class of tRNAs explains well their preferential utilisation in protein synthesis. The synthesis and accumulation of T54-lacking tRNAs in the nucleus of *D. discoideum* in early developmental stages suggests that they play a crucial role in the expression of tRNA genes at this stage. This suggestion is based on the results of Söll and co-workers (see this volume pp. 1–14) who studied the promotor regions of tRNA genes in eukaryotes. They provide experimental evidence that the promotor regions of tRNA genes are localized within the structural gene and involve DNA sequences complementary to conserved tRNA sequences in the D-loop and the TψC-loop. Alterations in the modification of the TψC sequence might change the expression of tRNA genes during developmental processes, a quantitative mechanism to adapt tRNA anticodons to particular codons in developmental mRNA.

Other possible mechanisms for the adaptation of tRNA anticodons to mRNA codons in differentiation and developmental processes might involve:

1. Selective aminoacylation of tRNA isoacceptors, as shown here for the transient, selective aminoacylation of $tRNA_2^{Asn}$ (Q34) in *D. discoideum* after the onset of development.
2. Alterations of the modification in the anticodon region of specific tRNAs, e.g., the conversion of G34 to Q34. Here we show that this tRNA modification plays an important role during the final steps of differentiation to stalk cells and spores in the slime mold. Furthermore, this modification is probably involved in the differentiation of the melanophoric system of the topminnow *Xiphophorus*.

Finally, I would like to emphasize that knowledge of the genetics of *Xiphophorus* will be of great help in elucidating why these adaptation and regulatory mechanisms are disturbed in neoplastic transformed cells.

Summary

To evaluate the role of the modified nucleosides in tRNA function, especially their involvement in regulatory mechanisms of development, differentiation, or neoplastic transformation we use the following organisms: eubacteria, the slime mold *D. discoideum,* the topminnow *Xiphophorus,* and mice.

Ribosylthymine, a common modified nucleoside at position 54 in tRNAs of prokaryotes and the major class of eukaryotic elongator tRNAs, is involved in the binding to the ribosomal A-site and is important for the proper functioning of tRNA during translation. Alterations in the extent of this modification occur early in the development of *D. discoideum.* The fully methylated species are found on polysomes, actively synthesizing protein. The partially methylated tRNAs accumulate in the nuclei, and might be involved in regulatory mechanisms at the transcriptional level.

The Q base, a modified deazaguanine derivative, is present at position 34, the first position of the anticodon of $tRNA^{Asn}$, $tRNA^{Asp}$, $tRNA^{Tyr}$, and $tRNA^{His}$. Alterations in the extent of this modification occur in corresponding tRNAs during the first minutes after the onset of development in *D. discoideum* and before final differentiation into spores, indicating that Q is important for developmental processes. Changes in the modification of G34 to Q34 in specific tRNAs of the melanophoric system of the topminnow *Xiphophorus* further support the view that Q is necessary in differentiation.

In plasmacytomas and in Ehrlich ascites tumor cells of mice, the amount of unmodified G34 in corresponding tRNAs is correlated to the growth rate, density, or age of the tumor cells.

Abbreviations

U, uridine; ψ, pseudouridine; *C,* cytidine; N^+, unidentified uridine derivative; *G,* guanidine; *Q,* queuosine (7-[(4,5-cis-dihydroxy-2-cyclopenten-1-ylamino)methyl]-7-deazaguanidine); *T* or m^5U, ribosylthymine. The abbreviations of all other methylated or modified nucleosides are given in the reference cited in the legend of Fig. 1a. $tRNA_f^{Met}$, formylmethionine tRNA; *Poly(Phe),* polyphenylalaline; *Poly(U),* polyuridylic acid; *Transglycosylase,* tRNA transglycosylase (E.C. 2.4.2.-); A_{260}*unit,* amount of material absorbing at 260 nm that gives an A_{260} of 1 when soluted in 1 ml (d = 1 cm).

References

Anders F, Diehl H, Scholl E (1980) Differentiation of normal melanophores and neoplastically transformed melanophores in the skin of fishes of genus Xiphophorus. Lennean Soc Symp Ser 9: 211–218

Barnes WM (1978) DNA sequence from the histidine operon control region: Seven histidine codons in a row. Proc Natl Acad Sci USA 75: 4281–4285

Bergmann JE, Lodish HF (1979) A kinetic model of protein synthesis. J Biol Chem 254: 11927–11937
Borek E (1977) Modification of nucleic acids in relation to differentiation. Trends Biochem Sci 2: 3–6
Cocucci SM, Sussman M (1970) RNA in cytoplasmic and nuclear fractions of cellular slime mold amebas. J Cell Biol 45: 399–407
Davanloo P, Sprinzl M, Watanabe K, Albani M, Kersten H (1979) Role of ribothymidine in the thermal stability of transfer RNA as monitored by proton magnetic resonance. Nucleic Acids Res 6: 1571–1581
Dingermann T, Pistel F, Kersten H (1980) Functional role of ribosylthymine in transfer RNA. Eur J Biochem 104: 33–40
Dingermann T, Ogilvie A, Pistel F, Mühlhofer W, Kersten H (1981) Reduced aminoacylation of asparagine-transfer RNA early in the developmental cycle of Dictyostelium discoideum. Hoppe Seylers Z Physiol Chem 362: 763–773
Gehrke CW, Kuo KC (1980) Chromatography of nucleosides. J Chromatogr 188: 129–147
Jacobson KB, Farkas WR, Katze JR (1981) Presence of queuine in drosophila melanogaster: correlation of free pool with queuosine content of tRNA and effect of mutations in pteridine metabolism. Nucleic Acid Res 9: 2351–2366
Jelenc PC, Kurland CG (1979) Nucleoside triphosphate regeneration decreases the frequency of translation errors. Proc Natl Acad Sci USA 76: 3174–3178
Kersten H (1981) Transfer RNA methylation, overview. In: Usdin E, Borchardt R, Creveling B (eds) Transmethylation. Elsevier North Holland, New York Oxford Shannon
Kersten H, Albani M, Männlein E, Praisler R, Wurmbach P, Nierhaus KH (1981) On the role of ribosylthymine and prokaryotic tRNA function. Eur J Biochem 114: 451–456
Ma DP, Merrick WC, Roe BA (1981) The ribothymidine content of mammalian elongator tRNAs modulates ternary complex ribosomal A site binding. In: Usdin E, Borchardt R, Creveling B (eds) Transmethylation. Elsevier North Holland, New York Oxford Shannon
Nishimura S (1979) Modified nucleosides and isoaccepting tRNA. In: Schimmel PR, Söll D, Abelson JN (eds) Transfer RNA: structure properties and recognition. Cold Spring Harbor Laboratory, Cold Spring Harbor, pp 59–79
Nishimura S, Kuchino Y (1979) Transfer RNA and cancer. Gan 24: 245–262
Ny T, Thomale J, Hjalmarsson K, Nass G, Björk GR (1980) Non-coordinate Escherichia coli. Biochim Biophys Acta 607: 277–284
Okada N, Shindo-Okada N, Sato S, Itoh YH, Oda Kl, Nishimura S (1978) Detection of unique tRNA species in tumor tissues by Escherichia coli guanine insertion enzyme. Proc Natl Acad Sci USA 75: 4247–4251
Praisler R, Männlein E, Richter H, Ott G, Kersten H (1981) Influence of modified nucleosides in tRNA on the efficiency of translation. Regard sur la Biochimie 3: 55 Tome 2.11
Rempeters G, Henze M, Anders F (1981) Carotenoids and pteridines in the skin of interspecific hybrids of Xiphophorus. Comp Biochem Physiol [B] 64: 91–98
Reyniers JP, Pleasants JR, Wostmann BS, Katze JR, Farkas WR (1981) Administration of exogenous queuine is essential for the biosynthesis of the queuosine-containing transfer RNAs in the mouse. J Biol Chem 256: 11591–11594
Roe BA, Tsen HY (1977) Role of ribothymidine in mammalian $tRNA^{Phe}$. Proc Natl Acad Sci USA 74: 3696–3700
Shindo-Okada N, Terada M, Nishimura S (1981) Changes in amount of hypomodified tRNA having guanine in place of queuine during erythroid differentiation of murine erythroleukemia cells. Eur J Biochem 115: 423–428

Effects of Cortisol on tRNA Methylase Activities in Rat Mammary Carcinoma

A. M. Leyman, P. Goddeeris, J. M. Lauwerijns, and W. De Loecker*

Afdelingen Biochemie en Histopathologie, Katholieke Universiteit Leuven, Campus Gasthuisberg, Herestraat, 3000 Leuven, Belgium

Introduction

Transfer RNA methyltransferases, which by methylating tRNA at a macromolecular level contribute to species and organ specificity, have been found to show greater activity in tumor tissue than in the corresponding normal adult tissue (Borek and Kerr 1972). It is possible that changes in the cellular content of tRNA methylases play a significant role in the development and growth of tumors. The differences in the degree of modifications of tRNA may be due to intrinsic differences in the specificity of tumor tRNA methylases, or may be the result of more simple factors inhibiting or stimulating the enzyme systems (Borek and Kerr 1972; Kaye and Leboy 1968; Pegg 1971).

When assaying the enzymes in various combinations over a wide range of concentrations of cations, e.g., ammonium and magnesium, the extent, rate, and pattern of methylation of *Escherichia coli* tRNA by different neoplastic and non-neoplastic sources depend greatly on ionic environment (Kaye and Leboy 1968; Leboy 1970, 1971; Pegg 1971). Apart from the ionic composition of the assay medium, the purification grade of the enzyme extracted from the crude tissue preparation also affects the methylation of bacterial tRNA under the influence of known natural inhibitors such as nicotinamide, glycine, and homocysteine. These natural inhibiting systems prove important in liver, pancreas, and kidney, organs containing significant levels of *S*-adenosylmethionine-synthesizing enzymes (Lombardini and Tallalay 1971). In tissues where these activities are low, for example brain and uterus, the tRNA appears to be controlled by other factors. In target organs as well as in tumor tissue tRNA methylation can be controlled by hormone action (Luck and Hamilton 1975; Sharma and Borek 1970; Munns et al. 1975; Turkington 1969). As these hormonal effects are sensitive to actinomycin D and cycloheximide, de novo enzyme synthesis has been suspected (Sheid et al. 1970; Turkington 1969). In order to approach the mechanism of hormone action on tumor tRNA methylases, we studied the effects of cortisol in experimental mammary carcinoma in rats.

* The authors are indebted to the Belgian National Foundation for Medical Research (F.G.W.O.) for a grant to the laboratory

Recent Results in Cancer Research. Vol. 84

Materials and Methods

Experimental mammary carcinomas were induced in several series of female, locally inbred, Sprague-Dawley rats at 50 days of age by two intragastric injections of 10 mg 7,12-dimethylbenz(a)anthracene (DMBA; Fluka, Buchs, Switzerland) dissolved in 0.5 ml sesame oil, the second injection 24 h after the first (Huggins et al. 1959). After 3–4 months, when tumors of 1–3 cm in diameter were present, the animals were adrenalectomized. For another 7 days they continued to be fed on an ad libitum Purina Chow diet with free access to pure drinking water and 0.9% NaCl solution. Subsequently a series of animals was treated with a daily intramuscular injection of 10 mg cortisol acetate (Cortril; Pfizer, New York) for 3 consecutive days. On the morning of the 4th day, the controls and treated adrenalectomized animals were killed and the mammary tumors removed and examined by light microscopy after fixation in Bouin-Hollande fluid and staining with routine hematoxylin-eosin.

The tumor tissue was homogenized in 2 vol 0.20 *M* sucrose/0.001 *M* dithiothreitol/0.01 *M* Tris-HCl buffer, pH 7.5. The homogenate was first centrifuged at 30000 *g* in a Sorvall RC-2 centrifuge (Dupont Co., Newtown, Connecticut), for 20 min at 4° C. The supernatant was recentrifuged at 105000 *g* for 90 min at 4° C (International Ultracentrifuge B-60-I.E.C., Needham Heights, Massachusetts). The obtained supernatant was further purified by fractionation and dialysis. The supernatant was adjusted to 30% saturation with $(NH_4)_2SO_4$ and centrifuged at 15000 *g* for 15 min at 4° C, then further saturated with $(NH_4)_2SO_4$ to 48%. The resulting precipitate after recentrifugation was dissolved in 0.2 vol 4 m*M* dithiothreitol/20% glycerol/0.01 *M* Tris-HCl buffer, pH 8.15. This solution was dialyzed against 2 liters 0.5 m*M* EDTA/10 m*M* 2-mercaptoethanol/0.05 *M* Tris-HCl buffer, pH 8.15, first for 2 h and further overnight against another 2 liters fresh buffer.

To measure total enzyme activity, fractions of 2 ml of this purified enzyme preparation were incubated for 1 h at 37° C with 800 μmol ammonium acetate, 10 μmol freshly prepared and neutralized reduced glutathione, 1 mg *E. coli* B tRNA (General Biochemical Corp. Chagrin Falls, Ohio), and 0.4 μCi neutralized *S*-adenosyl-L[methyl-^{14}C]methionine, specific radioactivity 55 mCi/mmol (Radiochemical Centre, Amersham) (Sheid et al. 1970). To stop the reaction 0.6 ml 6 *M* HCl and 10 ml 20% trichloroacetic acid were added. After centrifugation, the precipitate was successively washed with 85%, 75%, and 50% (v/v) ethanol in water and finally with ethanol/diethylether (3 : 1, v/v). The washed precipitate was dissolved in 3 ml Soluene-350 (Lumac Systems AG, Basel) and the radioactivity incorporated into 1 mg tRNA was counted in a liquid scintillation spectrometer (Rackbeta LSC; Wallac OY, Turku) and converted to nmol/mg tRNA/mg protein of the dialyzed enzyme extract (Leyman and De Loecker 1980).

Tissue protein concentrations were determined by the Folin phenol method (Lowry et al. 1951).

In an attempt to separate the different classes of tRNA methylases, 3-ml fractions of tumor enzyme preparation were introduced on a DEAE-Sephadex A50 column (K_{45} column, 30 cm × 1.5 cm; Pharmacia, Uppsala) equilibrated with EDTA/mercaptoethanol/Tris-HCl buffer pH 8.15 containing 0.10 *M* NaCl. The methylases were eluted in a three-step procedure, by 100 ml 0.10 *M* NaCl/Tris-HCl buffer followed by 100 ml buffer containing 0.14 *M* NaCl and finally by 280 ml of buffer containing a linear gradient of 0.14–0.22 *M* NaCl. Fractions of 7 ml were collected at an elution rate of 20 ml/h. Samples of 1 ml from the various fractions were incubated with 1 mg *E. coli* B tRNA. Optical densities at $A_{280\,nm}$ were determined for each fraction (spectrophotometer Beckman DB-GT, Beckman Instruments International SA, Geneva) (Glick and Leboy 1977).

To analyze the base composition, 1 mg *E. coli* tRNA was incubated with 2 ml of the different enzyme extracts containing the [^{14}C]CH_3-labeled tracer. After incubation for 1 h, tRNA precipitated with 67% ethanol containing 0.5 *M* NaCl was kept for at least 4 h at −15° C before being centrifuged for 10 min at 10000 *g*. The precipitate was resuspended in 3 ml 2 *M* NaCl, extracted for 5 min at room temperature, and recentrifuged at 10000 *g*. The tRNA present in the supernatant was reprecipitated by 2 vol cold 95% ethanol in water (Kaye and Leboy 1968). These tRNA samples, kept overnight at −15° C, were isolated after recentrifugation and hydrolyzed with 88% (v/v) formic acid at 180° C for 2 h in a sealed vial. After evaporation of the solvent in a nitrogen stream, the resulting purine and pyrimidine bases were dissolved in 60 μl 0.1 *M* HCl and separated by ascending two-dimensional thin-layer chromatography (TLC) (Munns et al. 1975).

Fractions of 30 μl were spotted on MN-300 cellulose plates (0.1 mm thick, 20 × 20 cm) (Polygram cel 300; Mackerey Nagel, Düren) and allowed to run in a first dimension in butan-1-ol/water (84 : 16, v/v) with ammonium as gas phase and in a second dimension in propan-2-ol/conc. HCl/water (170 : 44 : 36, v/v). Adequate separation was obtained by drying the cellulose plates after each run and repeating the chromatography a second time in the same direction. UV light allowed the different methylated compounds to be distinguished and to be compared with simultaneously run standards and methylated bases, uracil, cytosine, guanine, hypoxanthine, adenine, 3-CH_3-uracil, 5-CH_3-uracil, 6-CH_3-uracil, N^6-CH_3-adenine (Serva, Heidelberg), 3-CH_3-cytosine, 5-CH_3-cytosine, N^2,N^2-diCH_3-guanine, N^6,N^6-diCH_3-adenine (P. L. Biochemicals Inc., Milwaukee, Wisconsin), 1-CH_3-guanine, 7-CH_3-guanine, N^2-CH_3-guanine, 1-CH_3-hypoxanthine, and 1-CH_3-adenine (Sigma) (Fig. 1).

Autoradiography on X-ray films (Kodak X-omat R-films, 20 cm × 25 cm) of the hydrolyzed tRNAs allowed quantitative estimation of the [^{14}C]CH_3 groups present in each of the nucleic acid bases which were scraped from the cellulose plate and counted in a liquid scintillation spectrometer after the addition of 5 ml Aqualuma (Lumac Systems) (Leyman and De Loecker 1980).

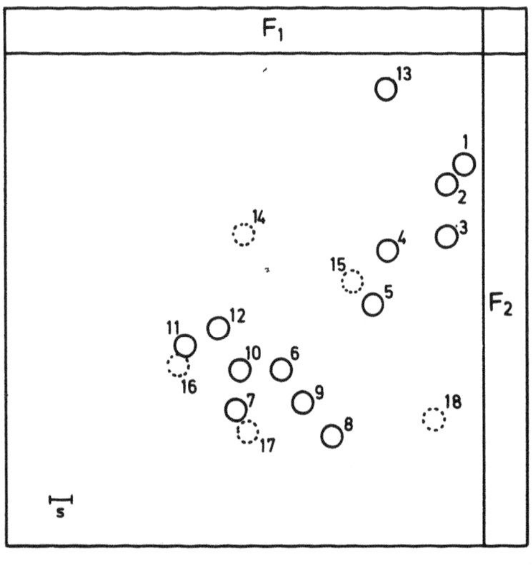

Fig. 1. TLC of methylated standard purine and pyrimidine bases, analysed as described in the text. *1,* 5-CH_3-uracil; *2,* 6-CH_3-uracil; *3,* 3-CH_3-uracil; *4,* 5-CH_3-cytosine; *5,* 3-CH_3-cytosine; *6,* 1-CH_3-guanine; *7,* 7-CH_3-guanine; *8,* N^2-CH_3-guanine; *9,* N^2,N^2-diCH_3-guanine; *10,* 1-CH_3-hypoxanthine; *11,* 1-CH_3-adenine; *12,* N^6-CH_3-adenine; *13,* N^6,N^6-diCH_3-adenine; *14,* adenine; *15,* cytosine; *16,* guanine; *17,* hypoxanthine; *18,* uracil

Results

All the glandular tumors examined presented a lobular or nodular architecture. The degree of differentiation of the various tumor structures varied only slightly in function of the cell density (Fig. 2), with some areas more specifically glandular in differentiation (Fig. 3) while others presented a more papillary growth (Fig. 4). The tumor cells had a rather quiet cytological aspect without any obvious nuclear

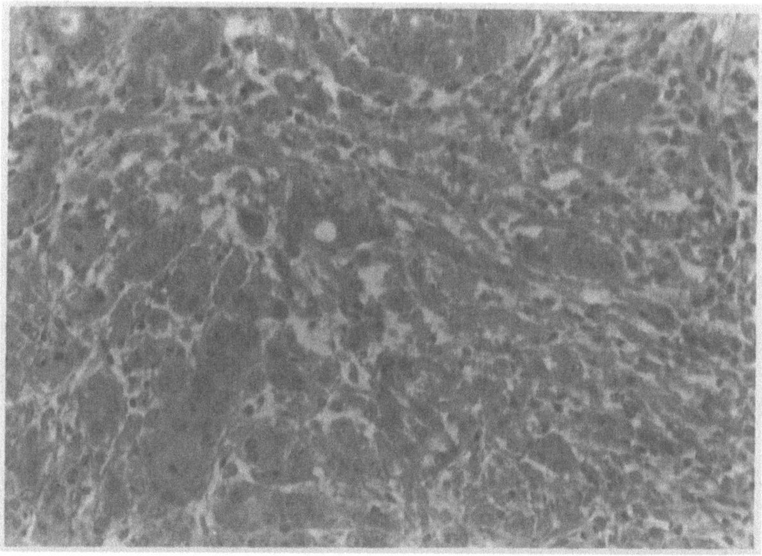

Fig. 2. DMBA-induced mammary carcinoma in female Sprague-Dawley rats: massive tumor with poorly differentiated areas. H & E, × 400

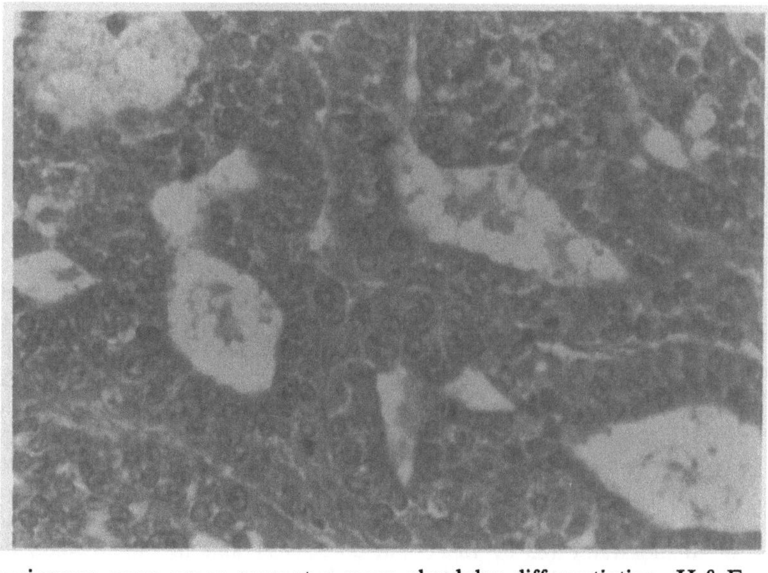

Fig. 3. Mammary carcinoma: some areas present a more glandular differentiation. H & E, × 640

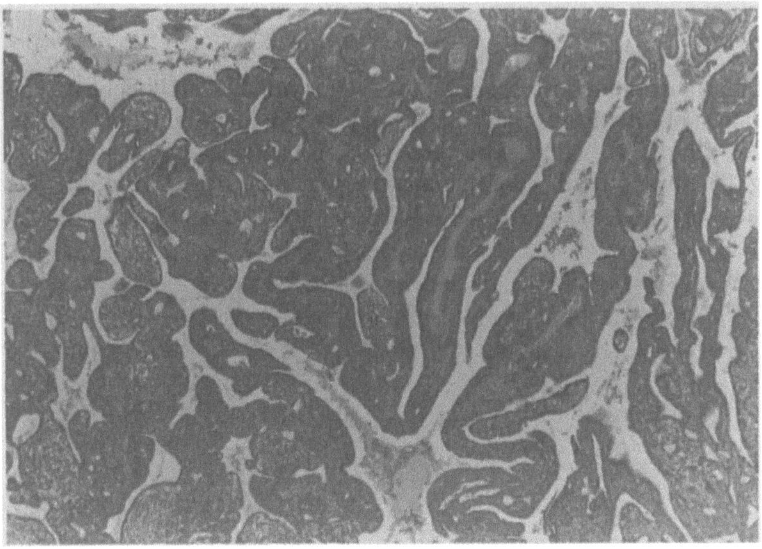

Fig. 4. Mammary carcinoma: other areas show papillary growth. H & E, × 64

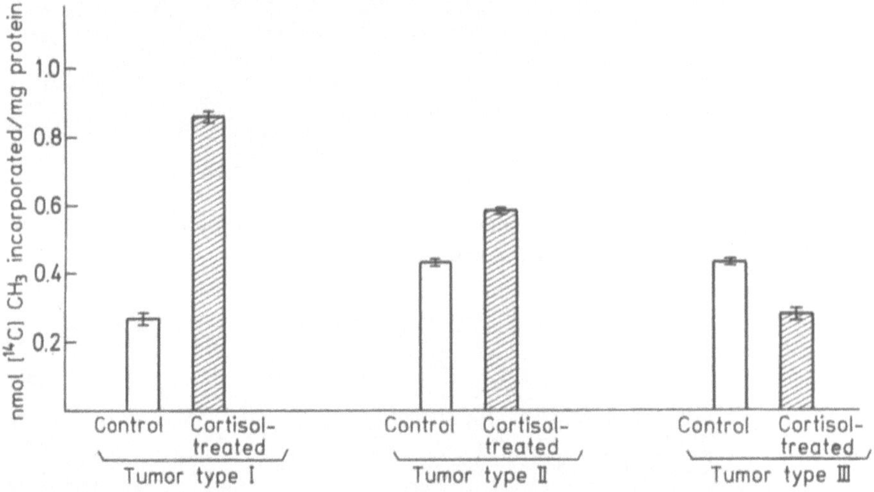

Fig. 5. Effect of cortisol treatment on tRNA methylase activity in different types of mammary carcinomas. Tumors of adrenalectomized control rats and those treated with 10 mg cortisol are homogenized in 2 vol 0.25 *M* sucrose/Tris-HCl buffer, pH 7.5. After centrifugation at 105000 *g* for 90 min the supernatant is purified by ammonium sulphate fractionation, first at a 30% saturation level and subsequently at a 48% saturation level. The resulting precipitate is dissolved in 0.2 vol 4 m*M* dithiothreitol/20% glycerol/0.05 *M* Tris-HCl buffer, pH 8.15. This solution is dialyzed against 2 liters 0.5 m*M* EDTA/10 m*M* 2-mercaptoethanol/0.01 *M* Tris-HCl buffer, pH 8.15, for 2 h and again overnight against 2 liters fresh buffer. This purified enzyme preparation (2 ml) is incubated with 800 μmol ammonium acetate, 10 μmol reduced glutathione, 1 mg *E. coli* B tRNA and 0.4 μCi neutralized *S*-adenosyl-L-[methyl ^{14}C] methionine. After 1 h at 38° C, 0.5 ml 3 *M* hydroxylamine (pH 7.2) is added and the incubation resumed for 10 min. The reaction is stopped by addition of 0.6 ml 6 *M* HCl and 10 ml 20% TCA. After successive washes in ethanol/water (85%, 75%, and 50%, v/v) and in ethanol/diethylether (3 : 1, v/v) the precipitate is dissolved in 3 ml Soluene-350 and after addition of 10 ml Lipoluma, counted in the liquid scintillation spectrometer. Each value represents the mean ± SEM of eight experiments

anomalies, although multiple mitoses were present. The nuclei were oval or rounded with a fine chromatine structure, mostly with one or two small nucleoli. The cytoplasm was always slightly eosinophilic and the nucleocytoplasmic index rather high.

Three groups of tumors were distinguished by macroscopic examination: Type I, hard and dense tumors without any obvious signs of necrosis (Fig. 2); Type II, tumors weaker in consistency and already showing signs of cellular necrosis and cystic degeneration; and Type III, lactating tumors containing white secretions without necrotic zones (Figs. 3, 4). Depending on still unknown factors, all the animals of one series, induced with DMBA under the same conditions, uniformly developed one of these three macroscopically distinguishable tumor types.

Histological analysis did not detect any significant differences in the control tumors from adrenalectomized rats before and after cortisol treatment. After cortisol treatment the total protein concentration (mg protein/g tissue) was decreased by 30% in tumor type I, by 26% in type II, and by 27% in type III.

Treatment of adrenalectomized tumor-bearing rats with 10 mg cortisol for 3 consecutive days resulted in different effects according to the tumor type described. The total tRNA methyltransferase activity was increased significantly in types I and II, by 200% ($P < 0.001$) and 37% ($P < 0.001$) respectively, while the enzyme activities of tumor extracts from type III were decreased by 35% ($P < 0.001$) compared to the adrenalectomized controls (Fig. 5).

The chromatographic profiles of the methyltransferases from tumor types I and II were characterized by seven distinct peaks, some of which seem to have disappeared or considerably decreased in tumor type III. In particular, the controls of tumor type II presented a very low activity profile. Treatment of tumor type I with cortisol reduced the first two fractions, while fractions 3, 5, and 7 were increased (Fig. 6). After

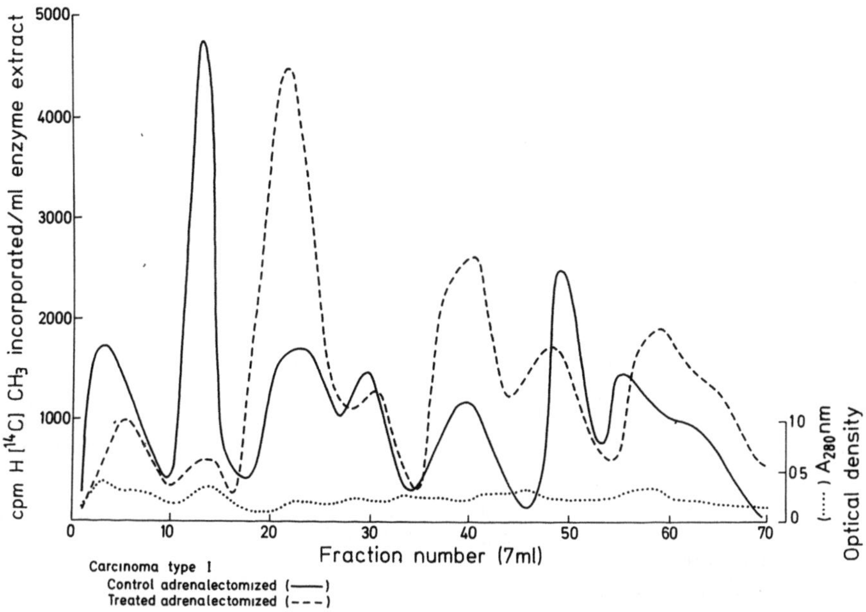

Fig. 6. tRNA methyltransferase activities of mammary carcinoma type I after chromatography on DEAE-Sephadex A50. Fractionated and dialyzed tumor enzyme extracts (3 ml) were eluted as described in the text. Each curve is the result of eight experiments

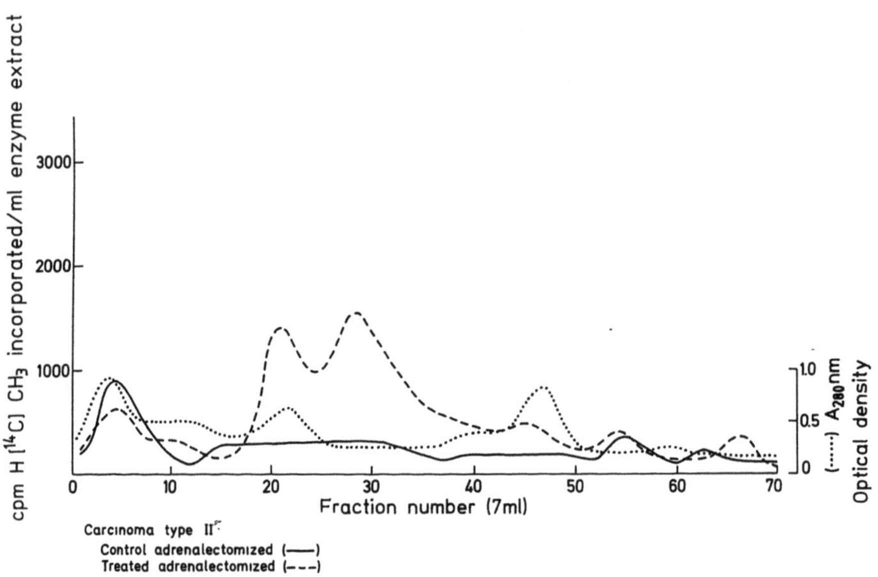

Fig. 7. tRNA methyltransferase activities of mammary carcinoma type II after chromatography on DEAE-Sephadex-A50. Fractionated and dialyzed enzyme extracts (3 ml) from treated and untreated animals are placed on a DEAE-Sephadex A50 column. The elution is performed as described for Fig. 5. Each curve is the result of eight experiments

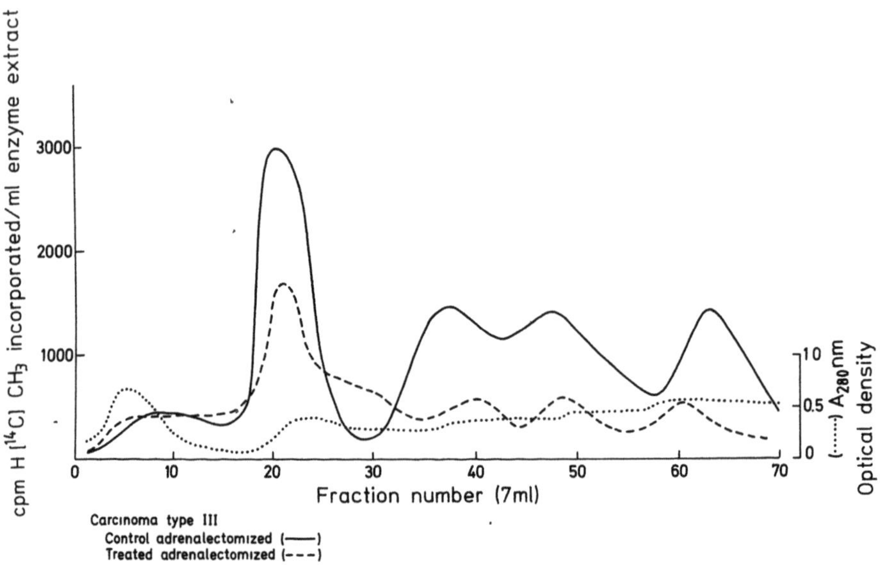

Fig. 8. tRNA methyltransferase activities of mammary carcinoma type III. Fractionated and dialyzed enzyme extracts (3 ml) from treated and untreated animals are placed on a DEAE-Sephadex A50 column. The elution is carried out as described for Fig. 5

Table 1. Distribution of the different methylated bases in hydrolyzed tRNA of DMBA-induced mammary carcinomas in rats after cortisol treatment

Methylated bases	Tumor type I		Tumor type II		Tumor type III	
	Controls (%)	Cortisol-treated (%)	Controls (%)	Cortisol-treated (%)	Controls (%)	Cortisol-treated (%)
5-CH_3-cytosine	13	60	2	4	14	5
1-CH_3-adenine, N^6-CH_3-adenine	12	30	20	28	14	9
N^6N^6-diCH_3-adenine	10	37	53	62	51	25
1-CH_3-guanine	10	34	–	–	2	2
7-CH_3-guanine	9	26	1	1	4	2
N^2-CH_3-guanine	14	20	12	7	5	5
N^2N^2-diCH_3-guanine	22	39	10	25	9	5
5-CH_3-uracil	10	60	2	3	1	1
Total enzyme activity	100	306	100	130	100	54

Methylated tRNA was analysed as described in the text

treatment with cortisol the methyltransferases present in fractions 3 and 4 of tumor type II were increased (Fig. 7), while treatment of tumor type III essentially reduced all the prominent peaks (Fig. 8).

Separation of the methylated bases obtained from tRNA molecules after hydrolysis indicated that the base-specific methyltransferase activities were not uniformly affected by cortisol treatment (Table 1).

In tumor type I the distribution of the methylated bases did not show any tumor-specific base. After treatment with 10 mg cortisol, the activities of all the base-specific enzymes seemed to increase, with a most striking stimulation of 5-CH_3-cytidine and 5-CH_3-uracil methyltransferases. Tumor type II presented high concentrations of CH_3-adenine methyltransferases, which were stimulated with cortisol treatment together with the N^2,N^2-diCH_3-guanine methyltransferases. Tumor type III again contained CH_3-adenines and N^2,N^2-diCH_3-guanine as the most important methylated components. These fractions were significantly decreased after cortisol treatment. The individual contribution of the various methylated adenines is difficult to determine in absolute values, due to structural artifacts which occur during acid hydrolysis and even give rise to the formation of N^6,N^6-diCH_3 adenine. These quantitative recovery data corresponded to the values of total enzyme activities (Fig. 5). After separation on DEAE-Sephadex A 50, the enzymes responsible for methylating cytosine, adenine, guanine, and uracil were recovered over a range of elution fractions; 0–12, 13–40, 25–55, and 45–63 respectively.

Discussion

Differentiation between the three types of carcinoma seems indicated in view of the different metabolic responses of the tumors. Although it is difficult to prove histologically, tumor type I seems the most proliferative, while in tumor type II signs of necrosis, probably induced by a more glandular differentiation, may affect the metabolic pattern. Tumor type III belongs to a group with specific lactation characteristics obviously controlled by interfering hormonal effects (Griswold et al. 1966; Middleton 1965; Teller et al. 1966). Each of these tumors, however, reacts to cortisol treatment, which affects the tRNA methyltransferases in different ways. Other contributing hormonal interactions by estrogens, progestogens, and prolactin may well be responsible for the final cortisol effect, resulting in the observed modifications of the methyltransferase activities. As cortisol treatment essentially inhibits protein synthesis and stimulates catabolism, a stimulatory effect on the methylases seems to suggest that increased methylation may well contribute to an inhibition of tumor growth (De Loecker and Stas 1973), while in different circumstances a similar effect could be ascribed to reduced methyltransferase levels.

Although these methylating reactions are supposed to be exclusive for one or several amino-acid-specific tRNA molecules, hormonal treatment affects simultaneously, but to different degrees, a great number of methylating systems (Klyde and Bernfield 1973; Sharma and Borek 1970). Multiple methylation sites are indeed likely to be involved in the regulatory function on protein metabolism (Sharma and Borek 1976). However, modified tRNA methylases are not necessarily involved during changes in growth rate. In regenerating liver the methyltransferase activity does not differ essentially from that in normal adult liver tissue (Rodeh et al. 1967). Although presenting a stimulated enzyme activity, no changes of in vitro methylated nucleoside pattern are detected in chemically induced rat kidney and mouse colon tumors (Pegg and Hawks 1974; Stewart and Pegg 1972). Furthermore, the use of bacterial tRNA in monitoring mammalian methylating enzymes does not allow methylation to be interpreted in terms of direct biological effects.

Even after purification of the enzyme preparation, inhibitory and stimulatory contaminants are not always eliminated, and corticosteroids may well, by affecting the ionic conditions, induce or accentuate certain changes in enzyme activity (De Loecker et al. 1978; Kaplay and Sanadi 1974; Sharma and Borek 1970; Turkington and Riddle 1970).

Some quantitative differences in the modification of total tRNA of hepatoma compared to normal liver have been observed, however, without any evidence of the formation of new modified bases (Randerath et al 1974). Mammary adenocarcinomas of mice contain elevated levels of some methylated purines in the tRNA (Berquist and Matthews 1962). The increased levels of 7-CH_3-guanine present in neoplastic mammary cells of mice and rats are not found in extracts of normal mammary tissue (Turkington and Riddle 1970). Cortisol treatment simultaneously affects 5-CH_3-cytosine, the N^2,N^2-diCH_3-guanine, and several adenine methyltransferases, which are either stimulated or inhibited depending on the tumor type examined. The 5-CH_3-uracil, 1-CH_3-guanine, 7-CH_3-guanine, and N^2-CH_3-guanine methyltransferases are significantly stimulated only in tumor type I and are almost unaffected in the other types. These hormonal effects may be the result of increased activity of existing transferases, but the synthesis of new or modified methylases can not be excluded.

The identification of the methyltransferases distributed over the various enzyme peaks may elucidate some of these problems, although it seems likely that each of the enzyme peaks represents several enzyme systems. The distribution of the methylated bases in the adrenalectomized control tumors is difficult to compare, as each of the three different types of tumor, particularly type III, presents its own individual distribution pattern. The present data suggest that the effects of cortisol on tRNA methyltransferases vary according to the tumor cell type examined, insofar that the hormone effects may be conditioned by the biological function of the cell type. The effects of cortisol seem simultaneously to be distributed over a wide range of different methyltransferases, with as yet no sure signs of specificity.

Summary

Mammary carcinomas induced in rats by DMBA were divided into three types: I, hard proliferating tumors; II, tumors presenting from an early stage the first signs of cystic degeneration; III, lactating tumors. In all three types, cortisol reduced the protein content by 26%–30%. The already high tRNA methyltransferase activity in type I increased by 200% after cortisol treatment. Hormonal treatment of type II increased the previously reduced control methyltransferases by 37%. In the type III lactating tumors, the total tRNA methyltransferases were inhibited by 35% after cortisol treatment. The methyltransferases of types I and II were separated chromatographically into seven analogous peaks, while the enzymes from type III presented a modified pattern. In each case, cortisol treatment affected the activities of several methyltransferases simultaneously without obvious specificity.

References

Berquist PL, Matthews REF (1962) Occurrence and distribution of methylated purines in the ribonucleic acids of subcellular fractions. Biochem J 85: 305–313

Borek E, Kerr SJ (1972) Atypical tRNA's and their origin in neoplastic cells. Adv Cancer Res 15: 163–190

De Loecker W, Stas ML (1973) Effect of cortisol treatment on free amino acid levels in rats. J Endocrinol 59: 57–63

De Loecker W, Leyman AM, De Wever F (1978) The effects of cortisol on transfer ribonucleic acid methylase activity and protein metabolism in cancer tissue. Biochem Soc Trans 6: 1237–1238

Glick JM, Leboy PS (1977) Purification and properties of tRNA/adenine-1 methyltransferase from rat liver. J Biol Chem 252: 4790–4795

Griswold DP, Skipper HE, Laster WR Jr, Wilcox WS, Schabel FM Jr (1966) Induced mammary carcinoma in the female rat as a drug evaluation system. Cancer Res 26: 2169–2180

Huggins C, Briziarelli G, Sutton H (1959) Rapid induction of mammary carcinoma in the rat and the influence of hormones on tumors. J Exp Med 109: 25–42

Kaplay SS, Sanadi DR (1974) Regulation of tRNA methylases by thyroxine in rat liver. Endocrinology 95: 1185–1188

Kaye AM, Leboy PS (1968) Methylation of RNA by mouse organs and tumors: ionic stimulation in vitro. Biochim Biophys Acta 157: 289–302

Klyde BJ, Bernfield MR (1973) Rate of serine transfer ribonucleic acid synthesis during estrogen-induced phosphoprotein synthesis in chick liver. Biochemistry 12: 3757–3762

Leboy PS (1970) Stimulation of soluble ribonucleic acid methylase activity by polyamines. Biochemistry 9: 1577–1584

Leboy PS (1971) Influence of polyamines and salts on changing patterns of tRNA methylations. FEBS Lett 16: 117–120

Leyman AM, De Loecker W (1980) Hormone effects on transfer ribonucleic acid methylases in rat liver. Biochem Soc Trans 8: 733–734

Lombardini JB, Thallalay P (1971) Formation, functions and regulatory importance of S-adenosyl-L-methionine. Adv Enzyme Regul 9: 349–384

Lowry OH, Rosebrough NJ, Farr AL, Randall RJ (1951) Protein measurement with folin phenol reagent. J Biol Chem 193: 265–275

Luck DN, Hamilton TH (1975) Early oestrogen action: stimulation of the synthesis of methylated ribosomal and tRNA's. Biochim Biophys Acta 283: 23–29

Middleton PJ (1965) The histogenesis of mammary tumours induced in the rat by chemical carcinogens. Br J Cancer 19: 830–839

Munns WT, Sims FH, Katzman PA (1975) Effects of estradiol on uterine ribonucleic acid methylation. Biochemistry 14: 4758–4763

Pegg AE (1971) The effects of diamines and polyamines on enzymatic methylation of nucleic acid. Biochim Biophys Acta 232: 630–642

Pegg AE, Hawks AM (1974) Further investigation of the increased transfer ribonucleic acid methylase activity in tumours of the mouse colon. Biochem J 137: 229–238

Randerath E, Chia LL, Morris H, Randerath K (1974) Transfer RNA base composition studies in Morris hepatomas and rat liver. Cancer Res 34: 643–653

Rodeh R, Feldman M, Littauer UZ (1967) Properties of soluble ribonucleic acid methylases from rat liver. Biochemistry 6: 451–460

Sharma OK, Borek E (1970) Hormonal effect on transfer ribonucleic acid methylases and on serine transfer ribonucleic acid. Biochemistry 9: 2507–2513

Sharma OK, Borek E (1976) Modulation of the synthesis in vitro of a hormone-induced protein by transfer RNA. Nature 262: 62–63

Sheid B, Billik E, Biempica L (1970) Estrogen-mediated enhancement of rat liver S-RNA methylase activity. Arch Biochem Biophys 140: 437–442

Stewart BW, Pegg AE (1972) Changes in tRNA-methylase activity of rat kidney following administration of the carcinogen dimethyl nitrosamine. Biochim Biophys Acta 281: 416–424

Teller MN, Stock CD, Stohr G, Merker PC, Kaufman RJ, Escher GC, Bowie M (1966) Biologic characteristics and chemotherapy of 7,12-dimethylbenz(a)anthracene-induced tumors in rats. Cancer Res 26: 245–252

Turkington RW (1969) Hormonal regulation of transfer ribonucleic acid and transfer ribonucleic acid-methylating enzymes during development of the mouse mammary gland. J Biol Chem 244: 5140–5148

Turkington RW, Riddle M (1970) Transfer RNA-methylating enzymes in mammary carcinoma cells. Cancer Res 30: 650–657

An Approach to Inhibition of Viral Replication: Inhibition of mRNA Methylation

B. B. Goswami, O. K. Sharma, and E. Borek

Department of Molecular Biology, AMC Cancer Research Center and Hospital, Lakewood, CO 80214, USA

Modification of mRNA

Several eukaryotic viral and cellular mRNAs contain at their 5′ terminus blocked methylated structures (often referred to as a "cap") of the type m^7GpppN′mpN″mp. . . (Fig. 1). Additional methylation of several mRNAs occurs internally between their 5′ cap and the 3′-poly(A) end, yielding 6-methyladenosine or 5-methylcytosine (Shatkin 1976). The 5′-terminal 7-methylguanosine in mRNAs is apparently required for their efficient translation in vitro (Both et al. 1975; Muthukrishnan 1978), and is also implicated in protection of mRNA against degradation by exonucleases. The enzymatic mechanisms involved in the synthesis of the cap structure have been worked out in detail by Moss and his co-workers with vaccinia virus (Moss et al. 1976) and by others (Furuichi et al. 1976). It involves (a) the transfer of a GMP residue from GTP to the 5′-diphosphate end of mRNA by GTP:mRNA guanylyltransferase to form the blocked structure GpppN . . ., (b) methylation of the 5′-terminal guanosine in the 7 position by mRNA (guanine-7-)-methyltransferase to form m^7GpppN . . ., and (c) subsequent methylation of the penultimate nucleoside by mRNA(nucleoside-2′-)-methyltransferase to form m^7GpppNm. All three enzymatic activities have been purified from vaccinia virus.

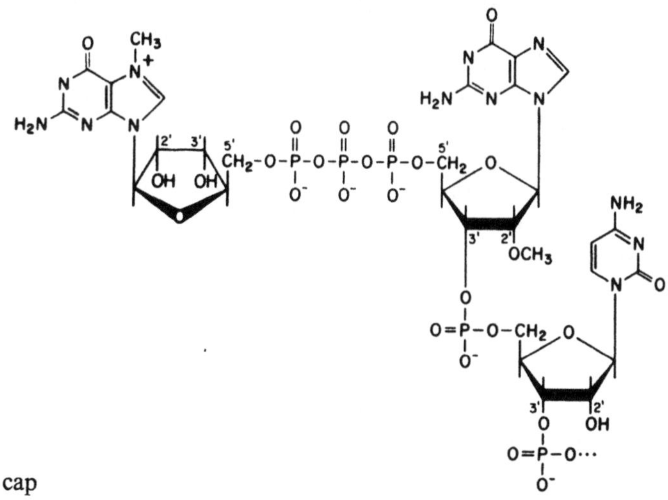

Fig. 1. Structure of mRNA cap

Recent Results in Cancer Research. Vol 84

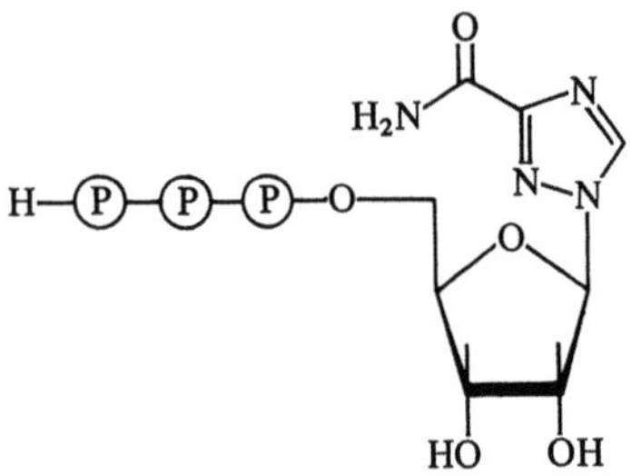

Fig. 2. Structure of ribavirin 5′-triphosphate

Mechanism of Action of Ribavirin

The broad spectrum antiviral agent ribavirin (1-β-D-ribofuranosyl-1,2,4,-triazole-3-carboxamide) (Virazole) is active against both DNA- and RNA-containing viruses (Smith and Kirkpatrick 1980). The precise mechanism of its antiviral activity was obscure until recently, but from studies it has become apparent that it involves the metabolism of some guanine derivative because its antiviral action in tissue culture can be overcome by high levels of guanosine.

The structure of the drug (Fig. 2) suggested to us the possibility that ribavirin may interfere with the cap guanylation of mRNA. This would explain its inhibitory activity against both RNA and DNA viruses, many of which produce mRNAs which are capped. Moreover, the drug is ineffective against EMC and polio virus replication, and it is known that EMC and polio virus do not produce capped mRNAs. We tested our hypothesis with the vaccinia virus system. This is an ideal system because the enzymes needed for the synthesis of the viral mRNA and its post-transcriptional modifications are present in the virion and by appropriate manipulation of experimental conditions mRNAs can be synthesized in vitro, free of the blocked methylated structures, and thus can serve as an ideal substrate for enzymatic studies. If vaccinia DNA is transcribed in the presence of high concentrations of *S*-adenosylhomocysteine and low concentrations of GTP, the product is partially unguanylated.

We studied the effect of ribavirin on the guanylation of in vitro synthesized, partially capped mRNAs with soluble enzymes isolated from vaccinia cores. Ribavirin 5′-triphosphate was found to be a potent inhibitor of the capping reaction (Table 1). The inhibition was competitive (Fig. 3), the K_m for guanylyltransferase for GTP was 22 μ*M*, and an inhibitor constant (K_i) of 32 μ*M* for ribavirin 5′-triphosphate was found (Goswami 1979).

Although earlier studies showed inhibition of methylation of terminal guanosine by rather high concentrations of ribavirin triphosphate, recent studies with purified viral enzymes indicate that ribavirin 5′-triphosphate is an effective inhibitor of vaccinia mRNA(guanine-7-)-methyltransferase (unpublished observation).

We investigated whether the RNA synthesized in vivo in the presence of ribavirin was deficient in methylation. RNA was labeled in vaccinia-infected L cells simultaneously with [^{3}H]methionine and [^{32}P]phosphate; poly(A)-containing RNA was isolated by affinity chromatography on oligo(dT) cellulose. Vaccinia-virus-specific RNA was isolated by hybridization to vaccinia viral DNA immobilized on nitrocellulose filters. Ribavirin inhibited methylation of vaccinia-specific poly(A)-containing RNA by 33%–42% (Goswami et al., to be published). Under similar conditions, there was a 58%–64% inhibition of protein synthesis. An analysis of the proteins synthesized by SDS polyacrylamide gel electrophoresis revealed that synthesis of both early and late

Table 1. Effect of ribavirin 5′-triphosphate on 5′-guanylation of in vitro synthesized vaccinia mRNA by GTP:mRNA vaccinia guanylyltransferase

Reaction mixture	[^{3}H]GMP Incorporated[a]
Complete	(100)
+ Ribavirin, 1 m*M*	100
+ Ribavirin 5′-monophosphate, 1 m*M*	100
+ Ribavirin 5′-triphosphate, 50 μ*M*	48

[a] Expressed as percentage of incorporation by the complete system, which in this experiment was 12 pmol

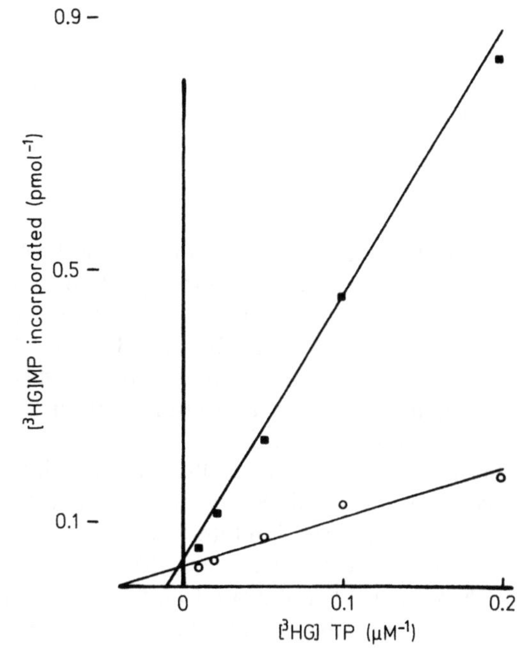

Fig. 3. Lineweaver-Burk plots showing competitive inhibition of viral guanylyltransferase by ribavirin 5′-triphosphate (RTP). ○–○, no RTP; ■–■, 100 μ*M* RTP (Goswami et al. 1979)

proteins was inhibited to the same extent (unpublished observation). Inhibition of proper modification of the 5′ terminus of mRNAs by ribavirin may be a mechanism of the antiviral action of this agent against those viruses which give rise to capped mRNAs and of its ineffectiveness against viruses which yield mRNAs that are not capped, such as polio and encephalomyocarditis (EMC) virus.

Inhibition of Vaccinia mRNA Methylation by 2′,5′-Linked Oligo (Adenylic Acid) Triphosphate

A low-molecular-weight inhibitor of protein synthesis is found in extracts of interferon-treated mouse L cells incubated in the presence of double-stranded RNA and ATP (Kerr and Brown 1978). Kerr and his colleagues have isolated this inhibitor and characterized it as a 2′-5′-linked oligo (adenylic acid) 5′-triphosphate,

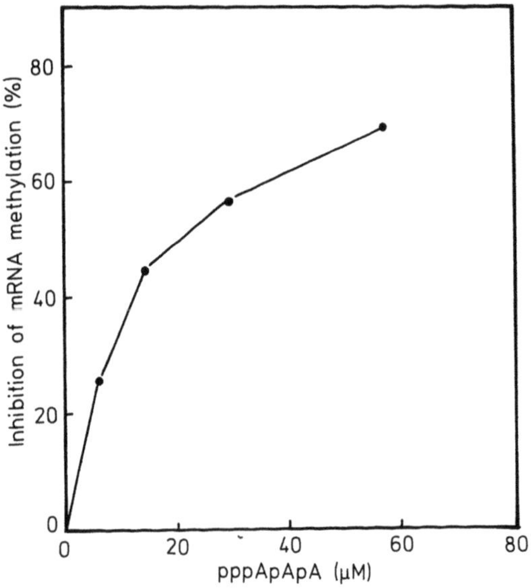

Fig. 4. Inhibition of vaccinia mRNA methyltransferase activity by 2-5A. (Sharma and Goswami 1981)

ppp(A2′p5′)$_n$A($n = 2-4$) referred to as 2-5A. The major component is a trinucleotide pppA2′p5′A2′p5′A. In cell-free protein-synthesizing systems, nanomolar concentrations of 2-5A inhibit protein synthesis by activating an endonuclease which degrades both cellular and viral RNA (Baglioni 1979). The introduction of 2-5A into permeabilized cells results in enhanced levels of endonuclease activity (Williams et al. 1979) concurrent with transient inhibition of protein synthesis. EMC virus production is also inhibited by 2-5A.

On the other hand, in L cells treated with low doses of interferon and infected with vaccinia virus, significantly more viral RNA is transcribed, whereas viral protein synthesis is severely inhibited as early as 20 min after infection (Joklik and Merigan 1966; Metz and Esteban 1972; Metz et al. 1975). Thus the degradation of vaccinia mRNA by a 2-5A-activated endonuclease seems highly unlikely.

A variety of other effects of interferon in eukaryotic cells have been described; however, they are not relevant to the investigations we are about to describe. They can be found in appropriate review articles (Vilcek et al. 1980).

In a search for an explanation of the inability of several apparently normal viral mRNAs to form polyribosomes in interferon-treated cells, it occurred to us that all these viral mRNAs, unlike the EMC viral RNA, are capped, i.e., they contain a 5′-terminal structure of the type m^{7}GpppNm. Since it is now recognized that the cap structure is important for binding to initiation factors and ribosomes (Muthukrishnan et al. 1978; Moss et al. 1976), we began to explore the possibility that 2-5A might in some way inhibit the formation of the cap structure of viral RNAs, thereby restricting their ability to form polyribosomes. We showed that 2-5A strongly inhibits in vitro methylation of vaccinia mRNA (Sharma and Goswami 1981). A 50% inhibition is observed with 21μM 2-5A (Fig. 4). Since the 2-5A we used in our initial experiment was a commercial product, we have rigorously established its authenticity by comparing it with enzymatically synthesized 2-5A. The commercial preparation and the biosynthetic material are identical with respect to chromatographic properties, nuclease sensitivities, inhibition of in vitro protein synthesis, and inhibition of

Table 2. Inhibition of vaccinia mRNA methyltransferase by 5′-mono- and triphosphate of adenosyl-(2′-5′)-adenylyl-(2′-5′)-adenosine

Additions	[^{3}H]Methyl incorporation (cpm)	Inhibition (%)
None	25000	0
pppA2′p5′A2′p5′A (28 μM)	7500	70.0
pA2′p5′A2′p5′A (28 μM)	9400	62.4
pA3′p5′A3′p5′A (28 μM)	24500	2.0
A2′p5′A2′p5′A (28 μM)	22500	10.0
A3′p5′A3′p5′A (28 μM)	24000	4.0
2′-AMP (30 μM)	24000	4.0
3′-AMP (30 μM)	25000	0
5′-AMP (60 μM)	24300	2.8
3′:5′-cyclic AMP (60 μM)	24600	1.6
2′:5′-cyclic AMP (60 μM)	24800	0.8
5′-GMP (60 μM)	22800	8.8
3′:5′-cyclic GMP (60 μM)	23900	4.4
2′:5′-cyclic GMP (60 μM)	23900	4.4

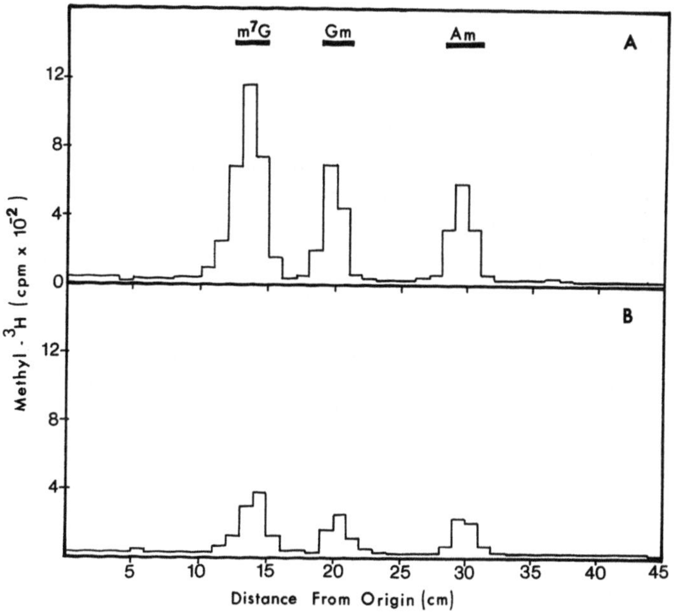

Fig. 5. Analysis of methylated nucleosides of vaccinia mRNA methylated in vitro by vaccinia mRNA methyltransferase in the absence (**A**) and presence (**B**) of 2-5A. (Sharma and Goswami 1981)

vaccinia-methylating enzymes. 2′-5′-Oligo(adenylic acid) 5′-mono- and triphosphate are equally effective inhibitors (Table 2). The requirement for 2′, 5′ linkage for inhibition was absolute. The 3′-5′-linked tri- and tetra (adenylic acid) 5′-monophosphate isolated by limited digestion of poly(A) had no inhibitory activity. In addition,

2′-AMP, 3′-AMP, 5′-AMP, 2′:5′-cyclic AMP, 3′:5′-cyclic AMP, 2′:5′-cyclic GMP, and 3′:5′-cyclic GMP also had no inhibitory activity.

2-5A inhibited both the methylation of the 5′-terminal G at the 7 position and the 2′-*O*-ribose methylation of the penultimate A and G (Fig. 5). The methylation of 5′-terminal G at the 7 position and the 2′-*O*-ribose methylation of the penultimate A and G residues in vaccinia virus is accomplished by two different enzymatic activities (Barbosa and Moss 1978). However, the methylation of the 5′-terminal G by vaccinia viral enzyme is a prerequisite for the 2′-*O*-ribose methylation of the penultimate A and G, which would account for the inhibition of the synthesis of Am and Gm in the cap.

Recently deFerra and Baglioni (1981) have reported that in HeLa cells treated with interferon and infected with VSV, the amount of viral RNA not associated with polyribosomes is significantly elevated compared to untreated infected cells, and that much of the nonpolysomal poly(A) RNA is not methylated at the terminal G. This may explain the inability of seemingly intact viral mRNAs to participate in polysome formation in vivo. Should cellular mRNA (guanine-7-)-methyltransferase be different from the viral counterpart in its sensitivity towards 2-5A, it may also explain why in several instances cellular mRNAs are normally translated in interferon-treated, virus-infected cells, whereas viral RNAs are not.

Clinical Significance

It has been shown that ribavirin inhibits viral reproduction in cells in tissue culture. It was also shown by Kerr and Brown (1978), that 2-5A inhibits replication of EMC virus in L cells. We have now observed that both of these agents inhibit methylation of virally derived mRNA. The significance of these findings in the design and testing of other antiviral agents is obvious. As a preliminary approach new substances may be tested in vitro as potential inhibitors of methylation of virally derived mRNA prior to testing in vivo. It is possible that agents will be found which are specific inhibitors of mRNA methylation derived from the virus and are at the same time innocuous to the methylation of host mRNA. The toxicity of such reagents to the host may thereby be substantially reduced. 2-5A has two drawbacks for practical use against viral infections at the present time: it is labile to a variety of nucleases present in cells, and moreover is not permeable into most eukaryotic cells. These two disadvantages could be remedied by chemical modifications. Such attempts are worth pursuing.

Summary

Eukaryotic mRNAs and most viral mRNAs contain very extensive modification on the 5′ end, consisting of the cap, part of which is a guanine methylated in the 7 position. It is quite well established that the methylated cap is essential for the efficient translation of mRNA.

In a search for an effective chemotherapeutic agent, Dr. Roland Robins synthesized the compound ribavirin, which turned out to be an extraordinarily effective virostatic agent against both RNA and DNA viruses. Given the capping of the mRNAs produced by both types of virus, and given the structure of ribavirin, it seemed to us

that it may be fruitful to explore whether this drug might act in both cases by blocking the capping reaction. Such a mechanism indeed turned out to be a reality.
We have shown that ribavirin triphosphate acts as a competitive inhibitor for the capping of mRNAs. We and others have shown that uncapped mRNAs are poorly translated. An interesting corollary confirmation of these findings is that EMC and polio virus generate mRNAs which are not capped, and ribavirin is innocuous to these viruses.
Another agent which acts as an inhibitor of mRNA methylation emerged from subsequent efforts. It is known from the work of Kerr and Brown (1978) that extracts of interferon-treated cells in the presence of double-stranded RNA synthesize a unique 2′-5′-linked oligo (adenylic acid) 5′-triphosphate, a small trinucleotide of unusual structure which inhibits protein synthesis. We have explored its effect on the methylation of mRNA and found it to be a potent inhibitor of methylation of the cap.
Thus two agents are known which inhibit methylation of mRNA. They may serve as prototypes for designing other such inhibitors, with a view to specific inhibition of mRNAs foreign to the host.

References

Baglioni C (1979) Interferon-induced enzymatic activities and their role in the antiviral state. Cell 17: 255–264

Barbosa E, Moss B (1978) mRNA (nucleoside-2′-)-methyltransferase from vaccinia virus: characteristics and substrate specificity. J Biol Chem 253: 7698–7702

Both GW, Banerjee AK, Shatkin AJ (1975) Methylationdependent translation of viral messenger RNAs in vitro. Proc Natl Acad Sci USA 72: 1189–1193

deFerra F, Baglioni C (1981) Viral messenger RNA unmethylated in the 5′-terminal guanosine in interferon-treated HeLa cells infected with vesicular stomatitis virus. Virology 112: 426–435

Furuichi Y, Muthukrishnan S, Tomasz J, Shatkin AJ (1976) Caps in eukaryotic mRNAs: mechanism of formation of reovirus mRNA 5′-terminal m^7GpppG_mC. Progr Nucleic Acid Res Mol Biol 19: 3–20

Goswami BB, Borek E, Sharma OK, Fujitaki J, Smith RA (1979) The broad spectrum antiviral agent Ribavirin inhibits capping of mRNA. Biochem Biophys Res Comm 89: 830–836

Goswami BB, Sharma OK, Borek E, Smith RA (to be published) Inhibition of methylation of vaccinia virus specific mRNA by the broad spectrum antiviral agent Ribavirin. Proceedings of XIIth International Congress of Chemotherapy, Florence, Italy

Joklik WK, Merigan TC (1966) Concerning the mechanism of action of interferon. Proc Natl Acad Sci USA 56: 558–565

Kerr IM, Brown RE (1978) $pppA^{2'}p^{5'}A^{2'}p^{5'}A$: An inhibitor of protein synthesis synthesized with an enzyme fraction from interferon-treated cells. Proc Natl Acad Sci USA 75: 256–260

Metz DH, Esteban M (1972) Interferon inhibits viral protein synthesis in L-cells infected with vaccinia virus. Nature 238: 385–388

Metz DH, Esteban M, Danielescu G (1975) The effect of interferon on the formation of virus polyribosomes in L-cells infected with vaccinia virus. J Gen Virol 27: 197–209

Muthukrishnan S, Moss B, Cooper JA, Maxwell ES (1978) Influence of 5′-terminal cap structure on the initiation of translation of vaccinia virus mRNA. J Biol Chem 253: 1710–1715

Moss B, Martin SA, Ensinger MJ, Boone RF, Wei CM (1976) Modification of the 5′-terminals of mRNAs by viral and cellular enzymes. Progr Nucleic Acid Res Mol Biol 19: 63–81
Shatkin AJ (1976) Capping of eucaryotic mRNAs. Cell 9: 645–653
Sharma OK, Goswami BB (1981) Inhibition of vaccinia mRNA methylation by 2′, 5′-linked oligo (adenylic acid) triphosphate. Proc Natl Acad Sci USA 78: 2221–2224
Smith RA, Kirkpatrick W (eds) (1980) Ribavirin: a broad spectrum antiviral agent. Academic Press, New York
Vilcek J, Gresser I, Merigan TC (eds) (1980) Regulatory functions of interferons. Ann NY Acad Sci 350
Williams BRG, Golgher RR, Kerr IM (1979) Activation of a nuclease by $pppA^{2'}p^{5'}A^{2'}p^{5'}A$ in intact cells. FEBS Lett 105: 47–52

*Specific Effects of 5-Fluoropyrimidines and 5-Azapyrimidines on Modification of the 5 Position of Pyrimidines, in Particular the Synthesis of 5-Methyluracil and 5-Methylcytosine in Nucleic Acids**

K. Randerath, W.-C. Tseng, J. S. Harris, and L.-J. W. Lu

Department of Pharmacology, Baylor College of Medicine, Texas Medical Center, Houston, TX 77030, USA

Introduction

Drug effects on nucleic acids may entail the incorporation of drugs or their metabolites, thereby altering the sequence of the four major bases, or involve postsynthetic modifications, e.g., methylations of nucleic acid constituents. While in the past the incorporation of drugs such as purine or pyrimidine analogs into tRNA and other nucleic acids has been recognized as a major effect of these compounds, during the past 5 years our laboratory has presented evidence for pronounced, sometimes highly selective effects of drugs on modifications of nucleic acids. This will be the main subject of this chapter.

In 1975 we wondered whether the ^{3}H-labeling procedure for base analysis of RNA (Randerath et al. 1972) might be useful in studies on the incorporation of chemotherapeutically active base and nucleoside analogs into RNA. In addition, as a major action of 5-fluorouracil is the inhibition of the thymidylate synthetase-catalyzed methylation of dUMP to dTMP, an important biological methylation, we wondered whether 5-fluorouracil and perhaps related compounds such as 5-azapyrimidines might also affect the modification of the 5 position of pyrimidines in nucleic acids.

We therefore treated normal mice and mice bearing a 7,12-dimethylbenz(a)anthracene-induced, transplantable mammary carcinoma with various doses of 5-fluorouracil or 5-fluorouridine, and isolated tRNA from normal and cancerous tissues after various intervals. The fluorogram shown in Fig. 1 was obtained by two-dimensional thin-layer chromatography (TLC) on cellulose of a ^{3}H-labeled digest of tRNA (Randerath et al. 1972, 1974) from livers of mice that had received 100 mg/kg 5-fluorouridine once daily for 4 days (Lu et al. 1976a). The presence of the trialcohol derivative of 5-fluorouridine (FU′) (see Fig. 1) provided evidence for the incorporation of 5-fluorouridine into tRNA.

As shown in Fig. 2, base composition analysis of tRNA after administration of 5-fluorocytidine to mice (one injection daily of 50 mg/kg for 4 consecutive days) showed not only 5-fluorocytidine but also 5-fluorouridine to be present in liver tRNA of the treated mice (Fig. 2b). This suggested the in vivo conversion of 5-fluorocytidine derivatives to 5-fluorouridine derivatives. Extensive incorporation of 5-fluorocytidine into liver tRNA was observed (Lu et al. 1979).

* Work from our laboratory was supported by USPHS Grants CA 13591 and CA 10893 (P8)

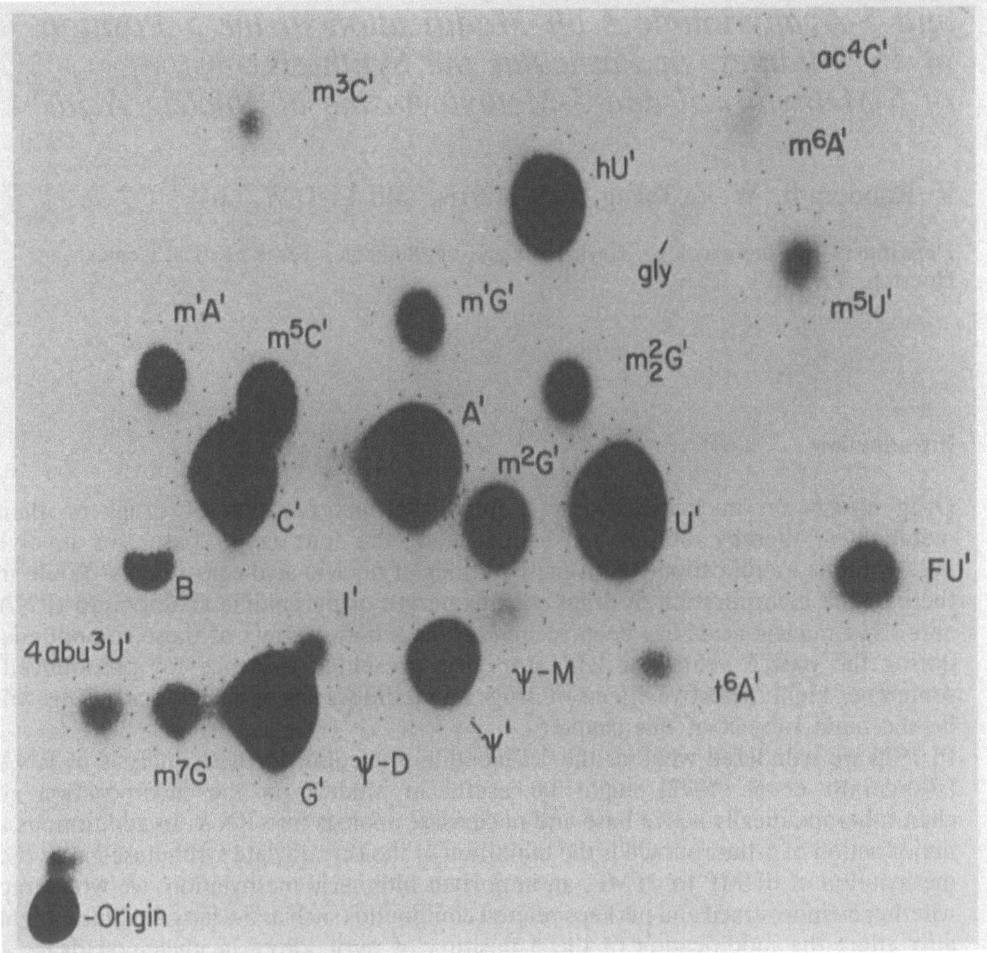

Fig. 1. Map of ^{3}H-labeled digest of liver tRNA from mice treated with 5-fluorouridine. *gly*, glycerol; *ψ-D*, decomposition product of pseudouridine; *ψ-M*, pseudouridine monoaldehyde; *B*, Background spot (not from RNA)

The fluorogram shown in Fig. 3 was obtained from liver tRNA of mice that had received 32 mg/kg 5-azacytidine once daily for 4 days (Lu et al. 1976b). This fluorogram looks normal except for a marked reduction of the intensity of the spot of 5-methylcytidine trialcohol (m^{5}C′), as can be seen, for example, by comparison with Fig. 2A.

Quantitative Analysis of Effects of Pyrimidine Analogs on tRNA Base Composition

5-Fluorouracil and 5-Fluorouridine

Most of our studies were conducted with 5-fluorouracil, but effects of 5-fluorouridine appeared to be closely similar to those of 5-fluorouracil. The following observations were made (Tseng et al. 1978; Lu et al. 1976b):

1. Drug incorporation was dose-dependent.

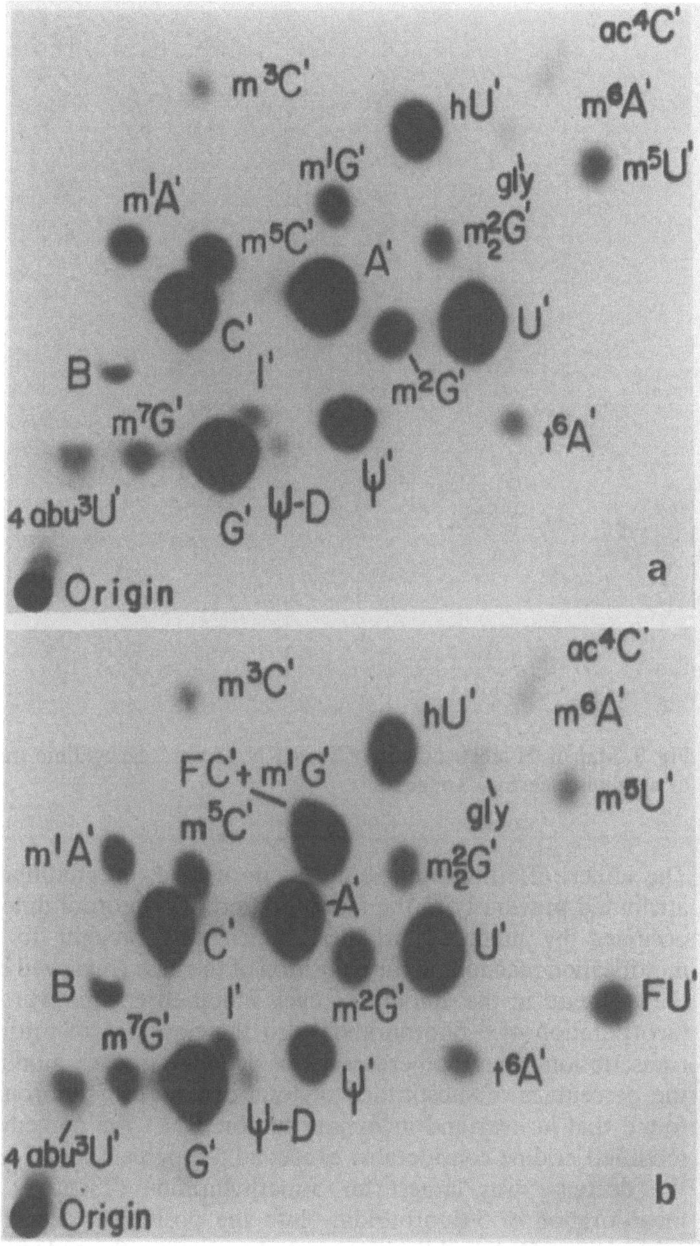

Fig. 2a, b. Maps of ^{3}H-labeled digests of liver tRNA obtained from normal mice (**a**) and 5-fluorocytidine-treated mice (**b**). *FC'*, trialcohol of 5-fluorocytidine. For other symbols, see Fig. 1 legend

2. There was no dose-related effect on purines (major and modified) or cytosine derivatives in tRNA.
3. There was a dose-dependent reduction in the levels of uridine derivatives modified in the 5 position of the pyrimidine ring (5-methyluridine, pseudouridine, and 5,6-dihydrouridine), while the sum of uridine and its derivatives remained unaffected at all doses of 5-fluorouracil or 5-fluorouridine examined.

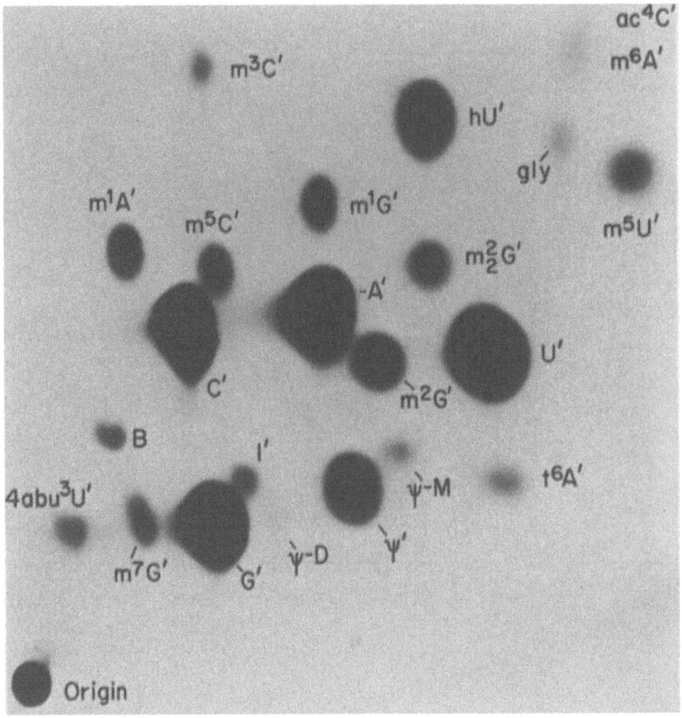

Fig. 3. Map of ^{3}H-labeled digest of liver tRNA from 5-azacytidine-treated mice. For explanation of symbols, see Fig. 1 legend

The effects of 5-fluorouracil and its derivatives on modified uridines in RNA were attributed previously to the incorporation of 5-fluorouridine into positions normally occupied by modified uridines, which was thought to prevent physically the modification reactions at the 5 position of the base (reviewed by Heidelberger 1975). If the decrease in the amount of each modified uridine were due simply to random incorporation of 5-fluorouridine into the positions of uridine in pre-tRNA during transcription, then the percentage of decrease in each modified uridine would equal the percentage of substitution of total uridine by 5-fluorouridine. However, it was found that in liver and mammary tumor tRNA the percentage of decrease in each modified uridine considerably exceeded the percentage of substitution at each dose; the decrease was largest for 5-methyluridine (Tseng et al. 1978). Preferential incorporation of 5-fluorouridine into the positions normally occupied by modified uridines in tRNA had been suggested to explain the reduction of 5-methyluridine in tRNA from 5-fluorouracil-treated *Escherichia coli* (Baliga et al. 1969). This mechanism would imply that the total decrease in modified uridines should not exceed the amount of 5-fluorouridine incorporated into tRNA following treatment with any 5-fluorouracil dose. However, as shown in Fig. 4, it was found in tRNA from both normal and mammary tumor tissue that the amount of incorporated 5-fluorouridine was smaller than the decrease in modified uridines, even if 5-methyluridine was excluded from the calculation (Tseng et al. 1978). This was a clear indication of the inhibition by 5-fluorouracil or derivative(s) of this analog of enzymatic modification reactions responsible for converting uridine to 5-methyluridine, pseudouridine, and

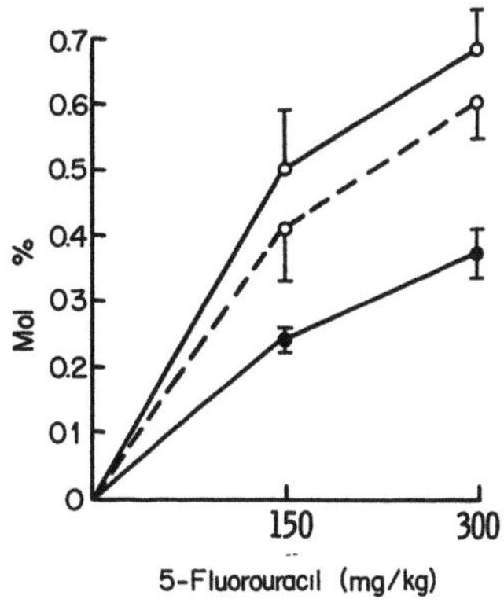

Fig. 4. Effects of 5-fluorouracil dose on 5-fluorouridine incorporation and amounts of modified uridine derivatives in liver tRNA isolated 24 h after treatment with a single dose of 5-fluorouracil. O———O, decrease in the sum of 5-methyluracil + pseudouridine + 5,6-dihydrouridine; O— — —O, decrease in the sum of pseudouridine + 5,6-dihydrouridine; ●———●, 5-fluorouridine incorporation; *bars*, standard deviations

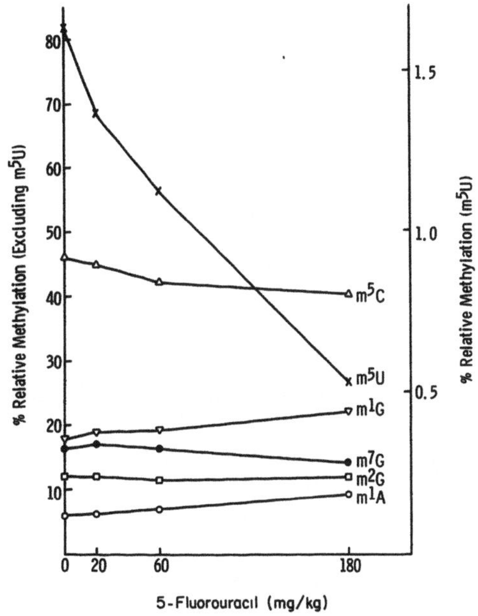

Fig. 5. In vitro methylation of individual nucleosides in partially methyl-deficient liver tRNA by enzymes extracted from liver 24 h after treatment with single doses of 5-fluorouracil

5,6-dihydrouridine during tRNA maturation, in addition to the physical replacement of uridine by 5-fluorouridine during tRNA transcription.

To obtain direct evidence for an effect of 5-fluorouracil on tRNA-modifying enzymes, we determined the tRNA methyltransferase activities of extracts from normal and drug-treated tissues using *Mycoplasma hominis* or homologous methyl-deficient tRNA [induced by ethionine treatment (Lu et al. 1976c)] as substrates. Figure 5 shows the distribution of methyl groups accepted by partially methyl-deficient mouse liver tRNA during in vitro methylation by enzyme extracts from livers of 5-fluorouracil-treated mice. Methyl incorporation into each base was calculated as a percentage of methylation relative to total methyl radioactivity recovered from identified methylated products. Only 5-methyluridine formation showed a sharp dose-dependent reduction; the other methylated nucleosides remained approximately the same. The degree of methylation of individual nucleosides did not parallel the actual methyl deficiency induced by ethionine treatment (Lu et al. 1976c). For example, in vitro methylation of

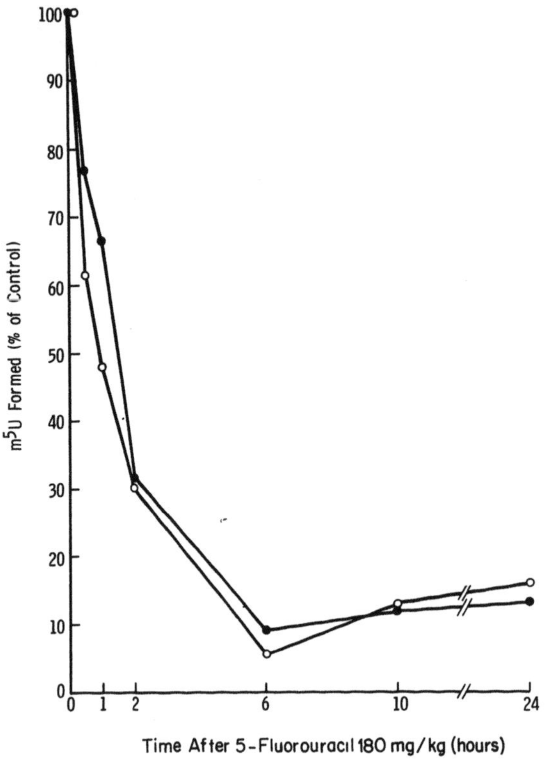

Fig. 6. Time course of inhibition of tRNA uracil-5-methyltransferase in liver (○) and mammary tumor (●) after treatment with a single dose of 5-fluorouracil (180 mg/kg). 5-Methyluracil formed by dialyzed enzyme extracts with *Mycoplasma hominis* tRNA as the substrate was calculated as percentage of control

the most deficient nucleoside, N^2,N^2-dimethylguanosine, was barely detectable, while a relatively large amount of the least deficient nucleoside, 1-methylguanosine, was formed by in vitro methylation.

Figure 6 illustrates the time course of inhibition of tRNA uracil-5-methyltransferase after a single i.p. dose of 5-fluorouracil (180 mg/kg). The enzyme activity in liver and mammary tumor was reduced very rapidly after treatment, and over 90% of the activity was lost after 6 h. The enzyme activity had recovered very little after 24 h, indicating prolonged inhibition (Tseng et al. 1978).

Thus the in vitro methylation assays demonstrated a specific, rapid, and prolonged decrease in the activity of tRNA uracil-5-methyltransferase in liver and mammary tumor following treatment with 5-fluorouracil. In addition, base composition analysis of tRNA from 5-fluorouracil-treated tissues indicated that the reduction of the amounts of pseudouridine and 5,6-dihydrouridine was also due, at least in part, to the inhibition of post-transcriptional modification reactions. These experiments, together with parallel experiments employing 5-fluorocytidine and 5-azacytidine (described below), firmly established fort the first time that pyrimidine analogs modified in the 5 position inhibited enzymes catalyzing normal modification reactions at the 5 position of pyrimidines of nucleic acids.

5-Fluorocytidine

Analogous observations were made for 5-fluorocytidine (Lu et al. 1979). In addition to drug incorporation (Fig. 2), the activities of tRNA cytosine-5-methyltransferase and

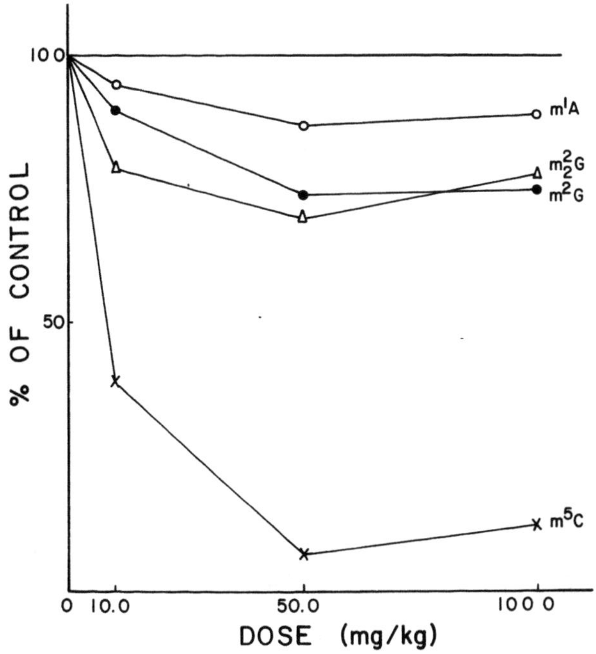

Fig. 7. Effects of a single dose of 5-fluorocytidine on activities of individual mouse liver tRNA methyltransferases

tRNA uracil-5-methyltransferase were strongly inhibited after administration of 5-fluorocytidine to mice. There were no consistent changes of tRNA purine-specific methylases. As shown in Fig. 7, the decrease in tRNA cytosine-5-methyltransferase was dose-dependent. The inhibition was very prolonged (over 72 h).

5-Azacytidine

Effects on tRNA. In 1975, shortly after the initial experiments with 5-fluorouracil outlined above were carried out, we observed that the administration to mice of another pyrimidine nucleoside analog modified in the 5 position, i.e., 5-azacytidine, resulted in a marked reduction of the 5-methylcytidine content of liver tRNA (Lu et al. 1976b). As shown in Fig. 8, this effect was found to be dose-dependent and specific for the methylation of the 5 position of cytosine. The drug had no effect on 3-methylcytidine, 5-methyluridine, 5,6-dihydrouridine, or modified purines in tRNA (see also Fig. 8). In our first paper describing this effect (Lu et al. 1976b) we hypothesized that 5-azacytidine might also inhibit the formation of 5-methylcytosine in other RNAs and in DNA. The latter prediction has been confirmed recently in several laboratories (see also below).

In contrast to 5-fluorouracil, 5-fluorouridine, and 5-fluorocytidine, incorporation of 5-azacytidine into mammalian tRNA was found to be extremely low. A calculation showed that the maximum extent of replacement of cytidine by 5-azacytidine was less than 1 in 50 cytidine residues.

To elucidate the mechanism underlying the effect, tRNA methyltransferases from drug-treated tissues were analyzed. The ability to catalyze the formation of 5-methylcytidine in substrate tRNA in vitro was greatly reduced in tRNA

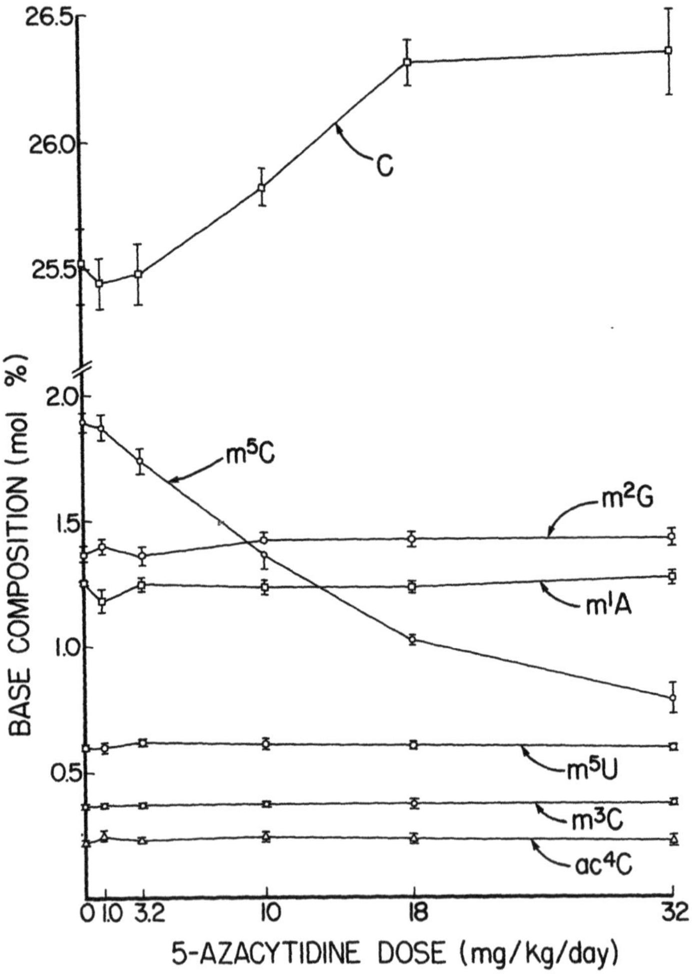

Fig. 8. Effect of 5-azacytidine treatment on the base composition of mouse liver tRNA. *Bars,* standard deviations

methyltransferase preparations from 5-azacytidine-treated liver. The inhibition of tRNA cytosine-5-methyltransferase activity was dose-dependent (Fig. 9) and prolonged. This inhibitory effect could be detected as early as 20 min after the administration of 18 mg/kg 5-azacytidine to mice. A minimum of enzyme activity was found at 4–7 h, at which time it was barely detectable.

While tRNA cytosine-5-methyltransferase activity was inhibited at all time points, the drug had no effect on tRNA purine-specific methyltransferases during the first few hours of exposure. However, 12 h after drug administration, 1-methyladenosine, N^2-methylguanosine, and N^2,N^2-dimethylguanosine tRNA methyltransferase activities (Fig. 9) were found to increase rapidly, peaking at about 24 h.

In Table 1, effects of 5-fluorouracil, 5-fluorouridine, 5-fluorocytidine, and 5-azacytidine on mammalian tRNA and tRNA modification have been summarized. Although there are differences, these drugs have much in common. Perhaps the most striking differences are the extensive incorporation of 5-fluorocytidine into tRNA and

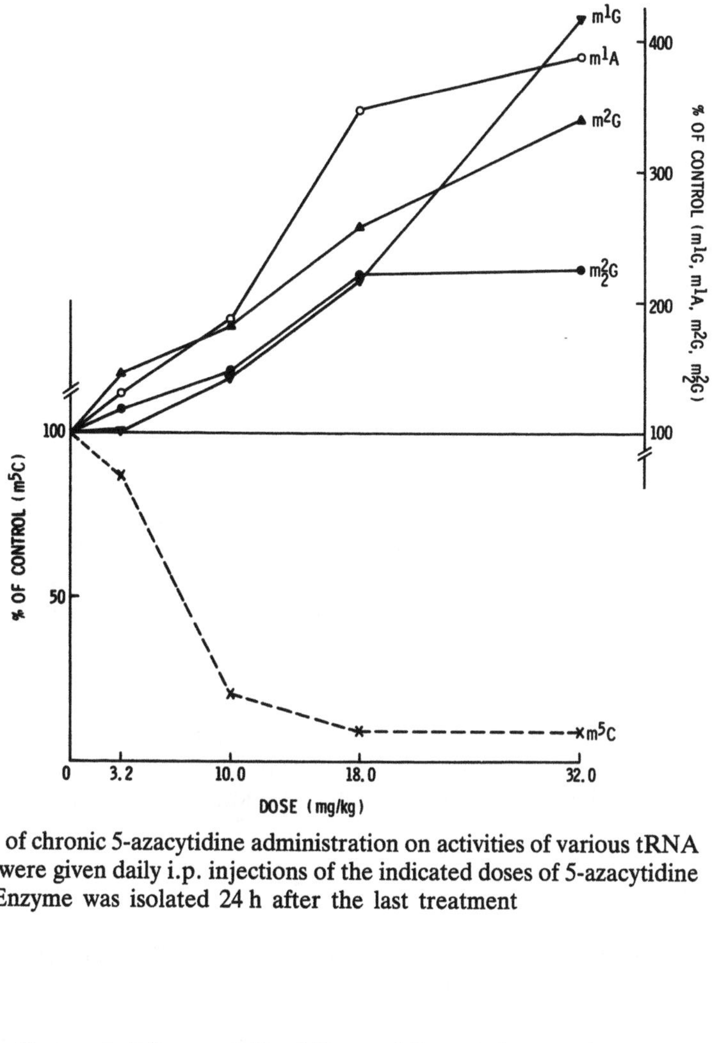

Fig. 9. Differential effects of chronic 5-azacytidine administration on activities of various tRNA methyltransferases. Mice were given daily i.p. injections of the indicated doses of 5-azacytidine for 4 consecutive days. Enzyme was isolated 24 h after the last treatment

Table 1. Summary of effects of 5-fluorouracil, 5-fluorouridine, 5-fluorocytidine, and 5-azacytidine on tRNA and tRNA modification

Analog	Incorporation	Inhibitory effects on			
		m^5C	m^5U	Ψ	hU
5-fluorouracil and 5-fluorouridine	+ +	–	+ + + +	+ + +	+
5-fluorocytidine	+ + + +[a] + +[b]	+ + + +	+ + +	+ +	+
5-azacytidine	(+)[c]	+ + + +	–	–	–

[a] Incorporation of 5-fluorocytidine
[b] Incorporation of 5-fluorouridine
[c] Very low (< 1 in 50 C residues)

the low level of incorporation of 5-azacytidine. All four drugs specifically cause the inhibition of modification reactions at the 5 position of pyrimidines in tRNA, 5-fluorouracil and 5-fluorouridine being specific inhibitors of uracil modifications and 5-azacytidine being a specific inhibitor of the methylation of cytosine. 5-Fluorocytidine affects all these reactions, which in part appears to be due to its biotransformation to 5-fluorouracil derivatives. From these data one may conclude that of the four drugs investigated, 5-fluorocytidine is the most powerful agent in terms of both qualitative and quantitative effects on tRNA.

Effects on DNA. Several laboratories have reported on the inhibition of DNA methylation by 5-azacytidine in *E. coli* (Friedman 1979), Ehrlich ascites tumor cells (Tanaka et al. 1980), and mouse embryo cells (Jones and Taylor 1980, 1981). We have analyzed the 5-methylcytosine content of DNA in regenerating rat liver and in mouse L1210 leukemic cells after exposure to 5-azacytidine. When rats were treated with 15 mg/kg 5-azacytidine 24 h and again 48 h after partial hepatectomy, the 5-methylcytosine content of DNA isolated 24 h after the second drug treatment was 80% of control. This decrease was statistically significant ($P < 0{,}001$). When mice bearing L1210 cells were treated with different doses of 5-azacytidine (4–32 mg/kg) for varying lengths of time, DNA methylation was found to be affected at all dose levels studied, with maximum inhibition detectable 24–48 h after drug treatment. Lower doses were more effective than higher doses. At 24 h after treatment with 4 mg/kg the 5-methylcytosine content of DNA of L1210 cells was reduced to 78% of control. DNA methylase activity was not detectable at 4 h after administration of this dose.
Our work thus shows that 5-fluoropyrimidines and 5-azapyrimidines have as their common targets a variety of enzymes responsible for modification reactions involving the 5-position of pyrimidines in both nucleic acid precursors and nucleic acids (Lu et al. 1979).

Mechanism of Inhibition of Pyrimidine Modifications by 5-Fluoro- and 5-Azapyrimidines

To elucidate the mechanism of the inhibition of nucleic-acid-modifying enzymes by 5-fluoro- and 5-azapyrimidines, effects of various inhibitors of RNA and protein synthesis on the inhibitions were studied and isolation of inhibitor(s) from drug-treated cells or tissues was also attempted. Most studies were conducted with 5-azacytidine (Lu and Randerath 1980). In view of the observed structure-activity relationships however, we suspect, that the basic mechanisms underlying the described effects are identical or very similar. We first observed that analog bases or analog nucleosides themselves exhibited no or very weak inhibitory activity on the modification reactions in vitro. Likewise, mononucleotide derivatives of the analogs were without effect. This suggested that perhaps drug incorporation was required, leading to the synthesis of fraudulent nucleic acids capable of binding to and thus inactivating the modifying enzymes. If drug incorporation into nucleic acid was required, then one would expect that interference with their synthesis would counteract the effects of the pyrimidine analogs on the modifying enzymes. This was indeed found to be the case (Randerath 1979; Lu and Randerath 1980). The possibility existed also that inhibition of protein synthesis by the pyrimidine analogs might be involved. Therefore it was of interest to investigate whether inhibiting RNA or protein synthesis had any effect on tRNA methyltransferases. This, however, was not observed (Randerath 1979). Thus it appeared unlikely that inhibition of RNA or protein synthesis per se was involved in the effects of the pyrimidine analogs on nucleic acid modification. However, it was found that inhibitors of RNA synthesis such as actinomycin D, α-amanitin, 3-deazauridine, and D-galactosamine reversed the effects of the drugs on tRNA uracil-5-methyltransferase (Randerath 1979) and tRNA cytosine-5-methyltransferase (Lu and Randerath 1980), respectively. Inhibitors of protein synthesis, on the other hand, did not affect the inhibition of the enzymes. Therefore RNA synthesis appears to be required for the inhibitions to occur, and it may be hypothesized that inhibition of the enzymes is a consequence of drug incorporation into nucleic acid. To establish this more clearly, we have fractionated RNA from 5-azacytidine-treated tissue by sucrose gradient centrifugation and tested various RNA fractions obtained for inhibitory activity (Lu and Randerath 1980). A slowly sedimenting (4–7 S) RNA from the livers of mice treated with 5-azacytidine, when present in an in vitro tRNA methyltransferase assay, was found to decrease the activity of tRNA cytosine-5-methyltransferase specifically without having an effect on other methylases. The inhibition of tRNA cytosine-5-methyltransferase by such added RNA is shown in Fig. 10. Figure 11 illustrates that the extent of inhibition of 5-methylcytosine formation depended on the amount of drug-treated RNA added. It was also found that the pretreatment of mice with actinomycin D or D-galactosamine prior to the administration of 5-azacytidine effectively prevented the formation of such inhibitory RNA, as determined by in vitro tRNA methyltransferase assay (Lu and Randerath 1980). The 4–7 S RNA fraction is known to consist mainly of tRNA and pre-tRNA. The most plausible explanation of these results is that after drug administration 5-azacytidine is incorporated into pre-tRNA and tRNA. Some of this incorporation will occur at the sites normally destined to be modified to 5-methylcytosine. The enzyme presumably binds strongly to such sites without being able to methylate them. In view of the prolonged effects seen in vivo, it may be postulated that this interaction between fraudulent nucleic acid and modifying enzyme is irreversible.

Similar observations were recently made by us with DNA preparations isolated from L1210 cells that had been treated in vivo with 10 or 100 mg/kg of 5-azacytidine for 4 h. (Such DNAs contained almost normal amounts of 5-methylcytosine.) The DNA exposed to 10 mg/kg of drug inhibited DNA methylase in vitro to 75% of control; the reduction amounted to 50% for DNA exposed to 100 mg/kg of drug. These data are consistent with a direct inactivation of DNA methylase by DNA containing incorporated 5-azacytidine.

The possibility, demonstrated here, that fraudulent nucleic acids may play an active role in modulating the activities of enzymes involved in normal nucleic acid metabolism deserves further investigation. The functional properties of drug-altered nucleic acids also need to be explored. Work in our laboratory (Harris and Randerath 1978) has shown that 5-methylcytidine-deficient tRNA can be aminoacylated normally, suggesting that 5-methylcytosine may be involved in different functions of tRNA which have yet to be determined. Drug-altered nucleic acids may thus become important tools for probing the functions of modified constituents in nucleic acids. The relevance of the observed inhibitory effects for the antineoplastic actions of the pyrimidine analogs also needs to be explored. However, in view of increased methylase activities in cancerous cells and the functional importance of the modified

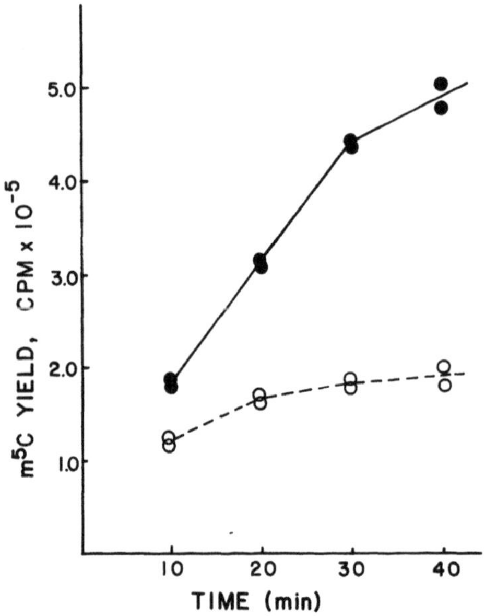

Fig. 10. Time course of 5-methylcytosine formation in *E. coli* B tRNA by normal mouse liver enzyme in the presence of mouse liver 4–7-S RNA isolated from control mice (●) or mice treated with 5-azacytidine (32 mg/kg) for 2 h (○). Thirty micrograms RNA were added to the in vitro assay

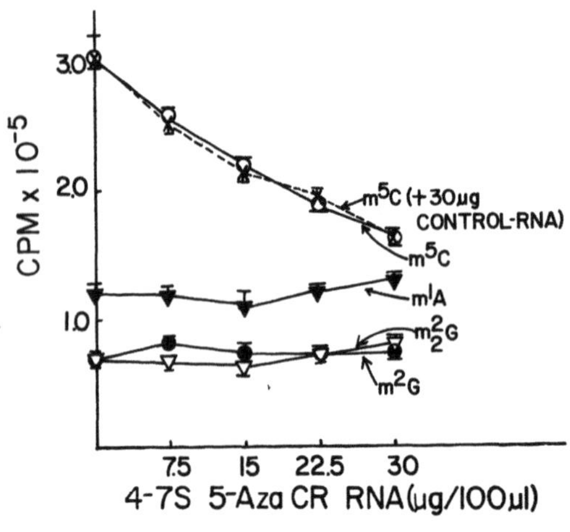

Fig. 11. Concentration-dependent inhibition of tRNA 5-methylcytosine formation by 4–7-S RNA from 5-azacytidine-treated tissue. RNA was isolated from mice treated for 2 h with 5-azacytidine (32 mg/kg). ○, 5-methylcytosine yield in the presence of varying amounts of drug-treated RNA. ×, radioactivity incorporated into 5-methylcytosine of *E. coli* B tRNA in the presence of 30 µg control RNA and varying amounts of drug-treated RNA as indicated. The formation of 1-methyladenosine, N^2-methylguanosine, and N^2,N^2-dimethylguanosine in the presence of drug-treated RNA has also been indicated

nucleosides, it appears likely that the pyrimidine analogs, at least in part, exert their antitumor actions by interfering with nucleic acid modification reactions.

As indicated schematically in Fig. 12, various processes may lead to the formation of undermodified tRNA in the cell. It may be speculated that this results in two major effects: increased degradation of tRNA due to reduced stability and perhaps activation of nucleases, and an overall increase in the synthesis of modifying enzymes. Increased degradation in turn gives rise to increased excretion of modified nucleosides in the urine, which has been well documented (Borek and Kerr 1972; Kerr 1978; Gehrke et al. 1979). Increased synthesis of modifying enzymes may be regarded as a response of the cell to the presence of undermodified tRNA. Our observation that 5-azacytidine on the one hand causes a severe reduction of the amount of 5-methylcytosine in tRNA, and on the other hand leads to greatly increased activities of several tRNA-modifying

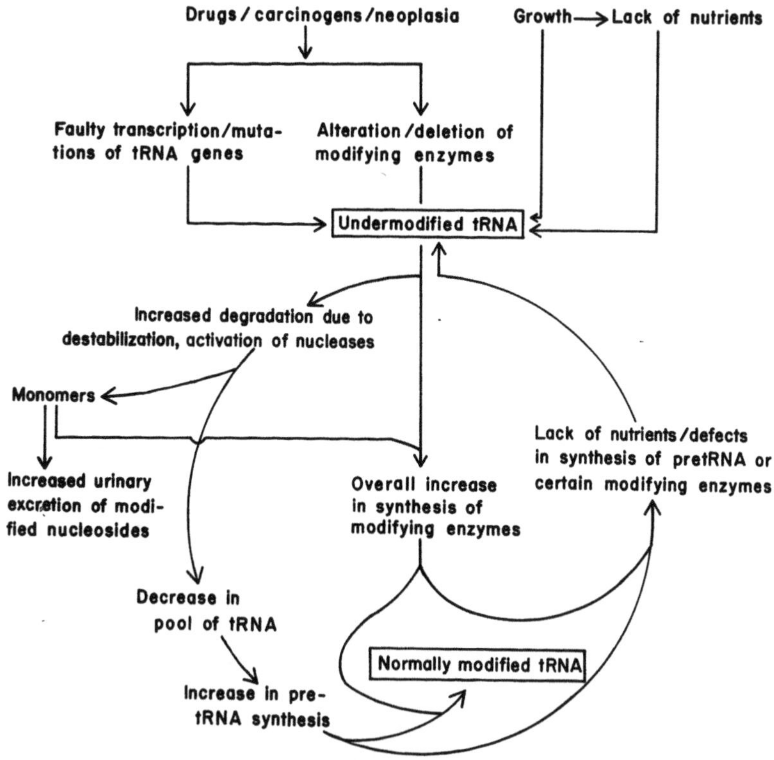

Fig. 12. Possible relationships between undermodified tRNA, induced by a variety of factors as indicated, and increases in tRNA turnover, urinary excretion of modified nucleosides, and levels of tRNA modifying enzymes

enzymes, would be in line with this assumption. Increased degradation of tRNA results in reduced intracellular tRNA concentrations which in turn would stimulate enhanced pre-tRNA synthesis. If the factors that caused tRNA undermodification no longer exist, then normally modified tRNA would be synthesized, as indicated in Fig. 12. However, if lack of nutrients or defects in synthesis of pre-tRNA or of certain modifying enzymes persist, then the newly synthesized tRNA again would be undermodified. Thus a permanent increase in tRNA turnover would be established, as well as a permanent increase in synthesis and levels of modifying enzymes. This scheme links three phenomena frequently observed in neoplastically transformed cells and neoplastic tissues, i.e., the presence of undermodified tRNA, increased tRNA turnover, and increased levels of modifying enzymes.

The scheme also suggests that the reduction in the excretion of modified nucleosides brought about by the administration of antineoplastic agents to cancer-bearing hosts may be due to the inhibition of transcription of tRNA genes. This would lead to decreases in synthesis and levels of undermodified tRNA, thereby interrupting the cycle depicted in Fig. 12. Furthermore, the scheme postulates a new role for modified nucleosides in tRNA, i.e., their participation in the regulation of tRNA turnover.

It would be of interest to explore relationships between these phenomena during carcinogenesis. Several carcinogens such as 5-azacytidine (Lu and Randerath 1979), ethionine (Hancock 1968; Wainfan et al. 1977), 2-acetylaminofluorene (Wainfan et al. 1978), and aflatoxin B_1 (Busby et al. 1976) were found to induce elevated tRNA methylase activities in animal systems, an effect that may conceivably be mediated by the induction of undermodified tRNA.

Summary

5-Fluoropyrimidines and 5-azapyrimidines were found in our laboratory to be specific inhibitors of modification reactions taking place at the 5 position of pyrimidines in nucleic acids. Thus, 5-fluorouracil and 5-fluorouridine specifically inhibit the formation of 5-methyluracil, pseudouridine, and 5,6-dihydrouracil in tRNA. 5-Fluorocytidine, which is partially biotransformed to 5-fluorouracil derivatives in mammalian cells, inhibits the formation of 5-methyluracil, pseudouridine, 5,6-dihydrouracil, and 5-methylcytosine, and 5-azacytidine is a specific inhibitor of the formation of 5-methylcytosine in tRNA and DNA.

Inhibitory effects on tRNA modifications require RNA synthesis, as shown by the observation that various inhibitors of RNA synthesis block the drug effects. An inhibitory low-molecular-weight (4–7 S) RNA, consisting mainly of tRNA and pre-tRNA, was isolated from livers of mice after treatment with 5-azacytidine. This RNA, when added to an in vitro tRNA methyltransferase assay, specifically interfered with the formation of 5-methylcytosine in substrate tRNA. Similarly, a DNA inhibiting the synthesis of 5-methylcytosine in an in vitro DNA methylation assay was isolated from L1210 leukemic cells treated with a high dose of 5-azacytidine for a short time.

Our data are consistent with the hypothesis that incorporation of 5-azacytosine into positions that are normally occupied by C residues destined to become methylated is required for the inhibition to occur, and a similar situation probably applies to the 5-fluoropyrimidine analogs. Analog base moieties occupying such sites are likely to bind strongly, perhaps irreversibly, to the active sites of the particular modifying enzymes. All our observations with the 5-fluoro- and 5-azapyrimidines are in accord with this hypothesis.

It was also observed that administration of 5-azacytidine to mice led to strong inhibition of tRNA cytosine-5-methyltransferase, while at the same time the activities and capacities of purine-specific tRNA methyltransferases became strongly elevated after an initial lag period. We speculate that such increases may represent a response of the cell to the methylation defect induced by the drug. Undermodified tRNAs present in neoplastic cells may also trigger an increased synthesis of modifying enzymes. A scheme has been presented which explains increased tRNA turnover and increased activities of modifying enzymes in neoplastic cells as a consequence of a primary defect in tRNA modification.

References

Baliga BS, Hendler S, Srinivasan PR (1969) Incorporation of 5-fluorouracil into the transfer RNA of *Escherichia coli* $K_{12}W_6$ and its effects on the methylation of uracil. Biochim Biophys Acta 186: 25–32

Borek E, Kerr SJ (1972) Atypical transfer RNAs and their origin in neoplastic cells. Adv Cancer Res 15: 163–190

Busby WF Jr, Paglialunga S, Newberne PM, Wogan GN (1976) Transfer RNA methylase activity and capacity during aflatoxin B_1-induced hepatocellular carcinogenesis. Cancer Res 36: 2013–2018

Friedman S (1979) The effect of 5-azacytidine on *E. coli* DNA methylase. Biochem Biophys Res Commun 89: 1328–1333

Gehrke CW, Kuo KC, Waalkes TP, Borek E (1979) Patterns of urinary excretion of modified nucleosides. Cancer Res 39: 1150–1153

Hancock RL (1968) Ethionine induced sRNA neomethylase activity. Biochem Biophys Res Commun 31: 77–81

Harris JS, Randerath K (1978) Aminoacylation of undermethylated mammalian transfer RNA. Biochim Biophys Acta 521: 566–575

Heidelberger C (1975) Fluorinated pyrimidines and their nucleosides. In: Handbook of experimental pharmacology, vol 38. Springer, Berlin Heidelberg New York, pp 193–231

Jones PA, Taylor SM (1980) Cellular differentiation, cytidine analogs and DNA methylation. Cell 20: 85–93

Jones PA, Taylor SM (1981) Hemimethylated duplex DNAs prepared from 5-azacytidine-treated cells. Nucleic Acids Res 9: 2933–2947

Kerr SJ (1978) tRNA methyltransferases. In: Busch H (ed) Methods in cancer research. Academic Press, New York, pp 163–185

Lu L-JW, Randerath K (1979) Effects of 5-azacytidine on transfer RNA methyltransferases. Cancer Res 39: 940–948

Lu L-JW, Randerath K (1980) Mechanism of 5-azacytidine-induced transfer RNA cytosine-5-methyltransferase deficiency. Cancer Res 40: 2701–2705

Lu L-JW, Chiang GH, Tseng W-C, Randerath K (1976a) Effects of 5-fluorouridine on modified nucleosides in mouse liver transfer RNA. Biochem Biophys Res Commun 73: 1075–1082

Lu L-JW, Chiang GH, Medina D, Randerath K (1976b) Drug effects on nucleic acid modification. I. A specific effect of 5-azacytidine on mammalian transfer RNA methylation in vivo. Biochem Biophys Res Commun 68: 1094–1101

Lu L-JW, Chiang GH, Randerath K (1976c) Effects of DL-ethionine on mouse liver tRNA base composition. Nucleic Acids Res 3: 2243–2253

Lu L-JW, Tseng W-C, Randerath K (1979) Effects of 5-fluorocytidine on mammalian transfer RNA and transfer RNA methyltransferases. Biochem Pharmacol 28: 489–495

Randerath K (1979) Drug effects on tRNA. In: Busch H, Crooke ST, Daskal Y (eds) Effects of drugs on the cell nucleus. Academic Press, New York, pp 275–299

Randerath E, Yu C-T, Randerath K (1972) Base analysis of ribopolynucleotides by chemical tritium labeling. A methodological study with model nucleosides and purified tRNA species. Anal Biochem 48: 172–198

Randerath K, Randerath E, Chia LSY, Nowak BJ (1974) Base analysis of ribopolynucleotides by chemical tritium labeling: An improved mapping procedure for nucleoside trialcohols. Anal Biochem 59: 263–271

Tanaka M, Hibasami H, Nagai J, Ikeda T (1980) Effect of 5-azacytidine on DNA methylation in Ehrlich's ascites tumor cells. Aust J Exp Biol Med Sci 58: 391–396

Tseng W, Medina D, Randerath K (1978) Specific inhibition of transfer RNA methylation and modification in tissues of mice treated with 5-fluorouracil. Cancer Res 38: 1250–1257

Wainfan E, Tscherne JS, Maschio FA, Balis ME (1977) Time dependence of ethionine-induced changes in rat liver transfer RNA methylation. Cancer Res 37: 865–869

Wainfan E, Randle SS, Relyea NM, Balis ME (1978) Effects of 2-acetylaminofluorene on transfer RNA methyltransferases of rat organs. Cancer Res 38: 1852–1856

Session III

Modified Nucleosides: Type and Concentration in Body Fluids and Relevance for Cancer Therapy of Tumor-Bearing Individuals

New Applications of Urinary Nucleoside Markers

E. Borek[1], O. K. Sharma[1], and T. P. Waalkes[2]

[1] Department of Molecular Biology, AMC Cancer Research Center and Hospital, Lakewood, CO 80214, USA; [2] The Oncology Center, The Johns Hopkins University, Baltimore, MD 21205, USA

Introduction

Progress in our understanding of the functions of modification of nucleic acid has been frustratingly slow. There are two reasons for this, of which the first is obvious. Very soon after we announced the existence of methyl-deficient tRNA, a number of investigators entered the field and drew some false negative conclusions from artifact-laden experiments. Methyl-deficient tRNA was used in a variety of simple in vitro experiments. To anyone knowledgeable in this field, it was obvious that these simplistically designed experiments were meaningless.

Methyl deficiency was only partial. The organisms that produced the methyl-deficient tRNA had to be grown to a substantial density in the presence of methionine in order to provide enough tRNA after the starvation. Therefore, at best, half the tRNAs that were used in early experiments were methylated and the other half unmethylated.

Experiments that were incredibly inept were run in systems for in vitro synthesis of protein. The effect of the addition of tRNAs, both fully methylated and partially unmethylated, on protein synthesis was tested in synthesizing conditions that were not tRNA-dependent. The ribosomes that were used were still saturated with the tRNAs of the original host cell.

From these unfortunate reports, it was concluded and accepted that the modification of tRNA has no function whatsoever. These early negative conclusions, accepted by many, inhibited investigators from entering this field. But there is a more subtle reason for rejecting conceptually any role for these modifications. Most of these modifying moieties are hydrophobic structures.

We have been programmed from studies of classical enzymology to believe that interactions among biomolecules must be covalent. We are the slaves of organic chemistry. We teach our students that enzymes make and break covalent bonds. tRNA does not fulfill many of its functions by covalent interactions. The only known covalent bonding of tRNA is its charging by the appropriate enzyme with its cognate amino acid. All of its other reactions must of necessity be transient. Consider its role in interaction with rRNA and mRNA. This must be transient, for once its amino acid is released into a growing peptide chain, the tRNA must be ejected from the site of the protein assembly. Its regulatory function in transcription of DNA sequences must also be achieved by transient interaction.

Recent Results in Cancer Research Vol. 84

Transfer RNA is a cardinal component of the molecular biology of every cell. It is the most complex biomacromolecule in both structure and function. It has a large variety of known functions, and probably others remain to be revealed. The function discovered first, transport of amino acids to the assembly site of proteins, has dominated our thinking for a long time. However, it was subsequently demonstrated in a number of laboratories that tRNA is, as predicted from the species specificity of its structure, a regulatory molecule. It regulates at all levels (Borek 1980). It can regulate gene expression at the transcription level. It can regulate translation of mRNA during protein synthesis, providing an additional control of gene expression. A tRNA molecule is a requirement for reverse transcriptase, which transcribes RNA into DNA. Furthermore, tRNA has been shown to regulate the biosynthesis of its cognate amino acid.

The Structure of tRNA in Normal and Malignant Tissues

Perhaps to enable it to perform its many functions, tRNA is endowed with an extraordinarily complex structure. Its primary sequence consists of about 80 of the four major bases found in other RNAs: adenine, cytosine, guanine, and uracil. In addition to these major bases, tRNA contains a large variety of modified bases that are unique to it. The modifications may be as simple as a methyl group or may be much more complex.

The total synthesis of tRNA is extraordinarily complex. The synthesis of its primary sequence probably requires only one enzyme, DNA-dependent RNA polymerase. The completion of its structure, for effectiveness and efficiency in its variety of functions, is extremely intricate. Of the over 50 modifications that are known, in some cases only one enzyme is required, such as for the introduction of a methyl group to a specific base. However, even these methylations can require several enzymes because the enzymes are specific for bases, positions in bases, and indeed positions in tRNA. At a conservative estimate, as many as 200 different enzymes are needed for the completion of the structure of tRNAs.

Of these enzymes, the ones that methylate tRNA turned out to be quantitatively aberrantly hyperactive and qualitatively different from those of the normal tissue counterpart in all malignant tumor tissues (Borek and Kerr 1972). This is evidently a universal attribute of all malignant tissues. The only exceptions are some benign tumors of the human ovary; in these, the tRNA-methylating enzymes are normal (Sheid et al. 1974).

In turn, every malignant tumor contains a few tRNAs which are different in structure from the tRNAs in the normal tissue counterpart (Borek and Kerr 1972; Kuchino and Borek 1978). Again, there is no exception. These are the first qualitatively different biochemical components of every malignant cell, not more or fewer, but different tRNAs.

It had been known for a long time that all normal subjects excrete in their urine several modified purines and pyrimidines. The origin of these modified bases in the urine, long a puzzle in kidney physiology, became obvious once the method of their synthesis in nucleic acids was discovered. Since modified bases must be positioned with extraordinary accuracy by highly specific enzymes, in order to prevent their reinsertion into forbidden sites after release by tRNA turnover, the kinases needed to convert the modified base nucleoside or deoxynucleoside into the appropriate triphosphate are lacking from mammalian cells. Therefore, since these bases are very stable and cannot be metabolized or recycled, they must be excreted.

There is an apparent teleological reason for the need to eliminate the methylated purines. It was shown recently by Kerr and her associates that the methylated purines m^1G and m^7G are toxic at physiological concentrations on prolonged incubation of cells in tissue culture. After passages, the cells become transformed; moreover, some of these cells are oncogenic when implanted in the nude mouse (Trewyn and Kerr 1978).

It was observed in several laboratories that cancer patients excrete elevated levels of modified bases in their urine. Whether the methylated purines and pyrimidines originate from the death of massive numbers of cells or from specific turnover of tRNA in which they are most numerous was debatable until resolved by two methods. One was a rather sophisticated use of isotopes (Borek et al. 1977); the other, much simpler method emerged from quantitative studies of the excretion levels of some markers which originate exclusively from tRNA breakdown. A normal adult excretes about 2 mg N^2-m^2_2G in a day. A woman with cancer of the breast may excrete as much as 20 mg. From a simple calculation of the amount of this substance per tRNA molecule (ca. 0.6 mol/mol) and the amount of tRNA in human liver (ca. 1 g/kg) we can calculate what weight of wet tissue would yield 20 mg m^2_2G (ca 6 kg). Therefore, the product obviously originates from specific tRNA breakdown and not from tissue destruction.

Earlier we had studied with Drs. T. Phillip Waalkes of the NCI (now at Johns Hopkins University) and Charles W. Gehrke of the University of Missouri the excretion levels of nucleic acid breakdown products in 24-h urine samples from normal and cancer patients. The obvious drawbacks of these early determinations were twofold: collection of 24-h samples is inconvenient and patients are often unreliable. We therefore changed the research strategy to try to overcome both of these disadvantages. We undertook an extensive study to determine whether the levels of the modified nucleosides in spot samples of urine could be related to another urinary component whose level is also a function of body mass. The obvious choice, creatinine, proved to be an extraordinarily reliable baseline for such comparisons (Gehrke et al. 1979). The excretion of marker levels relative to the creatinine level was determined in males ranging in age from 19 to 58 years and females ranging from 20 to 81 years. Table 1 shows pseudouridine (ψ) levels in spot samples collected at 8 *AM*, 10 *AM*, and 3 *PM* and in the total voided in 24 h. In the $\bar{x}$ column of the table, we present the ratio of the concentrations of modified nucleosides (in nmol) to the concentration of creatinine (in µmol). It is evident that the ratios in spot samples are remarkably similar to that in the 24-h sample (Gehrke et al. 1979).

Similar findings were obtained on the constancy of the excretion of other modified nucleosides relative to the diurnal excretion of creatinine. The excretion of the modified nucleosides is constant, not episodic, indicating an endogenous process as their source. In Table 2 we present data on the levels of excretion of markers in a large number of normal males and females (age ranges as for Table 1). The number whose excretion levels exceed the mean by more than 2 SD is what is expected from a Poissan distribution. The levels of excretion are also constant from day to day in the same subject. In Fig. 1 we present data on the excretion levels of markers in the urine of a normal adult male on 5 successive days. The range of excretion of these markers is very narrow relative to creatinine content in normal subjects. There were very small variations (not greater than SD) with respect to age and diet in this study; in general the marker levels were higher in females than in males.

Table 1. Excretion by normal males of pseudouridine relative to creatinine

Time	n	Pseudouridine (nmol/μmol creatinine) $\bar{x}$	SD	RSD%	$\bar{x}/\bar{x}_{24}$ [a]
8 AM	10	22.8	2.60	11.4	1.02
10 AM	10	22.9	1.65	7.2	1.02
3 PM	10	22.5	2.98	13.2	1.01
24 h	10	22.3	1.30	5.83	1.00
Total[b]	40	22.6	2.16	9.6	1.01

Random samples and urine voided during 24 h were collected and frozen. On aliquots of each, pseudouridine and creatinine were determined. RSD%, relative standard deviation (Gehrke et al. 1979)

[a] Ratio for the average value of each (random or total) collection to the average value of a 24-h total collection

[b] Combination of all data for random and 24-h samples

Table 2. Excretion patterns of tRNA breakdown products by normal populations of males and females

Nucleoside	$\bar{x}$ + 2 SD (nmol Nucleoside/μmol creatinine)		Number of normal samples having nucleoside values above $\bar{x}$ + 2 SD per total number of samples	
	Male	Female	Male	Female
ψ	26.6	35.7	2/57	1/73
m^1A	2.35	2.72	1/55	0/29
PCNR	1.33	1.57	2/59	1/35
m^1I	1.62	1.96	1/59	0/31
m^2G	0.48	0.65	2/59	1/29
m^2_2G	1.50	2.20	2/59	0/34
BAIB	8.13	14.03	3/125	2/120

PCNR, 2-pyridone-5-carboxamide-*N'*-ribofuranoside; *BAIB*, β-aminoisobutyric acid

The conclusions on the usefulness of parallel determinations of the markers and creatinine are valid only if the latter is specifically and accurately determined. In the Jaffee reaction with alkaline picrate, in complex sources, some nonspecific chromogens slowly accumulate. Therefore the color development must be quantitated within 5–15 s of the addition of the reagent. We use a "dedicated" creatinine analyzer manufactured by Beckman Instruments which reads out values within 15 with a precision of 1%. It should also be pointed out that these are somewhat sophisticated analytical procedures, and therefore cannot be entrusted to low-level technicians in the blood chemistry laboratory. However, it should be noted that the estimations of marker levels will be invalid in subjects with syndromes that interfere with the creatinine output. We should point out a caveat in interpretation: infants and young children excrete very high levels of the markers (Table 3). This is a consequence of low

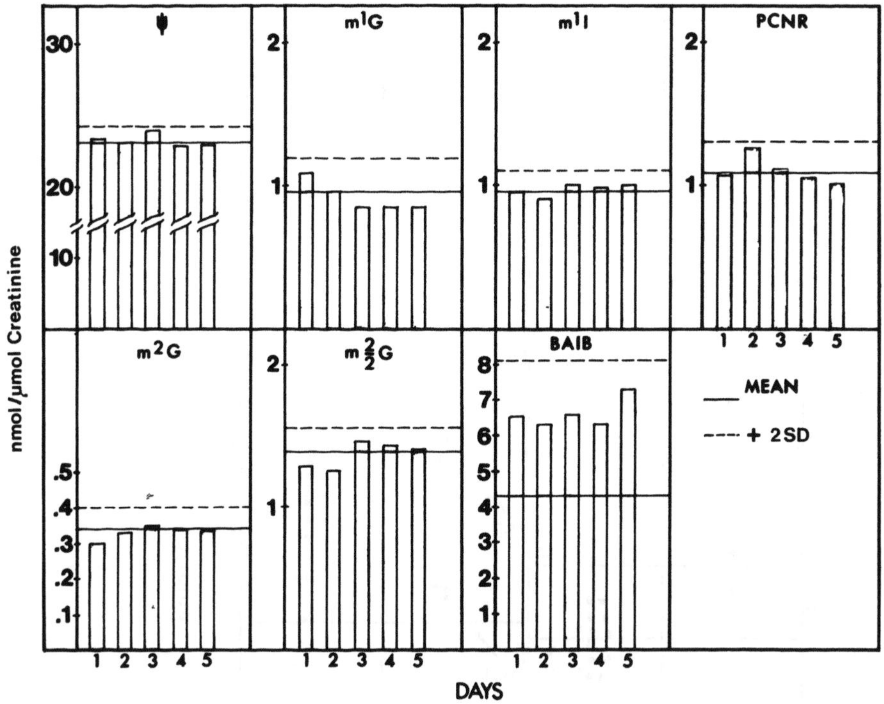

Fig. 1. Excretion of Urinary tRNA breakdown products by a normal male on 5 successive days

Table 3. Excretion of tRNA breakdown products by normal children and infants

Sex	Age (years)	ψ	m^1A	PCNR	m^1I	m^1G	m^2G	m^2_2G	BAIB
Normal adults									
Male		22.4	1.77	0.87	1.15	1.06	0.35	1.2	4.27
		±´2.10	±0.29	±0.25	±0.27		±0.07	±0.15	±1.93
Female		26.7	1.76	1.05	1.18	1.07	0.41	1.44	5.8
		± 4.5	±0.48	±0.26	±0.39		±0.12	±0.38	±4.11
Male									
	5	48.6	3.30	2.13	2.0	1.71	0.77	2.29	3.8
	9	33.5	2.47	1.63	1.43	1.19	0.52	1.63	4.1
Female									
	1	138.0	9.02	1.71	10.68	5.05	2.93	8.33	41.0
	1	96.5	6.60	1.54	5.94	3.10	2.29	5.34	82.0
	1	98.7	6.84	2.17	7.82	4.78	3.25	6.95	164.0
	8	30.4	1.44	1.20	1.35	0.96	0.45	1.28	13.0
	11	48.7	2.97	1.70	2.0	1.29	0.72	2.3	3.3
	12	23.1	1.74	1.05	1.25	1.06	0.53	1.30	7.3

Values expressed as nmol/μmol creatinine

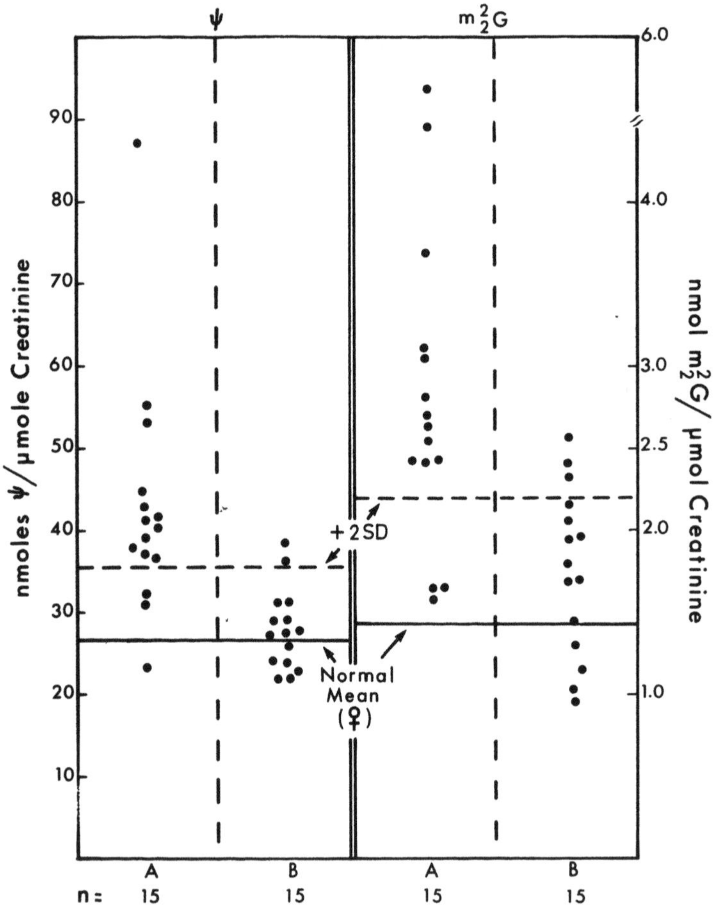

Fig. 2. Studies of urinary excretion levels of ψ and m$^2_2$G in 30 women with cancer of the breast after mastectomy. The two marker levels were highly elevated in both groups A and B prior to mastectomy. Group A had nodal involvement, group B had no nodal involvement

creatinine output. Pregnant women also excrete elevated levels of some of these markers.

In a recently completed study, we found that one or more of seven breakdown products of tRNA were elevated in 26 of 27 patients with 13 different malignancies (Speer et al. 1979). The one patient who had no elevated excretion was on high supplemental thyroxin therapy, which may have caused a spurt of creatinine excretion. In earlier feasibility studies of the usefulness of these markers, the urine of 62 patients with diseases other than cancer was analyzed (Waalkes et al. 1975). The disease syndromes were hepatitis, obstructive lung disease, cirrhosis, acute cholecystitis, acute pancreatitis, regional enteritis, rheumatoid arthritis, ulcerative colitis, and psoriasis. Three of the markers which are most frequently elevated in cancer patients were determined. ψ was elevated by 2 SD only in one of this group, m$^2_2$G was elevated in seven, and m'I was elevated in ten. Interestingly, the elevations were very low in these patients and in none of them were all three markers elevated. It is obvious, of course, that any possible contribution to elevation of the markers must be borne in mind in

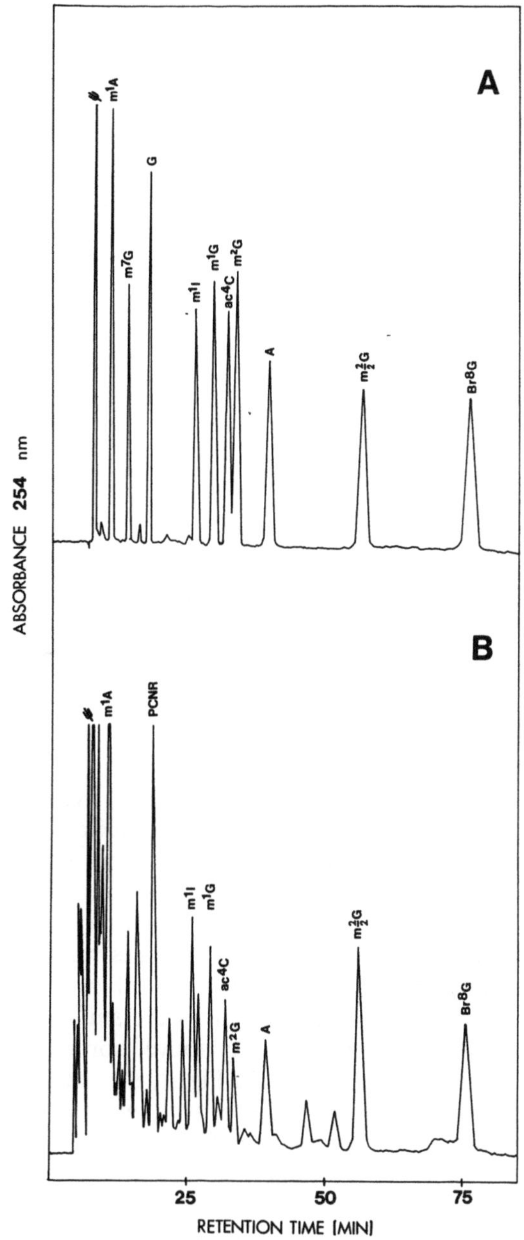

Fig. 3A, B. Reversed-phase HPLC isocratic separation of nucleosides. **A** Standards: 2 nmol ψ, 0,25 nmol γ-bromoguanosine (Br^8G), and 0,2 nmol each of other standards. **B** Nucleosides from urine. Column, μ Bondapak C_{18} (4 × 300 mm); buffer, $0.01M$ $NH_4H_2PO_4$ (pH 5.1) with 5% v/v methanol; flow rate, 1.0 ml/min; detector, 254 nm 0.02 AUFS; temperature, 30° C. The nucleosides were quantitated by the internal standard method, using Br^8G

every diagnostic approach in a cancer patient. Possible interference from the variety of medications which the subjects are apt to be taking must also be borne in mind. However, the fractionation by HPLC is so exquisitely discriminating that interfering urinary components are readily recognized during the analysis. The reason for the variation in the elevations of different modified nucleosides in cancer patients is unclear. It may result from the selective breakdown of some tRNAs, or some of the modified nucleosides may be metabolized by the bacterial flora of the genitourinary tract.

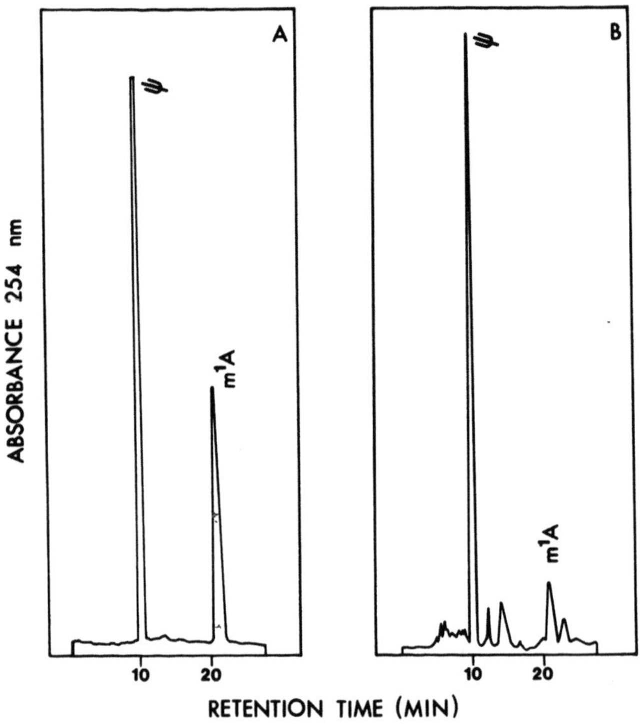

Fig. 4A, B. Reversed-phase HPLC isocratic separation of ψ and m'A. **A** standards; **B** ψ and m'A from urine. 2 nmol ψ, 0.2 nmol m'A. Experimental details were as described in Fig. 3, except that the elution buffer consisted of 1% methanol and quantitation was done by the external standard method

In collaboration with Drs. T. Phillip Waalkes and Charles W. Gehrke, we studied the excretion levels of five modified nucleosides by 15 women with cancer of the breast. (The markers determined have since been increased to seven.) All but one patient excreted elevated levels of one or more nucleosides. Unfortunately, no clinical data was available to us on the one exception.

To ascertain whether the markers return to normal levels after surgery for breast cancer as they do after surgical intervention in other malignancies, 30 female candidates for mastectomy, were studied before and after surgery. Prior to surgery, they were all excreting above normal levels of the two markers, ψ and m_2^2G (dimethylguanosine). In Fig. 2, the excretion levels of the two markers are indicated after surgery in subjects with no nodal involvement and in subjects with nodal involvement. Among the subjects with no nodal involvement, there were only two who excreted higher than 2 SD ψ and three who excreted m_2^2G at significantly elevated levels. Among those with nodal involvement, there were 12 who continued to excrete ψ and 12 who continued to excrete high levels of m_2^2G.

Since several contributors to this volume are highly knowledgeable about marker methodology and have extensive accumulated experience, the reader might be referred to the chapter (Gehrke et al.) by those colleagues who improved and extended our methodologies (Fig. 3 and 4 show reversed-phase HPLC separation of modified nucleosides.) We would therefore like to restrict our contribution to some of the novel findings which have emerged in our laboratory in the recent past. At least two of them appeared as gifts from the goddess of serendipity.

We noted very early that after effective chemotherapy the nucleoside markers return to normal very soon after the commencement of therapy (Fig. 5). The mechanism of

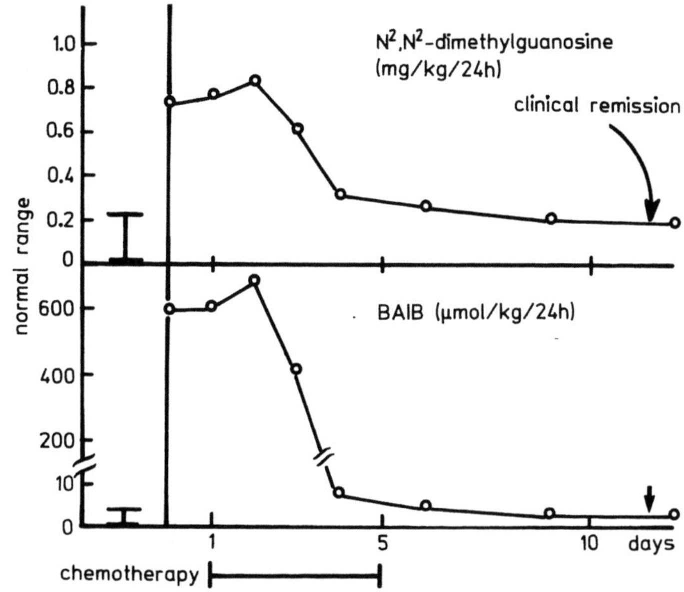

Fig. 5. The 24-h urinary excretion of m_2^2G and BAIB by a patient with Burkitt's lymphoma before, during, and after chemotherapy

the phenomenon is utterly baffling. For example, in Burkitt's lymphoma, where the original observations were made, there is some residual tumor mass 5 days after the commencement of therapy. Therefore we must assume that chemotherapeutic agents intrude somehow into the malignant metabolic process. The mechanism bears exploration.

We turned our attention to determine the generality, if any, of the cessation of excretion after effective chemotherapy. Children's acute leukemia is known to respond well to chemotherapy. Therefore we followed the excretion levels of the nucleosides in three children with acute T-cell lymphocytic leukemia (Odom and Borek, to be published). The purine and pyrimidine markers, as well as β-amino-isobutyric acid (BAIB), returned to normal levels 10 days after commencement of therapy. However, let us focus only on an unexpected phenomenon with the excretion of BAIB.

After 90 days, BAIB levels in the urine of all three children spiked enormously (Fig. 6). Since fortunately all three showed the effect, we could rule out some trivial technical problem. Inquiry to the pediatric oncologist revealed that all three children received around that time enormous doses of X-irradiation to their crania to control so-called sanctuary remnants of tumor cells. Upon receipt of this intelligence, the origin of the BAIB became obvious to a former radiation biologist (Borek and Ryan 1973). X-irradiation, as well as others, inflicts damage on the DNA, and repair enzymes are mobilized by the so-called SOS phenomenon. Large segments are excised and these are degraded by exonucleases. Hence the high excretion of BAIB, which, of course, stems from the degradation of thymine (Fig. 7).

We were not aware of any similar observation in the literature, but fortunately the same phenomenon was pointed out to us during a lecture in Copenhagen by Dr. Fliedner, who was part of a research team investigating some people exposed in 1958 in Oak Ridge Atomic Energy Laboratories to large doses of radiation because of an accidental assembly of a critical geometry of uranium. One worker was killed, but

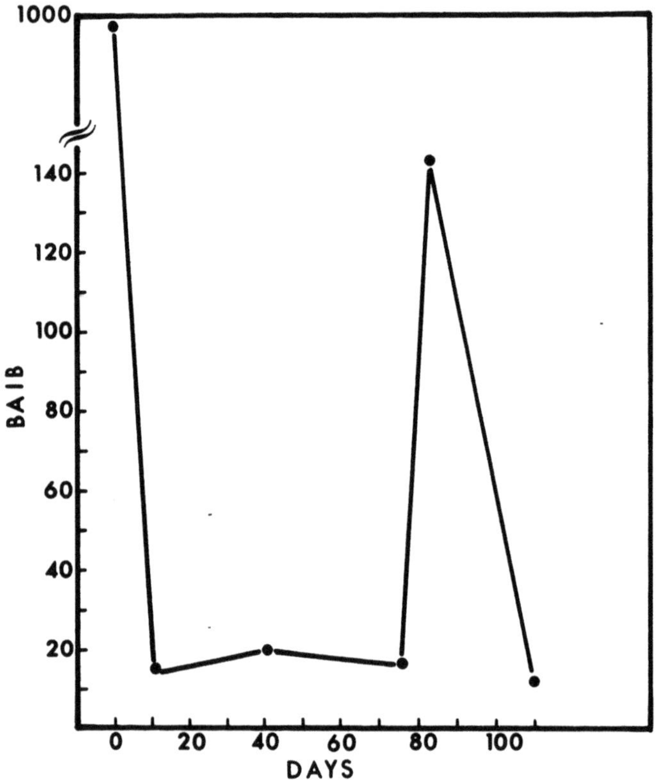

Fig. 6. The urinary excretion pattern of BAIB relative to creatinine of a child with T-cell acute lymphocytic leukemia before (day 0) and after chemotherapy and X-ray therapy. The spiking at day 82 followed extensive X-ray exposure of the cranium to reach sanctuary remnants of tumor cells beyond the blood-brain barrier

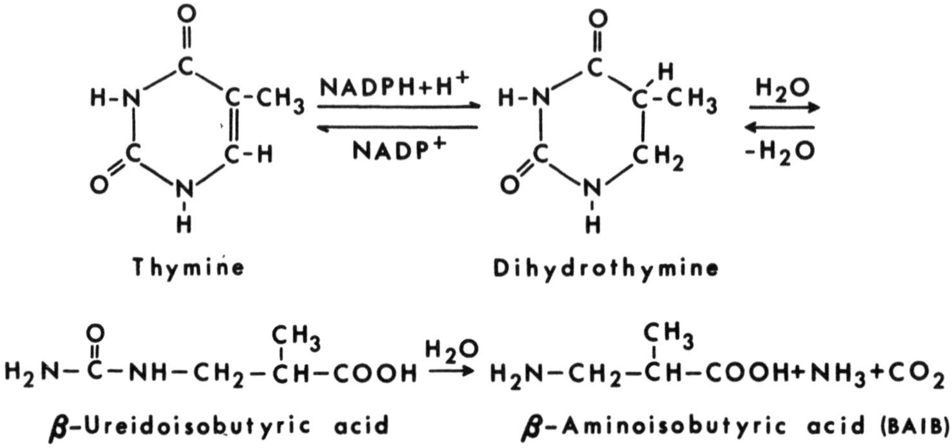

Fig. 7. The pathway of degradation of thymine to BAIB

eight others survived. Depending upon their position relative to the source of neutron and gamma irradiation, they received from 21 to 276 rads. BAIB was identified in their urine in excretion levels approximately proportional to the radiation received (Table 4).

Table 4. Urine BAIB excretion following radiation exposure based on 10-ml aliquots

Early estimated exposure (rads)	Patient							
	A	B	C	D	E	F	G	H
Neutrons	66	45	55	57	39	14	8	4
Gamma	210	143	175	182	114	43	34	17
Total	276	188	230	239	153	57	42	21
Final estimate exposure (rads)	365	270	339	327	236	68.5	68.5	22.8
BAIB level								
Day 3	+ +	0	+	+ +	±	+	0	0
Day 4	+ + +	+	+ +	+ +	+	0	0	0
Day 5	+ +	±	+	+	±			
Day 6	+ +	±	+	+	0			
Day 7	+	±	+	+	±			
Day 8	+	±	+	±	±			

0 = 0–50 μM/liter
± = 50–75 μM/liter
+ = 75–125 μM/liter
+ + = 125–250 μM/liter
+ + + = 250–500 μM/liter
Rubini et al. (1959)

In collaboration with Dr. Edward Gillette, Professor of Veterinary Oncology at the Colorado State University, we have repeated the phenomenon with dogs. In a few simple experiments, we have obtained data which indicate that BAIB excretion is indeed proportional to the irradiation dose.

A normal dog excretes 3 nmol BAIB/μmol creatinine. A dog under therapy for squamous cell carcinoma excreted 4.3 nmol of BAIB/μmol creatinine upon receipt of 375 rads to the afflicted area. After a cumulative dose of 1125 rads, it excreted 5.3 nmol. After a cumulative dose of 1875 rads, it excreted 8 nmol.

When fully explored, the determination of BAIB in the urine of subjects may offer certain advantages. For example, it might serve as a reliable biological dosimeter of radiation. The extent of cell destruction by irradiation may be assessed in individual patients by the level of BAIB excreted.

In radiation therapy, we have no quantitative guidelines which can be sued for following the effect of a given radiation dose on a subject. Essentially, the guideline is the cumulative experience the radiologist gained through therapy of previous patients. We may be able to begin a more individualized approach to the need of a patient.

Another use of the determination of this marker may be to assess damage from accidental release of radiation. In the case of a minor accident such as the one at Oak Ridge in 1958 or a catastrophic accident releasing large doses of radiation over a community, within 3–4 days of the accident, BAIB level, determined very easily by an amino acid analyzer, might reveal the radiation burden received by specific individuals.

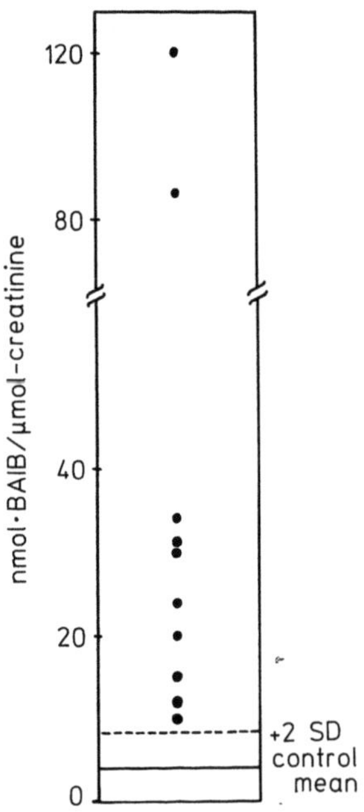

Fig. 8. Elevated urinary BAIB levels (free and conjugated) in subjects with diagnosed lead poisoning

Of course, to achieve either of these goals, we must have accurate dosimetry in humans. This obviously cannot be done experimentally, but we are undertaking such correlations in patients receiving therapeutic radiation.

Still another novel application of these urinary markers emerged serendipitously from collaborative studies with Drs. Irving Selikoff and Alf Fishbein of the Mount Sinai School of Medicine in New York.

Our initial project was to explore how early we could diagnose premalignant conditions in populations at high risk of cancer. Dr. Selikoff, one of the world's foremost experts on cancer in asbestos workers, has a large group of such subjects organized for a variety of studies. We have been analyzing the urine of asbestos workers, and part of these studies will be described later in this chapter.

The physician in charge, Dr. Fishbein, selected patients, had urine collected, and shipped the specimens to our laboratory. The work was done completely double-blind so that we received only code numbers. After our determination, the code and our findings were compared. Dr. Fishbein, properly, included some normal subjects and some patients with a variety of other syndromes. Data obtained on the urine of two subjects arrested our attention. They had no elevated levels of any of the markers except BAIB. We had shown in earlier studies that BAIB can originate from the thymine of either DNA or RNA, but if there were excessive breakdown of tRNA to produce the elevated levels of BAIB, some other markers stemming from tRNA would also be expected to be elevated. Relay of our information to Dr. Fishbein resolved the conundrum. The two subjects were both suffering from severe lead poisoning. Whether lead poisoning produces chromosomal breaks in humans has been disputed vehemently among toxicologists and pathologists. The excretion of BAIB was a clear indication to us that lead poisoning breaks DNA, with the consequent mobilization of repair enzymes and the excretion of BAIB from thymine, which is a product of the exonucleases.

We have repeated these findings in several other patients with lead poisoning, still double-blind of course. In Fig. 8, we show the results of our determinations of excretions of BAIB in ten patients (A. Fishbein et al., in preparation). This observation again raises a number of questions as to the practical use to which such a determination may be put. How early and at what dose level of lead would the excretion become elevated? Dosimetry as a relation between the level of intoxication and the level of excretion must be correlated. Obviously this cannot be done on humans, but fortunately we were able to elicit the cooperation of Dr. Walter Farkas of the University of Tennessee, who is one of the foremost experts on the molecular effects of lead poisoning. The marmoset is the experimental animal of choice in such studies, and we have already found in preliminary studies that the marmoset does indeed excrete BAIB upon lead poisoning. Therefore we have an experimental animal as a model for studies which we are pursuing in collaboration with Dr. Farkas.

Clinical Studies

We are exploring several areas for the applicability of the measurement of markers in unusual situations where other diagnostic methods are either difficult or unreliable. As stated earlier, we are exploring the possibility of early diagnosis in subjects who are at high risk of developing cancer. We have been analyzing the urine of asbestos workers who have no clinical symptoms. Also included were some who have a condition which is known as asbestosis, but is not considered to be a malignancy or even a premalignant condition. In 8 of 13 asbestos workers, we found some of the markers elevated. For the time being these observations are meaningless, but the subjects will be examined by CAT scan. Should that diagnostic method also reveal small loci of cancer, then the value of determination of markers on large numbers of such subjects becomes obvious. A routine screening of thousands of workers by CAT scan is, of course, out of the question, on economic as well as other grounds. However, routine screening of large numbers by the determination of urinary markers with CAT follow-up of those who are positive appears to be a highly valuable and certainly feasible approach.

During the course of these studies, another possible useful diagnostic method emerged. Dr. Fishbein sent us, again double-blind, specimens of urine from nine patients with definitely diagnosed mesothelioma. It ought to be added that mesothelioma is difficult to diagnose. It is impossible to diagnose by simple bronchoscopy, and does not appear until the very late stages on X-ray. Therefore a rib resection must be done to allow removal of tissues for examination by cytological means. We found very high elevation of two or more of the markers in the urine of these patients (Table 5), but unexpectedly ψ was very high in each (I. Selikoff et al., in preparation). A similar pattern was observed in advanced cases of small-cell carcinoma of the lung (Waalkes et al. 1981). Why the lung cells, when they become malignant, should excrete so much ψ is of course unknown to us at the present time. However, the method may still be useful in a patient with symptoms of lung morbidity; if small-cell carcinoma is eliminated by simple bronchoscopy, the source of the markers, especially of high ψ, could be mesothelioma.

The urinary nucleoside markers, unlike other markers, are cleared very rapidly after the removal of the source of malignancy. We have been studying with Dr. John Brewer, a gynecologist at the Northwestern University, the possibility of achieving early diagnosis of hydatidiform moles on the verge of becoming invasive. Hydatidi-

Table 5. Elevation of urinary markers in subjects with diagnosed mesothelioma

Sex	ψ	m^1A	PCNR	m^1I	m^1G	m^2G	m^2_2G	BAIB
Controls								
Male	22.4 ± 2.10	1.77 ±0.29	0.87 ±0.25	1.15 ±0.27	1.06	0.35 ±0.07	1.2 ±0.15	4.27 ±1.93
Female	26.7 ± 4.5	1.76 ±0.48	1.05 ±0.26	1.18 ±0.39	1.07	0.41 ±0.12	1.44 ±0.38	5.8 ±4.11
Patients with diagnosed mesothelioma:								
Male	41.1	1.84	1.74	2.85	1.20	0.44	2.26	4.0
Male	114.5	4.85	3.75	5.50	3.76	1.46	4.32	21
Female	48.3	2.78	1.02	1.63	1.30	0.40	1.44	9.4
Male	37.4	3.00	1.66	2.15	1.33	0.65	1.85	30
Male	38.6	2.89	1.76	2.68	1.14	0.67	2.08	2
Male	31.5	2.57	1.16	1.84	1.07	0.61	1.65	7
Male	36.9	2.45	1.57	2.10	1.13	0.74	1.68	6
Male	40.8	3.84	1.82	2.20	2.82	0.59	2.59	6
Male	38.6	2.97	1.90	2.16	NR	0.53	1.96	30

Values expressed as nmol/μmol creatinine. Underlining indicates elevation of values to 2 SD above normal. *NR*, not resolved

form mole is a benign affliction of the uterus in humans. Most remain benign, but a certain proportion become malignant and invasive. It would be of tremendous help to the gynecologist in deciding when to perform a hysterectomy if we could predict the invasiveness of some hydatidiform moles. We have made two significant observations in this area. Patients with incipient invasive hydatidiform moles excrete high levels of the markers. But perhaps even a more valuable observation emerged. Normal therapy for a hydatidiform mole which begins to be invasive is evacuation followed by dilatation and curettage. In seven women who had such treatment, the HCG levels remained high when the nucleoside markers returned to normal levels. These women received no other therapy and were followed up for 2 years. They were symptom-free and several have had uncomplicated deliveries (Brewer et al., in preparation). Thus the source of the markers is cleared very early and excretions return to normal. This could be a very valuable indicator, sparing the patient unnecessary chemotherapy. In our opinion, the most valuable application of these markers may be the assessment of the effectiveness of new therapeutic modalities, and also monitoring the therapy of patients, so that unlike heretofore the therapy of patients will not be based on the collective experience of the therapist. A particular advantage is that the subject serves as his own control prior to therapy.

Summary

In order to extend the usefulness of the quantitation of urinary nucleoside markers, studies were undertaken to explore the adaptability of such determinations for early detection in cancer-prone populations such as asbestos workers. Another study was aimed at exploring the usefulness of therapy in individual patients. During these studies, two heretofore unknown phenomena serendipitously emerged which expand the versatility of the marker determinations: (a) radiation damage in animals and humans causes an excretion of urinary BAIB which from preliminary studies appears to be proportional to the irradiation burden, and (b) lead poisoning in the human also produces BAIB excretion. Some of the practical uses of these determinations are self-evident.

Among 13 asbestos workers without clinical symptoms, eight were found to have significant elevations of the marker levels. Nine asbestos workers with diagnosed mesothelioma all excreted two or more markers at high levels. Some of the ψ levels were the highest seen. Currently the diagnosis of mesothelioma is difficult and painful, requiring a rib resection; however, an asbestos worker with such elevations – provided small cell carcinoma of the lung is ruled out – can be seriously suspected of having mesothelioma.

In a study of the usefulness of the markers in following therapy of trophoblastic disease, these markers were determined in women with incipient invasive hydatidiform mole. After curettage, the nucleoside markers indicated absence of residual disease but the usual marker, HCG, was still markedly elevated. The women were followed up for 2 years and were found to remain symptom-free. Therefore the source of the nucleoside markers is cleared more rapidly than that of HCG.

References

Borek E (1980) Transfer RNA and its by-products as tumor markers. In: Sell S (ed) Cancer markers. The Humana Press, Clifton, New Jersey, pp 445–462

Borek E, Kerr SJ (1972) Atypical tRNAs and their origin in tumor tissue. Adv Cancer Res 15: 163–190

Borek E, Ryan A (1973) Lysogenic induction. Prog Nucleic Acid Res Mol Biol 13: 249–300

Borek E, Baliga BS, Gehrke CW, Kuo KC, Belman S, Troll W, Waalkes TP (1977) High turnover of RNA in tumor tissue. Cancer Res 37: 3362–3366

Gehrke CW, Kuo KC, Waalkes TP, Borek E (1979) Patterns of urinary excretion of modified nucleosides. Cancer Res 39: 1150–1153

Gehrke CW, Kuo KC, Davis GE, Suits RD, Waalkes TP, Borek E (1978) Quantitative high-performance liquid chromatography of nucleosides in biological materials. J Chromatography 150: 455–476

Kuchino Y, Borek E (1978) Tumor-specific phenylalanine tRNA contains two supernumerary methylated bases. Nature 271: 126–129

Kuo KC, Cole TF, Gehrke CW, Waalkes TP, Borek E (1978) Dual-column, cation-exchange chromatographic method for beta-aminoisobutyric acid and beta-alanine in biological samples. Clin Chem 24: 1373–1380

Kuo KC, Gehrke CW, McCune RA, Waalkes TP, Borek E (1978) Rapid, quantitative high-performance liquid column chromatography of pseudouridine. J Chromatography 145: 383–392

Rubini JR, Cronkite EP, Bond VP, Fliedner TM (1959) Urinary excretion of beta aminoisobutyric acid (BAIBA) in irradiated human beings. Proc Soc Exp Biol NY 100: 130–133

Sheid B, Lu T, Nelson JH Jr (1974) Transfer RNA methylase activity in benign human ovarian neoplasms. Cancer Res 34: 2416–2418

Speer J, Gehrke CW, Kuo KC, Waalkes TP, Borek E (1979) tRNA breakdown products as markers for cancer. Cancer 44: 2120–2123

Trewyn RW, Kerr SJ (1978) Altered growth properties of Chinese hamster cells exposed to 1-methylguanine and 7-methylguanine. Cancer Res 38:2285–2289

Waalkes TP, Gehrke CW, Zumwalt RW, Chang SY, Lakings DB, Tormey DC, Ahmann DL, Moertel CG (1975) The urinary excretion of nucleosides of ribonucleic acid by patients with advanced cancer. Cancer 36:390–398

Waalkes TP, Abeloff MD, Ettinger DS, Woo KW, Gehrke CW, Kuo KC, Borek E (to be published) Biological markers and small cell carcinoma of the lung

Multivariate Analysis of Urinary RNA Catabolites in Malignancies: Cross-Sectional and Longitudinal Studies

J. Müller, N. Erb, G. Heller-Schöch, H. Lorenz, K. Winkler, and G. Schöch*

Universitäts-Kinderklinik und -Poliklinik, Martinistrasse 52, 2000 Hamburg 20, FRG

Introduction

It is well known that the mammalian organism handles modified ribonucleosides to a great extent as one-way products. They are liberated in the turnover of RNA molecules. Any reutilization of modified ribonucleosides is basically excluded. Systematic investigations of the degradation of modifying groups are largely lacking. It can be assumed, however, that modified ribonucleosides are mostly excreted into the urine (Mandel et al. 1966; Schöch and Heller-Schöch 1977).

We were previously able to show that the amount of urinary RNA catabolites in children is directly correlated to growth velocity. The excretion of RNA catabolites in relation to creatinine shows a maximum in early infancy, a steep decline in the following years of childhood, and a further increase during puberty, which in boys begins approximately 2 years later than in girls. Thus the slope of the curve corresponds perfectly to the growth velocity, as a function of the age (Schöch et al. 1981). Correlation with age-standardized normal values is therefore a prerequisite for the investigation of urinary RNA catabolites in children. With the help of a regression equation calculated for all RNA catabolites which we have determined so far in correlation to the creatinine content of a urine sample examined, it can be seen whether the excretion of single RNA catabolites by a child suspected to be ill falls into the normal range (Schöch et al. 1981).

Furthermore, we know that the pattern of mean values of urinary RNA catabolites changes in the course of growth (Schöch and Heller-Schöch 1977). We interpret this age dependence of the excretion of RNA catabolites as follows. Protein synthesis is largely organ-specific; for example, an erythrocyte produces almost exclusively hemoglobin, whereas a liver cell produces a broad spectrum of humoral and cellular proteins. Thus the RNA must be organ-specific. It can therefore be assumed that each organ, depending on the intensity of growth and metabolism, contributes specifically to the total balance of urinary RNA catabolites. As we know, during childhood single organs grow at different rates, for instance, in the postnatal period particularly the

* We are indebted to Privatdozent Dr. H. Becker, Prof. Dr. G. Trams, and Prof. Dr. K. von Windheim for the specimens, to Agnes Holtgrewe, Hilma Wolf-Doettinchem, and Gisa Ziemer for excellent technical assistance, and to Sabine Weiland for programming. This work was supported by the Bundesministerium für Forschung und Technologie, Bonn, FRG

brain develops rapidly, later the muscles, and finally the gonads. The total balance of urinary RNA catabolites should be modified correspondingly.
Due to the interference of a seemingly infinite number of metabolic processes, we can safely expect for each single analysis a broad range of deviation around the pertinent mean value. However, as we were able to show for the excretion values of single RNA catabolites, there are in fact remarkably constant and largely nutrition-independent normal ranges, according to age (Schöch et al. in preparation). The existence of relatively stable normal ranges dependent on growth velocity and therefore on age represents an important prerequisite for a mathematical interpretation of the excretion of RNA catabolites.
We are especially interested in the question of whether people with malignancies have an excretion pattern of RNA catabolites different from that of healthy people.

Multiple Univariate Analysis of Cross-sectional Studies

Our analytical methods have been published (Schöch and Heller-Schöch 1977; Schöch et al. 1980), but one fundamental point should be mentioned. A modified module of a RNA molecule will be excreted preponderantly as a modified ribonucleoside (Gehrke et al. 1979). On the other hand, however, m^7Gua is found almost exclusively as a free base. Finally, some RNA catabolites could behave in an intermediary way. We have therefore always taken care to analyse nucleosides as well as nucleobases. With our previous procedure (Schöch and Heller-Schöch 1977) this is achieved by splitting nucleosides with perchloric acid, so that finally the sum of corresponding nucleosides and nucleobases is determined as an uniform fraction of nucleobases.

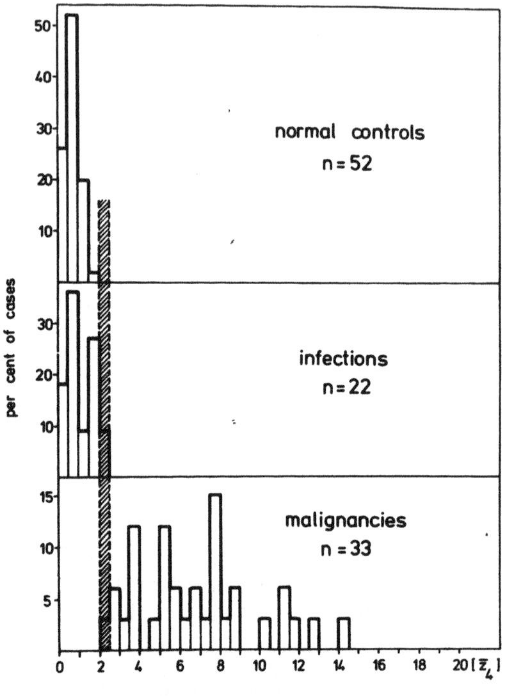

Fig. 1. Distribution of the urinary excretion values of RNA catabolites (measured as m^1Gua, m^2_2Gua, m^7Gua, and m^2Gua) of healthy children and those suffering from infections or malignancies. The shaded bar represents the overlap region between the sets. The z values are explained in the text. Schöch et al. 1979a

By this procedure we determined the excretion of the RNA catabolites m^1Gua, m_2^2Gua, m^7Gua, m^2Gua, and Ade. At first, as is common practice, we compared analytical values of people with malignancies with the range of distribution of RNA catabolites of healthy subjects (Schöch et al. 1979a). For the sake of easy comparison we decided to display our results in z-values.

We expressed the deviation of each measured value from the respective age-correlated mean value of healthy people in multiples of the pertinent standard deviations of healthy people.

A preliminary comprehensive representation of the single RNA catabolite values of a subject can then be given as the mean $\bar{z}$ of all single z-values.

Figure 1 shows that if we observe the mean $\bar{z}$ for the z-values of m^1Gua, m_2^2Gua, m^7Gua, and m^2Gua we can distinguish healthy children from children with infections and from those with malignancies with reasonable certainty.

Multiple Univariate Analysis of Longitudinal Studies

The z-values are especially suitable for clear representation of sequential analyses in the course of a disease. Figure 2 shows the course of urinary RNA catabolites, measured as nucleobases, in an adult patient suffering from CML (Schöch et al. 1979b). The columns correspond to the number of leukocytes. One can distinguish two active phases and a decrease of the number of leukocytes down to leukopenic values during the administration of cytotoxic drugs. The open circles symbolize the z-values for the excretion of m_2^2Gua, which somewhat parallels the course of the number of

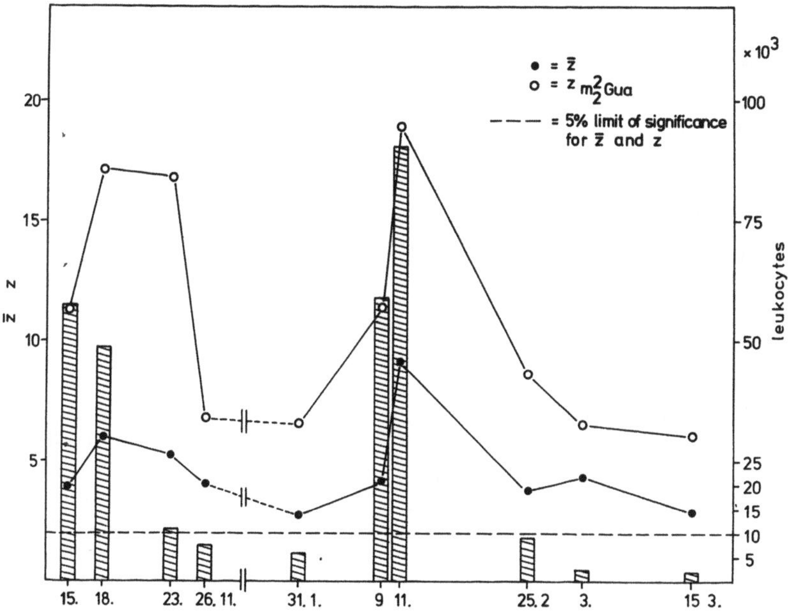

Fig. 2. Mean excretion of RNA catabolites ($\bar{z}$) (measured as m^1Gua, Gua, m_2^2Gua, m^7Gua, m^2Gua, Ade) and of m_2^2Gua in correlation to the number of leukocytes in the course of CML. The z-values are explained in the text. Schöch et al. 1979b

cells. However, even if the cell number is extremely decreased in seemingly clinical remission, the z-values for m_2^2Gua remain elevated far above the 5% limit of significance, which corresponds to z = 2. The solid circles represent the mean z-values of all measured RNA catabolites. As can be seen, the curves are considerably damped if the mean of the z-values is taken. In CML the contributions of the other RNA catabolites are therefore markedly smaller than that of m_2^2Gua. However, even in remission they too remain clearly pathological.

Figure 3 shows a corresponding typical follow-up in a case of ALL in a child. Initially, we find pathologically elevated levels of leukocytes and significantly increased values for the urinary RNA catabolites m_2^2Gua and m^7Gua. After the onset of an efficient cytotoxic treatment the number of cells decreases dramatically. At the same time m_2^2Gua and m^7Gua decrease, m^7Gua to a value below the minus 2 SD limit. Simultaneously, however, Gua increases markedly to 46 z, elevating the mean $\bar{z}$ of all z-values. Whereas in CML, even at low cell counts, the excretion of RNA catabolites remains highly elevated, in ALL, in the course of the clinical remission, complete normalization of the urinary values of all RNA catabolites takes place.

We are convinced that these findings offer a useful new check on the effects of different therapeutic measures and a sensitive new means for early detection of relapse.

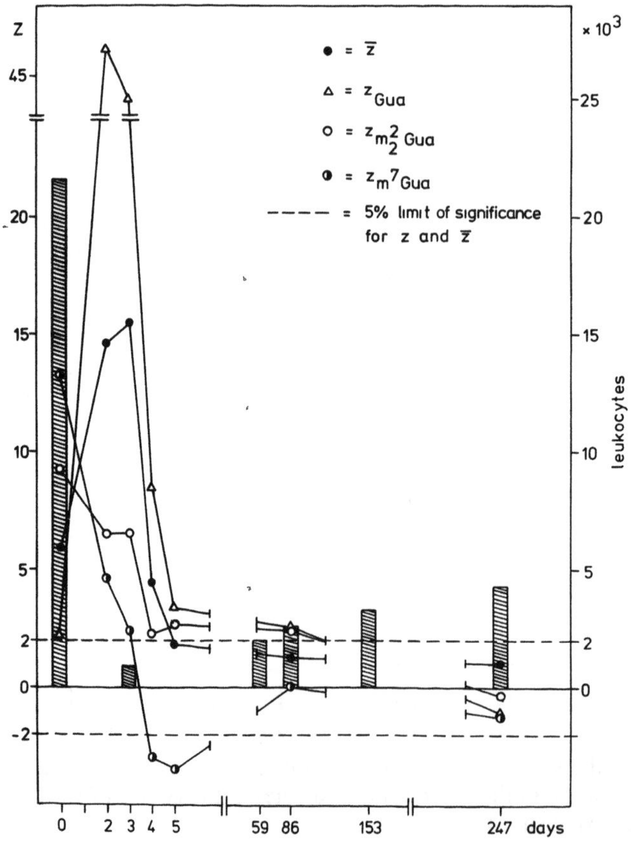

Fig. 3. Mean excretion of RNA catabolites ($\bar{z}$) (measured as m^1Gua, Gua, m_2^2Gua, m^7Gua, m^2Gua, Ade) and of Gua, m_2^2Gua, and m^7Gua in correlation to the number of leukocytes in the course of ALL in a 2.9-year-old girl. The z-values are explained in the text

Multivariate Analysis of Cross-sectional Studies

Automated Evaluation of RNA Catabolites

For systematic clinical application of the analysis of RNA catabolites it became necessary to improve the above-mentioned analytical pilot procedure so that it could be used for serial analyses. By coupling of ion exchange and affinity chromatography it is now possible to analyze nucleosides and nucleobases separately. A detailed description and critical evaluation of this procedure has recently been published (Schöch et al. 1980).

Figure 4 shows the complete configuration of our automated equipment for analysis and evaluation of RNA catabolites. There is one HPLC apparatus available for nucleosides and one for nucleobases. The analog raw data produced by the photometers are recorded by two programmable plotting integrators which also output retention times and peak values. From the integrators the measured values are transmitted alternately to a computer.

Peak values are normalized and retention times adjusted by internal standards in order to identify peaks. The final computation is done according to the external standard procedure, including the simultaneous correlation to creatinine. Results are expressed as nmol substance/μmol creatinine and stored. Personal data of the patients are entered via a terminal. Both sets of data are transferred into a clinical data bank system. With the help of a logical query language any desired group can be described as a matrix, the elements of which are the nucleosides and nucleobases and, in future,

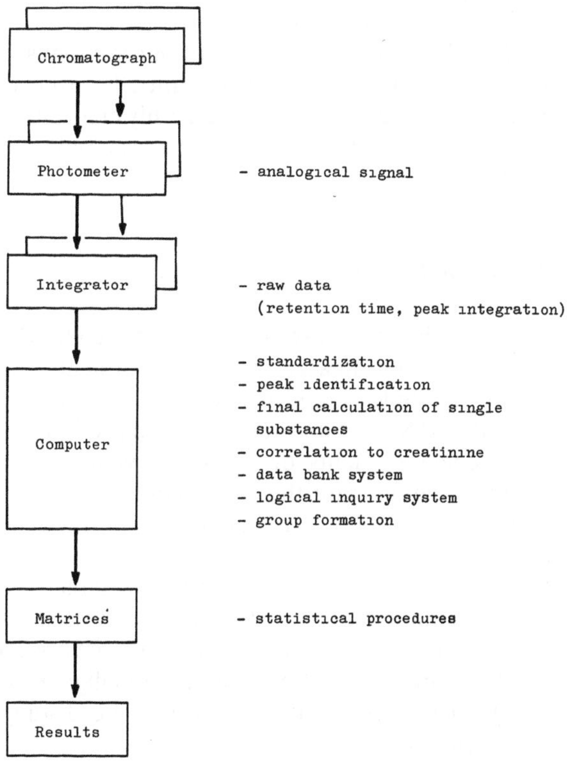

Fig. 4. Configuration of the automated equipment for separate analysis and evaluation of nucleosides and nucleobases

Table 1. Test sample (adults)

	Healthy	Tumor suspected	Tumor diagnosed	Diagnosis (*n*)
Females	41	17	8	Advanced carcinoma of the breast (4) Early carcinoma of the breast (4)
Males	23	19	14	Carcinoma of the prostate (5) Carcinoma of the lung (7) Carcinoma of the kidney (1) Non-Hodgkin's lymphoma (1)

additional clinical data. These matrices are processed using various statistical procedures.

Composition of the Sample

When we designed the above-mentioned largely automated analysis and evaluation procedure our hope was to be able to complete the system in a considerably shorter time than we actually needed. Accordingly, the presented number of random samples is much smaller than would be needed to comply with normal statistical requirements. We hope nevertheless that we will be able to demonstrate some interesting and sufficiently reliable results.

Table 1 shows the composition of our random sample. We used 41 healthy women. In 17 cases a malignant tumor was initially suspected, but this diagnosis was confirmed according to the clinical criteria in only eight cases, four advanced and four early breast cancers. In the remaining nine cases (not listed) benign tumors were clinically proven.

Analytical Results

Figure 5 shows a scattergram of the eight RNA catabolites so far automatically identified and evaluated in a sample of healthy and diseased adult males (there is, of course, a whole series of additional substances in the chromatograms). The eight evaluated RNA catabolites of each analysis are included in a vector which consists of eight single elements or analytical values. In each pair of columns the left-hand numbers denominate the frequency of measured values of healthy persons and the right-hand numbers correspond to the frequency of values measured in malignancies.

We have shown that children with malignancies very often exhibit deviations of values far above the range of 2 SD, but in contrast to this, one can see here predominantly values of malignancies which are within the normal range. One reason for this could be the different proliferation kinetics of malignancies in children and adults. Adults with malignancies could only occasionally be distinguished with the help of the z-value transformation.

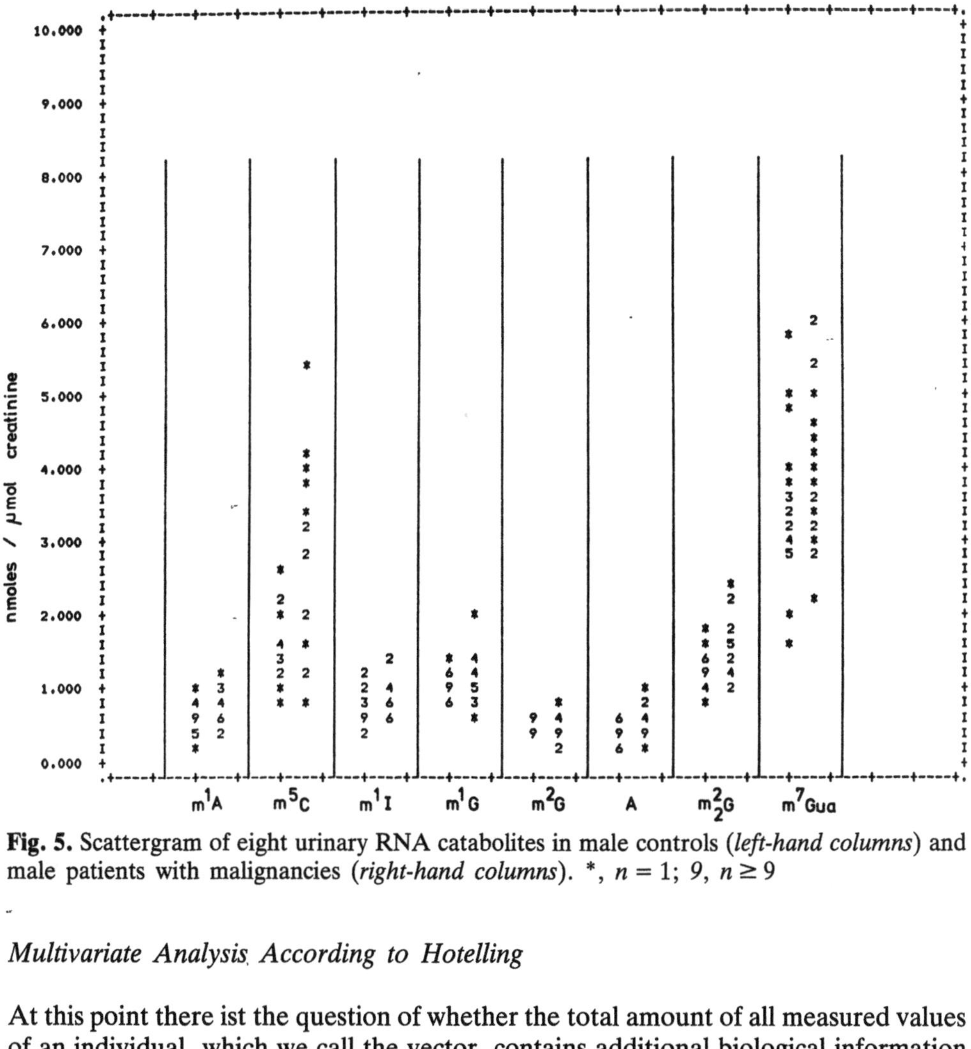

Fig. 5. Scattergram of eight urinary RNA catabolites in male controls (*left-hand columns*) and male patients with malignancies (*right-hand columns*). *, $n = 1$; 9, $n \geq 9$

Multivariate Analysis According to Hotelling

At this point there ist the question of whether the total amount of all measured values of an individual, which we call the vector, contains additional biological information which could be extracted through application of statistical models suitable for discrimination between healthy and pathological. Kendall (1957) has formulated this hypothesis as follows: "The variates are dependent on themselves so that we cannot split off one or more from the others and consider it by itself. The variates must be considered together."

We have, therefore, the univariate description of the normal range expanded to a multivariate one. Here we have to realize that the measured values as vector components span a multidimensional space (Cooley and Lohnes 1971). Subsequently it was explored whether vectors of carriers of malignancies are located outside this range. In other words, we have with the help of the eight elements of the vectors produced a point cloud in a maximally eight-dimensional space and computed an enveloping surface inside which – based on the test sample – 95% of all healthy persons should be located.

For a merely two-dimensional example, the pairwise projection of the elements m^1G and m^2_2G excreted by healthy men is shown in Fig. 6. It can be assumed that the normal

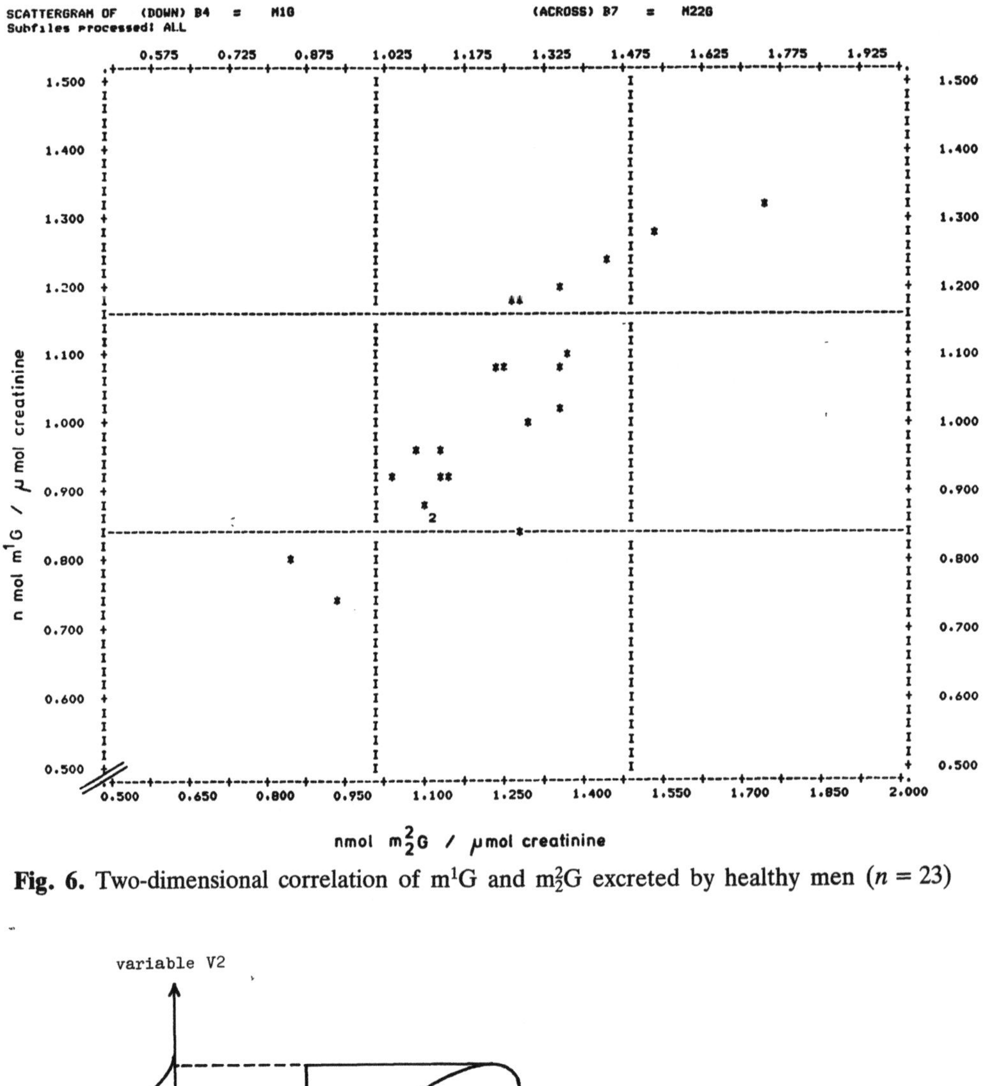

Fig. 6. Two-dimensional correlation of m[1]G and m_2^2G excreted by healthy men ($n = 23$)

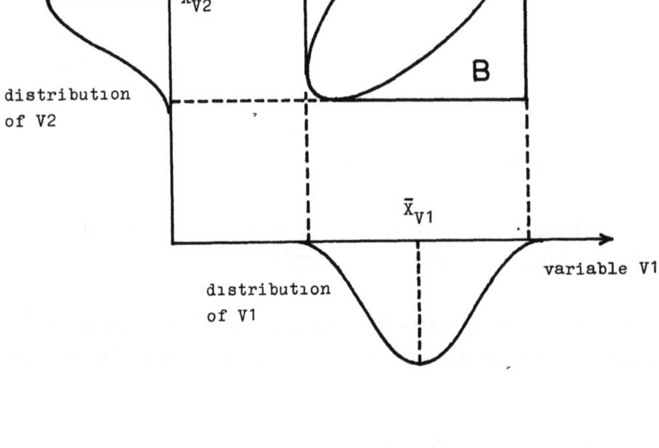

Fig. 7. Illustration of multivariate space of normal vectors according to Hotelling: 95% of all pairs (V1, V2) of a normal population are located within an ellipse. *A*, *B*: areas in which V1 and V2 are located within $\bar{X} \pm 2$ SD although pathological

Table 2. Pearson correlation coefficients (healthy male controls)

	m^1A	m^5C	m^1I	m^1G	m^2G	A	m^2_2G	m^7Gua
m^1A	1.0000 (n = 23)	0.2726 (n = 15) P = 0.326	−0.5010 (n = 23) P = 0.015[a]	0.5076 (n = 23) P = 0.013[a]	0.4201 (n = 23) P = 0.046[a]	0.2027 (n = 23) P = 0.345	0.5757 (n = 23) P = 0.004[a]	0.1263 (n = 23) P = 0.566
m^5C		1.0000 (n = 15)	−0.6279 (n = 15) P = 0.012[a]	−0.0583 (n = 15) P = 0.836	−0.0979 (n = 15) P = 0.729	0.0453 (n = 15) P = 0.873	0.0103 (n = 15) P = 0.971	−0.1667 (n = 15) P = 0.553
m^1I			1.0000 (n = 23)	−0.3511 (n = 23) P = 0.100	−0.3439 (n = 23) P = 0.108	0.2012 (n = 23) P = 0.357	−0.2287 (n = 23) P = 0.249	0.3323 (n = 23) P = 0.121
m^1G				1.0000 (n = 23)	0.7798 (n = 23) P = 0.000[a]	0.3281 (n = 23) P = 0.126	0.8598 (n = 23) P = 0.000[a]	0.0534 (n = 23) P = 0.809
m^2G					1.0000 (n = 23)	0.3376 (n = 23) P = 0.115	0.5749 (n = 23) P = 0.004[a]	−0.0017 (n = 23) P = 0.994
A						1.0000 (n = 23)	0.3156 (n = 23) P = 0.142	0.3384 (n = 23) P = 0.114
m^2_2G							1.0000 (n = 23)	0.2165 (n = 23) P = 0.231
m^7Gua								1.0000 (n = 23)

[a] Statistically significant

Table 3. Two-dimensional analysis (according to Hotelling) of male cancer patients

Patient	Histologic diagnosis	Stage	T_1	Constellation of variables outside 95% range of confidence
1	Carcinoma of renal parenchyma	$T_3\ N_0\ M_0$	3.31	Yes
2	Adenocarcinoma of the prostate	$T_3\ N_X\ M_0$	3.94	Yes
3	Adenocarcinoma of the prostate	$T_3\ N_X\ M_0$	5.54	Yes
4	Adenocarcinoma of the prostate	$T_2\ N_0\ M_0$	2.73	Yes
5	Adenocarcinoma of the prostate	$T_2\ N_1\ M_0$	1.04	No
6	Adenocarcinoma of the prostate (postoperative examination)	$T_0\ N_0\ M_X$	1.55	No
7	Squamous cell lung carcinoma	$T_2\ N_2\ M_X$	6.01	Yes
8	Squamous cell lung carcinoma	$T_2\ N_2\ M_0$	4.92	Yes
9	Squamous cell lung carcinoma	$T_3\ N_0\ M_X$	3.04	Yes
10	Squamous cell lung carcinoma	$T_2\ N_1\ M_0$	3.26	Yes
11	Squamous cell lung carcinoma	$T_2\ N_0\ M_X$	6.12	Yes
12	Undifferentiated lung carcinoma	$T_1\ N_0\ M_0$	5.04	Yes
13	Small cell lung carcinoma	$T_2\ N_1\ M_0$	2.60	No
14	Immunoblastic non-Hodgkin's lymphoma	IV B	5.04	Yes

Controls: $n = 23$
Variables tested: m^1G and m_2^2G
Level of significance: 5%
Cut-off point: $T_0 = 2.70$

range is represented by an ellipse. From this it follows that these two variables correlate.

Rehpenning (Rehpenning et al. 1979), extending Hotelling (1931), has investigated and described in great detail how these correlations can be utilized for the solution of our mathematical problem. Figure 7 represents in an idealized form the assumed ellipse from Fig. 6. Also shown are the frequency distributions for the two displayed variables V1 and V2, by the pairwise representations of which the ellipse is produced. Any constellation of the two variables outside the areas A and B lies, referring to V1 and/or V2, outside the 2 SD range of the normal distribution curve of both individual variables which comprises 95% of all cases. Values which fall into the area of the 2 SD range of V1 as well as V2 are located within the rectangle composed of the ellipse and the areas A and B. Once again the ellipse represents the range which comprises 95% of all normal constellations of V1 and V2. Value pairs in A or B are therefore located outside the common normal range. In analogy to the 5% significance level of the one-dimensional distribution, they are defined as pathological. When using more than two vector elements, multivariate correlations are to be expected and to be calculated accordingly.

Following this principle we were able in about 30% of all cases to confirm statistically a correlation of the measured vector elements in a two-dimensional test (Table 2). Correlation coefficients were observed in the ranges $r = 0.4-0.9$ for males and $r = 0.3-0.7$ for females on a level of significance of $P \leq 0.05$.

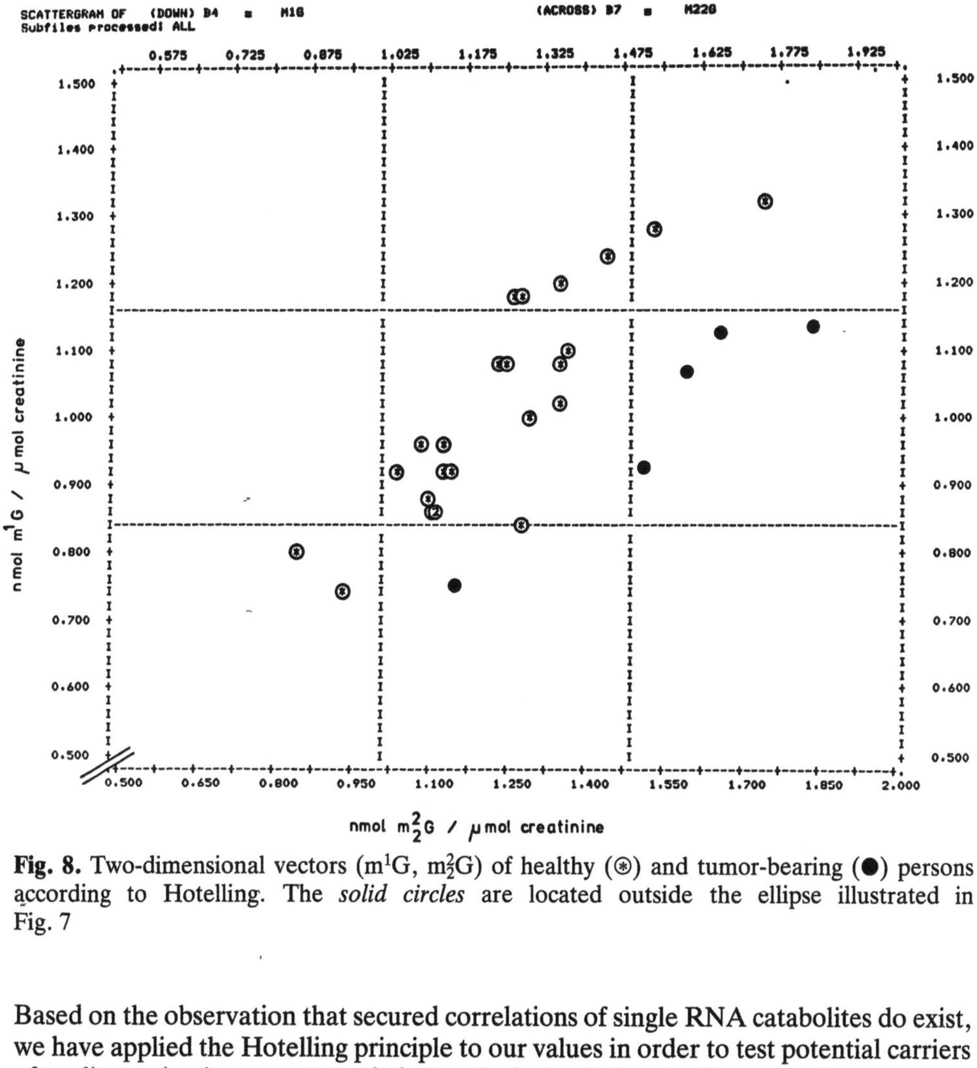

Fig. 8. Two-dimensional vectors (m^1G, m_2^2G) of healthy (⊛) and tumor-bearing (●) persons according to Hotelling. The *solid circles* are located outside the ellipse illustrated in Fig. 7

Based on the observation that secured correlations of single RNA catabolites do exist, we have applied the Hotelling principle to our values in order to test potential carriers of malignancies in respect to their topological relation to the normal range.
Table 3 shows that following the view of Hotelling we were able to demonstrate that 11 of 14 patients with malignancies did fall outside the two-dimensionally determined 95% range of confidence of healthy persons. Again, m^1G and m_2^2G were used as vector elements.
Figure 8 shows the elliptically distributed pairs of elements m^1G and m_2^2G of healthy persons, indicated by open circles. The five solid circles represent pathological pairs of values. According to Hotelling's principle (Fig. 7), these five two-dimensional vectors would be located in area B. If interpreted only one-dimensionally, these values would therefore be accepted as normal. In the case of six further pairs of values in our sample (not shown), at least one of the two elements is located outside the pertinent 2 SD range.
Figure 9 shows the already-demonstrated histogram of all vector elements measured in normal and malignancy-bearing men. In addition, we have marked the complete vector elements of two patients who, using Hotelling's principle, would fall into the

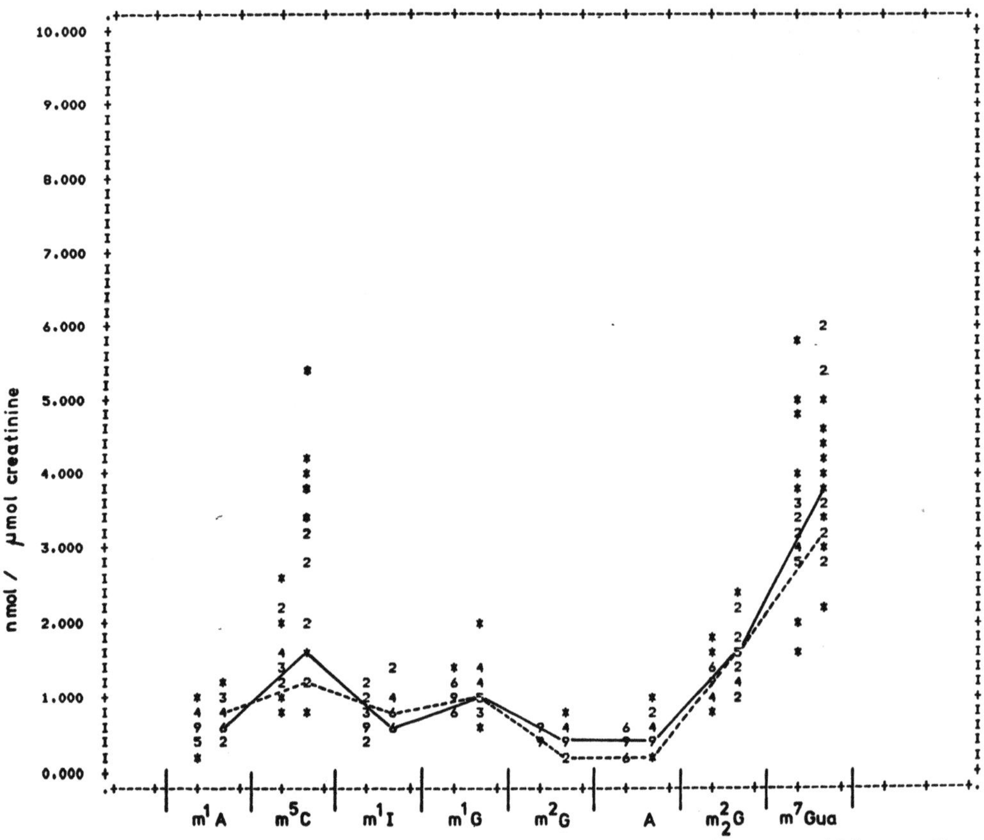

Fig. 9. Two examples of vectors with eight elements from tumor-bearing men, which according to Hotelling are recognized as pathological although all single elements lie within the normal range

pathological area B. As can easily be seen, we have chosen two vectors whose elements, without exception, fall into the range of healthy controls. Therefore the analysis of vectors based on multiple correlations carries decisive diagnostic advantages. Elements which without exception fall into the normal range when viewed in one dimension suddenly turn out to be part of a pathological vector when tested for their two-dimensional constellation.

More-dimensional evaluations produce hit rates of equal or better quality. However, a prerequisite is a stable normal range. The necessary number of normal people should be equal to at least the square of the number of vector elements, that is the number of values measured in each single urine sample. Accordingly, because of our relatively small number of samples we were not able to improve our test results markedly by introducing more variables.

Discriminant Analysis

An extension of statistical evaluation results from the following reflection. So far, we have defined the normal range only by prototypes of healthy controls. By analogy, it

Table 4. Results of classification of permutated samples from a control group (1) and a myeloproliferative syndrome group (2) before and after transformation with $1/\sqrt{x}$

	Group of origin			
	Native variables (%)		Transformed variables (%)	
	1	2	1	2
Group 1	82 (n = 14)		100 (n = 17)	
Group 2	18 (n = 3)	100 (n = 20)		100 (n = 20)

should also be possible to calculate more-dimensional distribution ranges for one or more homogeneous groups of patients suffering from other diseases. This would make possible the use of discriminant analysis (Nie et al. 1975). This method offers the advantage that no correlation of the vector elements is needed. Mainly, though, it enables quantification of the probability for the accuracy of the classification of a given vector into one of the predefined groups.

We have applied this procedure to the largest homogeneous group of patients at our disposal (Schöch et al. 1979b). This group consisted of 17 patients suffering from myeloproliferative syndrome, which comprises CML, osteomyelofibrosis, osteomyelosclerosis, polycythemia vera, and special forms of peripheral pancytopenia with hypercellular bone marrow.

Because of the low number of cases, we simulated ungrouped cases not included in the computation of the discriminant function by permutation of both the control group and the group of patients with malignancies as follows: We have in 37 (20 + 17) discriminant runs extracted another respective test vector from the total number of cases and recomputed the discriminant function each time. After the calculation of the weight factors, the 37 previously isolated respective test vectors were allocated on the basis of the respective calculated decision functions (Müller et al. in preparation).

As Table 4 shows, using native variables a correct classification of an ungrouped vector could be achieved in 82% of cases in the control group and in 100% of cases in the disease group. After transformation of the variables by $1/\sqrt{x}$, 100% correct classification could be achieved in all cases.

Summary

Urinary RNA catabolites, especially modified nucleosides and nucleobases, have turned out to represent valuable new criteria for diagnosis and follow-up of malignancies. Here we show for the first time that multivariate analysis of urinary RNA catabolites can distinguish between tumor carriers and controls who, if examined by univariate procedures, would remain undifferentiated. Two such models have been demonstrated. We hope that a continuation of this work will support primary clinical diagnostic procedures, the control of therapy effects, and the long-term follow-up of patients, which should be regarded as special medical applications of the general principles of molecular biology.

Abbreviations

ALL, acute lymphocytic leukemia; *CML*, chronic myelocytic leukemia; *HPLC*, high-performance liquid chromatography; *A*, adenosine; m^1A, 1-methyladenosine; m^5C, 5-methylcytidine; m^1G, 1-methylguanosine; m^2G, N^2-methylguanosine; m_2^2G, N^2,N^2-dimethylguanosine; m^1I, 1-methylinosine; *Ade*, adenine; *Gua*, guanine; m^1Gua, 1-methylguanine; m^2Gua, N^2-methylguanine; m_2^2Gua, N^2,N^2-dimethylguanine; m^7Gua, 7-methylguanine.

References

Cooley WW, Lohnes PR (1971) Multivariate data analysis. Wiley, New York
Gehrke CW, Kuo KC, Waalkes TP, Borek E (1979) Patterns of urinary excretion of modified nucleosides. Cancer Res 39:1150–1153
Hotelling H (1931) The generalization of Student's ratio. Ann Mathemat Statist 2:360–378
Kendall MG (1957) A course in multivariate analysis. Griffin, London
Mandel LR, Srinivasan PR, Borek E (1966) Origin of urinary methylated purines. Nature 209:586–588
Müller J, Heller-Schöch G, Garbrecht M, Schöch G (in preparation) Einsatz eines multivariaten Auswerteverfahrens für die Unterscheidung von Normalpersonen und Patienten mit myeloproliferativen Syndromen auf der Basis ausgewählter RNA-Kataboliten im Urin.
Nie NH, Hull CH, Jenkins JG, Steinbrenner K, Bent DH (1975) Statistical package for the social sciences (SPSS), 2nd edn. McGraw-Hill, New York
Rehpenning W, Harm K, Domesle A, Voigt KD (1979) Falsch positive Werte bei der Vielfachanalyse: Die Abschätzung ihrer Häufigkeit mit der Sylvesterschen Formel und ihre Reduktion durch eine multivariate Testgröße. J Clin Chem Clin Biochem 17:565–572
Schöch G, Heller-Schöch G (1977) Molekularbiologie und klinische Bedeutung des Stoffwechsels normaler und modifizierter Nucleobasen. Helv Paediatr Acta [Suppl] 38:7–171
Schöch G, Winkler K, Heller-Schöch G, Baisch H (1979a) Die Analyse von normalen und methylierten Nucleobasen im Urin als neues Kriterium für Diagnose und Verlauf von Malignomen. Klin Pädiatr 191:197–204
Schöch G, Garbrecht M, Heller-Schöch G, Baisch H, Leifer W (1979b) Die Ausscheidung von normalen und modifizierten Nucleobasen im Urin bei chronischen myeloproliferativen Syndromen. Blut 38:391–396
Schöch G, Thomale J, Lorenz H, Suberg H, Karsten U (1980) A new method for the simultaneous analysis of unmodified and modified urinary nucleosides and nucleobases by high performance liquid chromatography. Clin Chim Acta 108:247–257
Schöch G, Lorenz H, Heller-Schöch G, Baisch H, Clemens P (1981) Die Altersabhängigkeit der normalen und modifizierten Nucleobasen im Urin als Ausdruck der Wachstumsgeschwindigkeit. Monatsschr Kinderheilkd 129:29–33
Schöch G, Heller-Schöch G, Müller J, Heddrich M, Grüttner R (in preparation) The excretion of normal and modified RNA catabolites and of creatinine under different dietary regimen in children

*Evaluation of Carcinoembryonic Antigen, Tissue Polypeptide Antigen, Placental Alkaline Phosphatase, and Modified Nucleosides as Biological Markers in Malignant Lymphomas**

T. Rasmuson[1], G. R. Björk[2], L. Damber[3], S. E. Holm[4], L. Jacobsson[5], A. Jeppsson[6], B. Littbrand[1], T. Stigbrand[6], and G. Westman[1]

[1] Department of Oncology, The Regional Hospital, 901 85 Umeå, Sweden; [2] Department of Mikrobiology, University of Umeå, 901 87 Umeå, Sweden; [3] Oncological Center, The Regional Hospital, 901 85 Umeå, Sweden; [4] Department of Bacteriology, University of Umeå, 901 87 Umeå, Sweden; [5] Department of Clinical Chemistry, The Regional Hospital, 901 85 Umeå, Sweden; [6] Department of Physiological Chemistry, University of Umeå, 901 87 Umeå, Sweden

Introduction

Elevated levels of biological markers for cancer in various body fluids can play a role in diagnosis and in assessment of response to treatment. In recent years several new substances have been evaluated as biological markers. The usefulness of carcinoembryonic antigen (CEA) as a marker for cancer in the gastrointestinal tract as well as in other malignant conditions has been established (Bacchus 1977). However, other markers are still in the process of evaluation. Modified nucleosides in the urine have been evaluated as biological markers for different types of cancer, and some positive correlations have been observed by Waalkes and Borek (1975), Schöch and Heller-Schöch (1977), and Gehrke et al. (1979). During these early studies the analytical methods used were cumbersome and not suitable for routine analysis. However, with the recent development of high-performance liquid chromatography (HPLC), fast methods with great precision have been presented (Gehrke et al. 1978), and a more extensive study of the clinical use of modified nucleosides as biological markers can therefore be performed. Tissue polypeptide antigen (TPA) and placental alkaline phosphatase (PLAP) are proteins in the serum which may serve as markers in different malignant diseases (Björklund 1980; Holmgren et al. 1978). The aim of the present study was to evaluate the above-mentioned tumor markers individually and together in relation to tumor burden and stage of disease in a series of 63 patients with three different kinds of malignant lymphoma. The different types of biological markers assessed in this study are presented below in more detail.

The occurrence of tumor-specific antigen in human digestive cancer was described by Gold and Freedman (1965a, b). Material from gastrointestinal tumors were extracted

* This investigation was supported by grants from the Swedish Cancer Society (Project 1280) and the Research Foundation, Department of Oncology, University of Umeå, Sweden. Financial support was also given by the Folksam Insurance Company, Sweden. The authors are indebted to G. Lövdahl, M. Sjöberg, and R.-M. Nässlin for skilful technical assistance and to the clinical staff at the Oncological Department and at Vårdcentralen, Ålidhem, for the sample collection. The participation in the introduction of the analytical method for modified nucleosides by A. Byström, T. Hagervall, K. Hjalmarsson, and T. Ny in the initial phase of this investigation is gratefully acknowledged. The advice from K. Kjellin-Stråby during the study is also gratefully acknowledged, as is the critical reading of the manuscript and the continued interest in the project by Professor L.-G. Larsson

with perchloric acid (PCA) and further purified by chromatography and by preparative electrophoresis (Krupey et al. 1968). CEA was identified as a glycoprotein with a molecular weight of approximately 200000 daltons and a carbohydrate content of 50%–60%. To begin with, raised CEA levels were found in sera of patients with gastrointestinal cancer of endodermal origin. However, elevated CEA levels can also occur in neoplasms of different localization and histogenesis, as well as in several non-neoplastic disorders, as shown by the Joint National Cancer Institute of Canada-American Cancer Society Investigation (1972).

Björklund et al. (1973) and Björklund (1980) described TPA as a tumor marker present in the membrane structures of human cancer tissues and placenta, as well as in the endoplasmic reticulum. The molecular weight has been determined as 22500, but it is usually present as oligomers. The amino acid sequence is partly known and the isoelectric point is 4.4–4.6. TPA has been reported to be present in a wide variety of human tumors from different origins and it has also been demonstrated in tumors from other species. The presence of this antigen in serum and other body fluids from cancer patients regardless of type and site of cancer has also been reported. Increased levels of TPA may also be found in sera from patients with acute infections and other diseases (Björklund 1976).

Placental alkaline phosphatase is normally found in sera of pregnant women. It is produced by the syncytiotrophoblasts in the placenta. In 1968 Fishman first reported the appearance of an enzyme, (Regan isoenzyme) in the serum of a patient with squamous bronchogenic carcinoma. This enzyme was found to be similar to PLAP with respect to heat stability, electrophoretic mobility, and sensitivity to inhibition by L-phenylalanine. An immunological cross-reactivity with antisera to PLAP was also observed (Fishman 1969). The frequency of detectable activity of PLAP in sera from cancer patients ranges between 0% and almost 100% (Jacoby and Bagshawe 1972; Usategui-Gomez et al. 1973).

Transfer RNA plays a key role in protein synthesis in all organisms. When tRNA is synthesized in the cell, a polynucleotide is made of the four ordinary nucleosides, adenosine, guanosine, cytidine, and uridine. The polynucleotide acts as a substrate for many different tRNA-modifying enzymes, which change the ordinary polynucleotide by, for instance, substituting a hydrogen atom with a methyl group or an oxygen atom with a sulphur atom. Thus the biosynthesis of these modified nucleosides occurs on the polynucleotide level. More than 50 different modified nucleosides have been characterized so far (Nishimura 1980). It is known that triphosphate of modified nucleosides cannot be incorporated by DNA-dependent RNA polymerases. While the ordinary nucleosides can be reutilized, such recycling is not possible for the modified nucleosides. Thus in higher organisms they are excreted in urine. It has been suggested that the level of modified nucleosides in the urine is a measure of the rate of turnover of the tRNA molecule in the cell (Borek et al. 1977). Although tRNA is heavily modified, there are also other RNA molecules in the cell which contain modified nucleosides.

Materials and Methods

Reference Material

Eighty healthy adults, sampled at random, were used as a reference group. They were allotted to one of four age-groups, 15–30, 31–45, 46–60, and over 60 years, each group equally divided between men and women.

Table 1. Clinical material

Lymphoma	No. of patients			Age range (years)
	M	F	Total	
Histiocytic	13	8	21	33–77
Lymphocytic	12	7	19	47–78
Hodgkin's	13	10	23	20–83

Clinical Material

The patients with the different types of lymphoma were selected from those admitted to the University Hospital in Umeå. This is a regional hospital for northern Sweden and the treatment of patients with lymphoma is largely centralized to this hospital. The diagnoses were based upon histological as well as cytological and clinical examinations. The cases were histologically classified according to Rappaport (1966) in three different groups: (1) histiocytic lymphoma, (2) lymphocytic lymphoma, and (3) Hodgkin's disease. Patients with doubtful diagnoses were excluded.

Table 1 shows the age range and sex distribution within the three disease groups. Samples of serum and urine were taken consecutively from each patient at intervals of 1–3 months. Samples were collected before the treatment was initiated and later during the disease. A few samples were taken during radiotherapy, but we avoided sampling during ongoing cytostatic therapy and the week thereafter. Each patient was allocated to one of four clinical stages, largely according to a system described by Carbone et al. (1971): 1, no evidence of disease; 2, local manifestation; 3, regional manifestation; and 4, generalized disease with infiltration of bone marrow, spleen, or liver.

Determination of CEA

Blood specimens were collected in Vacutainer tubes containing EDTA. After centrifugation the supernate plasma was withdrawn and frozen (−80° C) until analyzed.

The determination of CEA was performed with the commercially available CEA assay marketed by Hoffmann-La Roche (Hansen et al. 1974). To remove PCA and equilibrate the sample in the final assay buffer, Sephadex G-50 medium (Pharmacia) columns were used according to Haagensen et al. (1978). CEA levels below 2.5 ng/ml were normally found in healthy nonsmoking subjects.

Determination of TPA

The serum samples were stored at −70° C until processed. The level of TPA in serum was determined by radioimmunoassay as described by Wiklund et al. (1979). The reagents from Sangtec Comp. (Bromma, Sweden) were used throughout the investigation. According to Björklund (1980) the normal level in serum is below 90 U/liter.

Determination of PLAP

The serum samples were stored at −70° C before analysis. Enzyme activity was measured spectrophotometrically at 505 nm and pH 9.8 with an assay described by Doellgast et al. (to be published). According to Stigbrand et al. (to be published) the normal level in serum is below 0.2 μmol/min × liter for males, which corresponds to an enzyme concentration of 1 μg/liter.

Analysis of Modified Nucleosides in Urine

Samples were frozen and stored at −80° C before analysis. The level of creatinine was determined immediately according to the Technicon procedure. Analysis of modified nucleosides was performed essentially according to Gehrke et al. (1978) and Kuo et al. (1978). The procedure includes purification of the urine on a boronate column and separation and quantitative determination of the modified nucleosides using HPLC. Pseudouridine (Ψ) and 1-methyl-adenosine (m^1A) were analyzed using 1% methanol in 0.01*M* ammonium phosphate buffer, pH 5.1, and the other modified nucleosides were analyzed using 6% methanol in the same buffer. The different modified nucleosides were routinely identified by retention time and absorbance at 260 nm and 280 nm. In the later stage of our investigation we utilized two integrators for the two different wavelengths, making identification easier and more reliable. Each week a spiked sample was analyzed and the retention time of the different modified nucleosides established. The same buffer was then used during the week to analyze the different urine samples.

Results

Reference Material

Figure 1 shows the distribution of the six modified nucleosides in urine from 80 normal adults. When our material was subdivided according to age and sex no essential difference between the groups was found, so all results are presented together. The distributions of the levels of Ψ, 1-methylinosine (m^1I), 1-methylguanosine (m^1G), and 2-methylguanosine (m^2G) were closely grouped and in order to characterize the limit of elevated levels, we excluded the three or four highest values. The same method was used for m^1A and 2-dimethylguanosine (m_2^2G), despite the fact that the values were more dispersed (Fig. 1). The average absolute levels, expressed as nmol/μmol creatinine, were 23.5 for ψ, 1.8 for m^1A, 1.2 for m^1I, 0.6 for m^1G, 0.3 for m^2G, and 0.8 for m_2^2G. These values were comparable to the values of 22.6 for ψ, 1.9 for m^1A, 1.3 for m^1I, and 1.2 for m_2^2G reported by Gehrke et al. (1979). This indicates that the analytical method is reliable and that the level of modified nucleosides in different populations is fairly constant.

The levels of PLAP and TPA in the control material is presented in Fig. 2. Only 2 of 79 normal healthy adults had increased levels of PLAP. For TPA the corresponding figure was 16 of 70 normal healthy adults, indicating a rather high frequency of values above the level defined as the upper limit. CEA was elevated in 3 of 80 individuals among the reference material. These three cases were all in the highest age-group, in agreement with an earlier report by Hansen et al. (1974).

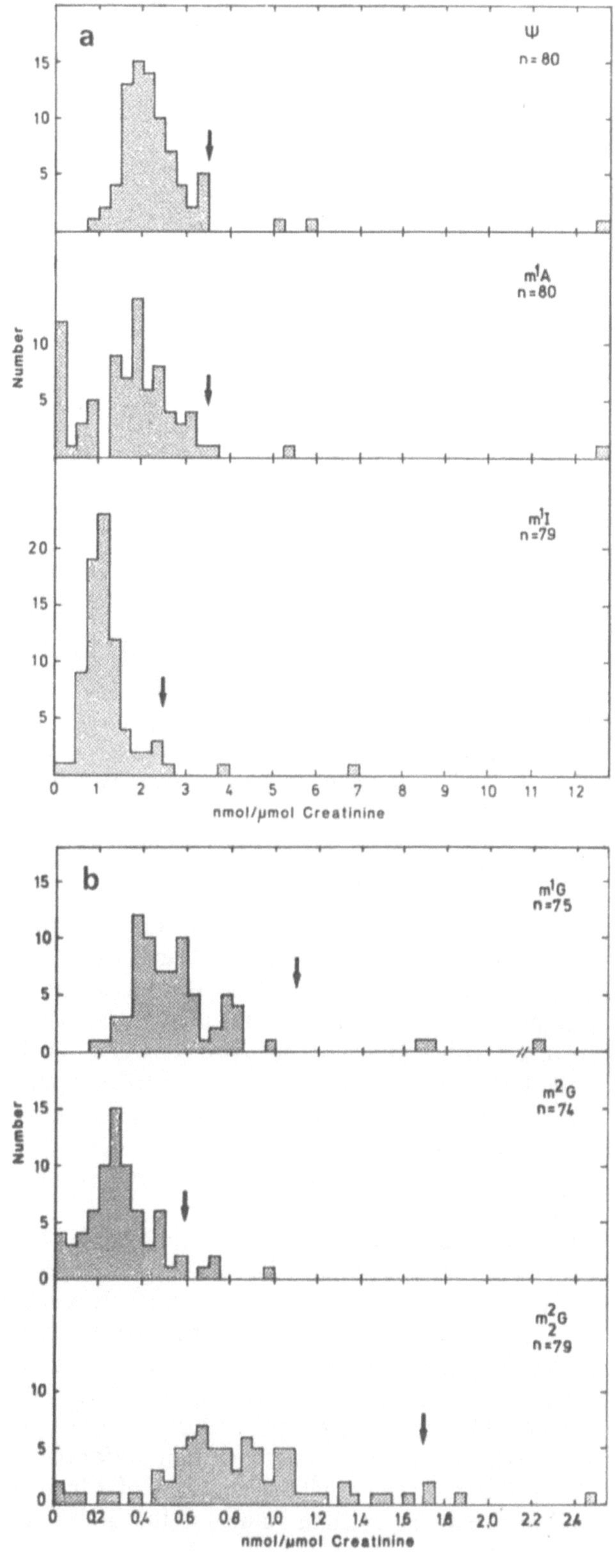

Fig. 1a, b. Distribution of modified nucleosides in urine from healthy adults. An average of 3–4 high values have been excluded and this limit is indicated by an *arrow*. The absolute value for *Ψ* is ten times higher than indicated

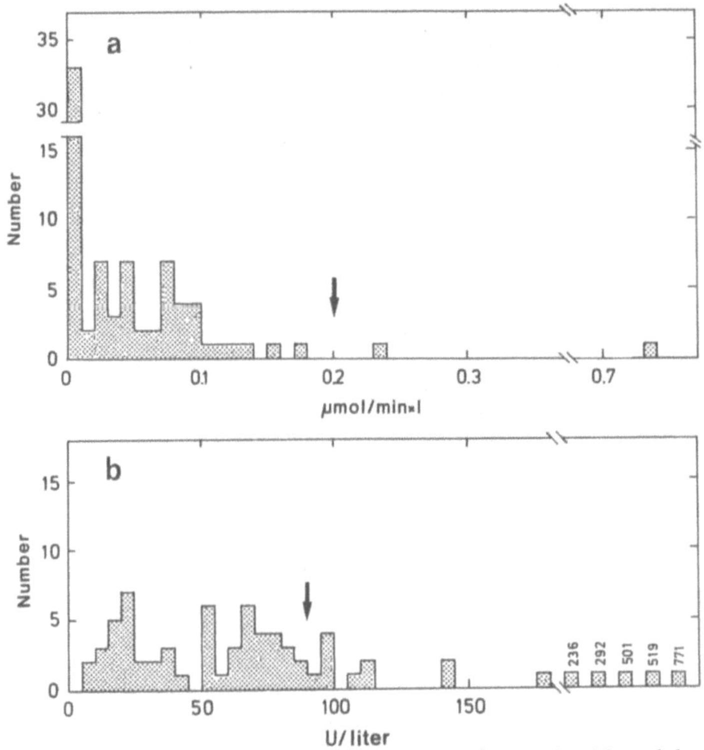

Fig. 2. Distribution of serum PLAP (*upper panel*) in 79 healthy adults and serum TPA (*lower panel*) in 70 healthy adults. *Arrows* indicate the limits for elevated values according to the literature data

Clinical Material

There was no correlation between elevated levels of TPA and PLAP to more advanced clinical stage (Table 2). On the contrary, for TPA a tendency of decreasing values in patients with generalized disease was observed. For PLAP a higher frequency of increased levels was noted than in the reference group, but the increase did not correlate with stages. We therefore conclude that TPA and PLAP have limited value as biological markers for lymphomas. CEA seemed to be positively correlated to stage 4 in Hodgkin's disease, but only 11 samples from four patients in stage 4 were analyzed and more material is needed for a definite conclusion. However, the level of ψ in urine showed a positive correlation to more advanced stages for all three types of lymphomas (Table 2).

The above results are based upon all samples analyzed, i.e., several samples may originate from one patient. Table 3 shows the results from individual patients. It can be seen that the incidence of elevated levels was higher than in normal adults for all modified nucleosides analyzed. Furthermore, there was a higher incidence of elevated levels in patients with more advanced disease. No systematic differences were observed between the different diagnoses for any of the six modified nucleosides, with the possible exception of m^1G in histiocytic lymphoma. Therefore, in this study the multitude of analyses did not give more information than, for instance, analysis of ψ alone. Figure 3 shows that the excretion of ψ increases when the disease is progressing and also that the median value for the different groups increases.

Table 2. Relative frequency (%) of samples with elevated levels of biological markers in lymphoma patients

Lymphoma	TPA clinical stage			PLAP clinical stage			CEA clinical stage			Ψ clinical stage		
	1	2 + 3	4	1	2 + 3	4	1	2 + 3	4	1	2 + 3	4
Histiocytic	41	16	11	26	22	0	4	17	14	33	55	67
Lymphocytic	53	27	24	36	6	11	14	9	2	21	11	61
Hodgkin's	51	30	60	8	17	17	7	24	55	22	7	77
Total patients (No. of)	48	23	26	22	16	10	8	16	14	25	27	67
Total samples (No. of)	81	44	31	102	58	59	203	63	66	125	55	63

The frequency of elevated levels in healthy adults was 23%, 4%, 3%, and 4% respectively for TPA, PLAP, CEA, and Ψ

Table 3. Relative frequency (%) of patients with elevated levels of modified nucleosides in urine

Nucleoside	Normal adults	Lymphoma											
		Histiocytic clinical stage			Lymphocytic clinical stage			Hodgkin's clinical stage			Total clinical stage		
		1	2 + 3	4	1	2 + 3	4	1	2 + 3	4	1	2 + 3	4
Ψ	4	14	56	63	8	18	58	18	8	67	14	31	62
m^1A	4	14	19	50	8	10	67	29	8	50	19	13	58
m^1I	4	14	6	38	8	9	33	11	9	33	11	8	35
m^1G	4	7	25	50	8	–	25	6	–	17	7	10	31
m^2G	5	29	25	63	8	18	42	19	33	33	19	26	46
m^2_2G	4	7	38	38	8	9	33	12	–	50	9	18	38
No. of patients		14	16	8	12	11	12	17	12	6	43	39	26

In patients with several observations in one stage the mean value for these have been compared to the limit value set (Fig. 1)

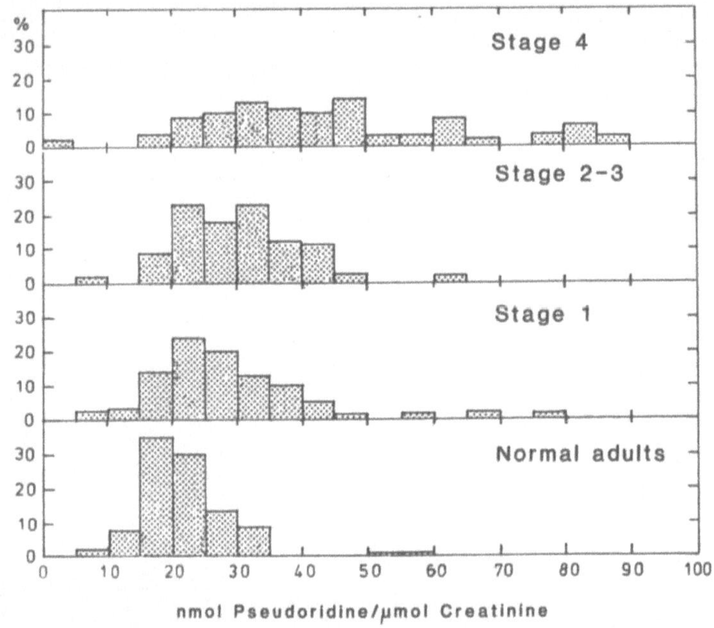

Fig. 3. Distribution of Ψ in all samples analyzed from patients with malignant lymphoma according to clinical stage and from the reference group of healthy adults. Sample number: normal adults 80, clinical stage (1), 125, clinical stage (2 + 3), 55, clinical stage (4), 63. The median values for these groups are: 21, 26, 30, and 40 nmol/μmol creatinine respectively

Case Reports

Biological markers can sometimes be of value in monitoring the result of treatment. To evaluate the modified nucleosides in this respect, samples were taken from patients during radiotherapy and cytostatic treatment and analyzed as described in Materials and Methods. Figure 4 shows two cases where a good correlation was observed between the levels of ψ and (less pronounced) m_2^2G and the clinical stage. Figure 4a shows a patient with a progressive disease and parallel increase of the level of modified nucleosides, while a decrease of the level of modified nucleosides was observed in another patient with a regression of the disease (Fig. 4b). However, we have also noticed some cases where a low level of modified nucleosides was found although the disease was generalized and progressing (Fig. 5b). Figures 5a and 6a show two cases where the patients went through cycles of different stages and corresponding changes in the level of modified nucleosides. Cytostatic therapy was successful and a marked decrease of ψ was observed parellel to the remission of the disease. Figure 6b, on the other hand, shows a patient who during intense radiation and cytostatic therapy still showed a progressing disease and increase in the level of ψ in the urine. Interestingly, the patients in Fig. 6a and b showed a lead time; the increase of ψ preceded the clinical manifestation by up to 3 months. The other four modified nucleosides behaved in a similar way to ψ and m_2^2G (data not shown). It should be emphasized that the levels of ψ and m^1A where analyzed on HPLC using a buffer containing 1% methanol, while m_2^2G and the other modified nucleosides were determined in a separate analysis using a buffer containing 6% methanol, but nevertheless there was a good correlation between the changes of all modified nucleosides analyzed.

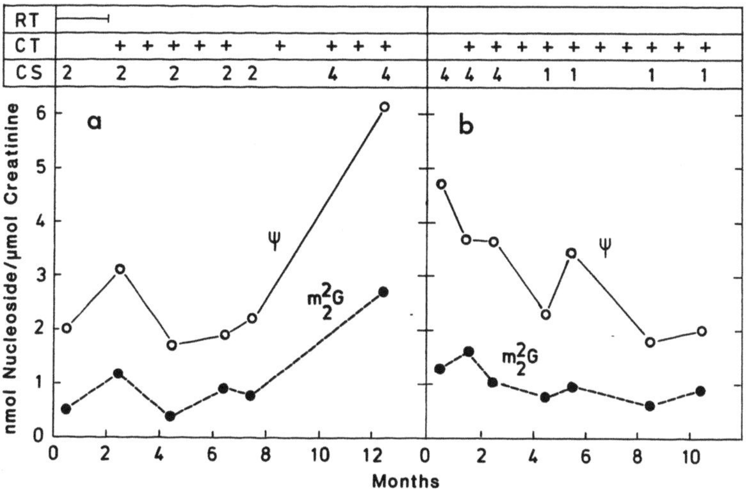

Fig. 4a, b. Levels of Ψ and m_2^2G in the urine in lymphocytic lymphoma. **a** A woman born in 1918. Abdominal manifestation in the ventricle and later in the pleura. Treatment was radiotherapy (*RT*) and cytostatic therapy (*CT*). *CS,* clinical stage. Levels of Ψ should be multiplied by a factor of 10. **b** A woman born in 1922. Manifestations in cervical, axillary, and inguinal lymph nodes. She was successfully treated with CT

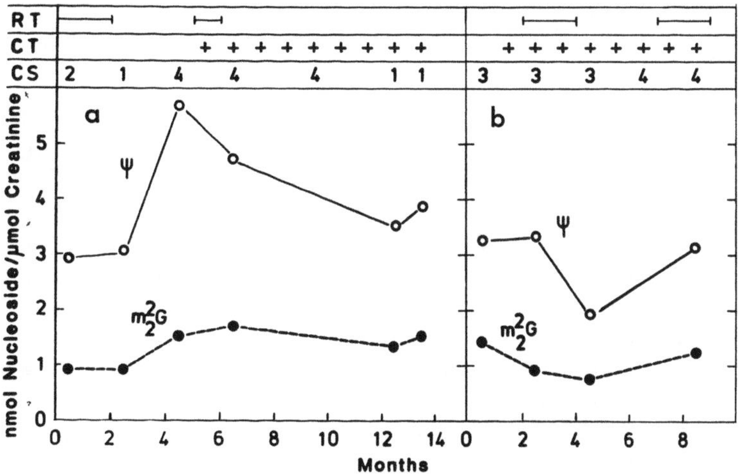

Fig. 5a, b. Levels of Ψ and m_2^2G in the urine in histiocytic lymphoma. **a** A male born in 1915. Histiocytic lymphoma initially localized in the maxilla. Later manifestations in the spine with paraparesis, successfully treated with RT and CT. Later generalization with pleural exudate and subcutaneous nodules. For further information see legend to Fig. 4. **b** A male born in 1934. Histiocytic lymphoma in the pancreatic region. Progressing disease with lymphoma in supraclavicular regions and in the inguae as well as subcutaneous infiltrates

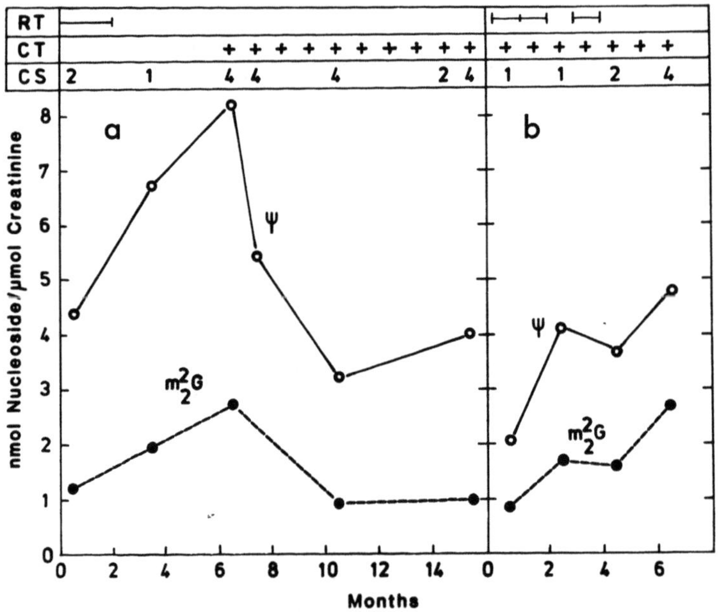

Fig. 6a, b. Levels of Ψ and m_2^2G in histiocytic lymphoma. **a** A woman born in 1917. Histiocytic lymphoma first manifested in a cervical lymph node treated with RT. Later abdominal manifestation with a palpable tumor in the epigastrium treated with CT with partial response. Note lead time with high level of Ψ 3 months before clinical manifestation. Also note marked reduction of Ψ levels after initiation of CT. For further information see legend to Fig. 4. **b** A male born in 1913. Histiocytic lymphoma localized in left thigh. In spite of intense RT and CT, progressing disease. Note lead time of 2 months between Ψ increase and clinical manifestation

Discussion

We have analyzed four different biological markers in 63 patients with different lymphomas. No evident correlation between the clinical stage and the level of the protein markers TPA and PLAP was observed (Table 2). For CEA a possible correlation with clinical stage was observed in Hodgkin's disease, although the material was too small for a definite conclusion (Table 2). In contrast, the level of modified nucleosides in urine correlated with clinical stage in all three types of lymphoma studied (Tables 2, 3; Fig. 3). The most pronounced increase at a more advanced clinical stage was observed for ψ, although the other nucleosides showed a similar pattern. Individual cases illustrated that the level of ψ often decreased after cytostatic therapy (Figs. 4b; 5a; 6a, b). In some cases the level of ψ increased up to 3 months before clinical manifestations were observed (Fig. 6, lead time).

The main conclusion concerning TPA and PLAP is that many patients with malignant lymphomas display significantly increased values, but that the levels do not seem to correlate to the clinical stage of the disease. Therefore these protein markers cannot be generally used as biological markers for malignant lymphomas. This is in contrast to the finding that PLAP seems to be a fairly good marker for seminomas, where 50% of the patients have been reported to have elevated levels (Wahren et al. 1979). TPA has been reported as a valuable marker both for several solid tumors and for lymphomas, but no information was given concerning the stage of the disease and the number of patients was low (Menendez-Botet et al. 1978; Björklund 1980). Our results are in contrast to the latter observation.

Besides as a marker for cancer in the gastrointestinal tract and in some other malignant conditions, elevated levels of CEA might be found in patients with chronic inflammation and with liver damage (Martin et al. 1976). We observed a moderate elevation of CEA in a small series of patients with generalized Hodgkin's disease. These patients often show systemic manifestations such as fever and weight loss. They also have a significantly greater tendency to succumb to certain types of infectious diseases and our observation may be a reflection of such a phenomenon.

Increased levels of modified nucleosides in the urine have been found in patients with various kinds of cancer. Of the lymphomas, only Burkitt's lymphoma has been previously studied and found to have increased excretion of Ψ (Waalkes et al. 1975). We have examined Hodgkin's disease and non-Hodgkin's lymphoma, the latter divided into histiocytic and lymphocytic types according to Rappaport (1966). In all types of lymphoma studied we have found an increase of modified nucleosides in stage 4 compared to stage 1 and the reference group. Using X-ray-induced leukemia in mice, a good correlation between manifestation of leukemia and a high level of various modified nucleosides in the urine was found (Thomale and Nass, this volume pp. 378–387). Thus, both spontaneous human tumors and induced animal tumors (Thomale and Nass, this volume pp. 378–387; Clark et al., this volume pp. 388–400) have shown a correlation between the disease and the level of modified nucleosides in the urine.

The aim of this investigation was to evaluate whether or not modified nucleosides in the urine could be used for diagnostic screening of lymphomas and/or as a biological marker during and after therapy. At present nothing supports the hypothesis that the measurement of these substances may be of value as a screening procedure. However, as a tool to monitor the effect of the treatment, the level of modified nucleosides might be of value. It should be pointed out that the well-established CEA is increased in 21% of stage 1 and in 92% of stage 4 colon carcinomas (our unpublished data). We have found that during storage of the urine samples at −80° C the ψ levels decreased by 25% in 5 months. Some of our samples were stored even longer, so our results might underestimate the incidence of elevated levels of modified nucleosides in the urine. In clinical routine analysis when the samples can be processed directly, the results from modified nucleosides in the urine in lymphoma might approach the results obtained by CEA in cancer of the colon.

As mentioned above, no more information was obtained by analyzing the other modified nucleosides than by the measurement of ψ and m^1A alone. The analysis of the latter two is made by HPLC using an isocratic elution with a buffer containing 1% methanol and is made within 30 min. The identification of ψ is simple and no impurities have been found in any samples. Analysis of ψ alone gave sufficient information in these three kinds of lymphomas, and the analytical technique is reliable, fast, and suitable for routine application. Therefore we consider measurement of ψ in urine of considerable clinical interest, especially for monitoring therapy, but more cases must be studied before final assessment can be made.

Summary

We have evaluated CEA, TPA, PLAP in sera from patients with three different kinds of malignant lymphomas. Six modified nucleosides, Ψ, m^1A, m^1G, m^1I, m^2G, and

m_2^2G were analyzed in the urine from the same group of patients. The histological diagnoses were histiocytic lymphoma (21 patients), lymphocytic lymphoma (19 patients) and Hodgkin's disease (23 patients). The patients were classified into four different clinical stages. Consecutive samples were analyzed before and during ongoing radiotherapy and chemotherapy and during the post-treatment period. Our results showed that TPA and PLAP had limited value as biological markers for patients with malignant lymphomas. For CEA a possible correlation with clinical stage was observed only in patients with Hodgkin's disease. The modified nucleosides, especially Ψ, showed a correlation with clinical stage for patients with all three diagnoses. Elevated levels of Ψ in urine were in healthy adults 4%, in patients in clinical stage 1 14%, and in patients with advanced disease 62%. Six cases showed a good correlation between the change in clinical stage upon treatment and the parallel change in the level of ψ in the urine. Our results suggest that modified nucleosides, especially Ψ, are valuable as biological markers for patients with malignant lymphomas.

References

Bacchus H (1977) Serum glycoproteins and malignant neoplastic disorders. Crit Rev Clin Lab Sci 8: 333–362

Björklund B, Wiklund B, Lundström R, Ekdahl PH, Hagbord L, Kaijser K, Eklund G, Lüning B (1973) A human tissue polypeptide related to cancer, I–III. In: Björklund (ed) Immunological techniques for detection of cancer. Bonniers, Stockholm, pp 133–187

Björklund B (1976) Tissue polypeptide antigen (TPA) in cancer and other conditions. In: Fishman WH, Sell S (eds) Onco-developmental gene expression. Academic Press, New York, pp 501–508

Björklund B (1980) On the nature and clinical use of tissue polypeptide antigen (TPA). Tumor Diagnostik 1: 9–20

Borek E, Baliga BS, Gehrke CW, Kuo CW, Belman S, Troll W, Waalkes TP (1977) High turnover rate of transfer RNA in tumor tissue. Cancer Res 37: 3362–3366

Carbone PP, Kaplan HS, Musshoff K, Smithers DW, Tubiana M (1971) Report of the committee on Hodgkin's disease staging classification. Cancer Res 31: 1860–1861

Doellgast GJ, Lemmons CC, Homesley HD (to be published) Placental type alkaline phosphatase in ovarian cancer fluids and tissues.

Fishman WH, Inglis NI, Stolbach LL, Krant MJ (1968) A serum alkaline phosphatase isoenzyme of human neoplastic cell origin. Cancer Res 28: 150–154

Fishman WH (1969) Immunological and biochemical approaches to alkaline phosphatase isoenzyme analysis: the Regan isoenzyme. Ann NY Acad Sci 166: 745–759

Gehrke CW, Kuo KC, Davis GE, Suits RD, Waalkes TP, Borek E (1978) Quantitative high-performance liquid chromatography of nucleosides in biological materials. J Chromatogr 150: 455–476

Gehrke CW, Kuo KC, Waalkes TP, Borek E (1979) Patterns of urinary excretion of modified nucleosides. Cancer Res 39: 1150–1153

Gold P, Freedman SO (1965a) Demonstration of tumor-specific antigens in human colonic carcinomata by immunological tolerance and absorption techniques. J Exp Med 121: 439–462

Gold P, Freedman SO (1965b) Specific carcinoembryonic antigens of the human digestive system. J Exp Med 122: 467–481

Haagensen DE, Easterday RL, Stolle CA, Wells SA (1978) Buffer-exchange column for rapid separation of carcinoembryonic antigen from perchloric acid. Clin Chem 24: 135–137

Hansen HJ, Snyder JJ, Miller E, Vandevoorde JP, Miller ON, Hines LR, Burns JJ (1974) Carcinoembryonic antigen (CEA) assay, a laboratory adjunct in the diagnosis and management of cancer. Hum Pathol 5: 139–147

Holmgren PÅ, Stigbrand T, Damber M, von Schoultz B, Wahren B (1978) Determination of placental alkaline phosphatase – Regan isoenzyme in cancer sera by a sensitive radioimmunoassay. Scand J Immunol 8: 515–518

Jacoby B, Bagshawe KD (1972) A radioimmunoassay for placental-type alkaline phosphatase. Cancer Res 32: 2413–2420

Joint National Cancer Institute of Canada-American Cancer Society Investigation (1972) A collaborative study of a test for carcinoembryonic antigen (CEA) in the sera of patients with carcinoma of the colon and rectum. Can Med Assoc J 107: 25–33

Krupey J, Gold P, Freedman SO (1968) Physiochemical studies of the carcinoembryonic antigens of the human digestive system. J Exp Med 128: 387–398

Kuo KC, Gehrke CW, McCune RA, Waalkes TP, Borek E (1978) Rapid, quantitative high-performance liquid column chromatography of pseudouridine. J Chromatogr 145: 383–392

Martin EW, Kibbey WE, DiVecchia L, Anderson G, Catalano P, Minton JP (1976) Carcinoembryonic antigen, clinical and historical aspects. Cancer 37: 62–81

Menendez-Botet CJ, Oettgen HF, Pinsky CM, Schwartz MK (1978) A preliminary evaluation of tissue polypeptide antigen in serum or urine (or both) of patients with cancer or benign neoplasms. Clin Chem 24: 868–872

Nishimura S (1980) Modified nucleosides in tRNA. In: Schimmel PR, Söll D, Abelson JN (eds) Transfer RNA: Structure, properties and recognition. Cold Spring Harbor, p 59

Rappaport H (1966) Tumors of hematopoietic system. Atlas of tumor pathology, sect III, fasc. 8. Armed Forces Institute of Pathology, Washington D.C.

Schöch G, Heller-Schöch G (1977) Molekularbiologie und klinische Bedeutung des Stoffwechsels normaler und modifizierter Nucleobasen. Helv Paediatr Acta, Suppl. 38, pp 7–171

Stigbrand T, Holmgren PÅ, Jeppsson A, Damber MG, von Schoultz B (to be published) On the value of placental alkaline phosphatase as a marker for gynecological malignancy. J Oncodevelopmental Biol Med

Usategui-Gomez M, Yeager FM, Fernandez de Castro A (1973) A sensitive immunochemical method for the determination of the Regan isoenzyme in serum. Cancer Res 33: 1574–1577

Waalkes TP, Borek E (1975) The biochemical assessment of the malignant status in man: Aspects related to tRNA modification. Excerpta Medica International Congress 375: 15–31

Waalkes TP, Gehrke CW, Bleyer WA, Zumwalt RW, Olweny CLM, Kuo KC, Lakings DB, Jacobs SA (1975) Potential biologic markers in Burkitt's lymphoma. Cancer Chemother Rep 59: 721–727

Wahren B, Holmgren PÅ, Stigbrand T (1979) Placental alkaline phosphatase alphafetoprotein and carcinoembryonic antigen in testicular tumors. Tissue typing by means of cytologic smears. Int J Cancer 24: 749–753

Wiklund B, Kallin E, Andersson K, Björklund B (1979) Radioimmunoassay of TPA versus hemagglutination techniques. In: Peters E (ed) Protein biological fluids, 27th Colloquium, Brugges. Pergamon, Oxford

Quantitative High-performance Liquid Chromatography Analysis of Modified Nucleosides in Physiological Fluids, tRNA, and DNA

C. W. Gehrke, R. W. Zumwalt, R. A. McCune, and K. C. Kuo

Department of Biochemistry and Experiment Station Chemical Laboratories, University of Missouri, Columbia, MO, USA

Introduction

This chapter will deal with the development of new research on the quantitative analysis of modified nucleosides in physiological fluids, tRNA, and DNA, with emphasis on precision and accuracy of measurement, selectivity, rapidity, and simplicity.

Our interest in the modified nucleosides began in the early 1970s as the United States' National Cancer Institute started its Biological Markers Program. Dr. Borek played a central role in the development of that program, along with Drs. Zubrod, Oliverio, Waalkes and others. At that time our laboratory was asked to develop a chromatographic method for measuring modified nucleosides in normal and cancer patient urine.

Investigations concerning the modified nucleosides, whether their presence is being studied in physiological fluids, tRNAs, other RNAs, or DNAs, are advanced by utilization of chromatographic techniques which provide accurate measurement of the wide array of these molecules, and our objective became the development of an accurate and sensitive method of analysis which would permit the rapid measurement of a number of different nucleosides indicative of tRNA turnover rates. We attained that objective, and that success has allowed us to make other advances in the chromatographic separation of modified nucleosides in tRNA and other nucleic acids. Here we present our recent studies on the analysis of modified nucleosides and illustrate applications of our analytical methods.

Four separate but closely related topics will be touched on:

1. RP-HPLC separation of modified nucleosides
2. Application of that method to the analysis of physiological fluids
3. Our studies on the quantitative enzymatic hydrolysis of tRNA and the HPLC analysis of the modified and major nucleosides resulting from hydrolysis
4. Development of a sensitive and accurate HPLC method for deoxyribonucleosides and analysis of modification of DNA

Our studies on HPLC separations allow more than 30 modified ribonucleosides to be analyzed in less than 2 h. For the analysis of physiological fluids, affinity chromatography is used to quantitatively isolate the ribonucleosides, followed by step-gradient separation of the isolated components.

Recent Results in Cancer Research. Vol. 84

We have also developed rapid hydrolysis methods which quantitatively hydrolyze tRNA to the component nucleosides, with no loss of the more labile nucleosides. The enzymatic hydrolysate can be completed in 2 h and directly placed on the HPLC column without further treatment.

The HPLC method described for the analysis of the major and modified nucleosides in DNA is rapid, extremely accurate, and allows analysis of as little as 1 μg DNA.

The HPLC Separation of Major and Modified Nucleosides

Figure 1 shows the result of our recent investigations on improved HPLC separation of an array of modified nucleosides (Kuo et al. to be published). More than 30 nucleosides can be separated and analyzed in ca. 2.5 h. In order to accomplish these separations and extend the separation technique to additional modified nucleosides, we conducted extensive studies on the effects of various parameters on the chromatographic behavior of the modified nucleosides (Gehrke et al. 1980). Those studies included the effect of methanol in the mobile phase, column temperature, and most importantly, the effect of mobile-phase pH on the retention of the modified nucleosides.

Figure 2 illustrates the effects observed from pH 4–7 for selected nucleosides. The effect of mobile-phase pH is the most pronounced in that changes in pH have the greatest effect on the retention of the modified nucleosides, and the changes in nucleoside polarity with pH provide considerable versatility for the separation technique. Also, as this effect is best understood, we can predict changes in separation with pH.

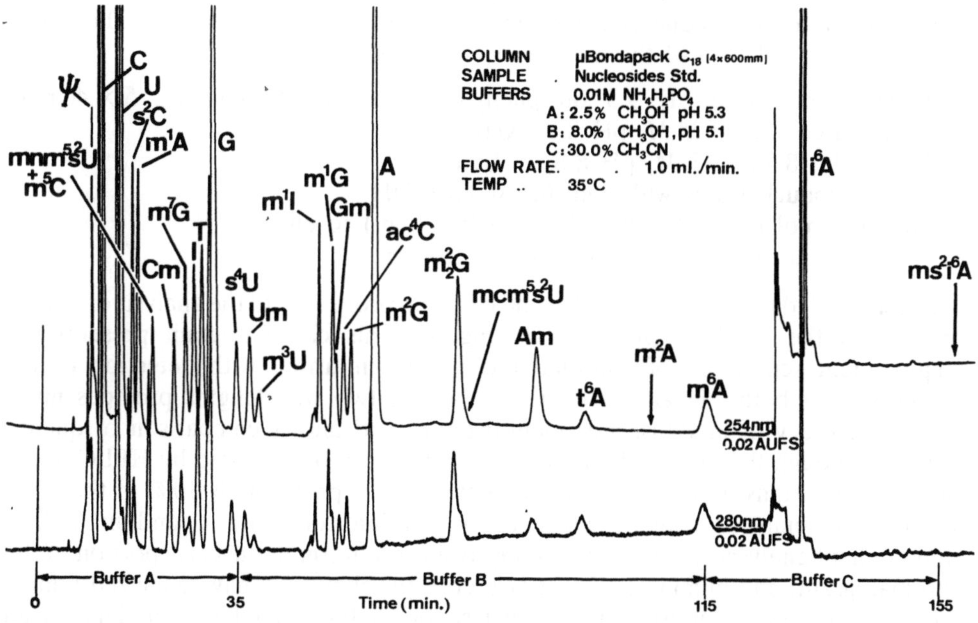

Fig. 1. RP-HPLC of major and modified nucleosides

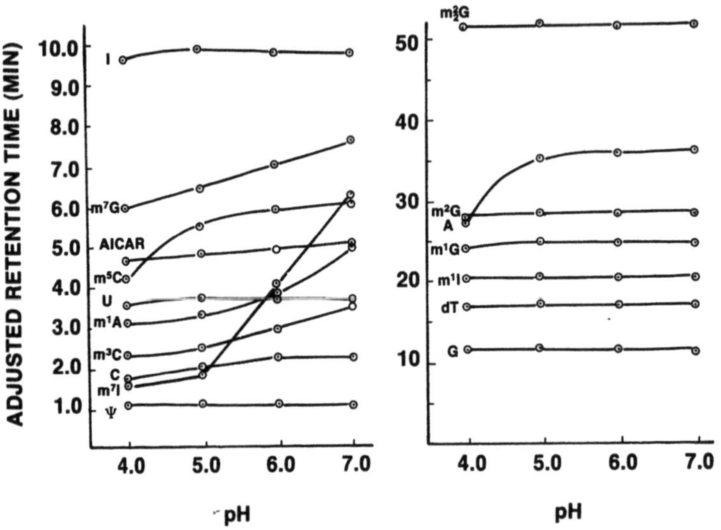

Fig. 2. Effect of buffer pH on HPLC retention times of nucleosides

Analysis of Physiological Fluids

After our earlier investigations (Gehrke et al. 1980) had shown the potential of HPLC for modified nucleoside analysis, our task was to utilize HPLC for the analysis of urine. Of course, such a complex matrix required a clean-up procedure, which we developed based on the work of Dr. Uziel at Oak Ridge National Laboratory with boronate gel affinity chromatography (Uziel et al. 1976). Figure 3 presents the structure of the boronate-derivatized polymer and the formation of the *cis*-diol complex. This affinity chromatographic technique is extremely selective for ribonucleosides. The actual procedure for isolation of the nucleosides is as follows:

1. Load 0.5 ml urine pH 9.5 on phenylboronate affinity column, 5 × 40 mm, equilibrated with 0.25 *M*, pH 8.8, NH_4Ac
2. Wash with 8 ml 0.25 *M*, pH 8.8, NH_4Ac
3. Elute ribonucleosides with 5 ml 0.1 *M* HCOOH
4. Add 20 nmol internal standard (Br^8G in 1.0 ml) to eluate
5. Inject 250 μl on μBondapak C18 HPLC column

We then applied the combined HPLC and clean-up procedure to the analysis of human urine, and the result is presented in Fig. 4. This chromatogram presents the step-gradient separation of modified nucleosides in urine, with detection of the nucleosides at both 254 and 280 nm. The use of two wavelengths provides much greater accuracy of analysis, aids identification, and allows comparison of quantitation. Although the modified nucleosides in urine can be analyzed by HPLC under isocratic conditions, our experience has shown that approximately 10% of the urine samples we analyzed contain substances which interfere with ψ and m^1A. The step-gradient analysis system provides improved resolution in the early portion of the chromatogram, and eliminates the interference problem. We have analyzed a large number of urine samples using the system described in Fig. 4 and have found it to be an excellent method for monitoring modified nucleosides in urine.

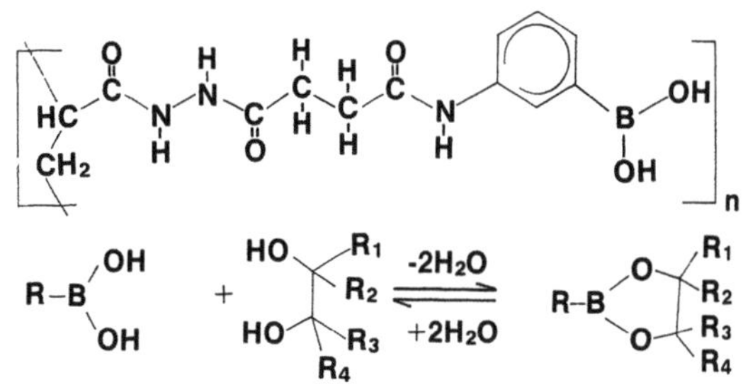

Fig. 3. Structure of boronate-derivatized polymer (*above*) and formation of *cis*-diol boronate complex (*below*)

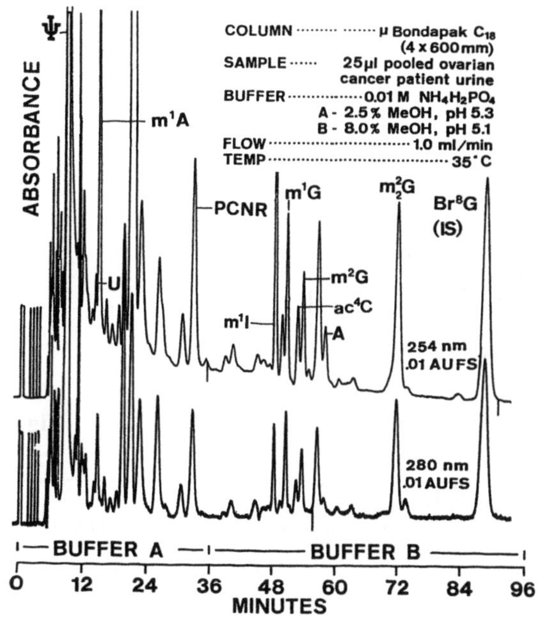

Fig. 4. RP-HPLC step-gradient separation of nucleosides in urine

An example of the versatility of this method is seen in Fig. 5, in which a rapid separation for m_2^2G is presented. This nucleoside is of particular interest in studies of tRNA turnover, and this separation allows quantitation of it in approximately 30 min. The application of this separation to urine is shown in Fig. 6. A similar rapid method for the analysis of urinary ψ has also been developed in our laboratory (Kuo et al. 1978); in addition, extensive data have been obtained showing the quantitative recovery of the nucleosides from the boronate gel clean-up procedure (Kuo et al. 1978).

Studies on the analysis of modified nucleosides in serum (Zumwalt et al. to be published) have shown that this isolation and analysis technique can successfully measure nucleosides present at widely differing and much lower concentrations than in urine. Table 1 illustrates the 100-fold concentration difference observed between ψ and m^1G. Recoveries of the nucleosides added to serum at very low levels was found to be quite good. In summary, we feel this method of isolation and HPLC analysis is currently the preferred technique for rapid and accurate measurement of the wide array of modified nucleosides in physiological fluids.

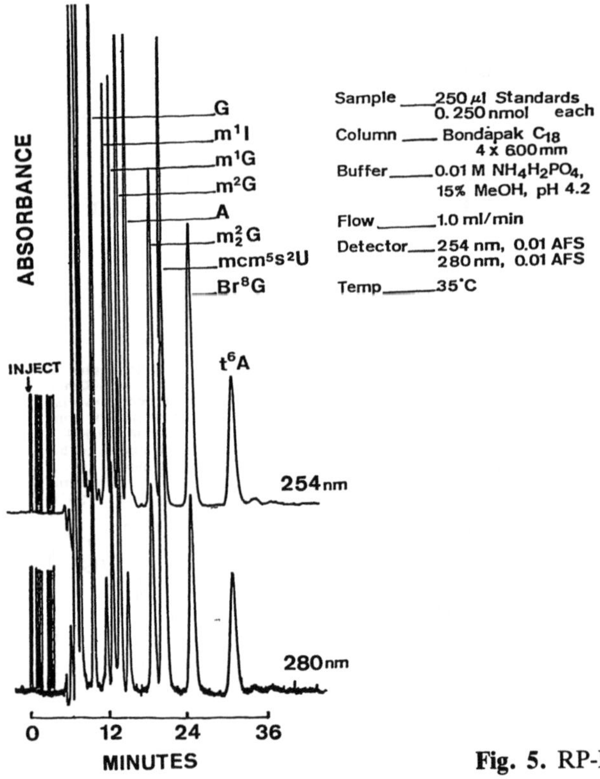

Fig. 5. RP-HPLC for m_2^2G, mcm^5s^2U, and t^6A

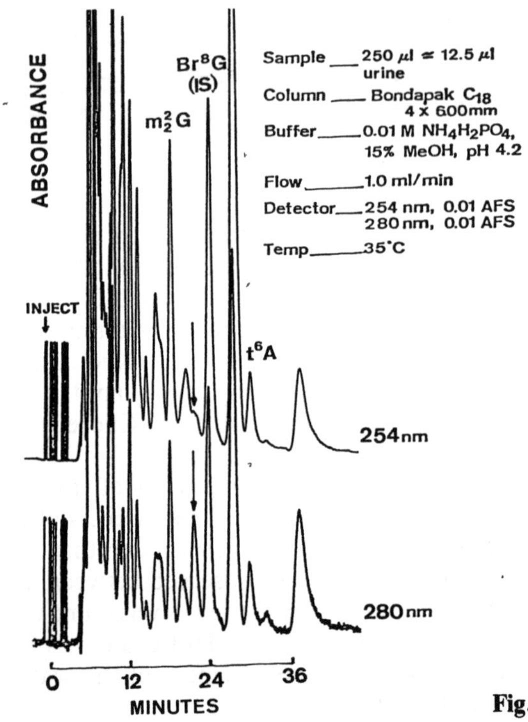

Fig. 6. RP-HPLC for urinary m_2^2G and t^6A

Table 1. HPLC analyses of nucleosides in serum

Analysis	Nucleoside levels (nmol/ml serum[a])					
	ψ	U	m^1I	m^1G	m^2G	m_2^2G
Pooled serum (n = 3)	3.99	5.57	0.108	0.032	0.170	0.101
	4.34	5.86	0.104	0.038	0.251	0.127
	4.17	5.75	1[b]	0.037	0.304	0.083
Average	4.17	5.73	0.106	0.036	0.242	0.104
Pooled serum "spiked"	6.90	5.61	0.298	0.087	0.417	0.160
	6.26	5.57	0.305	0.081	0.358	0.112
	6.67	5.59	0.293	0.094	0.387	0.205
Average	6.61	5.59	0.299	0.087	0.387	0.159
Spike added	2.51	0.00	0.175	0.052	0.051	0.063
Average recovery (%)	97		110	100	1[b]	88

[a] 1.66 ml serum injected
[b] Interference present

Enzymatic Hydrolysis and HPLC Analysis of Modified and Major Nucleosides in tRNA

Our investigations on the analysis of modified nucleosides naturally led us to consider tRNA. Dr. Randerath, of course, has developed elegant and extremely thorough techniques for studying the modified nucleosides in tRNA (Randerath et al. 1980); however, we decided to investigate a hydrolysis procedure especially suited to our HPLC chromatographic technique. Therefore, we undertook the study of nuclease P_1 and BAP for the enzymatic hydrolysis of tRNA. Figure 7 presents the HPLC analysis of yeast $tRNA^{Phe}$ after hydrolysis with nuclease P_1 and BAP for 1 h and 12 h respectively. We obtained all of the expected modified nucleosides, including Cm, Gm, and m_2^2G. hU is not detected at 254 and 280 nm, but its measurement at 214 nm is illustrated in Fig. 11.

We also analyzed hydrolysates resulting from treatment of $tRNA^{Phe}$ with the ribonucleases A and T_2 and BAP, as seen in Fig. 8. The 2′-*O*-methylated components were not observed, as expected, and the response of m_2^2G was half that obtained after hydrolysis with nuclease P_1 and BAP. The difference in m_2^2G levels apparently reflects differences in substrate specificity of the two enzyme systems and not differences in the specific activities, as they were compared over a wide range of incubation times. Of course, addition of snake-venom phosphodiesterase to the A and T_2 system gives results essentially identical to those for P_1. However, as hydrolysis with a single enzyme is more straightforward than use of a three-enzyme system, we chose to optimize the hydrolysis conditions for nuclease P_1.

Table 2 shows a comparison of nuclease P_1 and A and T_2 hydrolysates. Again, no Cm or Gm peaks were seen in the ribonuclease A, T_2 hydrolysates, and the value for m_2^2G was half of the nuclease P_1 value.

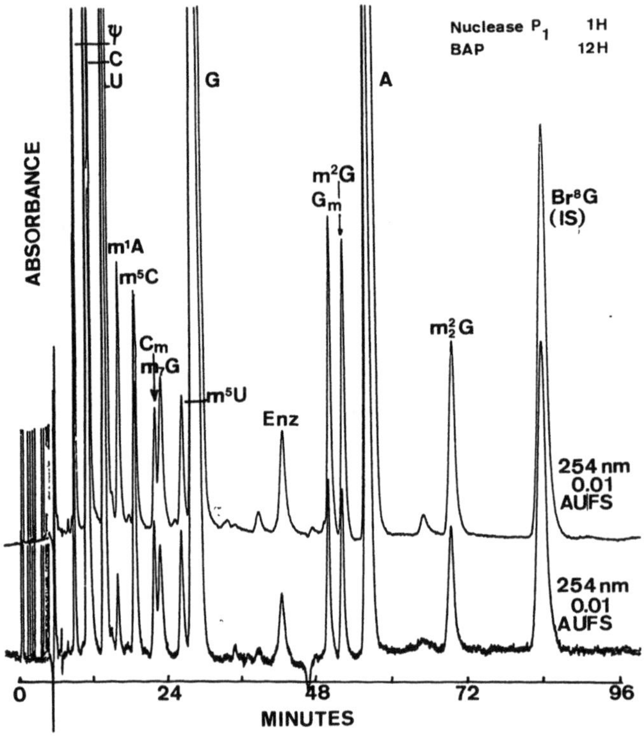

Fig. 7. Hydrolysis of tRNA^{Phe} with nuclease P_1 and BAP

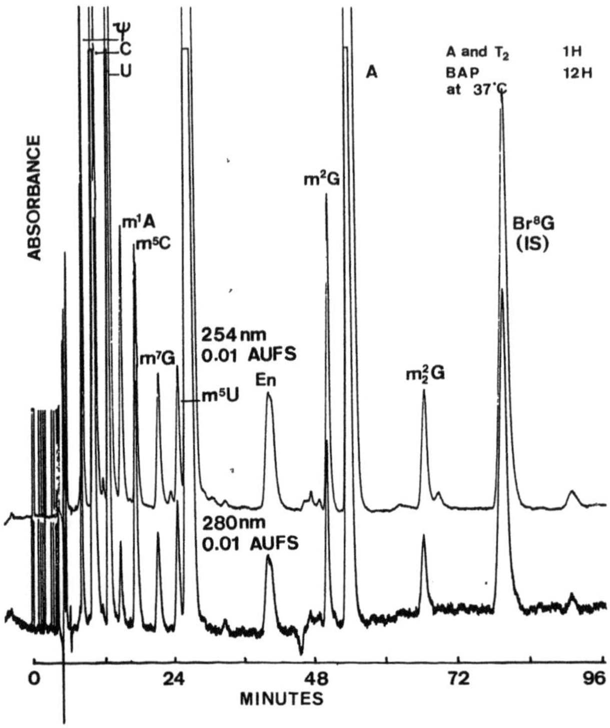

Fig. 8. Hydrolysis of tRNA^{Phe} with ribonuclease A,T_2, and BAP

Table 2. Hydrolysis of $tRNA^{Phe}$ from yeast

Nucleoside	Number of residues per molecule	
	Nuclease P_1 + BAP	Nuclease A,T_2 + BAP
ψ	2.1	2.1
C	16.2	16.4
U	11.6	11.0
m^1A	0.88	0.88
m^5C	1.68	1.70
Cm	0.74	Not found
m^7G	0.79	0.64
m^5U	0.93	0.92
G	18.8	19.0
Gm	0.97	Not found
m^2G	0.87	0.88
A	16.5	17.1
m^2_2G	0.90	0.49
Totals	73.00	71.00

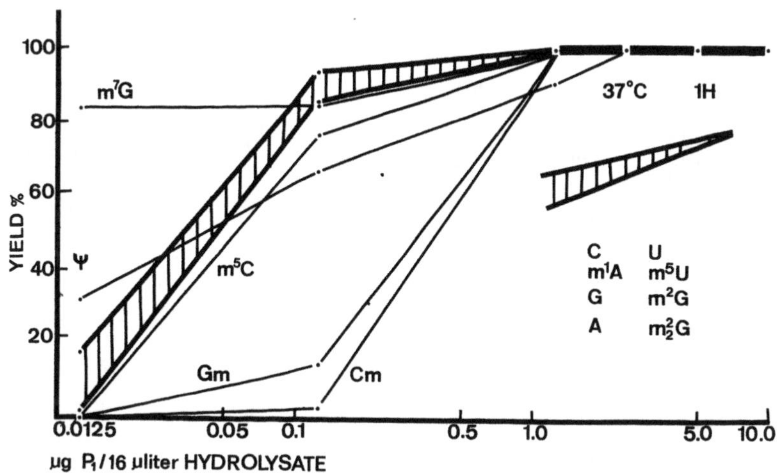

Fig. 9. Effect of nuclease P_1 concentration on hydrolysis of $tRNA^{Phe}_{yeast}$

Figure 9 summarizes our studies on the effect of nuclease P_1 concentration on hydrolysis of yeast $tRNA^{Phe}$ at 37° C for 1 h. Yields of the various modified nucleosides change with P_1 concentration, but the major point is that quantitative hydrolysis of all the modified nucleosides can be accomplished by operating on the far right portion of the curve.

A similar study using BAP is summarized in Fig. 10. Again, quantitative results are obtained at the concentration listed on the far right portions of the curve with a hydrolysis time of 1 h.

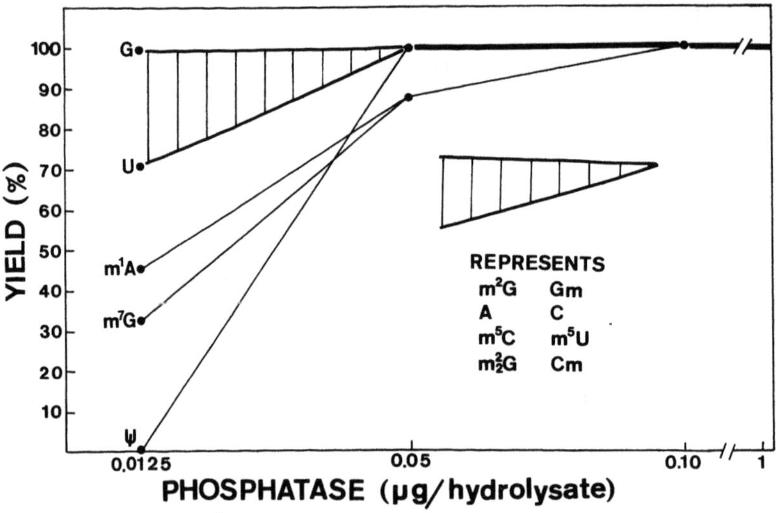

Fig. 10. Effect of phosphatase concentration on hydrolysis of $tRNA^{Phe}_{yeast}$

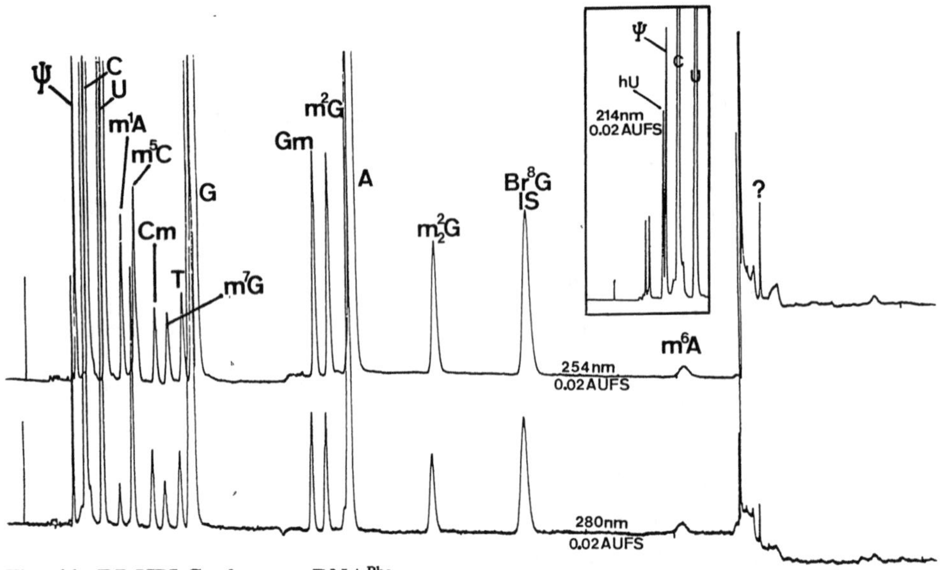

Fig. 11. RP-HPLC of yeast $tRNA^{Phe}$

Figures 11–15 show chromatograms of our analyses of tRNAs of known composition in order to evaluate our hydrolysis and HPLC analysis methods. Figure 11 presents the chromatogram of commercially obtained yeast $tRNA^{Phe}$, showing all the expected modifications. The insert at right shows our simultaneous detection of hU, which is monitored at 214 nm. The analysis of *Escherichia coli* $tRNA^{Phe}$ is shown in Fig. 12; again the tRNA was obtained commercially. The use of 30% acetonitrile is needed to elute the strongly retained ms^2i^6A; s^4U is also seen. Figure 13 is a chromatogram of *E. coli* $tRNA^{Glu}_2$, showing mnm^5s^2U, m^2A, and T. *E. coli* $tRNA^{Met}_f$ is shown in Fig. 14,

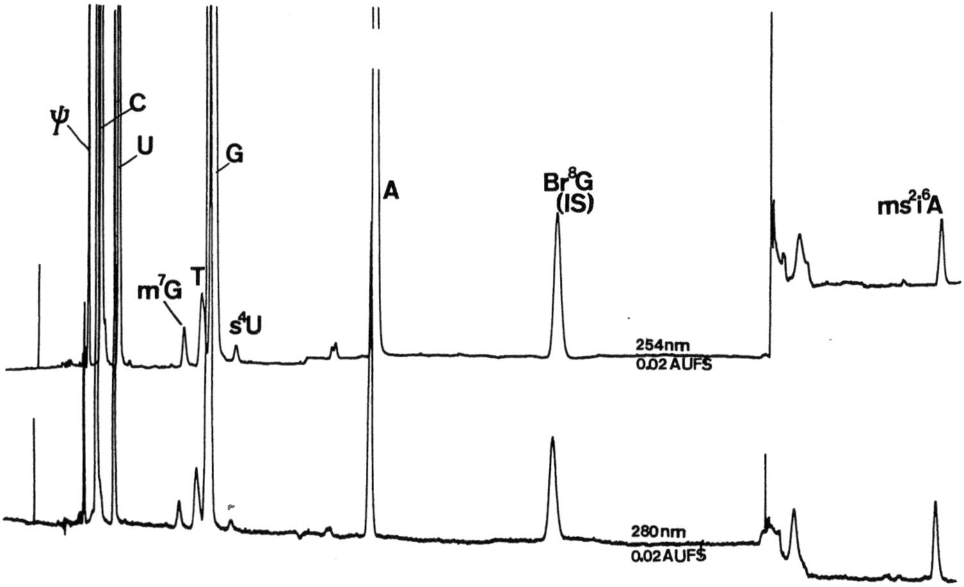

Fig. 12. RP-HPLC of *E. coli* $tRNA^{Phe}$

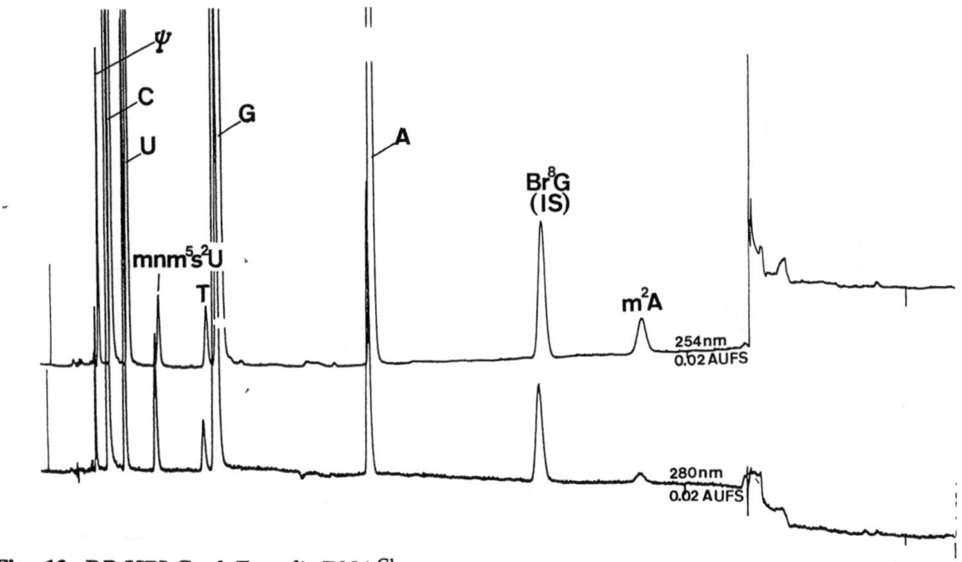

Fig. 13. RP-HPLC of *E. coli* $tRNA_2^{Glu}$

illustrating the *O*-methylated nucleoside Cm. Figure 15 shows analysis of *E. coli* $tRNA^{VaL}$ and its modifications.

Table 3 summarizes the data obtained from the previous five analyses. Some twenty different nucleosides are represented in those five samples. The agreement between our values and the values reported in the literature is generally excellent.

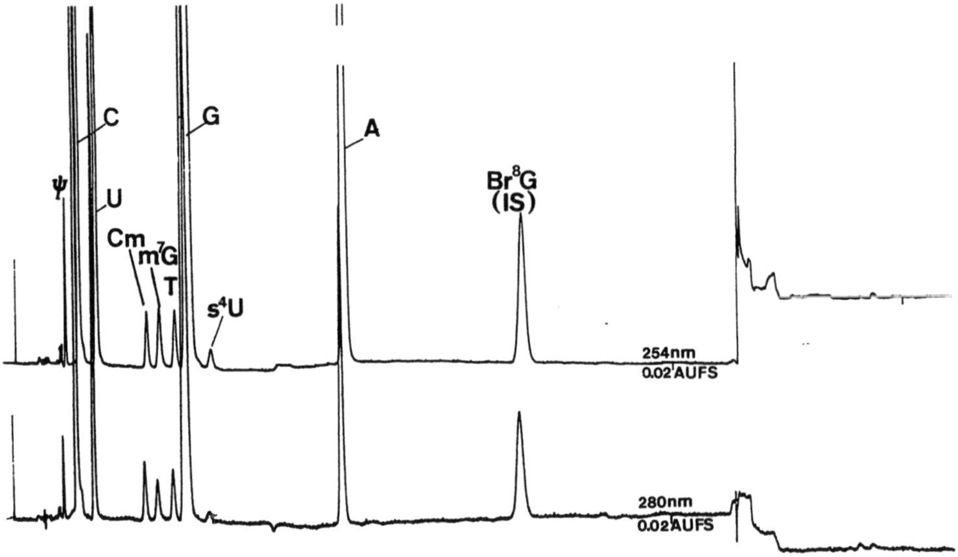

Fig. 14. RP-HPLC of *E. coli* $tRNA_f^{Met}$

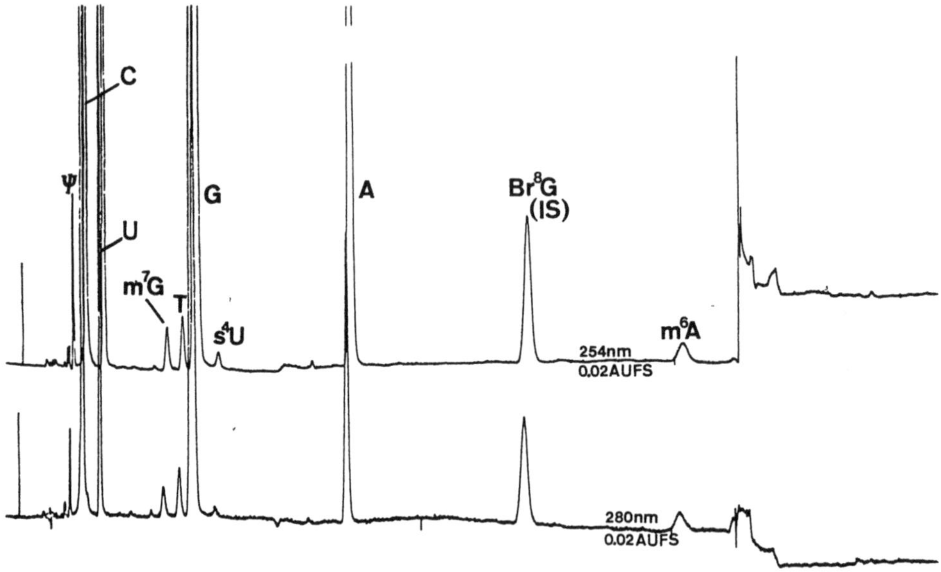

Fig. 15. RP-HPLC of *E. coli* $tRNA_1^{Val}$

This technique can be applied to the analysis of other RNAs, and the nucleoside compositions of mRNA and rRNA have been investigated in our laboratory. In summary, we have found the developed hydrolysis and HPLC methods for tRNA to be an excellent method for accurately determining the nucleoside composition of these complex macromolecules.

Table 3. Quantitative analysis of commercial tRNAs by RP-HPLC. Number of residues per 76 residues

	Yeast $tRNA^{Phe}$		*E. coli* $tRNA^{Phe}$		*E. coli* $tRNA^{Glu}$		*E. coli* $tRNA^{Met}_{f}$		*E. coli* $tRNA^{Val}$	
	Experimental	Theoretical	Experimental	Theoretical	Experimental	Theoretical	Experimental	Theoretical	Experimental	Theoretical
hU	2.16	2	2.39	2			1.08	1	1.05	1
ψ	2.05	2	2.80	3	2.02	2	1.00	1	1.18	1
C	15.8	15	20.6	21	27.1	27	25.1	25	23.2	23
U	12.1	12	8.8	8	9.0	9	8.3	8	10.1	9
m^1A	0.91	1								
mnm^5s^2U					1.24	1				
m^5C	1.98	2								
Cm	0.80	1					0.89	1		
m^7G	0.76	1	0.69	1			0.71	1	0.58	1
m^5U	1.01	1	1.01	1	1.00	1	1.00	1	1.00	1
G	18.3	18	22.8	23	21.9	22	23.6	24	22.1	23
s^4U			0.92	1			0.75	1	0.74	1
Gm	1.00	1								
m^2G	0.99	1								
A	16.0	17	14.0	14	12.9	13	13.6	14	13.8	14
m^2_2G										
m^2A					1.00[a]	1				
m^6A									1.00[a]	1
ms^2i^6A			1.01	1						
O^5U									1.00[b]	1

[a] Not quantitated: assumed to be 1.00 residue if present
[b] Not identified: assumed to be 1.00 residue

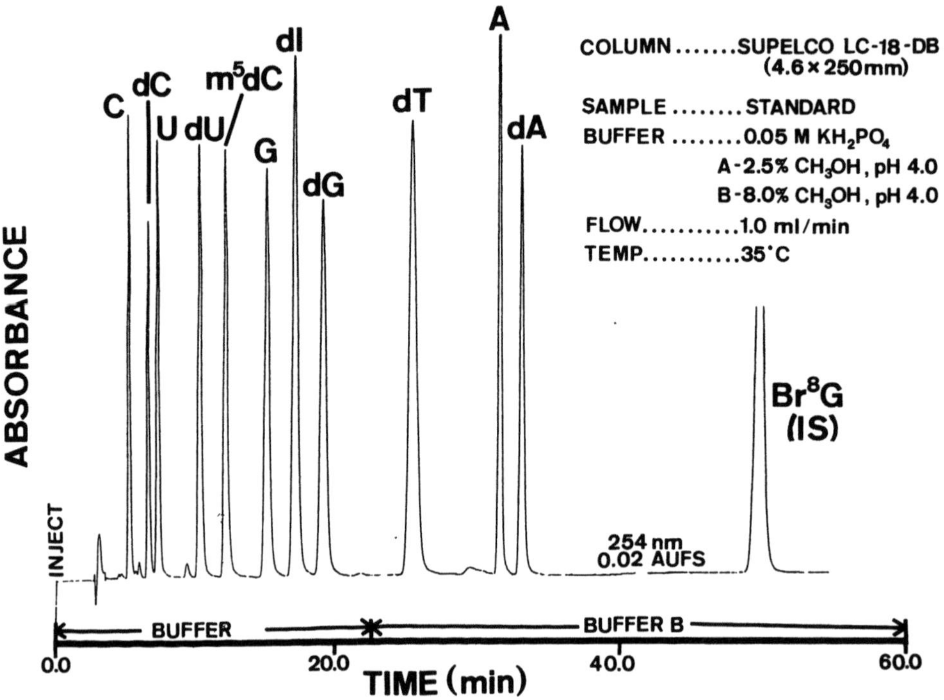

Fig. 16. RP-HPLC of deoxyribonucleosides

The HPLC Analysis of DNA

Our success in the analysis of ribonucleosides naturally led us to consider the deoxyribonucleosides as candidates for HPLC analysis with this system.

Figure 16 presents the results of our studies on the complete RP-HPLC separation of the deoxyribo- and ribonucleosides, including m^{5}dC, with a Supelco LC-18-DB column with an analysis time of less than 1 h (Gehrke et al. to be published). If desired, the analysis time can be reduced to approximately 20 min, as seen in Fig. 17. Also, if the investigator wishes to remove ribonucleosides from a sample containing the deoxyribonucleosides prior to analysis, use of the boronate gel is an efficient method for this purification step.

The automated aspects of our DNA analysis are particularly useful, in that a single chromatographic analysis of a hydrolyzed DNA sample is monitored at 254 and 280 nm. The amount of data from each channel is automatically reduced and the data appear in the desired format, in this case as both nmol nucleoside/hydrolysate and mole % of each nucleoside in the sample. Comparison of the 254-nm data with the 280-nm data is very useful in data evaluation. The 280-nm channel is particularly useful for analysis of m^{5}dC.

Precision data at four levels of injected sample are shown in Table 4. The center portion shows the major nucleoside data. On the right is the precision obtained for the analysis of m^{5}dC, which is quite good at these low levels of analysis. We have been interested in studying DNA modification, and thus we needed to know the long-term precision of the procedure. Table 5 presents data obtained over 6 months, and the SD

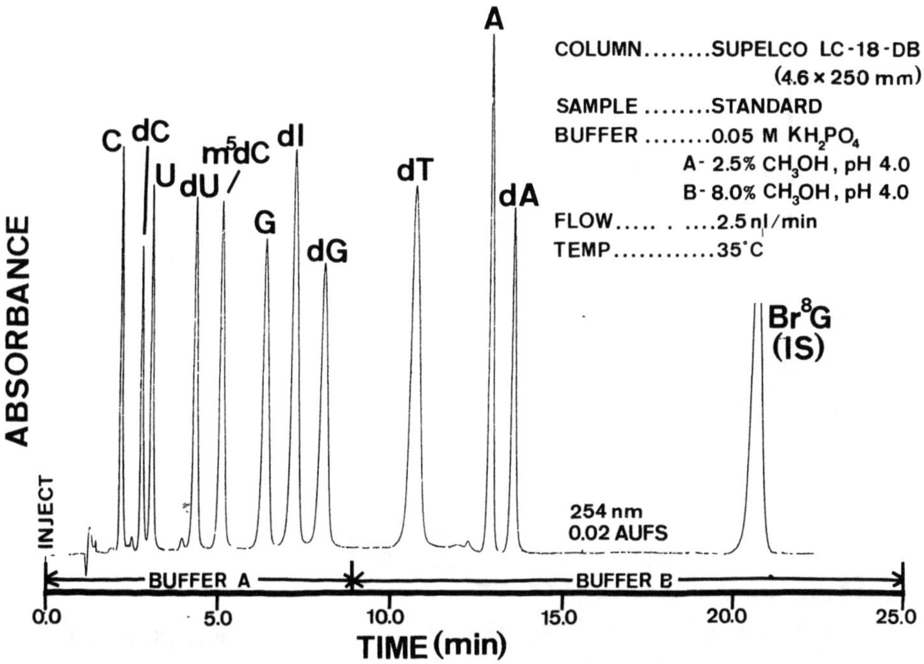

Fig. 17. Rapid RP-HPLC of deoxyribonucleosides

Table 4. Precision for HPLC analysis of calf thymus DNA

Weight injected (μg)	n[a]	Range of RSD (%)		RSD %	
		dC, dG, dT, dA		m^5dC	
		254 nm	280 nm	254 nm	280 nm
7.5	5	0.1–0.2	0.3–0.6	2.1	1.1
2.24	5	0.4–0.6	0.8–1.4	2.0	3.3
0.76	5	0.5–1.7	2.0–3.2	7.4	4.4
0.15	5	1.2–2.0	2.9–4.9	–	–

One microgram calf thymus contains ≃ 60 pmol m^5dC
[a] Replicate injection of one sample

Table 5. Long-term precision for HPLC analysis of human placenta DNA

Nucleoside	Mean mole %[a]	SD	RSD (%)
dC	19.5	0.14	0.7
m^5dC	0.76	0.02	3.1
dG	20.5	0.09	0.4
dT	29.7	0.12	0.4
dA	29.6	0.13	0.4

[a] These data represent 17 independent analyses over a period of 6 months. Approximately 10 μg DNA was used for each analysis

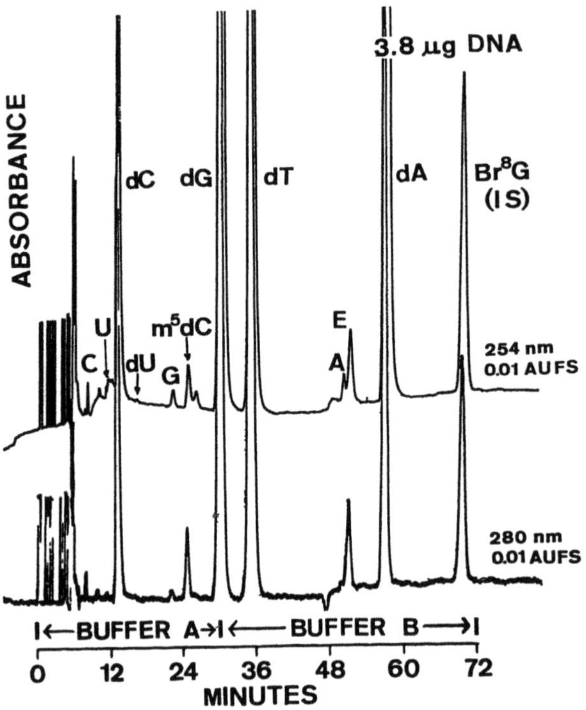

Fig. 18. RP-HPLC for hydrolysate of human liver DNA

and RSD data are quite good. Figure 18 simply shows an application of our method to human liver DNA.

Our laboratory has been involved in a collaborative research effort with Dr. Melanie Ehrlich at Tulane University in New Orleans, studying cancer and development of DNA and focusing on m^5dC in DNA. We have applied our technique to analyses of m^5dC in DNA from different tissues and cell populations, and the accuracy and precision of our analysis has allowed the detection of differences in m^5dC levels. We have also studied m^5dC levels in DNA from various tumor samples and have been able to detect differences in m^5dC levels. This will be of considerable value in studying the role of m^5dC in DNA and its significance in DNA function.

Conclusions

We have recently developed high-resolution chromatographic techniques and the research tools needed for the quantitative analysis of a wide array of modified nucleosides at the microgram level of RNAs. We feel that these methods will be of considerable value in the broad area of research on nucleic acid structure, function, and metabolism.

In our research we are now applying these high-resolution chromatographic methods to the analysis of oligonucleotides. We will also utilize our high-resolution mass spectrometric facility, and the mass spectrometric laboratory of Dr. David Stalling in these investigations.

Thus we are interested in, and will be pursuing, lines of research that could lead to unequivocal definition of the nature of modifications present in RNA and DNA oligonucleotides and fragments. We feel that the results of this research will have direct application to the definition of the roles of nucleic acid modification in neoplastic disease.

Abbreviations

RP-HPLC, reversed-phase high-performance liquid chromatography; *C,* cytidine; *U,* uridine; *G,* guanosine; *A,* adenosine; *T,* thymidine; *ψ,* pseudouridine; *s^2C,* 2-thiocytidine; *m^1A,* 1-methyladenosine; *mnm^5s^2U,* 5-methylaminomethyl-2-thiouridine; *Cm,* 2'-*O*-methylcytidine; *m^7G,* 7-methylguanosine; *I,* inosine; *s^4U,* 4-thiouridine; *Um,* 2'-*O*-methyluridine; *o^5U,* uridine 5-oxyacetic acid; *m^3U,* 3-methyluridine; *m^5U,* 5-methyluridine; *m^1I,* 1-methylinosine; *m^1G,* 1-methylguanosine; *Gm,* 2'-*O*-methylguanosine; *m^2G,* N^2-methylguanosine; *ac^4C,* N^4-acetylcytidine; *m^2_2G,* N^2,N^2-dimethylguanosine; *mcm^5s^2U,* 5-methylcarbonylmethyl-2-thiouridine; *Am,* 2'-*O*-methyladenosine; *t^6A,* N^6-threonyladenosine; *m^2A,* 2-methyladenosine; *m^6A,* N^6-methyladenosine; *i^6A,* N^6-(Δ^2-isopentenyl) adenosine; *ms^2i^6A,* 2-methylthio, N^6-(Δ^2-isopentenyl) adenosine; *hU,* dihydrouridine; *m^5dC,* 5-methyldeoxycytidine; *m^5C,* 5-methylcytidine; *Br^8G,* 8-bromoguanosine; *NH_4Ac,* ammonium acetate; *AUFS,* absorbance units full scale; *BAP,* bacterial alkaline phosphatase; *$tRNA^{Phe}$,* phenylalanine-accepting tRNA; *PCNR,* 2-pyridone-5-carboxamide-*N'*-ribofuranoside; *AICAR,* 5-aminoimidazole-4-carboxamide riboside.

References

Gehrke CW, Kuo KC, Zumwalt RW (1980) Chromatography of nucleosides. J Chromatogr 188: 129

Gehrke CW, McCune RA, Ehrlich M, Kuo KC (to be published) The chromatography of deoxyribonucleosides

Kuo KC, Gehrke CW, McCune RA (1978) Rapid quantitative high performance liquid chromatography of pseudouridine. J Chromatogr 145: 383

Kuo KC, McCune RA, Zumwalt RW, Agris PF, Gehrke CW (to be published) The chromatography of major and modified nucleosides

Randerath K, Gupta RC, Randerath E (1980) ^3H and ^{32}P derivative methods for base composition and sequence analysis of RNA. Methods Enzymol 45: 638–680

Uziel M, Smith LH, Taylor SA (1976) Modified nucleosides in urine: Selective removal and analysis. Clin Chem 22: 145

Zumwalt RW, Kuo KC, Phan D, Gehrke CW (to be published) HPLC analysis of nucleosides in serum

Zumwalt RW, Kuo KC, Agris PF, Ehrlich M, Gehrke CW (1982) High performance liquid chromatography of nucleosides in RNA and DNA. J Liquid Chromatogr 5, No. 11

*Modified Nucleosides in Body Fluids of Tumor-Bearing Patients**

F. Salvatore, A. Colonna, F. Costanzo, T. Russo, F. Esposito, and F. Cimino

Istituto di Chimica Biologica, II Facoltà di Medicina e Chirurgia, Università di Napoli, Via S. Pansini 5, 80131 Napoli, Italy

Formation of Modified Nucleosides and Their Content in Body Fluids

The multifunctional cellular role of tRNA is derived from its molecular structure, which is attained through a complex process of biosynthesis, including covalent modifications of many nucleosides (see Salvatore et al. 1982). In fact tRNA is the nucleic acid species which contains the highest and most varied number of modified nucleosides: among the tRNA species analyzed, more than 40 positions along the primary structure have been found occupied by a modified nucleoside (see Agris 1980). About 50 different types of modified nucleosides have been identified, and in a single tRNA species up to 15 of them can be present. In most cases, three or four are ψ residues and between four and ten are methylated nucleosides (see Dirheimer et al. 1979).

Several steps are involved in the catabolism of tRNA. By nuclease activity tRNA is converted into the four "major" nucleosides and all the variety of modified ones. As depicted in Fig. 1, while the four major nucleosides can be reutilized by various salvage mechanisms or further degraded to uric acid (purines) and β-alanine (pyrimidines), the modified nucleosides should be considered as end products. In fact no salvage mechanisms exist for their reutilization and no catabolic pathways are operative to degrade them further to uric acid and β-alanine. Furthermore, while uric acid and β-alanine are non-specific end products of the major nucleosides, deriving from all the species of nucleic acids, the modified nucleosides present in body fluids of mammals have essentially to be considered end products of tRNA, because of the high content of such compounds in tRNA compared to other nucleic acids (e.g., rRNA).

Due to the presence of so many salvage mechanisms for the major nucleosides and their closer metabolites, it is reasonable to expect their concentration in body fluids, especially in the urine, to be very low. In contrast, the concentration of the modified nucleosides should be higher, particularly in the urine, since their possible reabsorption at renal level would be meaningless. The data reported in Table 1 support

* Work in the authors' laboratory has been supported by research grants from the National Research Council, Rome: Progetto Finalizzato Controllo Crescita Neoplastica. The authors wish to thank Dr. C. W. Gehrke, University of Missouri, Columbia, MO, USA, for making available his unpublished results on HPLC methodology for estimation of nucleosides in body fluids

Recent Results in Cancer Research Vol. 84

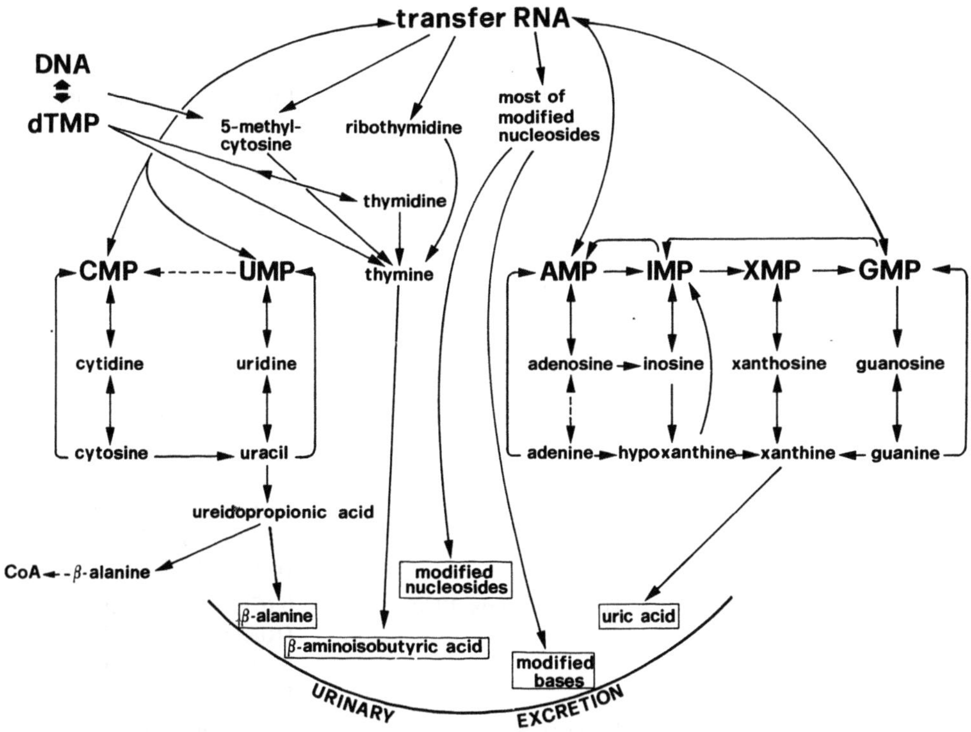

Fig. 1. Metabolic origin of the modified nucleosides present in body fluids

this interpretation, and are, to our knowledge, the only data available on the levels of modified nucleosides in both blood and urine in mammals; in some cases comparison is difficult because of the differences in the methods used for analysis. It is worth noting that ψ is present in both urine and blood at much higher concentrations than the other modified nucleosides. Its occurrence in quantity in all species of tRNA, as well as in rRNA, and in small nRNA does not appear to be sufficient to explain such high concentrations; a possible explanation is that while the other modified nucleosides can undergo cleavage at the *N*-glycosidic bond and then transformation into the corresponding bases, the unusual *C*-glycosidic linkage present in ψ is less susceptible to hydrolysis, as can be inferred from its stability properties (see Chambers 1966). Furthermore, it has also to be considered that a pseudouridylate synthetase activity has been reported to be present in *Tetrahymena pyriformis* (Heinrikson and Goldwasser 1964) and in *Agrobacterium tumefaciens* (Suzuki and Hochster 1966), as well as in calf thymus (Matsushita and Davis 1971). Such enzyme catalyzes the synthesis of ψMP from uracil and ribose-5-*P*. No data seem to be available in the literature on the behavior of this pseudouridylate synthetase in humans; however, its possible occurrence could be another factor explaining the high levels of ψ in body fluids. From the data reported in Table 1, considering that for a man of 70 kg the daily urinary volume derives from 180 liters glomerular filtrate, it is possible to conclude that ψ is not reabsorbed at tubular level: this is also confirmed by the fact that it shows a high clearance value, about 100 ml/min. On the contrary, the calculated clearance value of I, a compound which can be reutilized (Fig. 1), is about 12 ml/min.

Table 1. Nucleosides in body fluids of normal subjects

Nucleosides	Urinary excretion [mean ± 2 SD or range (nmol/μmol creatinine)]	Blood serum concentration [mean ± 2 SD or range (nmol/ml)]
Pseudouridine	17.77 ± 6.36 (HPLC) (Colonna et al. 1980) 13.74–20.21[a] (UV) (Chheda 1970) 22.6 ± 4.32 (HPLC) (Gehrke et al. 1979) 8.57–27.64[a] (GLC) (Tormey et al. 1980)	2.48 ± 0.13 (HPLC) (Russo et al. 1982) 1.72 ± 0.77 (RIA) (Levine et al. 1975)
Uridine	Trace (Chheda 1970)	1.9–8.4[b] (HPLC) (Karle et al. 1980) 2.54 ± 0.63 (HPLC) (Russo et al. 1982) 3.17 ± 1.11 (HPLC) (Hartwick et al. 1979)
Guanosine	Trace (Chheda 1970)	0.67 ± 0.27 (HPLC) (Russo et al. 1982) 0.88 ± 0.51 (HPLC) (Hartwick et al. 1979)
Adenosine	Trace (Chheda 1970)	0.11–0.56[b] (HPLC) (Pfadenhauer and Sun-de Tong 1979)
Cytidine	Trace (Chheda 1970)	n. d.
Inosine	0.05[a] (UV) (Chheda 1970)	0.35–2.2[b] (HPLC) (Pfadenhauer and Sun-de Tong 1979) 5.62 ± 2.87 (HPLC) (Hartwick et al. 1979)
1-Methylguanosine	0.96 ± 0.44 (HPLC) (Colonna et al. 1980)	n. d.
1-Methylinosine	1.04 ± 0.42 (HPLC) (Colonna et al. 1980) 1.15 ± 0.54 (HPLC) (Gehrke et al. 1979) 0–2.01[a] (GLC) (Tormey et al. 1980)	n. d.
1-Methyladenosine	4.32 ± 1.58 (HPLC) (Colonna et al. 1980) 1.77 ± 0.58 (HPLC) (Speer et al. 1979)	n. d.
N^2-Methylguanosine	1.29 ± 1.08 (HPLC) (Colonna et al. 1980) 0.35 ± 0.14 (HPLC) (Speer et al. 1979)	n. d.

Table 1. (Continued)

Nucleosides	Urinary excretion [mean ± 2 SD or range (nmol/μmol creatinine)]	Blood serum concentration [mean ± 2 SD or range (nmol/ml)]
N^2, N^2-Dimethylguanosine	1.36 ± 0.90 (HPLC) (Colonna et al. 1980) 1.20 ± 0.30 (HPLC) (Gehrke et al. 1979) 0.18–2.00[a] (GLC) (Tormey et al. 1980)	n. d.

[a] Calculated on the basis of creatinine mean urinary excretion: 12.3 mmol/24 h
[b] Quantitated on plasma sample

The very low concentration of the other modified nucleosides in the urine and blood is also due to transformation into the corresponding bases. Regarding the blood concentration of U, A, and I, the differences reported by various authors (see Table 1), as well as the absence of C, are evidently also due to the presence in blood serum of enzyme activities which convert A to I and C to U: this implies that great care must be taken in the handling of serum samples and in the timing of analysis after blood collection.

Factors Involved in the Alteration of Modified Nucleoside Formation in Tumor Tissues

In 1975 Waalkes, Gehrke, Borek, and their co-workers initiated a systematic study on the presence and quantitative analysis of several modified nucleosides in urine of cancer patients (Tormey et al. 1975; Waalkes and Borek 1975; Waalkes et al. 1975; Davis et al. 1977; Gehrke et al. 1978; Borek et al. 1979; Gehrke et al. 1979; Speer et al. 1979). The increased excretion of modified nucleosides appeared to be a rather frequent feature, thus indicating an alteration of the cellular process of their formation. The factors invoked as causing the altered excretion of modified nucleosides in urine have been either alterations of post-transcriptional modification enzymes, particularly tRNA methyltransferases, or increased turnover of tRNA, with special reference to specific subpopulations of such macromolecules in cancer cells.

Alteration of tRNA Methyltransferases in Tumor Tissues

In a comprehensive review, Borek and Kerr (1972) listed all the studies on the behavior of tRNA methylases in tumor cells. The impression gained from these studies was that an enhanced tRNA methylase capacity was a rather general phenomenon in tumor tissues. Since 1972 further observations have appeared which also indicate alterations in the activity of tRNA-modifying enzymes in tumor tissues, as reported in a review by Kerr (1978). Besides the previously mentioned results, other data have been obtained which also point to an increased rate and/or extent of tRNA methylation in tumor tissues (Table 2).

Table 2. Increased tRNA methyltransferase activities in tumor cells

Enzyme source	tRNA substrate	Authors
Carcinogen-induced hepatoma (monkey liver)	*E. coli* B (K_{12} B_6)	Lakings et al. (1977)
CEF (RSV); AMV	*E. coli* B *E. coli* K_{12}	Robert-Gèro et al. (1975) Vedel et al. (1978) Pierré et al. (1978)
Rat mammary tumors	*E. coli* MRE600 Single species *(E. coli)*	Brunke et al. (1980)
CEF (RSV)	Undermethylated *(E. coli)* Single species *(E. coli)*	Izzo et al. (1979) Salvatore et al.

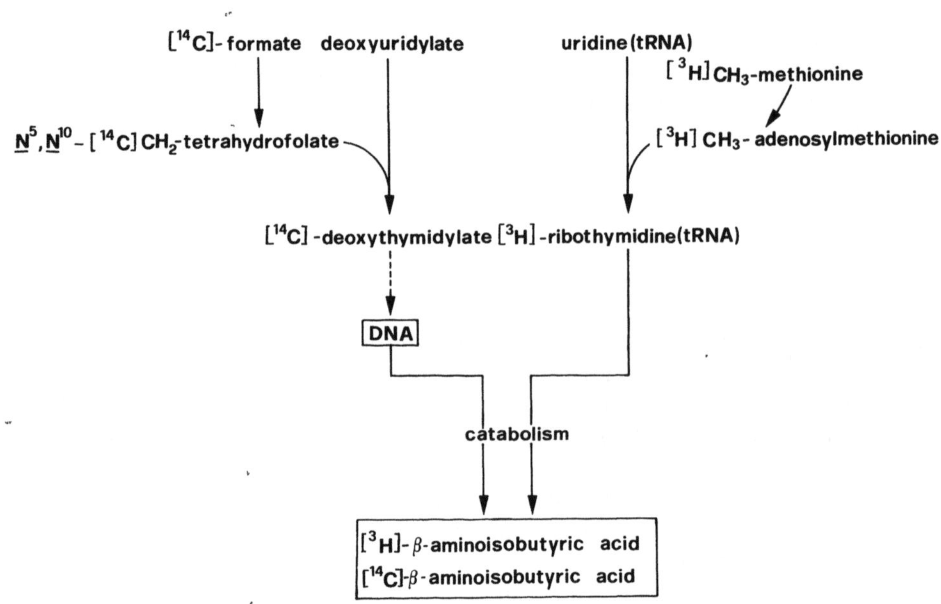

Fig. 2. Different metabolic origin of β-AIB from DNA and tRNA (from an experiment by Borek et al. 1977)

Altered Turnover of tRNA

An interesting observation has been presented by Borek et al. (1977), who showed a higher turnover rate of tRNA in tumor tissues than in normal tissues. β-AIB is the urinary excretion product deriving from thymine of both DNA and tRNA (see Fig. 1). Taking advantage of the difference in the methyl donor used for the biosynthesis of dTMP in DNA and of ribothymidine of tRNA (see Fig. 2), the authors administered [^{14}C]formate and [^{3}H]CH_3-methionine to normal rats and to rats with tumor of the bladder. They isolated β-AIB at different times from the urine and measured the ratio of the specific activity of the two labels. The results showed that the ratio was markedly decreased in tumor-bearing rats. This has been interpreted as being due to a greater turnover rate of tRNA in tumor tissue than in normal tissue: in fact the thymine deriving from the subpopulations of tumor tRNA is more diluted as far as the label is concerned, thus provoking a decrease of β-AIB-specific radioactivity.

The mechanism of the increased turnover of tumor tRNA has not yet been explained: one possibility proposed (Borek et al. 1977) is that specific "surveillance" RNases quickly eliminate aberrantly modified tRNA.

Isoaccepting tRNA Species and Aberrant Nucleoside Modifications in Tumor Cells

Many altered isoaccepting species of tRNA have been observed in tumor tissues and transformed cells. Several reviews have been published on these topics: we refer to the extensive ones by Sueoka and Kano-Sueoka (1970), Borek and Kerr (1972), and Littauer and Inouye (1973), as well as to the more recent one by Nishimura (1979). The general pattern arising from such studies, based on the analysis of changes in the chromatographic profiles of the amino acid acceptor activity, indicates the appearance of "new" isoaccepting tRNA species unique to tumor cells. A further observation is that the new species were only related to particular amino acids and not to all 20 of them. The most frequently altered were the isoaccepting species of phenylalanine, lysine, tyrosine, histidine, asparagine, and aspartic acid.

Only recently, by the refinement of analytical techniques and by skilful sequence analysis methodology, has the exact definition of the alterations present in some isoaccepting tRNA species been successfully achieved. Most of these studies are listed in Table 3. Hypomodifications have been detected in a number of cases, among which lack of the Y base next to the anticodon of $tRNA^{Phe}$ appears rather frequently, as does lack of the Q base at the first position of the anticodon in several tRNAs.

The first gene-prone alteration of tRNA in a tumor cell has been presented by Randerath et al. (see this volume pp. 103–120). In fact mitochondrial $tRNA^{Val}$ from Morris hepatoma has been found to possess an altered primary sequence, with G replacing U in the 5′-arm region, as compared with the same tRNA species from rat liver.

An interesting observation is that undermethylation has also been found (see Randerath et al. 1981) in other tumor nucleic acids (e.g., 5.8-S rRNA and DNA). It may therefore be inferred that undermethylation, or more generally undermodification, of nucleic acids is a rather general phenomenon, possibly involved in metabolic and regulatory derangements occurring in the neoplastic state. The described hypomodifications may be due to different factors, including the in vivo inhibition of methyltransferase enzymes from reacting at a proper time with the tRNA molecule or its precursor.

The apparent paradox between the increased activity of tRNA methylase enzymes from tumor cells and the hypomodification, particularly hypomethylation, of tRNA extracted from tumor tissues or cells may be due to the conditions for assay of in vitro tRNA methylases: use of heterologous tRNA or undermethylated tRNA as substrates, absence in vitro of specific inhibitors, and altered subcellular compartmentalization occurring during the preparation of cell extract.

Recently, in the authors' laboratory, Gionti et al. (1980) have studied the influence of oncogenic viral transformation of CEF on the cellular pattern of tRNA species. The experiments were performed as depicted in Fig. 3. The efficiency of 3′-OH-terminus

Table 3. Altered modifications of tRNA species in tumor cells

Species	System	Nucleoside hypomodification	Author(s)
$tRNA^{Phe}$	Rat hepatoma	Y base	Grunberger et al. (1975)
	SV40-transformed Balb 3T3		Katze (1975)
	Mouse neuroblastoma		Salomon et al. (1976)
	VERO cells		Pergolizzi et al. (1978)
$tRNA^{Phe}$	Novikoff hepatoma	m^1G in	Kuchino and Borek (1978)
	Ehrlich ascites tumor cells	place of Y;	Grunberger et al.
	Neuroblastoma cells	Cm_{32};	(this volume, 133–145)
		Gm_{34}	
$tRNA^{Asp}$	Rat ascites hepatoma	Q base	Okada et al. (1978)
$tRNA^{Asn}$	SV40-transformed mouse fibroblasts		Katze (1978)
$tRNA^{His}$	Walker 256 carcinosarcoma		Roe et al. (1979)
$tRNA^{Tyr}$	Murine erythroleukemia cells		Shindo-Okada (1981)
$tRNA_2^{Lys}$	SV40-transformed Balb 3T3	hU; t^6A; Tm	Raba et al. (1979)
$tRNA^{Val}$	Rat ascites hepatoma	Gm	Shindo-Okada et al. (see in Nishimura 1979)
$tRNA^{Ser}$	Morris hepatoma 5123D	Gm	Randerath et al. (1981)

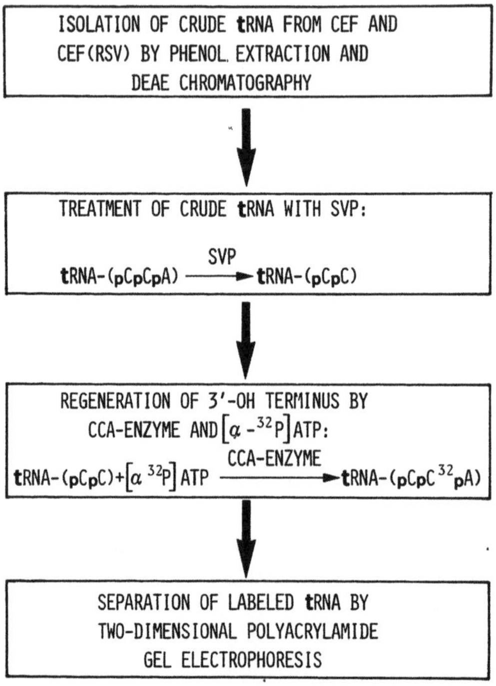

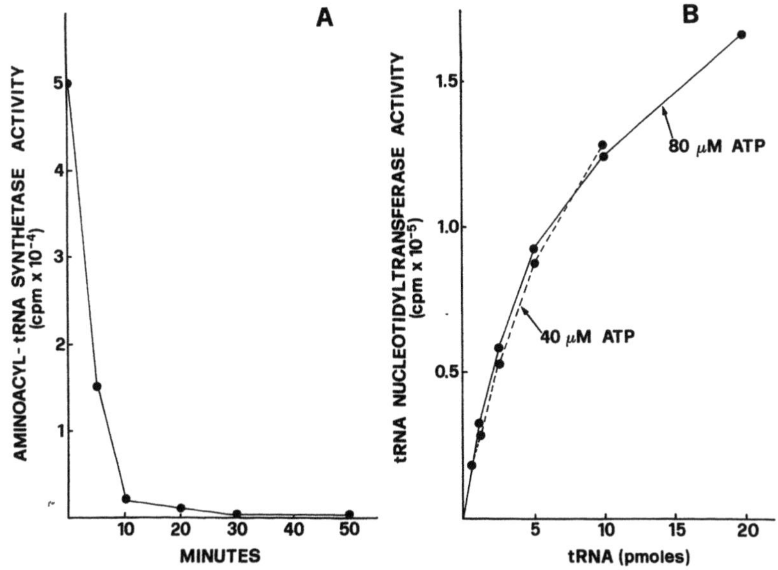

Fig. 4. Labeling of tRNA at 3′-OH terminus. tRNA 3′-OH digestion by SVP **(A)** was done in the following conditions: An aliquot of tRNA [from CEF or CEF(RSV)] was incubated with SVP (20 : 1) for 20 min at room temperature in 50 m*M* Tris-HCl, 10 m*M* Mg^{2+}, pH 8.0. After extraction with phenol-chloroform (1 : 1), tRNA was separated from 5′-mononucleotides on a Sephadex G-25 column (50 m*M* sodium acetate, 10 m*M* Mg^{2+}, pH 5.5). The effect of SVP treatment was evaluated by measuring the residual capacity of tRNA to incorporate tritiated valine, arginine, and lysine in a conventional aminoacylation reaction by running it for 20 min at room temperature in the presence of a partially purified aminoacyl-tRNA synthetase complex from rat liver. Optimal conditions for tRNA 3′-OH terminus regeneration **(B)** were studied as follows: Aliquots of tRNA previously treated with SVP were incubated with *E. coli* nucleotidyltransferase and [8-^{3}H]-adenosine 5′-triphosphate (22 Ci/mmol) at the indicated concentrations in 120 m*M* Tris-HCl, 40 m*M* KCl, 8 m*M* Mg^{2+}, 10 μ*M* CTP, pH 8.7. After 30 min at 37° C, the reaction was stopped with TCA and the radioactivity of TCA-insoluble material was collected on glass fiber filters and counted (Gionti et al. 1980)

Fig. 3. Analysis of tRNA pattern of normal and transformed CEFs. CEFs were prepared from CHF White Leghorn chicken embryos; their transformation was obtained by infection with Schmidt-Ruppin RSV. Subconfluent secondary CEF and CEF(RSV) were disrupted by homogenization and tRNA was extracted and purified according to Silbert et al. 1966. After deacylation at 37° C for 45 min in 1.8 *M* Tris-HCl pH 8.0, tRNA preparations were first treated with SVP and then incubated with *E. coli* nucleotidyltransferase (CCA-enzyme) and [α-^{32}P]ATP as described in the legend to Fig. 4. SVP treatment (20 min) caused complete (99.5%) digestion of tRNA at 3′-OH terminus (see Fig. 4A). The regeneration of 3′-OH terminus was about 100% when using the following conditions: 40 μ*M* ATP, 10 μ*M* CTP, 5 μ*M* tRNA, 8 m*M* Mg^{2+}, 120 m*M* Tris-HCl, pH 8.7 at 37° C for 30 min after preincubation of the nucleotide mixture (15 min at 37° C) in an ATP regenerating system containing 1.5 m*M* phosphoenolpyruvate and 2 units pyruvate kinase in 10 m*M* Tris-HCl pH 7.5. Separation of the labeled tRNA was performed as described in the legend to Fig. 5 (Gionti et al. 1980)

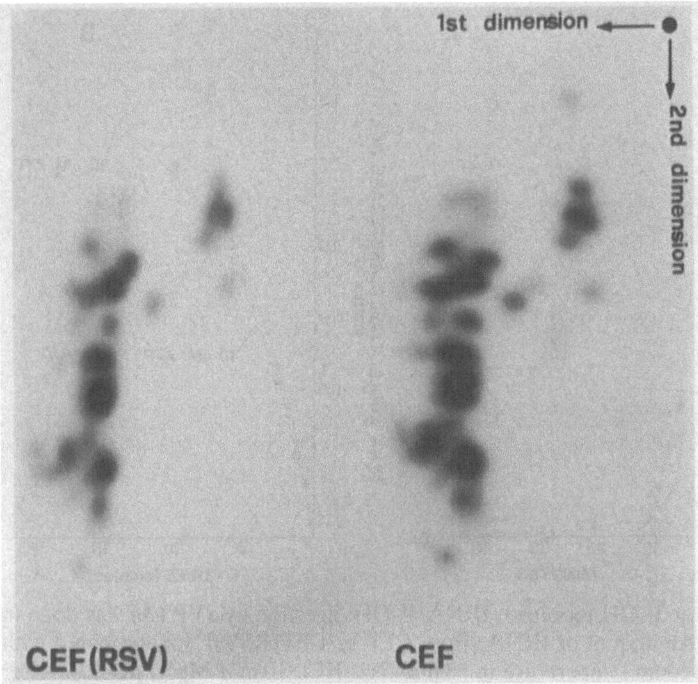

Fig. 5. tRNA patterns of normal (CEF) and transformed [CEF(RSV)] chick embryo fibroblasts (from Gionti et al. 1980). ^{32}P-labeled tRNA was prepared as described in the legend to Fig. 3. Two-dimensional polyacrylamide electrophoresis (0.3 × 20 × 40 cm) was done in the following conditions. First dimension: 10% polyacrylamide, 4 *M* urea, Tris-borate buffer, pH 8.3 (300 V, 20 h); second dimension: 20% polyacrylamide, 4 *M* urea, Tris-borate buffer, pH 8.3 (300 V, 90 h). Spots were revealed by conventional autoradiography

labeling with [α^{32}P]ATP is reported in Fig. 4. Figure 5 shows that the pattern of tRNA species present in both normal (CEF) and transformed [CEF(RSV)] cells includes about 40 spots and that in several areas of the gels both quantitative and qualitative differences appear. The most interesting of these differences seems to be in the area of high-molecular-weight tRNA (the upper right area of the gels) which have been eluted and analyzed by RPC, as illustrated in Fig. 6. It is worth noting that $tRNA^{Trp}$, the primer for replication of RSV, being a low-molecular-weight species, migrates in a very different region of the gel. The identification of the new species of tRNA appearing in the transformed cells (see Fig. 6) deserves further study, as does the definition of its real nature: a gene-specified new product or, more likely, a new tRNA species aberrantly modified or processed.

Analysis of Modified Nucleosides in Body Fluids

In the past few years, the development of HPLC has given a great boost to the study of the urinary excretion of modified nucleosides in tumor-bearing subjects. Numerous results have been accumulated in several laboratories and most of them appear to suggest a possible correlation between the increased excretion of modified nucleosides

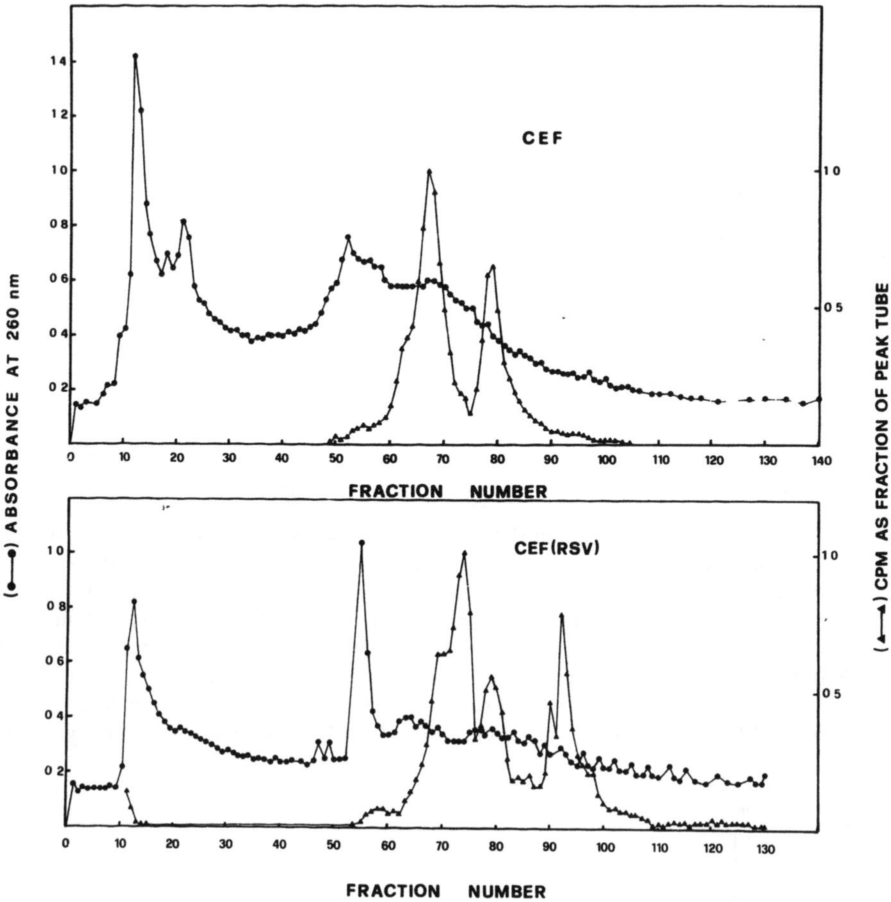

Fig. 6. Reverse phase chromatography (RPC-5) of high-molecular-weight tRNA from normal (CEF) and transformed [CEF(RSV)] chick embryo fibroblasts (Gionti et al. 1980). ^{32}P-labeled tRNAs were eluted from the upper right area of the gels shown in Fig. 5 at 37° C for 4 h in 0.5 *M* ammonium acetate, 0.1 *M* EDTA, 50% formamide, pH 4.5. Each eluate, added to 10 A_{260} units crude tRNA, was passed through an RPC-5 column (20 × 1 cm) equilibrated with 0.4 *M* NaCl, 10 m*M* Tris-HCl, 10 m*M* Mg^{2+}, 1 m*M* β-mercaptoethanol, pH 7.0. Elution was from 0.4–0.8 *M* NaCl. The flow-rate was 40 ml/h with a pressure of 150 psi

and neoplastic disease (Davis et al. 1977; Gehrke et al. 1978; Gehrke et al. 1979; Speer et al. 1979; Tormey et al. 1980; Colonna et al. 1980, 1981; Cimino et al. 1982).

The main steps of the procedure used in the authors' laboratory to separate, identify, and quantitate modified nucleosides and to purify the urine samples are detailed in the legends to Figs. 7 and 8.

Table 4 summarizes a study carried out on a group of 17 patients with different types of lymphomas, in whom levels of seven different modified nucleosides were determined before the onset of any therapeutic treatment. The compound most frequently and markedly increased was ψ: in 15 of 17 patients the urinary concentration of ψ was higher by at least 2 SD than in normal subjects. m^1A was elevated in more than 85% of

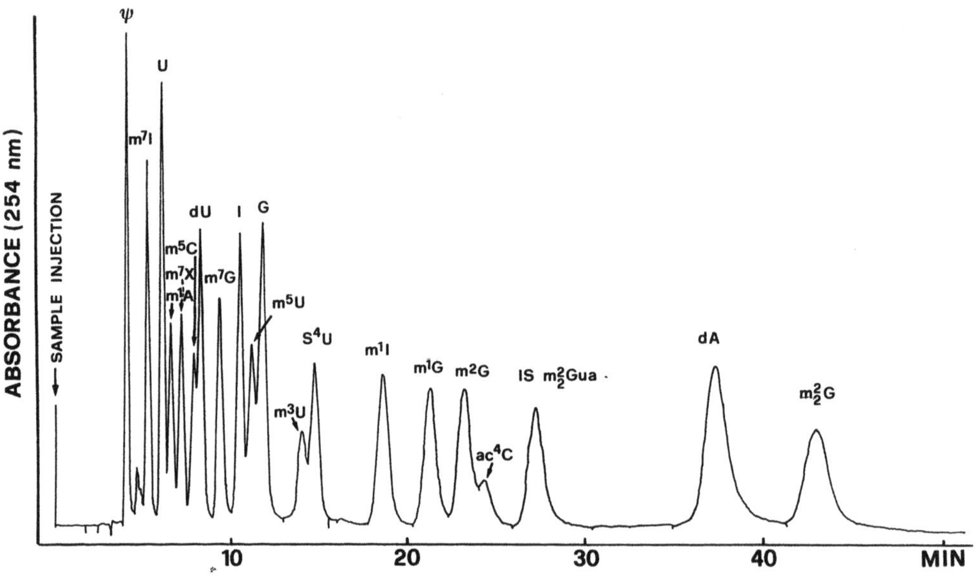

Fig. 7. HPLC separation of standard modified nucleosides. Experimental conditions: 250 pmol of each nucleoside was dissolved in a total volume of 25 µl H_2O and injected on a 4 × 300 mm µBondapak/C_{18} column (Waters Assoc., Mildford, Massachusetts). The analysis was performed on a Waters HPLC system composed of the Model 6000 A solvent delivery system, Model U6K injector, and Model 440 absorbance detector. Elution was performed at a flow rate of 1 ml/min with 0.01 *M* monobasic ammonium phosphate, pH 5.1, containing 6% methanol (v/v), at 36 ± 0.5° C. The mean operative pressure was 1000 psi. Absorbance was detected at 254 nm using 0.02 AUFS sensitivity. The integration of each peak area was done by using m_2^2Gua as IS

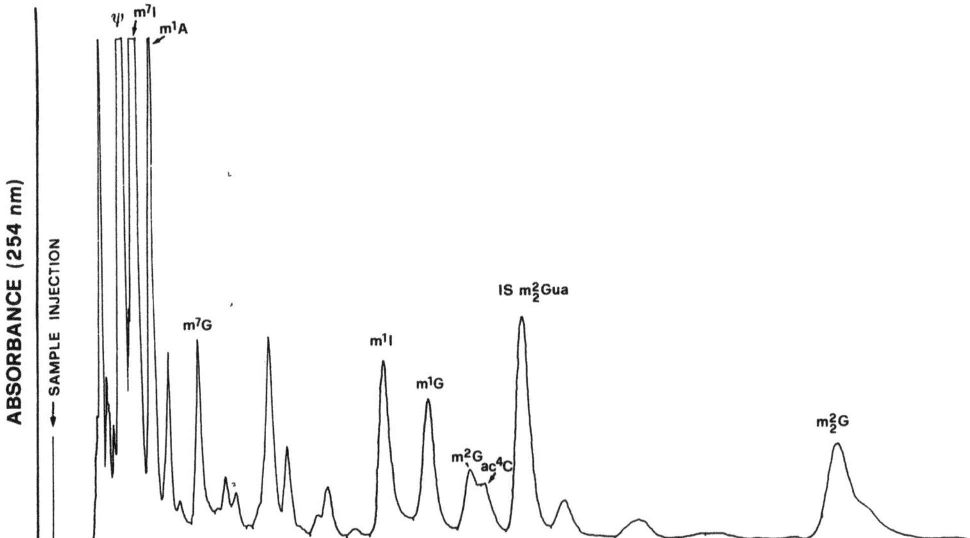

Fig. 8. Monitoring of urinary excretion levels of ψ in patients suffering from malignant lymphomas. *CVP*, combination chemotherapy with cyclophosphamide, vincristine, and prednisone; *MOPP*, combination chemotherapy with mechlorethamine, vincristine, procarbazine, and prednisone. Experimental conditions were those reported in the legends of Fig. 7 and 8

Table 4. Modified nucleosides in the urine of lymphoma-bearing patients

Disease	Stage	Nucleosides (nmol/μmol urinary creatinine)						
		ψ	m^1A	m^7G	m^1I	m^1G	m^2G	m^2_2G
Control mean + 2 SD		24.13	5.91	1.46	1.46	1.41	2.38	2.27
Hodgkin's disease n. s.	I A	40.62	9.37	1.40	2.02	1.16	1.25	1.40
Hodgkin's disease m. c.	II A	36.66	7.17	n. q.	2.94	2.14	3.15	2.25
Hodgkin's disease m. c.	II A	39.28	9.60	n. q.	0.69	0.27	n. q.	1.26
Hodgkin's disease l. p.	II B	61.10	n. q.	n. q.	2.20	2.05	n. q.	3.80
Hodgkin's disease n. s.	III A	32.00	n. q.	n. q.	1.16	0.64	n. q.	1.19
Hodgkin's disease m. c.	III B	36.00	12.00	2.76	0.45	0.43	n. q.	1.55
Hodgkin's disease n. s.	III B	29.57	7.19	n. q.	1.70	1.20	n. q.	2.60
Lymphocytic lymphoma, diffuse	II A	19.55	7.59	n. q.	0.27	0.35	n. q.	0.84
Lymphocytic lymphoma, diffuse	III A	44.88	8.96	n. q.	1.20	0.41	2.19	1.48
Lymphocytic lymphoma, diffuse	III B	28.87	n. q.	n. q.	0.64	0.49	0.26	0.83
Lymphocytic lymphoma, diffuse	IV	41.45	12.63	3.00	2.04	1.30	n. q.	2.18
Lymphocytic lymphoma, nodular	III A	82.64	19.00	1.17	1.65	1.47	1.25	1.35
Histiocytic lymphoma, diffuse	I E A	18.82	5.04	n. q.	0.91	0.41	1.80	1.13
Histiocytic lymphoma, diffuse	I E B	67.75	14.42	6.85	1.92	1.82	n. q.	2.42
Histiocytic lymphoma nodular	III B	37.86	10.40	n. q.	2.56	1.60	3.57	1.95
Histiocytic lymphoma nodular	III B	44.60	12.00	n. q.	3.58	2.27	3.75	2.53
Brill-Symmers disease	I	25.78	4.69	n. q.	0.50	0.37	1.71	0.99

Histopathologic classification was according to Rappaport (1966). The patients were staged as recommended by the Ann Arbor Conference (Carbone et al. 1971). HPLC experimental conditions were those reported in the legends of Figs. 7 and 8. Underlined values exceed control mean + 2 SD

n. q., not quantitated because of lack of complete resolution; *n. s.*, nodular sclerosis; *m. c.*, mixed cellularity; *l. p.*, lymphocyte predominant

cases, while m^7G, m^1I, m^1G, m^2G, and m^2_2G were increased in lower percentages of cases. The results, even if they do not permit any correlation with the type and stage of the tumor or the general prognosis of the disease, seem to indicate that among the seven nucleosides tested, ψ is the compound of choice for investigation in the follow-up of the neoplastic disease.

Examples of monitoring the effects of chemotherapy in lymphoma patients are reported in Fig. 9: in some cases it was possible to correlate the progression of the disease with the urinary excretion of ψ. In fact ψ urinary excretion correlates with the clinical behavior: exacerbation (upper left panel), remission (lower panel), and stationary conditions (upper right panel).

Very recently an HPLC method to measure ψ and other nucleosides in blood serum has been developed in the authors' laboratory (Colonna et al., to be published). The main advantages of this analysis are the easier normalization of serum constituents with respect to the urine and more accurate quantitation of ψ because of the less complex pattern as compared to the urinary one. Figure 10 (panel A) shows a typical profile of blood serum nucleosides in a normal subject. The presence in blood serum of adenosine deaminase and cytidine deaminase is a likely cause of the absence of the peaks corresponding to A and C. They may indeed be shown when serum samples are analyzed soon after the blood collection, or by addition of specific enzyme inhibitors (Koller et al. 1980). In addition, a proportional increase of I and U peaks may be

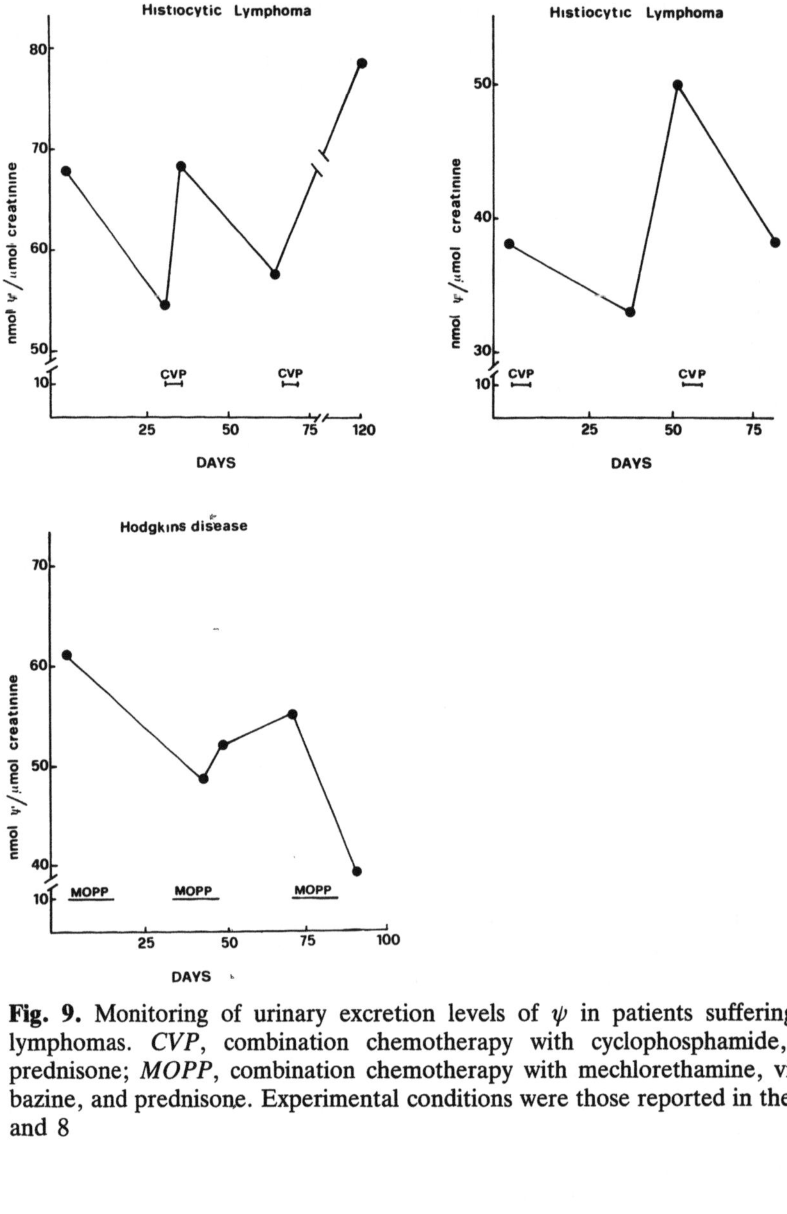

Fig. 9. Monitoring of urinary excretion levels of ψ in patients suffering from malignant lymphomas. *CVP*, combination chemotherapy with cyclophosphamide, vincristine, and prednisone; *MOPP*, combination chemotherapy with mechlorethamine, vincristine, procarbazine, and prednisone. Experimental conditions were those reported in the legends of Fig. 7 and 8

observed when proper amounts of A and C respectively are added to the serum sample (Colonna et al., to be published).

The profile reported in Fig. 10 (panel B) refers to a preliminary result obtained with the serum of a lymphoma patient. In this profile the presence of several not yet identified UV-absorbing compounds possessing *cis*-diol structure has been observed. The results reported in Fig. 11 show that in 10 of 14 subjects with various types of neoplasia, ψ concentration in serum exceeded normal mean value plus 2 SD. However, three of the four "normal" values pertained to tumor patients in clinical remission. These results strongly suggest that ψ estimation in blood serum can be exploited as a biochemical marker of the neoplastic disease.

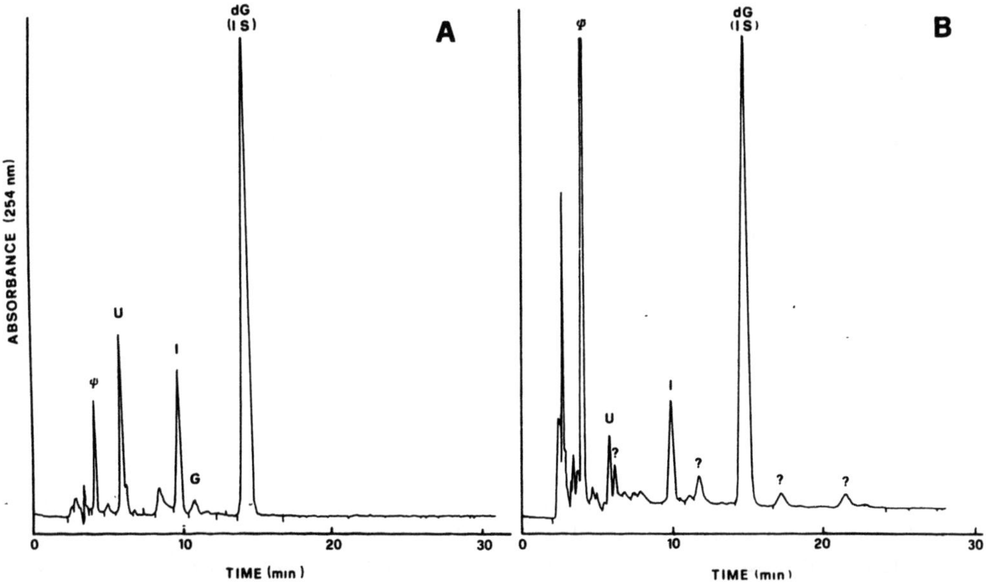

Fig. 10. Chromatographic profile of human serum nucleosides in a normal subject **(A),** and in a lymphoma-bearing patient **(B).** Serum sample purification and HPLC conditions were essentially those reported in legends of Fig. 7 and 8, with slight modifications. The amount of serum analyzed on HPLC corresponds to an original volume of 0.05 ml (Russo et al. 1982)

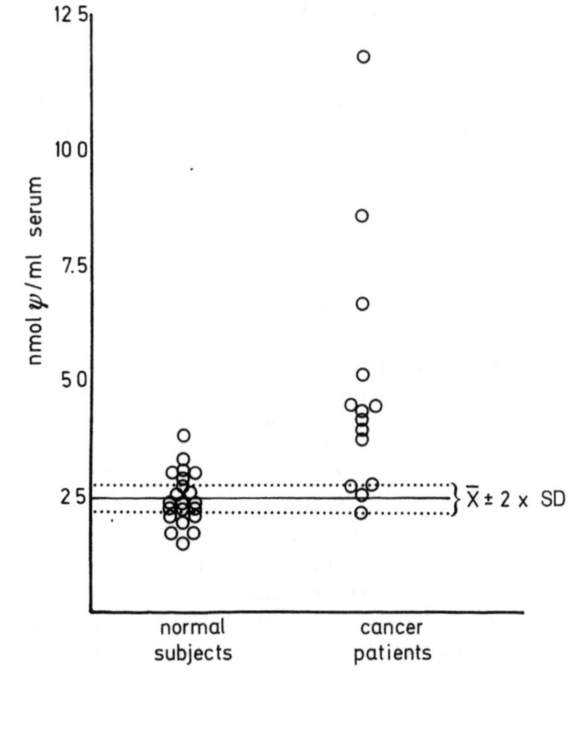

Fig. 11. Serum ψ levels in normal subjects and cancer patients. Diagnoses in the 14 cancer patients examined included breast cancer, lung cancer, non-Hodgkin's lymphoma, acute lymphoblastic leukemia, and hepatoma. HPLC experimental conditions were as reported in the legend to Fig. 10. $\bar{X} \pm 2$ SD refers to normal subjects (Russo et al. 1982)

Concluding Remarks

Attempts to find in biological fluids specific compounds whose concentration could correlate to the proliferative state of the cell are being pursued in many laboratories where tests for early diagnosis of cancer are sought. It must be said, however, that so far all the tests found have appeared useful mainly in following the progression of the disease or in showing a relapse in minimal residual disease.

On the basis of data reported in the literature and our data in urine and blood serum, it appears that among the various modified nucleosides, ψ may be suggested as a useful marker for following the progression of neoplastic disease and the response to tumor therapy.

Summary

The catabolism of nucleic acids, particularly tRNA, produces a variety of modified nucleosides which are not reutilized by mammalian cells. Investigation of these compounds in body fluids, mainly urine, has recently provided evidence of altered metabolic situations in tumor-bearing patients.

The factors involved in the alterations of modified nucleosides formation are connected with altered tRNA-modifying enzymes and/or altered turnover of subpopulations of tRNA. A common pattern in tumor cells or tissues is the presence of isoaccepting tRNA species containing aberrant nucleoside modifications.

Several modified nucleosides have been detected and quantitated by HPLC analysis of the urine of normal subjects and cancer patients. Results obtained, in the authors' laboratory, among others, indicate a possible correlation between urinary excretion of these compounds and the course of the disease, with implications for the follow-up of therapeutic treatment. Particular reference should be made to ψ, which appears to be a suitable marker for monitoring these subjects. The data from the authors' laboratory also show that the analysis of modified nucleosides in blood may be considered a useful tool in the search for proper markers associated with the cancer status. In this respect ψ is suggested as a biochemical indicator for cancer patients.

Abbreviations

β-AIB, β-aminoisobutyric acid; ψ, pseudouridine; *ψMP*, pseudouridine 5′-phosphate; m^7I, 7-methylinosine; *U*, uridine; m^1A, 1-methyladenosine; m^7X, 7-methylxanthosine; m^5C, 5-methylcytidine; *dU*, deoxyuridine; m^7G, 7-methylguanosine; *I*, inosine; m^5U, 5-methyluridine; *G*, guanosine; *A*, adenosine; *C*, cytidine; m^3U, 3-methyluridine; s^4U, 4-thiouridine; m^1I, 1-methylinosine; m^1G, 1-methylguanosine; m^2G, N^2-methylguanosine; ac^4C, N^4-acetylcytidine; m^2_2G, N^2,N^2-dimethylguanosine; *dA*, deoxyadenosine; *dG*, deoxyguanosine; *Cm*, 2′-*O*-methylcytidine; *Gm*, 2′-*O*-methylguanosine; *dTMP*, thymidine 5′-phosphate; *Tm*, 2′-*O*-methylribothymidine; *hU*, dihydrouridine; t^6A, N^6-threonyladenosine; *Y*, α-(carboxyamino)-4,9-dihydro-4,6-dimethyl-9-oxo-1H-imidazol[1,2-α]-purine-7-butyric acid dimethyl ester; *Q*, 7-(4,5-*cis*-dihydroxy-l-cyclopenten-3-ylaminomethyl)-7-deazaguanosine; m^2_2Gua, N^2,N^2-dimethylguanine; *IS*, internal standard; *AUFS*, absorbance units full scale; *psi*, pounds per square inch; A_{260} *unit*, quantity of material contained in 1 ml solution which has an absorbance of 1.0 at 260 nm when measured in 1-cm lightpath cell; *GLC*, gas-liquid chromatography; *RPC,* reverse-phase chromatography; *HPLC,* high-performance liquid chromatography; *RIA,* radioimmunoassay; *SVP,* snake venom phosphodiesterase; *TCA,* trichloracetic acid; *EDTA,* ethylenediaminetetraacetate; *CEF,* chick embryo fibroblasts; *CEF(RSV),* chick embryo fibroblasts transformed by Rous sarcoma virus; *AMV,* avian myeloblastosis virus; *VERO,* cell line derived from African green monkey kidney.

References

Agris PF (1980) The modified nucleosides in tRNA. Liss, New York

Borek E, Kerr SJ (1972) Atypical transfer RNA's and their origin in neoplastic cells. Adv Cancer Res 15: 163–190

Borek E, Baliga BS, Gehrke CW, Kuo KC, Belman S, Troll W, Waalkes TP (1977) High turnover rate of transfer RNA in tumor tissue. Cancer Res 37: 3362–3366

Borek E, Gehrke CW, Waalkes TP (1979) Aberrant methylation of tRNA in tumor tissue. In: Usdin E, Borchardt RT, Creveling CR (eds) Transmethylation. Elsevier North Holland Inc., New York Amsterdam Oxford, pp 457–464

Brunke KJ, Strickler G, Leboy PS (1980) Elevated methylation capacity of selected transfer RNA methyltransferases from 9,10-dimethyl-1,2-benzanthraceneinduced rat mammary tumors. Cancer Res 40: 417–423

Carbone PP, Kaplan HS, Musshoff K, Smithers DW, Tubiana M (1971) Report of the committee on Hodgkin's disease staging classification. Cancer Res 31: 1860–1861

Chambers RW (1966) The Chemistry of pseudouridine. Prog Nucleic Acid Res Mol Biol 5: 349–398

Chheda GB (1970) Purine and pyrimidine derivatives excreted in human urine. In: Sober HA (ed) Handbook of biochemistry, 2nd edn. The Chemical Rubber Co., Cleveland, Ohio, pp G-106–G-113

Cimino F, Costanzo F, Russo T, Colonna A, Esposito F, Salvatore F (1982) Modified nucleosides from transfer ribonucleic acid as tumor markers. In: Usdin E, Borchardt RT, Creveling CR (eds) Biochemistry of S-Adenosyl-methionine and related compounds. MacMillan, London, pp 409–412

Colonna A, Costanzo F, De Caterina M, Salvatore F, Cimino F (1980) High performance liquid chromatography of modified nucleosides in the urine of cancer patients, (abstr). Commun 1st Congress of the Italian Society of Clinical Biochemistry, Milan pp 330

Colonna A, Russo T, Cimino F, Salvatore F (1981) Modified nucleosides in biological fluids of cancer patients determined by high performance liquid chromatography. J Clin Chem Clin Biochem 19: 640

Davis GE, Suits RD, Kuo KC, Gehrke CW, Waalkes TP, Borek E (1977) High-performance liquid chromatographic separation and quantitation of nucleosides in urine and some other biological fluids. Clin Chem 23: 1427–1435

Dirheimer G, Keith G, Sibler AP, Martin RP (1979) The primary structure of tRNAs and their rare nucleosides. In: Schimmel PR, Söll D, Abelson JN (eds) Transfer RNA: Structure, properties and recognition. Cold Spring Harbor Laboratory, pp 19–41

Gehrke CW, Kuo KC, Davis GE, Suits RD, Waalkes TP, Borek E (1978) Quantitative high-performance liquid chromatography of nucleosides in biological materials. J Chromatogr 150: 455–476

Gehrke CW, Kuo KC, Waalkes TP, Borek E (1979) Patterns of urinary excretion of modified nucleosides. Cancer Res 39: 1150–1153

Gionti E, Arcari P, Costanzo P, Salvatore F, Cimino F (1980) Studies on tRNA patterns in normal and Rous Sarcoma virus transformed chick embryo fibroblasts. Embo-FEBS tRNA Workshop, Strasbourg, France

Grunberger D, Weinstein IB (1975) Deficiency of the Y base in a hepatoma phenylalanine tRNA. Nature 253: 66–67

Hartwick RA, Krstulovic AM, Brown PR (1979) Identification and quantitation of nucleosides, bases and other UV-absorbing compounds in serum using reverse-phase high-performance liquid chromatography-II. Evaluation of human sera. J Chromatogr 186: 659–676

Heinrikson RL, Goldwasser E (1964) Studies on the biosynthesis of 5-ribosyluracil 5′-monophosphate in *Tetrahymena pyriformis*. J Biol Chem 239: 1177–1187

Izzo P, Traboni C, Esposito F, Salvatore F, Cimino F (1979) Transfer RNA methylation in normal and transformed chick embryo fibroblasts. Special FEBS Meeting on Enzymes, Dubrovnik-Cavtat, Yugoslavia

Karle JM, Anderson LW, Dietrick DD, Cysyk RL (1980) Determination of serum and plasma uridine levels in mice, rats, and humans by high pressure liquid chromatography. Anal Biochem 109: 41–46

Katze JR (1975) Relation of cell type and cell density to the degree of posttranscriptional modification of $tRNA^{Lys}$ and $tRNA^{Phe}$. Biochim Biophys Acta 407: 392–398

Katze JR (1978) Relation of cell type and cell density in tissue culture to the isoaccepting spectra of the nucleoside Q containing tRNAs: $tRNA^{Tyr}$, $tRNA^{Hys}$, $tRNA^{Asn}$, $tRNA^{Asp}$. Nucleic Acids Res 5: 2513–2524

Kerr SJ (1978) tRNA methyltransferase. In: Busch H (ed) Methods Cancer Res 15: 163–185

Koller CA, Stetson PL, Nichamin LV, Mitchell BS (1980) An essay of deoxyadenosine and adenosine in human plasma by HPLC. Biochem Med 24: 179–184

Kuchino Y, Borek E (1978) Tumour-specific phenylalanine tRNA contains two supernumerary methylated bases. Nature 271: 126–129

Lakings DB, Waalkes TP, Borek E, Gehrke CW, Mrochek JE, Longmore J, Adamson RH (1977) Composition, associated tissue methyltransferase activity, and catabolic end products of transfer RNA from carcinogen-induced hepatoma and normal monkey livers. Cancer Res 37: 285–292

Levine L, Waalkes TP, Stolbach L (1975) Serum levels of N^2,N^2-dimethylguanosine and pseudouridine as determined by radioimmunoassay for patients with malignancy. J Natl Cancer Inst 54: 341–343

Littauer UZ, Inouye H (1973) Regulation of tRNA. Ann Rev Biochem 42: 439–470

Matsushita T, Davis FF (1971) Studies on pseudouridylic acid synthetase from various sources. Biochim Biophys Acta 238: 165–173

Nishimura S (1979) Modified nucleosides in tRNA. In: Schimmel PR, Söll D, Abelson JN (eds) Transfer RNA: Structure, properties and recognition. Cold Spring Harbor Laboratory, pp 59–79

Okada N, Shindo-Okada N, Sato S, Itoh YH, Oda KI, Nishimura S (1978) Detection of unique tRNA species in tumor tissues by *Escherichia coli* guanine insertion enzyme. Proc Natl Acad Sci USA 75: 4247–4251

Pergolizzi RG, Engelhardt DL, Grunberger D (1978) Formation of phenylalanine transfer RNA lacking the Wye base in VERO cells during methionine starvation. J Biol Chem 253: 6341–6343

Pfadenhauer EH, Sun-de Tong (1979) Determination of inosine and adenosine in human plasma using high-performance liquid chromatography and a boronate affinity gel. J Chromatogr 162: 585–590

Pierré A, Berneman A, Vedel M, Robert-Géro M, Vigier P (1978) Avian oncornavirus associated N^2-methylguanine transferase, location and origin. Biochem Biophys Res Comm 81: 315–321

Raba M, Limburg K, Burghagen M, Katze JR, Simsek M, Heckman JE, Rajbhandary UL, Gross HJ (1979) Nucleotide sequence of three isoaccepting lysine tRNAs from rabbit liver and SV40-transformed mouse fibroblasts. Eur J Biochem 97: 305–318

Randerath E, Gopalakrishnan AS, Gupta RC, Agrawal HP, Randerath K (1981) Lack of a specific ribose methylation at guanosine 17 in Morris hepatoma 5123 D $tRNA^{Ser1}_{IGA}$. Cancer Res 41: 2863–2867

Rappaport H (1966) Tumors of hematopoietic system, Atlas of tumor pathology, sec III, fasc 8. Washington DC, Armed Forces Institute of Pathology

Robert-Géro M, Lawrence F, Farrugia G, Berneman A, Blanchard P, Vigier P, Lederer E (1975) Inhibition of virus-induced cell transformation by synthetic analogues of S-adenosylhomocysteine. Biochem Biophys Res Comm 65: 1242–1249

Roe BA, Stankiewicz AF, Rizi HL, Weisz C, Di Lauro MN, Pike D, Chen CY, Chen EY (1979) Comparison of rat liver and Walker 256 carcinosarcoma tRNAs. Nucleic Acids Res 6: 673–688

Russo T, Colonna A, Esposito F, Salvatore F, Cimino F (1982) Detection and estimation of several modified nucleosides in serum of cancer patients. Ital J Biochem 31: 75–78

Salomon R, Giveon D, Kimhi Y, Littauer UZ (1976) Abundance of $tRNA^{Phe}$ lacking the peroxy Y-base in mouse neuroblastoma. Biochemistry 15: 5258–5262

Salvatore F, Izzo P, Traboni C, Esposito F, Cimino F (1982) Studies of transfer RNA methylation in cell transformation. In: Usdin E, Borchardt RT, Creveling CR (eds) Biochemistry of S-Adenosyl-methionine and related compounds. MacMillan, London, pp 389–397

Shindo-Okada N, Terada M, Nishimura S (1981) Changes in amount of hypo-modified tRNA having guanine in place of Queuine during erythroid differentiation of murine erythroleukemia cells. Eur J Biochem 115: 423–428

Silbert DF, Fink GR, Ames BN (1966) Histidine regulatory mutants in *Salmonella typhimurium*-III. A class of regulatory mutants deficient in tRNA for histidine. J Mol Biol 22: 335–347

Speer J, Gehrke CW, Kuo KC, Waalkes TP, Borek E (1979) tRNA breakdown products as markers for cancer. Cancer 44: 2120–2123

Sueoka N, Kano-Sueoka T (1970) Transfer RNA and cell differentiation. Prog Nucleic Acid Res Mol Biol 10: 23–55

Suzuki T, Hochster RM (1966) On the biosynthesis of pseudouridine and of pseudouridylic acid in *Agrobacterium tumefaciens*. Can J Microbiol 44: 259–272

Tormey DC, Waalkes TP, Ahmann D, Gehrke CW, Zumwalt RW, Snyder J, Hansen H (1975) Biological markers in breast carcinoma I. Incidence of abnormalities of CEA, HCG, three polyamines, and three minor nucleosides. Cancer 35: 1095–1100

Tormey DC, Waalkes TP, Gehrke CW (1980) Biological markers in breast carcinoma. Clinical correlations with pseudouridine, N^2,N^2-dimethylguanosine, and 1-methylinosine. J Surg Oncol 14: 267–273

Vedel M, Robert-Gèro M, Legraverend M, Lawrence F, Lederer E (1978) Inhibition of tRNA methylation *in vitro* and in whole cells by an oncostatic S-adenosyl-homocysteine (SAH) analogue: 5′deoxy 5′-S-isobutyladenosine (SIBA). Nucleic Acids Res 5: 2979–2989

Waalkes TP, Borek E (1975) The biochemical assessment of the malignant status in man: Aspects related to tRNA modification. In: Biological characterization of human tumours (6th International Symposium). Excerpta Medica, Amsterdam pp 15–31

Waalkes TP, Gehrke CW, Zumwalt RW, Chang SY, Lakings DB, Tormey DC, Ahmann DL, Moertel CG (1975) The urinary excretion of nucleosides of ribonucleic acid by patients with advanced cancer. Cancer 36: 390–398

Increasing Urinary Levels of Modified Nucleosides and Bases During Tumor Development in Mice

J. Thomale and G. Nass*

Zentrallabor für Mutagenitätsprüfung der Deutschen Forschungsgemeinschaft, Breisacher Strasse 33, 7800 Freiburg, FRG

Introduction

Since the first reports on altered urinary excretion patterns of nucleic acid catabolites by humans suffering from various diseases (Weissman et al. 1962, 1963; Mirvish et al. 1971; Pinkard et al. 1972), more and more evidence has accumulated that cancer patients excrete increased amounts of these compounds (Cooper et al. 1977; Schöch and Heller-Schöch 1977; Gehrke et al. 1978; Gehrke et al. 1979). The specificity in the increased excretion rates of the RNA catabolites is demonstrated by the fact that patients suffering from non-cancer diseases, such as acute infections and chronic pulmonary diseases, do not have altered excretion rates of modified RNA constituents (Waalkes et al. 1975; Schöch et al. 1979).

Experimentally, cancer can be induced by exposure to certain chemicals, viruses, or radiation. There are a few reports on the elevated excretion rate of some modified nucleosides by tumor-bearing animals. For example, increased excretion of methylated purines by hamsters bearing adenovirus-induced tumors (McFarlane and Shaw 1968) and altered excretion rate of modified nucleic acid catabolites in tumor-bearing monkeys (Lakings et al. 1977) have been described. However, since the methods for analysis of these nucleic acid catabolites have been dramatically improved during recent years (Schöch et al. 1980; Gehrke et al. 1981), the number of identified and analyzed compounds in body fluids of tumor-bearing individuals has steadily increased.

Our experiments were aimed at establishing the time course between the onset of the increased excretion rate of modified nucleic acid catabolites and the development of an experimentally induced tumor. The experiments were conceived with the rationale that if altered urinary excretion of those molecules occurs before a tumor is recognizable by other methods, our results could serve as a basis for the development of an early screening test for malignant diseases. We report here the results of two sets of experiments performed during the past year.

We routinely analyzed eight different modified nucleosides and four modified bases. As laboratory animals we used C57Bl mice, and as carcinogens MCA and X-ray

* We are very grateful to Privat-Dozent Dr. Arne Luz, Institut für Biologie der GSF, Abteilung für Pathologie, Neuherberg, for carrying out the histological examinations and interpreting the findings. We also wish to thank Petra Micheels for excellent technical assistance

Table 1. Mean values of urinary excretion of nucleosides and bases by adult male mice

Compound	nmol/24 h	SD (nmol)	RSD (%)
ψ	1560.0	143.0	9
m^1A	79.0	11.0	14
m^5C	29.9	3.5	11
m^1I	46.0	8.4	18
m^1G	45.0	7.2	16
ac^4C	21.0	2.5	12
m^2G	4.8	0.9	19
m^2_2G	9.9	0.8	8
m^1Gua	28.0	3.9	14
m^7Gua	76.0	13.0	17
m^2Gua	18.0	4.5	24
m^2_2Gua	8.2	1.9	23

The 24-h urines were collected and analyzed as described (Thomale and Nass 1982; Schöch et al. 1980). Mean values, SDs, and RSDs of eight modified ribonucleosides and four modified bases were calculated on the basis of 50 single determinations

treatment. The mice were kept in metabolic cages and exact 24-h urines were collected. Aliquots of urines were prefractionated and analyzed by HPLC (Thomale and Nass 1982; Schöch et al. 1980). Since there were no data available concerning the urinary excretion rate of modified nucleosides and bases in healthy mice, we first had to establish these basic values.

Table 1 summarizes our results for the eight modified nucleosides and four modified bases. Fifty 24-h urine samples were collected from 15 healthy, untreated adult (120-day-old) mice over a period of 4 weeks. The interindividual and week-to-week intraindividual variations of excretion were found to be slight for nucleosides, resulting in RSDs between 8% and 19%.

For the four methylated guanine bases RSDs were found to be somewhat greater, i.e., between 12% and 25%. This is probably due to the more complicated three-step prefractionation procedure required for the analysis of the bases and to the fact that the bases, in contrast to the ribonucleosides, can be derived from both RNA and DNA.

Urinary Excretion of Modified Nucleosides and Bases After MCA Treatment

In a first set of experiments we used the chemical carcinogen MCA, which induces fibrosarcomas at the site of its application.

Before determining the time course of the excretion of the modified RNA catabolites, we had to establish whether there is an elevated excretion rate of those compounds in mice with an existing malignant tumor. This we investigated in mice bearing MCA-induced tumors in an advanced stage (0.5–1 cm in diameter). Figure 1 shows the results for the modified nucleosides and bases. Values are given for five untreated control mice and five mice bearing MCA-induced tumors. It is evident that in tumor-bearing mice the excretion levels are far higher than the significance border determined for the controls. The concentrations of some modified compounds, such as

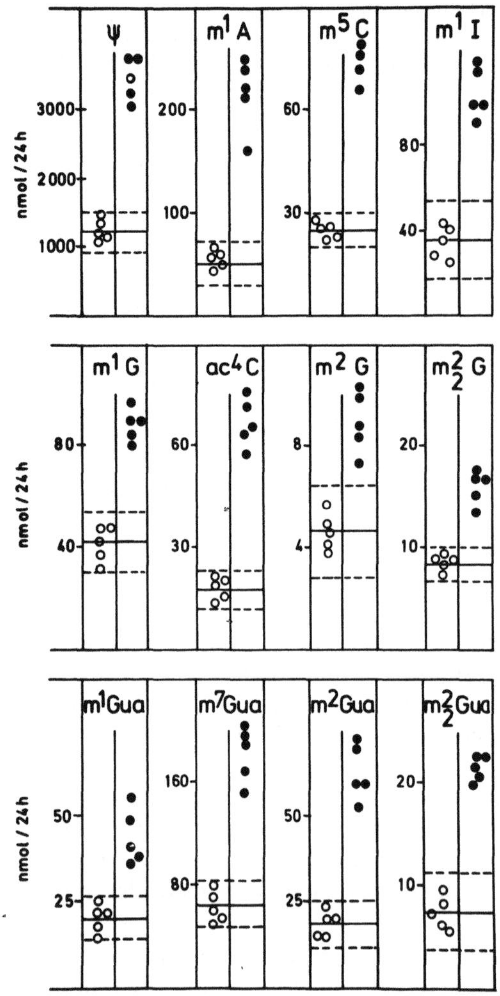

Fig. 1. Excretion of modified nucleosides and bases by tumor-bearing and control mice. The 24 h excretion values of eight modified ribonucleosides and four modified guanine bases, measured in five untreated control mice (○) and in five mice bearing MCA-induced tumors at advanced stages (●). All animals were male C57Bl mice between 300 and 350 days old at the time of measurement. The tumor was induced by a single dose of 100 μg MCA at an age of 120 days. Urine collection and analysis were achieved as described in Table 1. The horizontal *solid lines* represent the mean values of the control group and the *dotted lines* mark the ± 2 SD borders

ψ, ac^4C, m^5C, m^2Gua, and m^7Gua, are drastically increased, whereas others like m_2^2G and m^1Gua respond less.

To achieve our stated aim of correlating the time course of increased excretion with tumor development after tumor induction, we injected a single dose of 100 μg MCA into the ventral skin of each mouse and followed the excretion of the modified nucleosides and bases in ten treated mice. Five of the treated animals developed a tumor between 15 and 25 weeks after carcinogen injection and died after a further 6–8 weeks when bearing a hazelnut-sized, solid tumor. The other five animals did not respond to the MCA injection, even weeks later.

Figure 2 shows the time course of the urinary excretion values of five selected nucleosides during tumor development in an individual mouse. There is a nearly continuous increase of excretion from the 7th week after tumor induction until the death of the animal in the 23rd week. The earliest date of tumor diagnosis by palpation was the 16th week after MCA injection, when the tumor had reached a volume of 1 μl. The shapes of the excretion curves for the three modified nucleosides determined but

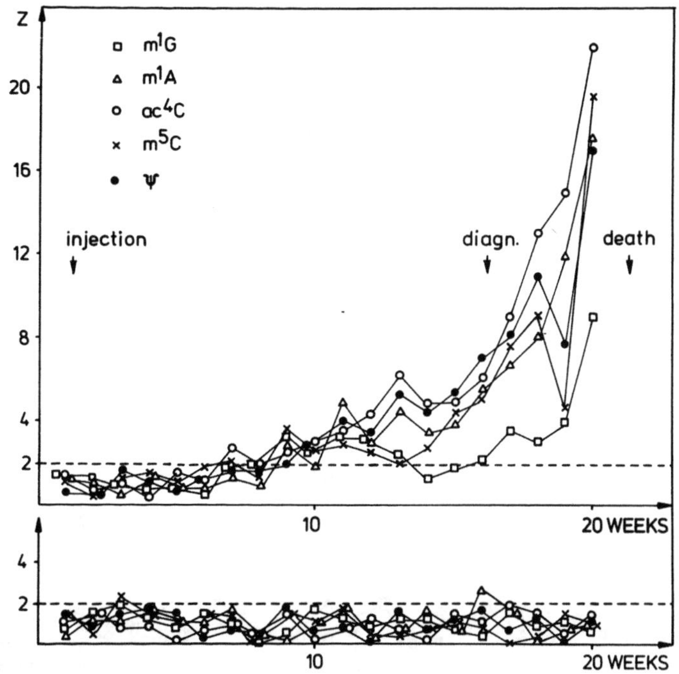

Fig. 2. Time course of urinary excretion of five modified nucleosides during tumor development. The *upper part* shows the individual excretion curves of a MCA-treated mouse from the week of injection over a period of 20 weeks until its death. *Diagn.* marks the first occurrence of a palpable tumor in the ventral skin of the mouse. Excretion is plotted as z-values, defined as differences to the mean values of the control group, expressed as multiples of SDs of the control group (Sachs 1979). The *dotted line* indicates the significant 2 SD border. The *lower part* shows the excretion curves for the same five nucleosides of an individual mouse from the corresponding control group

not shown (m^1I, m^2_2G, m^2G) were similar. Furthermore, the time courses of nucleoside excretion for the other animals which developed a tumor were similar to the one shown. The nucleoside excretion values of a mouse from the untreated control group, given for comparison in the lower part of Fig. 2, showed only little variability.

The determination of the excretion curves of the four methylated bases in the tumor-developing mouse gave similar results, as shown in Fig. 3. Again, excretion values of control mice varied only slightly. Not explicitly shown, but important, is the fact that all animals which failed to develop a tumor after treatment with MCA exhibited excretion values similar to those shown by the untreated control mice. This demonstrates the specificity of the increased excretion rate of the nucleic acid catabolites for the growth of a malignant tumor in mice.

Figure 4 summarizes the excretion values of the five tumor-developing mice at the point of diagnosis (a tumor of approximately 1 mm in diameter). Seven of 12 modified nucleosides and bases show even at this early stage urinary concentrations clearly above the 2 SD border of the control group. The other five compounds (m^1G, m^2G, m^2_2G, m^1Gua, and m^2_2Gua) exhibit a slight but not in all cases significant augmentation of excretion rate.

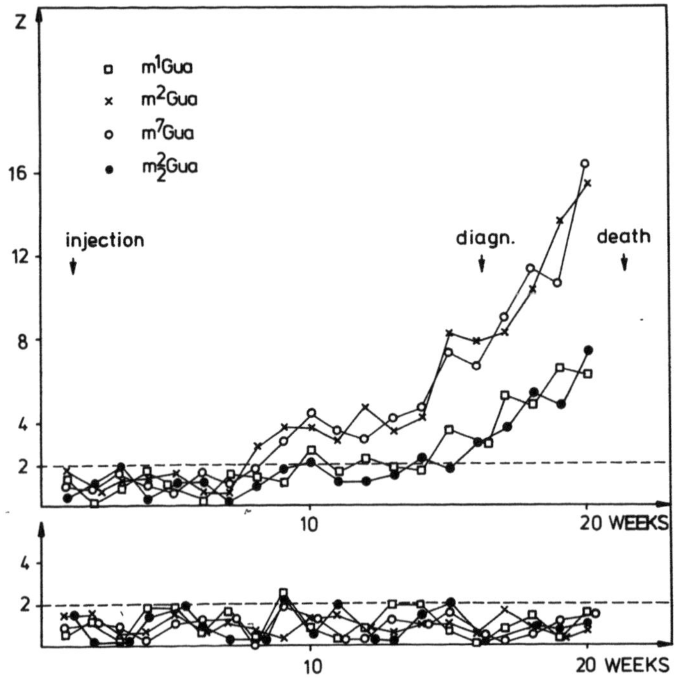

Fig. 3. Time course of urinary excretion of four methylated guanine bases during tumor development. Analysis of the bases' fraction was carried out as described in Fig. 2, using the same urine samples. The method of calculation and plotting is as described in Fig. 2, showing in the *upper part* excretion curves of the tumor-developing mouse and in the *lower part* those of an untreated control mouse

Excretion of Modified Nucleosides in Irradiated Mice

In this series of experiments we used X-ray irradiation as tumor initiator. The conditions were again chosen so that a single exposure to the carcinogen should result in cancer induction; leukemia should develop within 8 months after X-ray treatment (Upton et al. 1958). Ten C57Bl mice were irradiated with 300 rads each and their urinary excretion of modified nucleosides was monitored weekly thereafter. Nine months have now passed since irradiation, so we can give a progress report. The data so far obtained again indicate that increased excretion rate of modified nucleosides and bases is an early signal of cancer development.

Figure 5 shows the time course of excretion of five nucleosides in the only one of the 10 mice irradiated to die of leukemia so far. The excretion rate of the modified nucleosides began to increase about 20 weeks after irradiation, then declined under the significance border, and finally increased tremendously about 4 weeks before the mouse died.

We also followed the excretion rate of modified nucleosides in the other irradiated mice. So far the excretion of modified nucleosides has begun to increase in five of the ten irradiated mice in comparison to the untreated control mice. Three of them were killed so histological leukemic signs could be correlated to the urinary excretion rates of modified nucleosides. In addition, one of the irradiated mice which at this time did

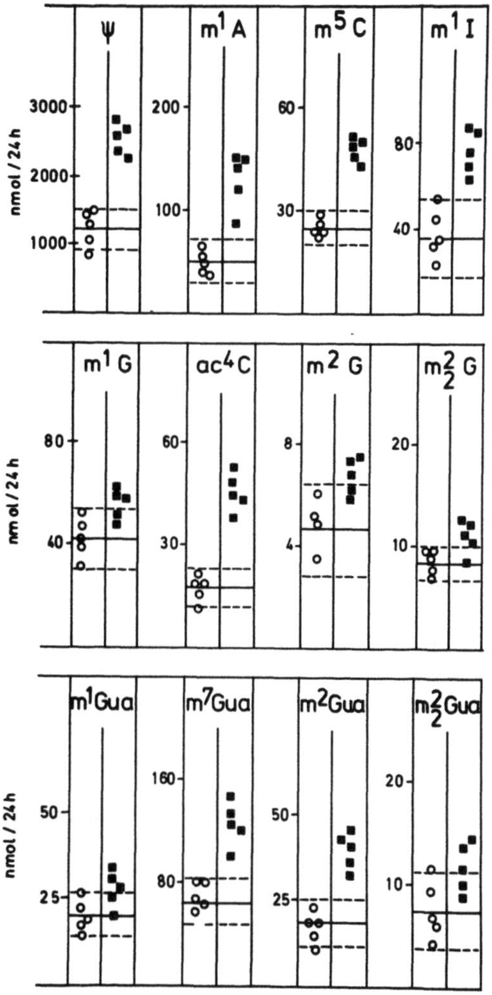

Fig. 4. Excretion rates of modified nucleosides and bases in early stages of tumor growth. The 24-h excretion values of five untreated control mice (○) and five tumor-developing mice (■) were determined and plotted as described in Fig. 1. At the time of determination, fibrosarcomas in the ventral skin had reached a diameter of 0.5–1.0 mm

not show any pathological urinary excretion values and one untreated control mouse were killed and investigated histologically.

Table 2 summarizes the results. The untreated control mouse exhibits normal nucleoside excretion and normal histological data. Mouse I, though irradiated, did not show any pathological excretion values at the time of killing and was also free of histological abnormalities. The other three irradiated mice (II–IV) excreted modified nucleosides at variously increased rates and exhibited preleukemic histological signs. Interestingly, the degrees of deviation of both criteria from normal values moved in parallel.

These results support our notion that an increased excretion rate of modified nucleosides precedes tumor manifestation and is thus suitable as a basis for the development of an early test for cancer diagnosis. We are also attempting to apply the determination of urinary modified nucleosides and bases as a relatively simple in vivo test for screening the carcinogenicity of compounds.

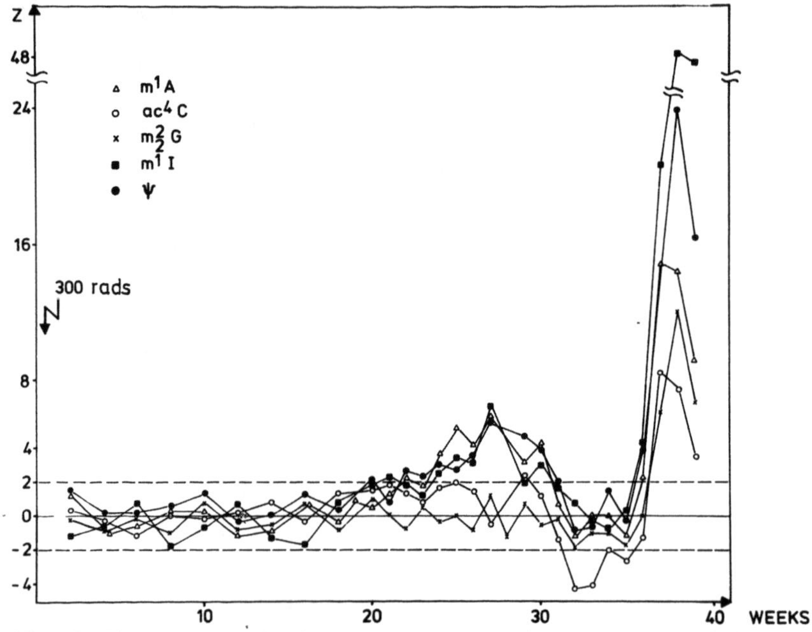

Fig. 5. Time course of urinary excreted modified nucleosides during irradiation-induced leukemia in a C57Bl mouse. The 150-day-old male animal was irradiated with a single dose of 300 rads (whole body). Excretion of urinary nucleosides was measured as described in Table 1 over a period of 40 weeks until the death of the mouse. Excretion values of five selected nucleosides are plotted as z-values as described in Fig. 2

Table 2. Urinary excretion of modified nucleosides and histological data of irradiated mice

Nucleoside	Control	Irradiated mice			
		I	II	III	IV
ψ	1.7	−0.4	2.8	7.7	8.3
m^1A	1.1	−2.1	2.0	5.4	4.9
m^5C	1.3	−1.5	4.4	7.2	7.1
m^1I	−0.2	−2.3	−0.9	8.5	6.2
m^1G	−0.4	−1.8	−1.9	6.6	5.1
ac^4C	−1.6	−1.4	−1.1	4.0	5.3
m^2G	1.5	0.8	−1.5	5.9	2.0
m^2_2G	1.3	1.1	−1.4	−0.7	4.3
Pathological criteria					
Spleen					
1. Loss of lymphocyte cuff of follicles	−	−	+	+	−
2. Accumulation of transformed lymphocytes	−	−	−	+	+
Lymph node					
3. Macroscopically enlarged	−	−	−	−	+
4. Loss of lymphocyte cuff of follicles	−	−	+	+	+
5. Paracortical hyperplasia	−	−	−	−	+

Radiation treatment and analysis of nucleosides were carried out as described in Fig. 5. Excretion values of the last week before death are given in z-values as defined in Fig. 2. Histological preleukemic features are listed in the lower part of the table

Considerations of the Meaning of the Increased Excretion rate of Modified Nucleosides and Bases During Tumor Development

The first question to be asked concerns the origin of the modified nucleosides and bases excreted at an increased rate in tumor-bearing individuals. When using methylated compounds like MCA as carcinogens, the methyl groups, of methylated nucleic acid catabolites, could at first sight be thought to be derived from the injected carcinogen. This possibility is easy to rule out by comparing the amount of potential methyl groups injected with a single dose of 100 μg MCA, the time elapsed after the onset of the increased excretion rate, and the amount of methylated nucleosides and bases excreted. A further indication that the methyl groups are not derived from the injected carcinogen stems from our finding that the mice which received MCA but did not develop a tumor excreted normal values of methylated nucleic acid catabolites throughout the experiment. Only in the cases where the amount of methylated nucleosides in urine increased within a few days after injecting the methylated carcinogen (Weyland et al. 1972; Chu and Lawley 1975; Hanski and Strehlik 1980) might the modifications of the nucleic acid catabolites be derived from the carcinogen itself.

The second question concerns the biological meaning of the increased excretion of these modified nucleic acid catabolites. From our data on the time course of modified nucleic acid catabolites excretion it can be deduced that several weeks have to pass after initiation of the tumor before pathological values are measurable, but they do appear before the tumor has reached 1 mm in diameter or leukemic features are found. Thus we believe that the increased excretion rate is not the result of tumor metabolism alone, although an increased turnover of tRNA in tumors has been reported (Borek et al. 1977). Our interpretation of the increased excretion rate of modified nucleosides and bases in tumor-bearing individuals is that it is an expression of an altered overall metabolism in the whole organism preceding and accompanying tumor growth.

Experimental support for this hypothesis also comes from results in plasmacytoma-bearing mice, in which not only the tRNAs of the tumor cells, but also those of the liver cells, showed an altered pattern of tRNA isoacceptors (Marini et al. 1979). However, other organs besides the liver should be analyzed for tRNA isoacceptors, since in mammals it is particularly the liver which is involved in the organism's anabolism and catabolism. Further evidence supporting our interpretation that the altered tRNA metabolism is not restricted to the tumor cells is seen in the fact that the energy metabolism of human cancer patients is altered (Weber 1977). Furthermore, it has recently been found that the energy metabolism in tumor-bearing mice changes specifically even before malignant cachexia begins (Burt et al. 1981).

Thus there is apparently a general alteration in the regulation of metabolism before tumor growth starts. For this reason, reports in the literature which document an elevated excretion rate of modified nucleosides a few days after inoculating tumor cells into an animal (Shimizu and Fujimura 1978) do not give information on the changes in RNA metabolism, immune system, etc. of the individual during the time after a tumor cell develops and tumor growth begins.

Another so far open question is that of the tumor specificity of different excretion patterns. In this regard, we want to draw attention to our data on ac^4C excretion in the fibrosarcoma and leukemic mice. The excretion rate of this modified nucleoside is little affected during the preleukemic stages and even sinks below the ± 2 SD region of the control mean value during manifestation of the leukemia (Fig. 5). In contrast, during growth of the MCA-induced solid skin tumor ac^4C is the most increased modified nucleoside (Fig. 2). These findings are in line with data obtained from human patients reported by Gehrke et al. in 1978. They found the excretion rate of ac^4C to be unaffected in patients suffering from leukemia, but significantly augmented in patients bearing solid tumors such as mammary or colonic carcinoma. Data obtained in the future will reveal whether an increased excretion rate of ac^4C, which so far has been found in eukaryotic tRNAs only in the D-stem of $tRNA^{Leu}$ and $tRNA^{Ser}$ (Gauss and Sprinzl 1981), signals the presence of organ-specific tumors.

Summary

Based on the fact that human cancer patients excrete increased amounts of various modified nucleosides and bases in their urine, we investigated whether the same phenomenon takes place in mice bearing experimentally induced tumors. We did indeed find that mice with MCA-induced skin tumors and mice exhibiting leukemia after X-ray irradiation excrete severalfold higher levels of modified nucleosides and bases than do untreated control mice.
Comparison of the time course of altered urinary excretion of these RNA catabolites with the appearance of a recognizable tumor after MCA application revealed that the onset of the altered excretion rate of these compounds precedes tumor diagnosis. At present, the time-course studies in our mice exposed to a single X-ray dose to induce lymphoblastic leukemia seem to indicate a similar situation. Mice exhibiting preleukemic histological features already excrete increased amounts of various modified nucleosides and bases. Confirmation of our results by analysis of further irradiation-exposed mice in our present detailed time-course studies and of tumors experimentally induced in other organs of mice and other species will be taken as a basis for developing an in vivo test for carcinogenicity. Furthermore, the results could provide a foundation for the setting up of a noninvasive, early screening method for cancer in human beings.

Abbreviations

MCA, 3-methylcholanthrene; *HPLC,* high-pressure liquid chromatography; *RSD,* relative standard deviation; *SD,* standard deviation; m^1A, 1-methyladenosine; ac^4C, N^4-acetylcytidine; m^5C, 5-methylcytidine; m^1G, 1-methylguanosine; m^2G, N^2-methylguanosine; m^2_2G, N^2,N^2-dimethylguanosine; m^1I, 1-methylinosine; ψ, 5-(β-D-ribofuranosyl)-uracil (pseudouridine); m^1Gua, 1-methylguanine; m^7Gua, 7-methylguanine; m^2Gua, N^2-methylguanine; m^2_2Gua, N^2,N^2-dimethylguanine.

References

Borek E, Baliga BS, Gehrke CW, Kuo KC, Belman S, Troll W, Waalkes TP (1977) High turnover of tRNA in tumor tissue. Cancer Res 37: 3362–3366

Burt ME, Lowry SF, Gorschboth C, Brennan MF (1981) Metabolic alterations in a noncachectic animal tumor system. Cancer 47: 2138–2146

Chu BCF, Lawley PD (1975) Increased urinary excretion of nucleic acid and nicotinamide derivatives by rats after treatment with alkylating agents. Chem Biol Interactions 10: 333–338

Cooper IA, Wray GR, Murphy TL (1977) Urinary excretory patterns of tRNA degradation products: A marker of Hodgkin's cell metabolism? Eur J Cancer 13: 1309–1312

Gauss DH, Sprinzl M (1981) Compilation of tRNA sequences. Nucleic Acids Res 9: r1–r23

Gehrke, CW, Kuo KC (1981) Major and modified nucleosides, RNA and DNA. In: Marton LJ, Kabra PM (eds) Liquid chromatography in clinical analysis. Humana Press, Clifton pp. 409–444

Gehrke, CW, Kuo KC, Davis GE, Suits RD, Waalkes TP, Borek E (1978) Quantiative high-performance liquid chromatography of nucleosides in biological materials. J Chromatogr 150: 455–476

Gehrke CW, Kuo KC, Waalkes TP, Borek E (1979) Patterns of urinary excretion of modified nucleosides. Cancer Res 39: 1150–1153

Hanski C, Stehlik G (1980) Increased concentration of 7-methylguanine and 1-methylhypoxanthine in urine of rats bearing Yoshida tumour. Cancer Lett 9: 339–343

Lakings, DB, Waalkes TP, Borek E, Gehrke CW, Mrochek JE, Longmore J, Adamson RH (1977) Composition, associated tissue methyltransferase activity, and catabolic end products of transfer RNA from carcinogen-induced Hepatoma and normal monkey livers. Cancer Res 37: 285–292

Marini M, Muldoon WP, Mushinsky JF (1979) Biochemical changes induced by tumors at distant sites: Altered transfer RNA profiles in liver of mice bearing plasmacytomas. Cancer Lett 9: 177–181

McFarlane ES, Shaw GJ (1968) Observed increase in methylated purines excreted by hamsters bearing adenovirus-12 induced tumors. Can J Microbiol 14: 185

Mirvish SS, Medalie J, Linsell CA, Yousuf E, Reyad S (1971) 7-Methylguanine and other minor urinary purines: values for normal subjects from Israel, Gaza, and Kenya, and for patients with cancer of various organs or cirrhosis of the liver. Cancer 27: 736–743

Pinkard PJ, Cooper IA, Motteram R, Turner CN (1972) Purine and pyrimidine excretion in Hodgkin's disease. J Natl Cancer Inst 49: 27–37

Sachs L (1979) Statistische Methoden. Springer, Berlin Heidelberg New York

Schöch G, Heller-Schöch G (1977) Molekularbiologie und klinische Bedeutung des Stoffwechsels normaler und modifizierter Nucleobasen. Helv Paediatr Acta [Suppl] 38: 7–171

Schöch G, Thomale J, Lorenz H, Suberg H, Karsten U (1980) A new method for the simultaneous analysis of unmodified and modified urinary nucleosides and nucleobases by high performance liquid chromatography. Clin Chim Acta 108: 247–257

Schöch G, Winkler K, Heller-Schöch G, Baisch H (1979) Die Analyse von normalen und methylierten Nucleobasen im Urin als neues Kriterium für Diagnose und Verlauf von Malignomen. Klin Pädiatr 191: 197–204

Shimizu M, Fujimura S (1978) Studies on the abnormal excretion of pyrimidine nucleosides in the urine of Yoshida ascites sarcoma-bearing rats. Increased excretion of deoxycytidine, pseudouridine and cytidine. Biochim Biophys Acta 517: 277–286

Thomale J, Nass G (1982) Elevated urinary excretion of RNA catabolites as an early signal of tumor development in mice. Cancer Lett 15: 149–159

Upton AC, Wolff FF, Furth J, Kimball AW (1958) A comparison of the induction of myeloid and lymphoid leukemias in X-radiated RF mice. Cancer Res 18: 842–848

Waalkes TP, Gehrke CW, Zumwalt RW, Chang SY, Lakings DB, Tormey DC, Ahmann DL, Moertel CG (1975) The urinary excretion of nucleosides of ribonucleic acid by patients with advanced cancer. Cancer 36: 390–398

Weber G (1977) Enzymology of cancer cells (part II). N Engl J Med 296: 541–551

Weissman S, Eisen AZ, Karon M (1962) Pseudouridine metabolism. II. Urinary excretion in gout, psoriasis, leukemia, and heterozygous oroticaciduria. J Lab Clin Med 59: 852–858

Weissman S, Lewis M, Karon M (1963) Pseudouridine metabolism. IV. Excretion of pseudouridine and other nitrogenous metabolites in chronic leukemia. Blood 22: 657–663

Weyland P, Gross HJ, Dannenberg H (1972) Ausscheidung von 7-Methylguanin im Harn von Ratten nach einmaliger Applikation verschiedener Carcinogene. Z Krebsforsch 77: 141–149

Comparison of Urinary Modified Nucleosides and Bases in Rats with Hepatomas and Nephroblastomas

I. Clark, J. W. MacKenzie, J. R. McCoy, and W. Lin*

Departments of Surgery, Biochemistry, and Pathology, CMDNJ-Rutgers Medical School, Piscataway, NJ, USA

Introduction

It has been known for more than 20 years that patients with cancer excrete greater than normal amounts of purine and pyrimidine derivatives in their urines (Adams et al. 1960; Park et al. 1962). The unmodified purine derivatives, adenine and guanine, are normally metabolized to uric acid, but in some instances they are not metabolized further and may be excreted or recycled into nucleic acids. The unmodified pyrimidine derivatives, cytosine and uracil, are usually degraded and excreted as ammonia and urea, but recycling and excretion may occur. It was not until the pioneering studies by Borek and his students on tRNA methyltransferases (Fleissner and Borek 1963) that the methylated nucleosides in the urine were shown to be derived from tRNA (Mandel et al. 1966). More recently, using more sensitive techniques, several groups of investigators have reported increased levels of modified nucleosides in urines from patients with cancer (Hogan et al. 1970; Waalkes et al. 1973; Mrochek et al. 1974; Senftleber et al. 1976; Davis et al. 1977; Gehrke et al. 1978; Speer et al. 1979; Hartwick et al. 1980). The increased levels of most modified nucleosides and bases in urine of hosts with neoplasms have been attributed to an increased rate of turnover of tRNA in cancer tissue (Borek et al. 1977). The evidence to date suggests that modified nucleosides or bases are not metabolized further and are quantitatively excreted into the urine (Weissman et al. 1962; Dlugajczyk and Eiler 1966). More than 20 modified nucleosides have been isolated from human urine (Chedda 1975).

Not only does the urine from man or animals with cancer contain higher levels of methylated nucleosides, but also tRNA methyltransferases extracted from tumor tissue have a significantly greater capacity for methylating heterologous tRNA than do extracts from normal tissue (Tsutsui et al. 1966; Hancock et al. 1967; Stewart and Pegg 1972; Hancock and Forrester 1973). Analyses of tRNAs from tumor tissue, however, have shown that some tRNAs are undermethylated (Randerath et al. 1974). Although enzyme extracts from several rat tissues contained the same tRNA methyltransferases, the activities of these enzymes varied from tissue to tissue. For example, m^1A tRNA methyltransferase from liver methylated *Escherichia coli* tRNA to a greater extent

* The authors are indebted to Mr. Jeffrey Turner for excellent technical assistance and to the American Cancer Society for supporting this work with the Herbert P. Clauberg Memorial Grant for Cancer Research

than did that from kidney (Clark and Trebilcock-Guzman 1979). Also, the effects of vitamin D deficiency on tRNA methyltransferase activities of bone and liver are different; it decreased them in bone while it increased them in liver (Bradford et al. 1972). These findings, that the activities of specific tRNA methyltransferases normally vary in different tissues and that the responses of these enzymes to pathologic changes also vary with the tissue, suggested that the quantitative profile of methylated nucleosides of liver tRNA might be different from that of kidney tRNA. If so, urinary excretion by animals with hepatomas might exhibit a different pattern of modified nucleosides than that by those with kidney neoplasms. Attempts to relate specific modified nucleosides to specific tumors, however, have not been successful. To test this hypothesis, we have induced hepatomas and kidney neoplasms in two strains of rats and analyzed their urines for modified nucleosides and bases.

Preparation of Animals

Aflatoxin Study

Fifty male Sprague-Dawley rats weighing 80–100 g were given orally 50 μg aflatoxin B_1 dissolved in DMSO for 22 days. Forty rats of the same age and sex served as controls and received the same volume of DMSO for the same length of time. Animals were killed monthly until the termination of the study 18 months after the last dose. No cancer was found in the few rats killed during the first 9 months, but several rats developed multinodular hepatocyte hyperplasia. Hepatocellular adenocarcinoma was first evident at the 11th month, and 24-h urines were collected monthly beginning at this time. All rats at the end of the study had hepatomas and 24-h urine collections were made prior to killing them.

Dimethylnitrosamine Study

One hundred and ten Wistar male rats weighing between 80 and 100 g were injected intraperitoneally with a single dose of dimethylnitrosamine (60 mg/kg body weight). For 5 days prior to injection, they were fed a protein-free diet (50% glucose + 50% sucrose) and drinking water containing 20% glucose. About half of the rats died during the first 2 weeks. Forty rats of the same sex and age served as controls. Two treated rats and one control rat were killed monthly. At the end of the study (8 months) all animals had nephroblastomas, first noted at 4 months. Twenty-four-hour urines of all rats were collected prior to killing.

Analytical Procedures

Urines were analyzed for nucleosides and bases using HPLC (Clark and Trebilcock-Guzman 1979). Figure 1 shows the UV absorption spectra of urines from a control rat and a hepatoma-bearing rat. Equal quantities of urine (10 ml) were added to a column of QAE Sephadex and the UV-absorbing material eluted with different concentrations of borate in a stepwise manner. Nucleosides and bases used as standards were also separated into six fractions and their individual location in the

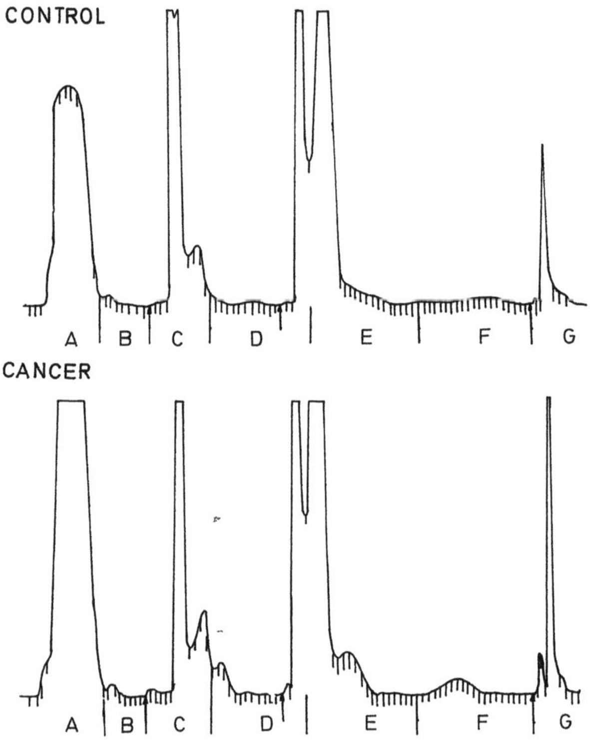

Fig. 1. UV absorption spectra of urine from a control rat and a rat with hepatoma. Ten milliliters of urine was added to a column (0.9 cm × 15 cm) of QAE Sephadex A25 and eluted with 0.01, 0.1, and 0.5 *M* H_3BO_3 in a stepwise fashion. *Fraction A,* 0.01 *M* H_3BO_3 for 28 min, flow rate 1.0 ml/min; *fraction B,* 0.01 *M* H_3BO_3 for 16 min, flow rate 4.0 ml/min; *fraction C,* 0.1 *M* H_3BO_3 for 24 min, flow rate 4.0 ml/min; *fraction D,* 0.1 *M* H_3BO_3 for 24 min, flow rate 4.0 ml/min, also 0.5 *M* H_3BO_3 for 12 min, flow rate 4.0 ml/min; *fraction E,* 0.5 *M* H_3BO_3 for 40 min, flow rate 6.7 ml/min; *fraction F,* 0.5 *M* H_3BO_3 for 40 min, flow rate 7.5 ml/min; *fraction G,* 0.1 *M* HCl for 20 min, flow rate 7.5 ml/min

different fractions established. The curves are similar except for the larger amounts of UV-absorbing materials excreted by the animal with the neoplasm. After removal of the boric acid, the fractions were made up to 1.0 ml and aliquots were injected into the HPLC apparatus. The components were separated on a reverse-phase Whatman Partisil ODS-3 column using an ammonium phosphate-methanol mobile phase. In the original method (Clark and Trebilcock-Guzman 1979) a Magnum Partisil SCX column was used.

Figure 2 shows a typical absorption curve of fraction B. Our usual procedure is first to introduce a sample into the HPLC and obtain its absorption spectrum. This is followed by a mixture containing the sample and standards known to be in that fraction. From the differences in peak heights the concentration of nucleoside or base in the urine may be calculated. We have not found retention time alone to be a satisfactory criterion for the identification of a nucleoside or base. To help establish the identity of the various nucleosides, urine fractions were also analyzed using a Whatman Partisil SCX column. In addition, ratios of UV absorption at 280 nm and 254 nm were determined for the

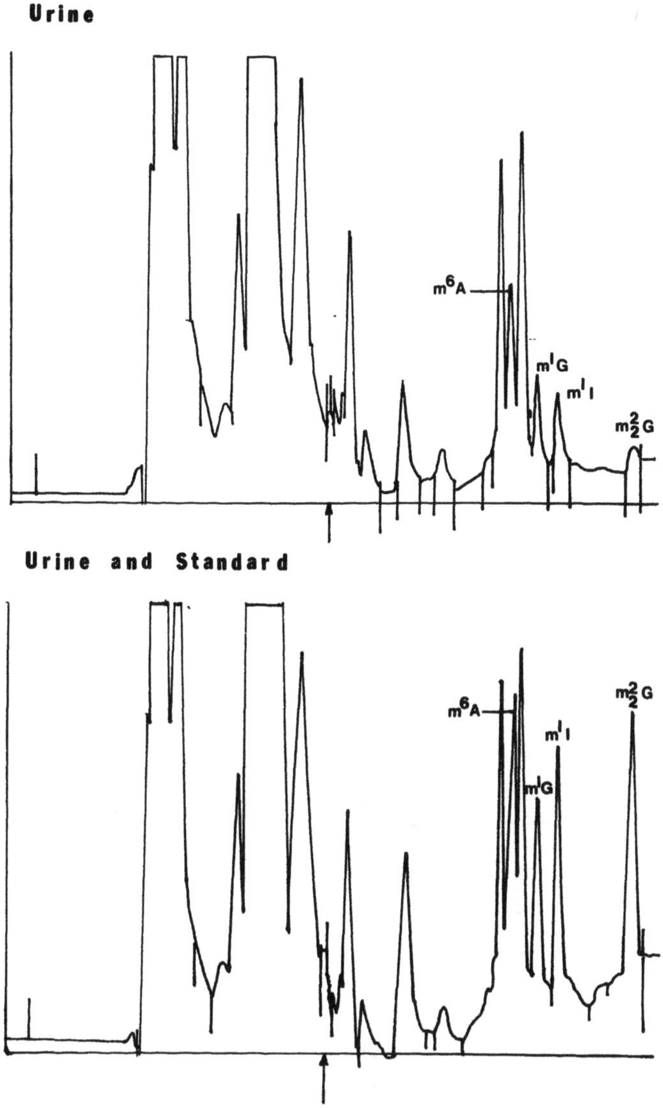

Fig. 2. UV absorption spectra of 50 μl fraction E, our most complicated fraction (equivalent to 0.5 ml urine), and 50 μl fraction E plus 50 μl standard solution containing 0.79 nmol ψ, 0.68 nmol m^6A, 0.66 nmol m^1G, 0.58 nmol m^1I and 2.19 nmol m^2_2G. The components were separated using a Whatman Partisil ODS-3 analytical column. The first mobile phase contained 0.125% methanol (v/v) and 0.11% H_3PO_4 (v/v) in 0.005 *M* $NH_4H_2PO_4$ at a flow rate of 0.5 ml/min for 15 min. The second mobile phase, introduced at the *arrow*, contained 10% methanol, 0.22% H_3PO_4 in 0.01 *M* $NH_4H_2PO_4$ at a flow rate of 1.5 ml/min for 16 min

urinary nucleosides and bases and compared with the ratios of known standards. The nucleosides and bases described in this report have been determined by these three methods.

Results and Discussion

Table 1 shows the 24-h control urinary excretion values of Sprague-Dawley and Wistar rats. The Wistar rats excreted significantly more of the specified substances than did the Sprague-Dawley rats. This undoubtedly reflects differences in the body weight, since the Wistar rats weighed almost twice as much as the other strain. When the body

Table 1. Control urinary modified nucleosides and bases of Sprague-Dawley and Wistar rats

	Sprague-Dawley (nmol/ 24 h)	Wistar (nmol/ 24 h)	*P*	Sprague-Dawley (nmol/ 100 g)	Wistar (nmol/ 100 g)	*P*
Ribonucleosides						
ψ	2118 (580)	3664 (640)	< 0.001	5.94 (1.85)	5.18 (0.88)	NS
m^1A	175 (61)	275 (91)	< 0.01	0.44 (0.17)	0.40 (0.11)	NS
m^1G	16 (6)	32 (11)	< 0.005	0.043 (0.014)	0.049 (0.017)	NS
m_2^2G	13 (3)	22 (6)	< 0.05	0.035 (0.007)	0.032 (0.008)	NS
m^1I	9.2 (3.5)	17.7 (4.0)	< 0.001	0.025 (0.007)	0.026 (0.009)	NS
m^2G	3.4 (1.0)	8.3 (3.2)	< 0.001	0.009 (0.003)	0.013 (0.004)	NS
m^3C	42 (15)	72 (22)	< 0.025	0.118 (0.045)	0.094 (0.028)	NS
m^6A	41 (13)	41.6 (13)	NS	0.11 (0.05)	0.063 (0.028)	<0.01
Um	32 (8)	50 (13)	< 0.005	0.089 (0.021)	0.076 (0.017)	NS
Bases						
m^7Gua	271 (90)	419 (98)	< 0.005	0.76 (0.28)	0.69 (0.17)	NS
m^1H	85 (47)	93 (21)	NS	0.24 (0.16)	0.13 (0.05)	NS
Ura	568 (162)	925 (120)	< 0.001	1.57 (0.42)	1.38 (0.24)	NS
Thy	84 (45)	114 (59)	NS	0.22 (0.17)	0.152 (0.087)	NS
Deoxyribonucleosides						
dT	29 (9)	27 (12)	NS	1.2 (3.15)	0.0393 (0.018)	NS

Average body weights: Sprague-Dawley = 362/Wistar = 662 g. The numbers in parentheses refer to the standard deviation from the mean

weights of the rats were taken into account there were no differences in the excretion of practically all the nucleosides and bases.

Table 2 shows a comparison of the excretion values of control rats and those with histologically proven hepatocellular adenocarcinoma. Examination of all other soft tissues in these rats showed no metastases or other primary lesions. The animals with hepatomas excreted significantly more of the ribonucleosides and m^7Gua, m^1H, and Ura than did the control rats. No significant differences were found in the excretion of Thy or dT, the latter nucleoside reflecting DNA metabolism. Analyses of several urines from these animals 11 months after administration of the carcinogen also showed significant increases in these nucleosides. However, since the rats were not

Table 2. Modified urinary nucleosides and bases in rats with hepatomas (nmol/24 h)

	Control	Hepatoma	*P*	Hepatoma/ control ratio
Ribonucleosides				
ψ	2118 [9] (581)	6978 [9] (2628)	< 0.001	3.29
m^1A	158 [9] (61)	527 [10] (174)	< 0.001	2.92
m^1G	16 [9] (6)	78 [8] (33)	< 0.001	4.96
m^2_2G	13.3 [4] (3.3)	44 [6] (24)	< 0.05	3.37
m^1I	9.1 [9] (3.5)	49 [8] (19)	< 0.001	5.35
m^2G	3.4 [9] (1.0)	13 [11] (11)	< 0.005	3.68
m^3C	42 [9] (14)	124 [9] (54)	< 0.001	2.59
m^6A	41 [9] (13)	108 [9] (33)	< 0.001	2.65
Um	32 [9] (8)	104 [9] (35)	< 0.001	3.24
Bases				
m^7Gua	271 [9] (90)	860 [9] (372)	< 0.001	3.16
m^1H	85 [9] (47)	151 [8] (71)	< 0.05	1.77
Ura	568 [9] (162)	1212 [8] (371)	< 0.001	2.13
Thy	65 [8] (45)	95 [7] (78)	NS	1.13
Deoxyribonucleosides				
dT	29 [8] (9)	41 [8] (25)	NS	1.42

Numbers in brackets refer to the number of animals per group, and numbers in parentheses refer to the standard deviation from the mean

killed at this time the magnitude or type of the lesions could not be determined. To date, all rats that developed hepatomas showed a gradual increase in the excretion of these nucleosides from month 11 until they were sacrificed at 18 months (to be published).

The hepatoma/control ratios of many of the urinary ribonucleosides (Table 2) are similar, further supporting the studies of Borek et al., 1977 which showed increased tRNA turnover in tumor tissue. However, the fact that the ratios are not all the same implies that perhaps certain tRNAs or precursor tRNAs may be turning over more rapidly or that some of the nucleosides may be derived from other RNA species in addition to tRNA.

Table 3. Concentrations of modified nucleosides and bases in liver and urine

	Liver[a] (molar ratios)	Liver[b] (molar ratios)	Liver[c] (molar ratios)	Urine (nmol/24 h)
ψ	3.61	2.99	4.3	2118
m^1A	1.30	0.90	1.6	175
m^1G	0.78	0.64	0.80	15.7
m^2G	1.25	0.95	0.40	13.3
m^2_2G	0.57	0.41	0.65	3.4
m^7G	0.79	0.58	+	271[d]
m^6A	–	–	–	40.8
Um	–	–	0.30	32.1
m^3C	0.343	0.23	+	42.2
m^1I	–	–	–	9.2
m^1H	–	–	–	85.0

[a] From Randerath et al. (1974)
[b] From Roe et al. (1979)
[c] From Garel et al. (1976)
[d] m^7Gua

Table 3 shows a comparison between the concentrations of modified nucleosides in the liver and those in control urine. The excretion of ψ, m^1A, m^1G, m^2G, and m^2_2G correlates reasonably well with their concentration in liver tRNA (Randerath et al. 1974; Garel et al. 1976; Roe et al. 1979). The concentrations of major modified nucleosides in tRNA of other mammalian tissues are probably similar to those of liver, since even the tRNA of Walker 256 carcinosarcoma contains the same relative concentrations as liver with only minor deviations (Roe et al. 1979). Thus the concentration of some modified nucleosides in the urine would reflect, to some extent, their levels in the tRNA of the various tissues in the body. The presence of relatively large amounts of m^6A in the urine, however, suggests that the turnover of mRNA may contribute to the excretion of modified nucleosides, since m^6A is not found in tRNA but in the internal structure of mRNA (Desrosiers et al. 1974; Rottman 1978). It is conceivable that the conversion of m^1A to m^6A, which occurs under certain conditions, may account for the presence of some m^6A in the urine. Also, the relatively large amounts of Um in the urine as compared to the small amount found in tRNA from liver or kidney (to be published) suggests that it too may be derived from other RNA species. Um is found in rRNA and also in the cap structure of mRNA (Shatkin 1976). Finally, we found no m^7G (or only traces) in rat urine, but large amounts of m^7Gua. m^7G is also found in the cap strucutre of mRNA and is linked differently to its neighboring nucleosides than it is in tRNA; the enzymatic hydrolysis of the cap structure in vivo is most likely different from that of tRNA and rRNA. Thus, although tRNA is the major source of urinary modified nucleosides and bases, some of them may also be derived from mRNA and rRNA. Since m^6A, m^7Gua, and Um are elevated in urines from rats with hepatomas, the possibility exists that there also may be increased turnover of mRNA and rRNA in tumor tissue. The relatively large amounts of m^1I and m^1H found in the urine may be metabolic products of m^1A, if it is metabolized in the same way as adenosine. We have no explanation for the large

Table 4. Modified urinary nucleosides and bases in rats with nephroblastoma (nmol/24 h)

	Control	Nephroblastoma	P	Nephroblastoma/ control ratio
Ribonucleosides				
ψ	3426 [8] (640)	8492 [12] (1971)	< 0.001	2.48
m^1A	268 [8] (91)	749 [12] (282)	< 0.001	2.72
m^1G	33 [8] (12)	74 [12] (32)	< 0.005	2.29
m^2_2G	21 [8] (6)	73 [12] (44)	< 0.005	3.25
m^1I	17 [8] (6)	42 [12] (14)	< 0.001	2.38
m^2G	9 [8] (3)	17 [12] (10)	< 0.05	2.07
m^3C	63 [8] (23)	190 [12] (38)	< 0.001	2.64
m^6A	39 [8] (13)	107 [12] (31)	< 0.001	2.70
Um	50 [9] (12)	143 [11] (119)	< 0.05	3.24
Bases				
m^7Gua	446 [8] (92)	1377 [11] (433)	< 0.001	2.85
m^1H	85 [8] (22)	278 [11] (182)	< 0.01	3.29
Ura	902 [8] (121)	2142 [11] (990)	< 0.001	2.56
Thy	102 [7] (59)	421 [9] (297)	< 0.025	4.13
Deoxyribonucleosides				
dT	26.0 [8] (12.0)	59.1 [9] (26.4)	< 0.01	2.04

Numbers in brackets refer to the number of animals per group, and numbers in parentheses to the standard deviation from the mean

amounts of m^3C in the urine or for the absence of m^5C. Although rat liver RNA also contains other modified nucleosides, we have not been able to detect them in our samples of urine. It may be that the quantities excreted are below our level of detection.

Table 4 shows the effects of nephroblastoma on the urinary excretion of modified nucleosides and bases. Rats with kidney neoplasms excrete significantly more of the same modified nucleosides as the animals with hepatomas. We have not as yet been able to find any qualitative differences between the urinary modified nucleosides and bases of the rats with hepatomas and those with nephroblastomas. Unlike those with hepatomas, the rats with nephroblastomas appear to excrete significantly more thymine than do control rats. There was a significant increase in urinary modified

Table 5. Modified urinary nucleosides and bases in rats with nephroblastoma (nmol/μmol creatinine)

	Control	Nephroblastoma	*P*
Ribonucleosides			
ψ	143 (26)	178 (66)	NS
m^1A	10.1 (2.3)	15.0 (3.4)	< 0.005
m^1G	1.26 (0.42)	1.94 (0.88)	NS
m_2^2G	0.85 (0.26)	1.55 (1.38)	NS
m^1I	0.66 (0.21)	0.97 (0.42)	NS
m^2G	0.34 (0.09)	0.35 (0.13)	NS
m^3C	2.51 (0.54)	3.68 (0.54)	< 0.001
m^6A	1.59 (0.62)	2.45 (0.87)	< 0.05
Um	1.91 (0.57)	2.73 (1.77)	NS
Bases			
m^7Gua	17.9 (4.3)	25.1 (13.6)	NS
m^1H	3.52 (1.46)	5.53 (3.07)	NS
Ura	37.6 (8.6)	39.1 (21.9)	NS
Thy	5.0 (3.4)	6.4 (6.7)	NS
Deoxyribonucleosides			
dT	1.05 (0.69)	1.25 (1.02)	NS

Numbers in parentheses refer to the standard deviation from the mean

nucleosides in one rat in which the only observable change was the appearance of a single small nodule in the kidney with no histologic evidence of cancer. Thus it is possible that precancerous changes may be detected by the appearance of increased modified nucleosides in the urine.

Table 5 shows that no significant differences in the excretion of most nucleosides and bases were observed between control rats and those with nephroblastoma when the data were expressed as nmol nucleoside/μmol creatinine, but as noted in Table 4, highly significant differences were found when the data were expressed as nmol/24 h. It appears that the rat behaves differently from the human, whose urinary nucleoside/creatinine ratio is constant throughout the day (Gehrke et al. 1979).

Table 6 compares neoplastic/control ratios of urinary nucleosides and bases from rats with hepatomas and rats with nephroblastomas. There are no significant differences in

Table 6. Modified urinary nucleosides and bases:

	Ratios		*P*
	Hepatoma/ control	Nephroblastoma/ control	
Ribonucleosides			
ψ	329 [9] (124)	231 [12] (54)	0.023
m^1A	292 [8] (50)	272 [12] (103)	NS
m^1G	496 [8] (211)	229 [12] (98)	0.0012
m_2^2G	337 [5] (196)	325 [12] (197)	NS
m^1I	535 [8] (209)	238 [12] (77)	0.001
m^2G	368 [11] (212)	207 [12] (122)	0.029
m^3C	259 [8] (79)	264 [12] (53)	NS
m^6A	265 [9] (80)	270 [11] (55)	NS
Um	324 [9] (107)	285 [11] (237)	NS
Bases			
m^7Gua	316 [9] (139)	285 [10] (60)	NS
m^1H	177 [8] (83)	329 [11] (215)	0.032
Ura	213 [8] (65)	256 [10] (96)	NS
Thy	113 [7] (94)	413 [9] (292)	0.044
Deoxyribonucleosides			
dT	142 [8] (86)	204 [9] (91)	NS

Numbers in brackets refer to the number of animals per group, and numbers in parentheses to the standard deviation from the mean

the urinary ratios of m^1A, m^6A, m_2^2G, m^3C, m^7Gua, Um, Ura, and dT; some ratios are even identical. However, the ratios for m^1G, m^2G, ψ, and m^1I of the rats with hepatomas are significantly higher and the ratios of m^1H and Thy are significantly lower than those of rats with kidney tumors. Preliminary data from a few rats that developed both hepatomas and leukemia show significant differences in patterns of excretion between them and the rats with hepatomas only. Thus it appears that rats with different neoplasms may excrete quantitatively different patterns of modified nucleosides and bases.

Conclusions

Hepatomas induced by aflatoxin B_1 and nephroblastomas induced by dimethylnitrosamine cause elevated excretion of modified nucleosides and bases. The urinary patterns of these excretory products by rats with the two neoplasms are qualitatively the same, but quantitatively are significantly different. Preliminary data indicate that the presence of other primary cancers or metastases alters the urinary pattern of rats with hepatomas. Also, they suggest that increases in urinary modified nucleosides may occur during the precancerous stage. There is a gradual increase in urinary modified nucleosides and bases with the development of the neoplasm. Unlike the human, the ratio of nucleoside excretion to creatinine excretion in the rats is not constant throughout a 24-h period. In addition to an increased rate of tRNA turnover in cancer tissue, the data suggest that there is increased turnover of mRNA and possibly rRNA. The data clearly support the ideas that urinary modified nucleosides may be used as an aid to diagnosis of cancer, in following the progression of the cancer, and in determining the effectiveness of chemotherapy or surgery.

Summary

Hepatomas were induced in rats with aflatoxin B_1, and nephroblastomas with dimethylnitrosamine. Microscopic examination of livers of aflatoxin-treated rats revealed multinodular hepatocyte hyperplasia at 8 months, and by 13 months all rats had hepatomas. Nephroblastomas were observed by 4 months and by 8 months all rats had developed them. The urinary excretion of several modified nucleosides and bases by normal rats is dependent on body weight and reflects, to a certain extent, their concentrations in tissue tRNA. Increased levels of several modified nucleosides and bases were found in all rats that had cancer. Rats with hepatomas excreted essentially the same modified nucleosides and bases as did those with nephroblastomas; the quantitative patterns of excretion were different, however, suggesting that the urinary modified nucleosides and bases may be used to differentiate between neoplasms. Although the increase in urinary modified nucleosides and bases by tumor-bearing animals results primarily from more rapid turnover of neoplastic tRNAs, the data indicate that increased turnover of mRNA and possibly rRNA may occur in neoplastic tissue. Preliminary data suggest that increases in urinary modified nucleosides and bases may occur during a precancerous stage. The urinary pattern of modified nucleosides and bases by rats with hepatomas is altered if another primary tumor is present. The results obtained from these studies support the use of modified nucleosides and bases in urine as biochemical markers of cancer.

Abbreviations

ψ, pseudouridine; *m^1A,* 1-methyladenosine; *m^1G,* 1-methylguanosine; *m^2_2G,* N^2_2dimethylguanosine; *m^2G,* 2-methylguanosine; *m^1I,* 1-methylinosine; *m^3C,* 3-methylcytidine; *m^5C,* 5-methylcytidine; *m^6A,* 6-methyladenosine; *Um,* 2'-*O*-methyluridine; *m^7Gua,* 7-methylguanine; *Ura,* uracil; *m^1H,* 1-methylhypoxanthine; *Thy,* thymine; *dT,* thymidine; *UV,* ultraviolet light; *DMSO,* dimethylsulfoxide; *HPLC,* high-pressure liquid chromatography.

References

Adams WS, Davis F, Nakatani M (1960) Purine and pyrimidine excretion in normal and leukemic subjects. Am J Med 28: 726–734

Borek E, Baliga BS, Gehrke CW et al. (1977) High turnover rate of transfer RNA in tumor tissue. Cancer Res 37: 3362–3366

Bradford DS, Hacker B, Clark I (1972) Transfer ribonucleic acid methylases of bone: Studies on vitamin A and D deficiency. Biochem J 126: 1057–1066

Chedda CB (1975) In: Fasman G (ed) The handbook of biochemistry and molecular biology, vol I. Chemical Rubber Co., Cleveland Ohio, p 251

Clark I, Trebilcock-Guzman M (1979) Improved separation of modified nucleosides from tRNA hydrolysate: The patterns of tRNA methylation in rat tissue. J Biochem and Biophys Methods 1: 287–298

Datta RK, Datta B (1969) Role of methylated nucleic acids in carcinogenesis. Exp Mol Pathol 10: 129–140

Davis GE, Suits RD, Kuo KC, Gehrke CW, Waalkes TP, Borek E (1977) High-performance liquid chromatographic separation and quantification of nucleosides in urine and some other biological fluids. Clin Chem 23: 1427–1435

Desrosiers R, Frederici K, Rottman F (1974) Identification of methylated nucleosides in messenger RNA from Novikoff Hepatoma cells. Proc Natl Acad Sci USA 71: 3971–3975

Dlugajczyk A, Eiler JJ (1966) Lack of catabolism of 5-ribosyluracil in man. Nature 212: 611–612

Dunn DB, Hall RH (1975) In: Fasman G (ed) The handbook of biochemistry and molecular biology, vol I. Chemical Rubber Co, Cleveland Ohio

Fleissner E, Borek E (1963) Studies on the enzymatic methylation of soluble RNA. Biochemistry 2: 1093–1100

Garel JP, et al. (1976) Structural studies on RNA from Bombyx mori L. I. Nucleoside composition of enriched tRNA species from posterior silk gland purified by counter current distribution. Biochimie 58: 1089–1100

Gehrke CW, Kuo KC, Davis GE, Suits RD, Waalkes TP, Borek E (1978) Quantitative high-performance liquid chromatography of nucleosides in biological material. J Chromatogr 150: 455–476

Gehrke CW, Kuo KC, Waalkes TP, Borek E (1979) Patterns of urinary excretion of modified nucleosides. Cancer Res 39: 1150–1153

Hancock RL, Forrester PI (1973) Increase of soluble RNA methylase activities by chemical carcinogens. Cancer Res 33: 1747–1753

Hancock RL, McFarland P, Fox RR (1967) sRNA methylase activity of embryonic liver. Experientia 23: 806–807

Hartwick RA, Krstulovic AM, Brown PR (1979) Identification and quantitation of nucleosides, bases and other UV absorbing compounds in serum, using reversed phase high performance liquid chromatography. II. Evaluation of human sera. J Chromatogr 186: 659–676

Hogan A, Creuss-Callaghan MB, Fenelly JJ (1970) Studies of pseudouridine changes in chronic lymphatic leukemia during therapy. Irish J Med Sci 3: 505–511

Mandel LR, Srinivasan PR, Borek E (1966) Origins of urinary methylated purines. Nature 209: 586–588

McFarlane ES, Shaw GJ (1968) Observed increase in methylated purines excreted by hamsters bearing adenovirus-12 induced tumors. Can J Microbiol 14: 185–187

Mrochek JE, Dinsmore SR, Waalkes TP (1974) Analytic techniques in the separation and identification of specific purine and pyrimidine degradation products of tRNA: application to urine samples from cancer patients. J Natl Cancer Inst 53: 1553–1563

Park RW, Holland JF, Jenkins A (1962) Urinary purines in leukemia. Cancer Res 22: 469–477

Randerath E, Chia LL, Morris HP, Randerath K (1974) Transfer RNA base composition studies in Morris hepatomas and rat liver. Cancer Res 34: 643–653

Roe BA, Stankiewicz AF, Rizi HL, Weisz C, DiLauro MN, Pike D, Chen C, Chen E (1979) Comparison of rat liver and Walker 256 carcinosarcoma tRNAs. Nucleic Acids Res 8: 673–688

Rottman FM (1978) In: Clark BFC (ed) International review of biochemistry, biochemistry of nucleic Acids II, Vol 17. Methylation and polyadenylation of heterogeneous nuclear and messenger RNA, pp 45–73

Senftleber FC, Halline AG, Veening H, et al. (1976) Reversed phase liquid chromatographic analysis of hemodialysate from uremic patients. Clin Chem 22: 1522–1527

Shatkin AJ (1976) Capping of eucaryotic mRNAs. Cell 9: 645–653

Speer J, Gehrke CW, Kuo KC, Waalkes TP, Borek E (1979) tRNA breakdown products as markers for cancer. Cancer 44: 2120–2123

Stewart BW, Pegg AE (1972) Changes in tRNA methylase activity of rat kidney following administration of the carcinogen dimethylnitrosamine. Biochim Biophys Acta 281: 416–424

Tsutsui E, Srinivasan PR, Borek E (1966) tRNA methylases in tumors of animal and human origin. Proc Natl Acad Sci USA 56: 1003–1009

Waalkes TP, Dinsmore SR, Mrochek JE (1973) Urinary excretion by cancer patients of the nucleosides N-dimethylguanosine, 1-methylinosine and pseudouridine. J Natl Cancer Inst 51: 271–274

Weissman S, Eisen AZ, Lewis M, Karon M (1962) Pseudouridine metabolism. III. Studies with isotopically labeled pseudouridine. J Lab Clin Med 60: 40–47

Characterization and Analysis of Oncofetal tRNA and Its Possible Application for Cancer Diagnosis and Therapy

S. Nishimura, N. Shindo-Okada, H. Kasai, Y. Kuchino, S. Noguchi, M. Iigo, and A. Hoshi

Biology Division, National Cancer Center Research Institute, Tsukiji 5-1-1, Chuo-ku, Tokyo, Japan

Nucleotide Sequence Analysis of Tumor-Specific tRNAs

In 1966 Borek and his co-workers reported that tumor cells have higher levels of tRNA-methylase activity than normal cells, and consequently tRNA from tumor cells is hypermodified (Tsutsui et al. 1966). They proposed that such hypermodified tRNA has a specific functional role in tumor cells (Tsutsui et al. 1966). Although the validity of their findings was brought into question from time to time by reports of contradictory results, their fascinating hypothesis stimulated much work in this field. During the past 15 years an enormous number of reports of the appearance of new isoacceptor tRNA species in tumor cells have been published (Nishimura 1979a, b). However, it should be mentioned that in most cases those reports are suggestive but not quite informative, since new isoaccepting tRNA species were only detected by changes in the chromatographic profile of particular amino-acyl-tRNAs in column chromatography, such as RPC-5 or benzoylated DEAE cellulose, and therefore it is not known whether those new isoaccepting tRNA species are derived by transcription of different tRNA gene(s) or by changes in post-transcriptional modification. It was difficult to obtain enough pure tRNA from tumor cells for structural study using conventional sequencing methods.

Recently several postlabeling techniques for RNA sequencing have been developed (Silberklang et al. 1977; Gupta and Randerath 1979; Tanaka et al. 1980). By adopting those procedures, it now becomes possible to obtain a total nucleotide sequence of tRNA quickly with a very small amount of material (~ 5 μg). Raba et al. (1979) have shown that $tRNA_4^{Lys}$, which appears specifically in SV40-transformed mouse fibroblasts, is a product formed by changes in the post-transcriptional modification of $tRNA_2^{Lys}$, which is the major isoaccpeting species for normal cells. Roe et al. (1979) showed that $tRNA^{Asn}$ from Walker 256 mammary carcinosarcoma only differs from normal rat liver $tRNA^{Asn}$ in having guanosine in place of queuosine in the first position of anticodon.

Table 1 shows the number of reports in the literature of isoaccepting tRNA species for particular amino acids found in tumor cells. It is evident that new isoaccepting tRNA species are not found for all amino acids. New isoaccepting tRNAs frequently found in tumor cells were for phenylalanine, tyrosine, histidine, asparagine, aspartic acid, and lysine.

Recent Results in Cancer Research Vol. 84

Table 1. Isoaccepting tRNA species detected in cancer cells by column chromatography

Amino acid	No. of reports in literature
Phenylalanine	15
Tyrosine	12
Histidine	6
Aspargine	3
Aspartic acid	8
Lysine	5
Valine	4
Serine	7
Leucine	3
Glycine	2
Glutamic acid	2
Alanine	1
Arginine	2

tRNAs for those amino acids in normal tissues are known to contain hypermodified nucleosides such as Y base (in $tRNA^{Phe}$), queuosine (in $tRNA^{Tyr}$, $tRNA^{His}$, $tRNA^{Asn}$, and $tRNA^{Asp}$), and ms^2t^6A (in $tRNA^{Lys}$). Since the presence of such hypermodified nucleosides in tRNA influences elution properties of tRNA in column chromatographies, it is very likely that tumor-specific tRNAs are all produced by the change of the formation of hypermodified nucleosides in post-transcriptional process. We have also developed a postlabeling procedure for tRNA sequencing (Kuchino et al. 1979b; Kuchino et al. 1980). The method is a modification of Stanley and Vassilenko's procedure (Stanley and Vassilenko 1978). By using nuclease P_1 instead of alkaline hydrolysis, the nucleotide at the 5′ end of oligonucleotide can be analyzed as 5′-nucleotide instead of nucleoside 3′,5′-diphosphate. Two-dimensional thin-layer chromatography was used instead of the original one-dimensional electrophoresis for identification of nucleotides. In this way modified nucleotides are better characterized.

Tumor-specific $tRNA^{Asp}$ from rat ascites hepatoma (AH7974) as well as normal rat liver $tRNA^{Asp}$ were purified by successive column chromatographies, followed by two-dimensional polyacrylamide gel electrophoresis (Okada et al. 1978), and their nucleotide sequences were determined (Kuchino et al. 1981). Figure 1 shows patterns of fragments derived from tumor-specific $tRNA^{Asp}$ and normal rat liver $tRNA^{Asp}$ by partial alkaline hydrolysis. The patterns of the bands of the two tRNAs were similar, indicating that their primary structures are quite similar. The only difference observed between the two $tRNA^{Asp}$ species was replacement of the queuosine located in the first position of the anticodon of normal rat liver $tRNA^{Asp}$ with guanosine in tumor-specific $tRNA^{Asp}$ (Figs. 2, 3). It should be mentioned that other modified nucleosides present in tumor-specific $tRNA^{Asp}$ are the same as normal $tRNA^{Asp}$, indicating that queuosine biosynthesis in tRNA is specifically restricted in tumor cells, but that of other modified nucleosides is not. Similarly, nucleotide sequences of AH7974-specific $tRNA^{Val}$ and normal rat liver $tRNA^{Val}$ were determined (Shindo-Okada et al. 1981a). As shown in Fig. 4, differences between the two were again only the changes of post-transcriptional modification. Gm_{18}, C_{32} and the unknown modified nucleoside N_{34} in normal rat liver $tRNA^{Val}$ were replaced by G_{18}, Cm_{32} and I_{34} in the case of AH7974 $tRNA^{Val}$.

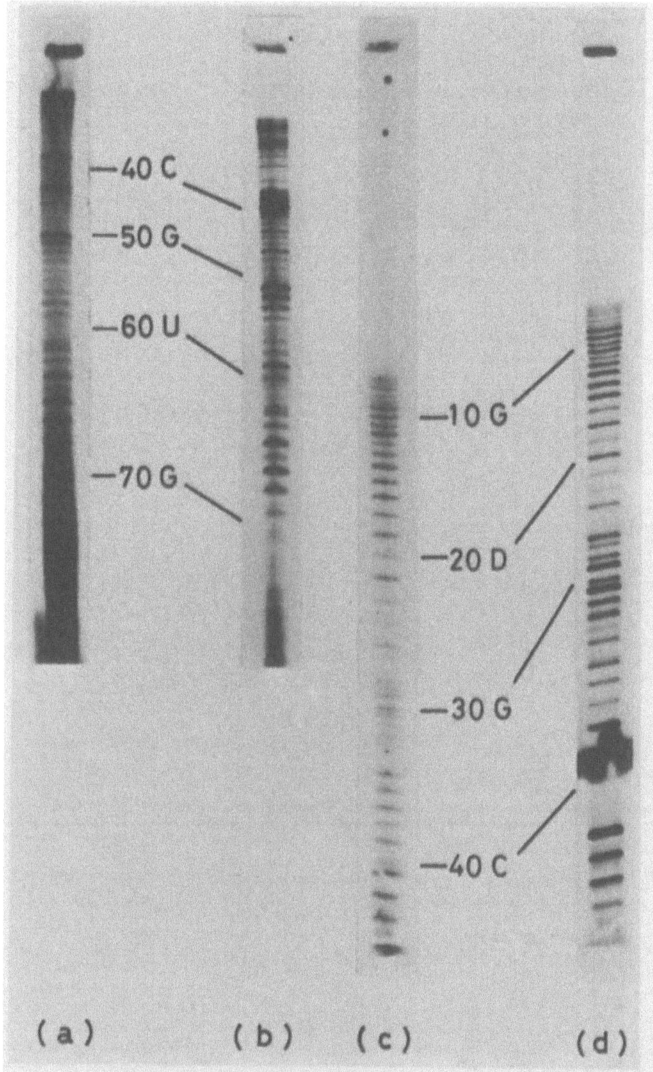

Fig. 1. Autoradiograms of 5′-labeld fragments of normal rat liver $tRNA^{Asp}$ (**a, c**) and ascites hepatoma $tRNA^{Asp}$ (**b, d**) produced by limited alkaline hydrolysis (Kuchino et al. 1981)

Therefore in the case of tumor-specific $tRNA^{Val}$, change of modification proceeds in both directions, i.e., hypomodification and hypermodification depending upon location of nucleotide residues.

Detection of the Undermodified Y Base (Y^*_{OH}) Present in Tumor-specific $tRNA^{Phe}$

As described by Dr. Grunberger (see this volume pp. 133–145), Ehrlich ascites tumor and neuroblastoma cells contained tumor-specific $tRNA^{Phe}$. The sequence analysis of these $tRNA^{Phe}$ species indicated that they contained either undermodified Y base (Y^*_{OH}) or m^1G in the position next to the anticodon in place of the fully modified Y base (Y_{OH}) present in normal $tRNA^{Phe}$, while their primary nucleotide sequences were

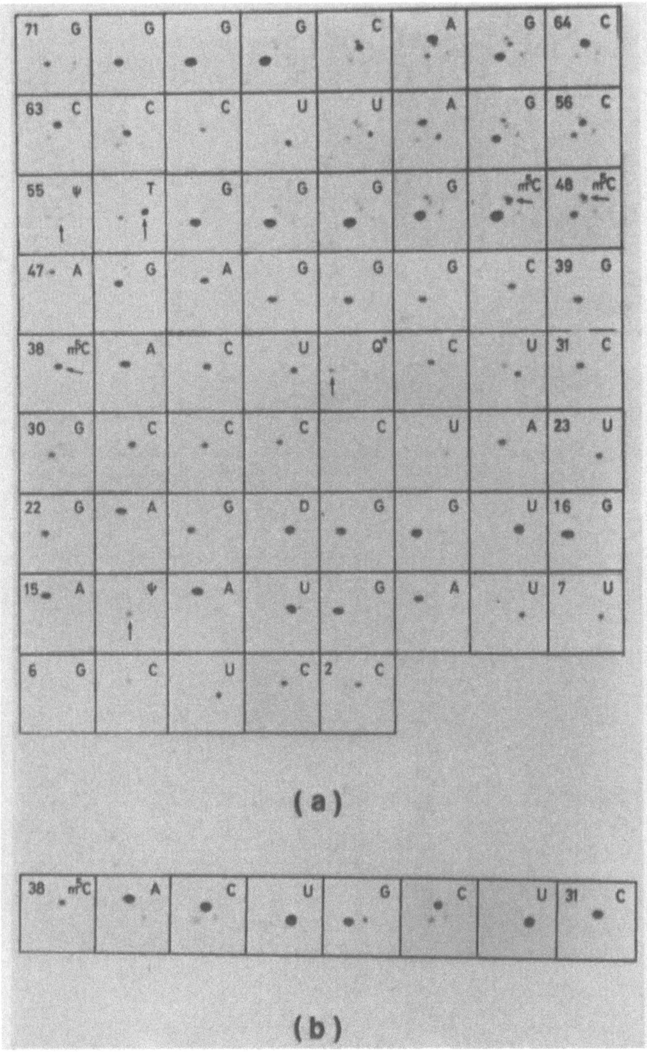

Fig. 2. Analysis of the 5′-terminal nucleotides of the fragments of normal rat liver $tRNA^{Asp}$ (**a**) and ascites hepatoma $tRNA^{Asp}$ (**b**) by two-dimensional thin-layer cellulose chromatography. The *arrows* indicate locations of modified nucleotides (Kuchino et al. 1981)

the same as that of normal $tRNA^{Phe}$ (Fig. 5) (Kuchino et al. 1979a; Y. Kuchino, D. Grunberger, E. Borek, JF, Mushinski, S. Nishimura, unpublished work). Thus it is possible to detect the presence of tumor-specific $tRNA^{Phe}$ simply by analyzing Y^*_{OH}. Sensitive and quantitative analysis of Y^*_{OH} can be carried out by the use of high-pressure liquid chromatography (HPLC) with a fluorescence detector. Approximately 1 A_{260} unit of unfractionated tRNA is treated with acid to liberate Y base. The Y base released is analyzed by HPLC using a column of μBondapak C_{18}. Y^*_{OH} and Y_{OH} are separated well by this procedure. Picomole amounts of Y base can easily be measured. It should be mentioned that approximately 100 mg tissue (net weight) is enough for the assay. Y^*_{OH} was detected in tRNA from Ehrlich ascites and Novikoff hepatoma cells, but not in tRNA from normal rat liver. The amount of Y^*_{OH} present in tumor tRNA varied in different types of tumor cell. This can be explained by the facts that the amount of tumor-specific $tRNA^{Phe}$ differs depending upon type of tumor cells and some tumor-specific $tRNA^{Phe}$ contains m^1G instead of Y^*_{OH}. Y^*_{OH} was not

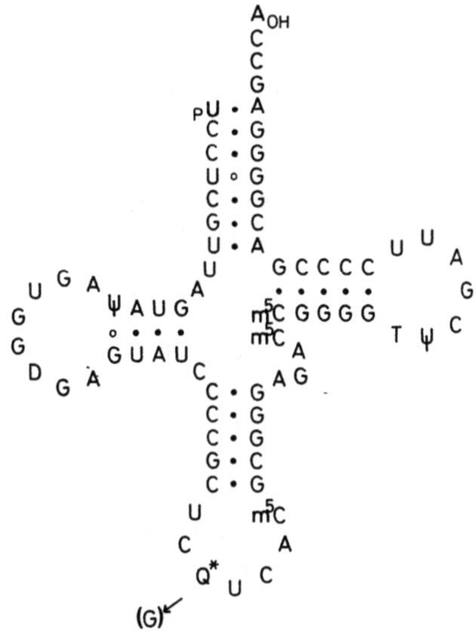

Fig. 3. Nucleotide sequence of ascites hepatoma $tRNA^{Asp}$ and normal rat liver $tRNA^{Asp}$. *Base in parentheses* is altered base found in ascites hepatoma $tRNA^{Asp}$. Q^* is mannose-containing queuosine (Kuchino et al. 1981)

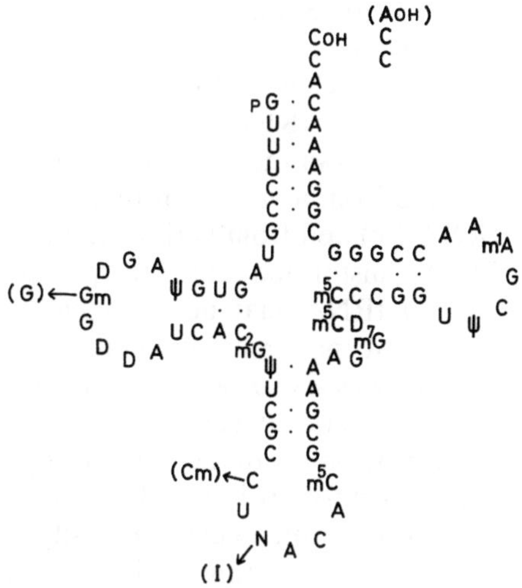

Fig. 4. Nucleotide sequence of ascites hepatoma $tRNA^{Val}$ and normal rat liver $tRNA^{Val}$. *Bases in parentheses* are altered bases found in ascites hepatoma $tRNA^{Val}$ (Shindo-Okada et al. 1981a)

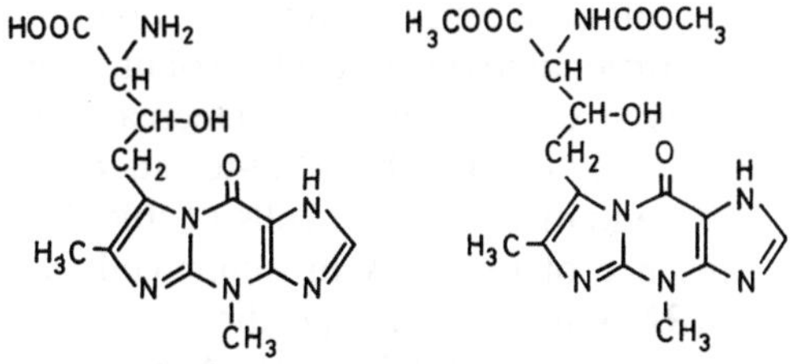

Y^{*}_{OH} Y_{OH}

Fig. 5. Structures of hydroxy Y base (Y_{OH}) and undermodified hydroxy Y base (Y^{*}_{OH}) (Kuchino et al. 1979a)

detected in normal rat kidney, spleen, and testis. The use of Y^*_{OH} analysis for cancer diagnosis would have the advantage that Y^*_{OH} is an unique compound found only in tumor cells, unlike other markers of modified nucleosides.

Detection of Q-Lacking tRNA (G-tRNA) by the Use of tRNA-Guanine Transglycosylase

Lack of queuosine in tRNA can easily be detected by analyzing incorporation of radioactive guanine into tRNA catalyzed by tRNA-guanine transglycosylase, the enzyme involved in queuosine biosynthesis in tRNA (Okada et al. 1978). It has been shown that queuosine biosynthesis in tRNA proceeds in unique fashion, quite unlike the biosynthesis of other modified nucleosides (Okada et al. 1976, 1979; Shindo-Okada et al. 1980; Katze and Farkas 1979). Queuine (the base of queuosine) or its precursors are synthesized without the participation of tRNA and then inserted into undermodified tRNA (G-tRNA) by an exchange reaction with guanine located in the first position of the anticodon of G-tRNA catalyzed by tRNA-guanine transglycosylase. In the case of *Escherichia coli,* the actual substrate for tRNA-guanine transglycosylase in vivo is likely to be a precursor of queuine, 7-(aminomethyl)-7-deazaguanine, while queuine itself seems to be a substrate in mammalian systems (Okada et al. 1979; Shindo-Okada et al. 1980; Katze and Farkas 1979). tRNA-guanine transglycosylase catalyzes incorporation of guanine, queuine, or queuine analogs into precursor tRNA that contains guanine in place of queuine (G-tRNA), but not into Q-containing tRNA (Okada et al. 1979; Shindo-Okada et al. 1980).

Table 2 shows the incorporation of radioactive guanine into unfractionated tRNAs isolated from a variety of tumor cells (Okada et al. 1978). It was demonstrated that tRNA isolated from various tumors, including slowly growing Morris hepatoma and SV40-transformed cells, incorporated a considerable amount of guanine catalyzed by *E. coli* tRNA-guanine transglycosylase, whereas tRNA isolated from all normal tissues except regenerating rat liver incorporated scarcely any. Slight incorporation of guanine was also observed with tRNA from undifferentiated cells such as rat fetal liver or rabbit reticulocyte.

For further study of the relationship between the presence of G-tRNA and the state of cells, Friend-virus-infected murine erythroleukemia cells in culture were chosen, since these transformed cells can easily be induced to differentiate into mature erythroid cells without altering their initial growth rate (Shindo-Okada et al. 1981b). The amounts of G-tRNA in murine erythroleukemic cells decreased markedly when the cells differentiated into mature erythroid cells. The decrease was detected at an early stage of erythroid differentiation; namely before any detectable increase in the percentage of cells containing hemoglobin. The amount of G-tRNA species was nearly proportional to the percentage of undifferentiated cells in the population, regardless of the type of inducer used. Decrease in the amounts of G-tRNA in the cells was effectively blocked by 12-*O*-tetradecanoxylphorbol 13-acetate (TPA), which inhibits differentiation of these cells (Table 3). These results clearly demonstrated that the presence of G-tRNA in tumor cells is not due merely to their fast growth rate.

G-tRNA is probably specific to cells in an undifferentiated state and thus can be termed oncofetal tRNA. tRNA-guanine transglycosylase with the same specificity was obtained in approximately equal amounts from tumor cells, such as rat ascites hepatoma cells, as from rat liver (Shindo-Okada et al. 1980). Thus it is possible that

Table 2. Incorporation of guanine into various tumor tRNAs by *E. coli* tRNA-guanine transglycosylase

Source of tRNA	Guanine incorporated ($pmol/A_{260}/h$)
AH7974 rat ascites hepatoma	18.1
Morris hepatoma 7794A	25.3
Ehrlich mouse ascites tumor	13.2
SN36 mouse ascites tumor	18.4
Sarcoma 180 mouse ascites tumor	6.9
MM46 mouse ascites tumor	8.8
SV40-transformed AGMK cells	40.7
Control AGMK cells	14.0
Regenerating rat liver (24 h after hepatectomy)	28.3
Regenerating rat liver (48 h after hepatectomy)	32.1
Rat fetal liver	1.5
Rabbit reticulocyte	1.0
Rabbit liver	< 0.3
Rat liver	< 0.3
Mouse liver	< 0.3
Rat kidney	< 0.3
Rat spleen	< 0.3
Rat testis	< 0.3

SN36 is a transplantable ascites tumor derived from mouse leukemia cells. MM46 is a transplantable ascites tumor derived from a spontaneous mammary carcinoma (Okada et al. 1978)

Table 3. Correlation between decrease of G-tRNA and extent of differentiation of murine erythroleukemic cells induced by different reagents

Inducer added	Guanine incorporated ($pmol/A_{260}$)	Hemoglobinized cells (%)
None (control)	17.5	< 0.5
Nicotinamide	9.4	60
DMSO	5.1	85
N^1-Methylnicotinamide	3.8	90~100
DMSO + TPA	8.9	22

The cells were harvested 5 days after addition of inducers (25 m*M* nicotinamide, 2% DMSO, 8 m*M* N^1-methylnicotinamide, 50 ng/ml TPA) (Shindo-Okada et al. 1981b)

queuine is limited in tumor cells, so that biosynthesis of Q in tRNA does not proceed fully. Another possibility is that a factor present in tumor cells inhibits the tRNA-guanine transglycosylase reaction.

Studies on an *E. coli* Mutant Lacking tRNA-Guanine Transglycosylase

The nature of tumor-specific tRNA is now well understood. However, it should be mentioned that its biological function in tumor cells is totally unknown. It may have the ability to read through a nonsense codon and lead to the formation of unique proteins that have a specific function in tumor cells (Bienz and Kubli 1981), or it may have a unique regulatory function which is not known thus far. It is difficult to study the function of queuosine in tRNA in mammalian cells, and therefore we have chosen an *E. coli* mutant which lacks tRNA-guanine transglycosylase. This mutant was isolated by random screening from a collection of *E. coli* mutants obtained by treatment with *N*-methyl-*N'*-nitro-*N*-nitrosoguanidine (S. Noguchi, Y. Nishimura, Y. Hirota, and S. Nishimura, unpublished work). The mutant's lack of tRNA-guanine transglycosylase activity demonstrated that the enzyme is actually involved in the biosynthesis of queuosine in tRNA. The defective gene, named *tgt*, was mapped at about 9 min on the *E. coli* chromosome. No clear biological defect was observed in the mutant, and in fact it grew slightly faster than the control isogenic strain. The only phenotypic change observed in the mutant thus far is marked reduction of viability when the cells are kept under unsuitable conditions for growth, suggesting that the presence of Q in tRNA is important to *E. coli* for survival in the natural environment.

Effect of Administration of Q Base on Tumor-Bearing Mice

Katze and Beck (1980) reported that injection of queuine into Ehrlich ascites tumor-bearing mice can restore queuine to tumor tRNA and consequently may inhibit tumor growth. They used natural queuine isolated from amniotic fluid, and therefore the amount of queuine available for further extensive studies is limited. In order to extend this interesting work, a large amount of optically active Q base was synthesized chemically through 31 steps by Drs. Akimoto and Nomura of the Takeda Pharmaceutical Co., Japan, according to the procedure developed by Goto and his co-workers (Okada et al. 1979). The Q base thus synthesized was injected intraperitoneally into BDF_1 mice at a dose of 100 mg/kg body weight/day for 5 days after transplantation of L-1210 or S-180 into the peritoneal cavities. No inhibition of tumor growth was observed in either case, contrary to the previous report by Katze and Beck (1980). It is necessary to perform more thorough work using other slowly growing tumors before coming to a definite conclusion whether Q base administration in tumor-bearing animals inhibits tumor growth.

At 24 h after the last intraperitoneal injection of Q base S-180 tumor tissues were removed from the tumor-bearing mice. Unfractionated tRNA was isolated from the tumor tissues, and the amount of G-tRNA was analyzed by incorporation of radioactive guanine catalyzed by *E. coli* tRNA-guanine transglycosylase. It was found that the S-180 tumor tRNA mice treated with Q base does not contain G-tRNA at all, indicating complete shift of G-tRNA to Q-tRNA in the in vivo reaction. The amount of Q base administered to the mice in this experiment was far more than that used by Katze and Beck (1980). This may be the reason why we got complete conversion of G-tRNA to Q-tRNA while Katze and Beck (1980) found that G-tRNA decreased, but still remained in small amounts in tumor tRNA after administration of Q base to Ehrlich ascites tumor-bearing mice.

Q Base Analogs Utilized in the tRNA-Guanine Transglycosylase Reaction

It is interesting to examine what type of Q base analogs can be inserted into G-tRNA. In the case of rat liver tRNA-guanine transglycosylase, 7-aminomethyl-7-deazagua-

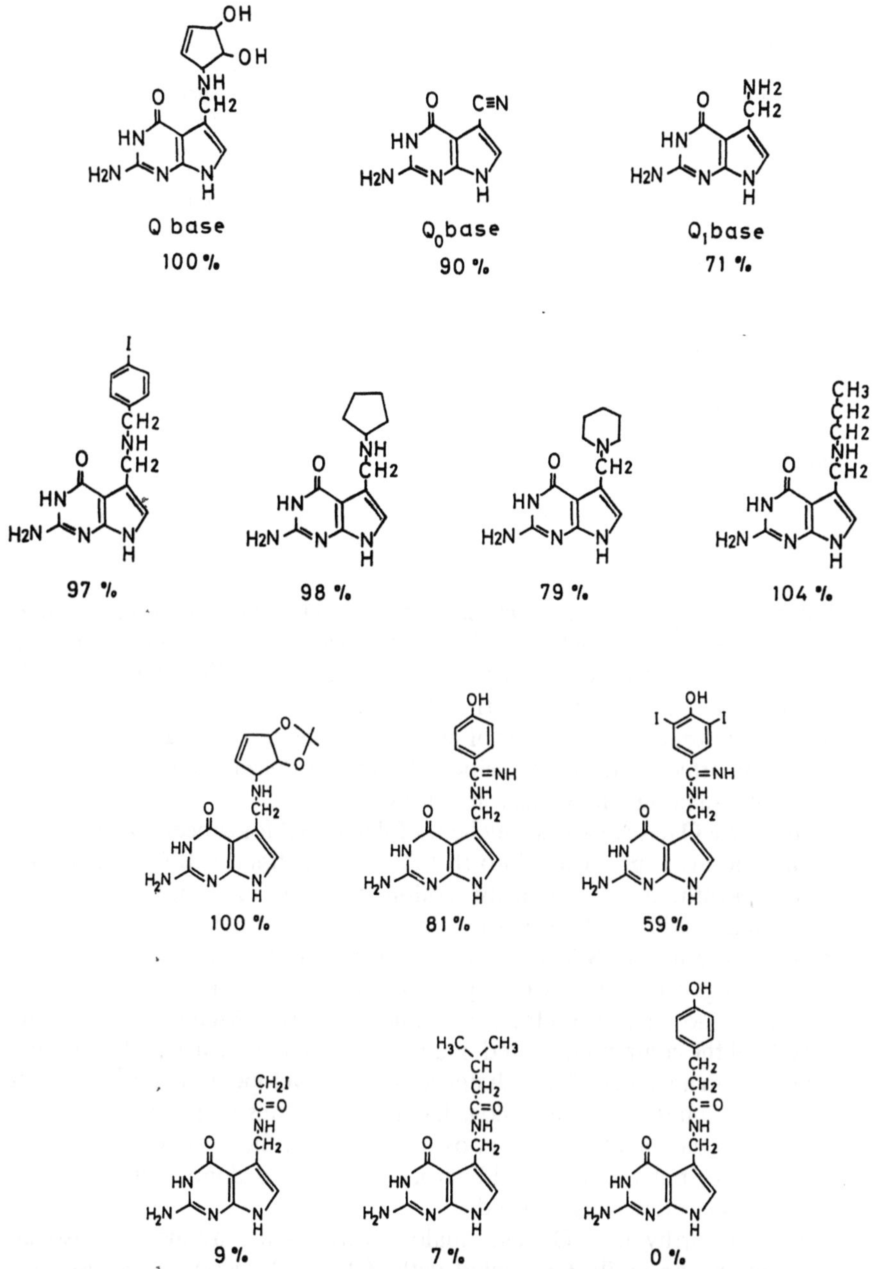

Fig. 6. Chemically synthesized Q base and its analogs tested as donors for rat liver tRNA-guanine transglycosylase. Percentages indicate efficiency of incorporation as compared with queuine

nine and 7-cyano-7-deazaguanine, which are known to be Q precursors in *E. coli* tRNA (Okada et al. 1979), were utilized as donors (Shindo-Okada et al. 1981). However, other guanine or queuine analogs, such as 7-deazaguanine, 7-methyl-7-deazaguanine, and 7-methylguanine, were not utilized at all (Table 4). It should be noted

Table 4. Incorporation of guanine or queuine analogs into rat ascites hepatoma AH7974 tRNA catalyzed by rat liver tRNA-guanine transglycosylase (Shindo-Okada et al. 1980)

Compounds	Incorporation ($pmol \times 10^{-3}/3.5\ A_{260}$ tRNA)
Guanine	4.9
Queuine	5.8
7-Cyano-7-deazaguanine	5.4
7-Aminomethyl-7-deazaguanine	2.6
8-Azaguanine	5.6
6-Thioguanine	3.9
7-Deazaguanine	0.6
7-Methyl-7-deazaguanine	0.2
6-Mercaptopurine	0
7-Methylguanine	0
Xanthine	0.1
Hypoxanthine	0

that artificial guanine analogs, such as 8-azaguanine and 6-thioguanine, were also incorporated into G-tRNA. 6-Mercaptopurine, hypoxanthine, and xanthine were inactive. The enzyme seems to recognize rather strictly the guanine or 7-deazaguanine structure. To be a substrate for tRNA-guanine transglycosylase, a compound seems to be required to have a lone pair of electrons in the nitrogen atom in the 7 position or a side chain attached to the 7 position, because 7-deazaguanine, 7-methylguanine, and 7-methyl-7-deazaguanine were not utilized.

Radioactive Q base analogs may be useful as a tool for cancer diagnosis, as they should be incorporated specifically into tRNA in tumor tissues. If Q base analogs can affect protein synthesis by changing codon recognition properties of tRNA or by cross-linking with protein-synthesizing machinery, such as ribosomes after they are incorporated into tRNA, they might also be useful as anticancer reagents. Many Q base analogs were chemically synthesized for this purpose, by Drs. Akimoto and Nomura, and their usefulness as donors for tRNA-guanine transglycosylase was tested. Of the compounds tested, many were found to be active donors (Fig. 6). Q base analogs with a variety of side chains in place of cyclopentenediol were as active donors as natural Q base. Q base analogs having side chains with amide linkage were almost inactive. Q base analogs with a positive charge in the nitrogen atom of the side chain were active, but this is not obligatory for being a donor, since 7-(cyano)-7-deazaguanine was effectively utilized.

It is noteworthy that Q base analogs with iodine atoms are also active. These compounds can easily be labeled with ^{125}I or ^{135}I. Since a Q base analog with an aliphatic side chain is active, it may be possible to synthesize an active Q base analog with an aliphatic side chain containing a cross-linking group.

Summary

We determined the primary structures of various tumor-specific tRNAs as well as of their normal counterparts by postlabeling RNA-sequencing procedures. The results clearly indicated that tumor-specific tRNAs are mostly formed by undermodification of hypermodified nucleosides located in the anticodon loop: no new tRNA transcripts have so far been found in tumor cells.

Among the modified nucleosides affected by tumorigenesis, queuosine and Y base are the most interesting. In various tumor $tRNA^{Phe}$ species, hydroxy Y base located next to the anticodon is undermodified to form hypomodified hydroxy Y base lacking methyl and carboxymethyl groups. This Y base analog should be a good marker for analyzing the state of cancer cells. Queuosine, located in the first position of the anticodon, is partly or completely replaced by guanosine in all tumor cells tested so far. The amount of G-tRNA decreased markedly when the cells differentiated into mature erythroid cells, with concomitant increase of Q-tRNA. This indicates that the presence of G-tRNA is closely related to the state of the cells, not merely to the fast growth rate of tumor cells. The enzyme tRNA-guanine transglycosylase, which is a key enzyme in biosynthesis of queuosine in tRNA (inserting Q base into tRNA by a transglycosylase reaction), is active in both tumor cells and normal cells. Administration of chemically synthesized Q base to tumor-bearing mice resulted in complete conversion of G-tRNA to Q-tRNA in tumor cells, indicating that exogenously added Q base is effectively incorporated into G-tRNA.

Various Q base analogs that can be used as substrates for tRNA-guanine transglycosylase were synthesized chemically. These compounds may be used for clinical cancer diagnosis, since they should be incorporated selectively into tRNA in tumor cells. In addition to use as cancer chemotherapeutic reagents, it should be possible to develop new Q base analogs that induce miscoding or blocking of protein synthesis after insertion into G-tRNA.

References

Bienz M, Kubli E (1981) Wild-type $tRNA_G^{Tyr}$ reads the TMV RNA stop codon, but Q base-modified $tRNA_Q^{Tyr}$ does not. Nature 294: 188–190

Gupta RC, Randerath K (1979) Rapid print-readout technique for sequencing of RNA's containing modified nucleotides. Nucleic Acids Res 6: 3443–3458

Katze JR, Beck WT (1980) Administration of queuine to mice relieves modified nucleoside queuosine deficiency in Ehrlich ascites tumor tRNA. Biochem Biophys Res Commun 96: 313–319

Katze JR, Farkas WR (1979) A factor in serum and amniotic fluid is a substrate for the tRNA-modifying enzyme tRNA-guanine transferase. Proc Natl Acad Sci USA 76: 3271–3275

Kuchino Y, Kasai H, Yamaizumi Z, Nishimura S, Borek E (1979a) Under-modified Y base in a $tRNA^{Phe}$ isoacceptor observed in tumor cells. Biochim Biophys Acta 565: 215–218

Kuchino Y, Kato M, Sugisaki H, Nishimura S (1979b) Nucleotide sequence of starfish initiator tRNA. Nucleic Acids Res 6: 3459–3469

Kuchino Y, Watanabe S, Harada F, Nishimura S (1980) Primary structure of AUA-specific isoleucine transfer ribonucleic acid from *Escherichia coli*. Biochemistry 19: 2085–2089

Kuchino Y, Shindo-Okada N, Ando N, Watanabe S, Nishimura S (1981) Nucleotide sequences of two aspartic acid tRNAs from rat liver and rat ascites hepatoma. J Biol Chem 256: 9059–9062

Nishimura S (1979a) Modified nucleosides in tRNA. In: Schimmel PR, Söll D, Abelson JN (eds) Transfer RNA: Structure, properties, and recognition. Cold Spring Harbor Laboratory, Cold Spring Harbor, N.Y., pp 59–79

Nishimura S (1979b) Transfer RNA and Cancer. In: Sugimura T, Endo H, Ono T, Sugano H (eds) Progress in cancer biochemistry. Japan Scientific Societies Press, Tokyo and University Park Press, Baltimore, Gann Monograph 24, pp 245–262

Okada N, Harada F, Nishimura S (1976) Specific replacement of Q base in the anticodon of tRNA by guanine catalyzed by a cell-free extract of rabbit reticulocyte. Nucleic Acids Res 3: 2593–2603

Okada N, Shindo-Okada N, Sato S, Itoh YH, Oda K, Nishimura S (1978) Detection of unique tRNA species in tumor tissues by *Escherichia coli* guanine insertion enzyme. Proc Natl Acad Sci USA 75: 4247–4251

Okada N, Noguchi S, Kasai H, Shindo-Okada N, Ohgi T, Goto T, Nishimura S (1979) Novel mechanism of post-transcriptional modification of tRNA. J Biol Chem 254: 3067–3073

Raba M, Limburg K, Burghagen M, Katze JR, Simsek M, Heckman JE, RajBhandary UL, Gross HJ (1979) Nucleotide sequence of three isoaccepting lysine tRNAs from rabbit liver and SV40-transformed mouse fibroblasts. Eur J Biochem 97: 305–318

Roe BA, Stankiewicz AF, Rizi HL, Weisz C, DiLauro NM, Pike D, Chen CY, Chen EY (1979) Comparison of rat liver and Walker 256 carcinoma tRNAs. Nucleic Acids Res 6: 673–688

Shindo-Okada N, Okada N, Ohgi T, Goto T, Nishimura S (1980) Transfer ribonucleic acid guanine transglycosylase isolated from rat liver. Biochemistry 19: 395–400

Shindo-Okada N, Kuchino Y, Harada F, Okada N, Nishimura S (1981a) Biological and structural differences between $tRNA^{Val}$ species isolated from rat ascites hepatoma cells and normal rat liver. J Biochem 90: 535–544

Shindo-Okada N, Terada M, Nishimura S (1981b) Changes in amount of hypomodified tRNA having guanine in place of queuine during erythroid differentiation of murine erythroleukemia cells. Eur J Biochem 115: 423–428

Silberklang M, Prochiantz A, Haenni A-L, RajBhandary UL (1977) Studies on the sequence of the 3′-terminal region of turnip-yellow mosaic-virus RNA. Eur J Biochem 72: 465–478

Stanley J, Vassilenko S (1978) A different approach of RNA sequencing. Nature 274: 87–89

Tanaka Y, Dyer TA, Brownlee GG (1980) An improved direct RNA Sequence method: its application to Vicia faba 5.8S ribosomal RNA. Nucleic Acids Res 8: 1259–1272

Tsutsui E, Srinivasan PR, Borek E (1966) tRNA methylases in tumors of animal and human origin. Proc Natl Acad Sci USA 56: 1003–1009

*Excretion of Polyamines by Children with Leukemia During Chemotherapy**

M. Mach[1], U. Schneider[2], and W. Kersten[1]

[1] Institut für Physiologische Chemie, Universität Erlangen-Nürnberg, Fahrstrasse 17, 8520 Erlangen, FRG; [2] Universitätskinderklinik, Universität Erlangen-Nürnberg, 8520 Erlangen, FRG

Introduction

During the past 10 years polyamines and modified nucleosides have both been suggested as useful tumor markers. Since the polyamine-synthetic pathway and nucleic acid methylation share the common cosubstrate *S*-adenosylmethionine, it is likely that the two metabolic routes have common regulatory features.

Many analyses of these compounds in various body fluids from ill and healthy people have been performed (Desser 1980; Speer et al. 1979). With respect to excretion of polyamines, it is now generally accepted that they do not fulfill the requirements of specific tumor markers. There is one exception: polyamines in the cerebrospinal fluid are the most sensitive markers for the detection of recurrent medulloblastomas (Marton et al. 1979). However, the measurement of polyamine excretion might still be useful to find out whether patients with particular malignant diseases respond to antitumor chemotherapy.

A prerequisite for basic clinical research is knowledge of the metabolism and function of polyamines within the cell. Accordingly, the two parts of this chapter present results from our laboratory showing a relationship between polyamine concentration and the methylation of tRNA and the results of polyamine analyses of the urine of children suffering from acute lymphocytic and acute myeloblastic leukemia (ALL and AML), including the response of polyamine excretion to chemotherapy.

Regulation of tRNA Methylation by Polyamines

Polyamines are essential in pro- and eukaryotes for optimal growth and development. The organic cations stabilize cells, membranes, DNA, and ribosomes. They associate with nucleic acids and proteins and stimulate the synthesis of DNA and RNA. In cell-free systems they can replace Mg^{2+} in the aminoacylation or methylation reaction of tRNA, they influence ribosome-dependent steps of protein synthesis, and they enhance the fidelity of translation (Tabor and Tabor 1976). During the synthesis of

* Work was supported by the Deutsche Forschungsgemeinschaft SFB 118 and the W. Sander Stiftung. The authors thank Mrs. L. Mutschler, Mrs. Stockhausen, and Mrs. U. Christel for their excellent technical assistance

polyamines *S*-adenosylmethionine decarboxylase produces *S*-methyl-adenosylhomocysteamine, from which spermidine synthetase transfers the propylamine residue to putrescine or spermidine to form spermidine or spermine respectively. *S*-Adenosylmethionine plays another vital role: It serves as a donor of methyl groups in almost all transmethylation reactions of tRNA.

Since the transfer of methyl groups from *S*-adenosylmethionine to tRNA was found to be enhanced by putrescine or spermidine in cell-free systems (Leboy 1970), the question was raised of whether the observed effects of polyamines on the methylation of tRNA in vitro might reflect a functional role of polyamines on tRNA methylation in vivo. In order to solve this question we have used *Dictyostelium discoideum* as a model system. Vegetative amoebae of this organism comprise relative high amounts of three polyamines: namely putrescine 10 m*M*, spermidine 1.6 m*M*, and the unusual 1.3-diaminopropane (Mach et al. 1982). Two inhibitors of polyamine synthesis were applied to reduce the intracellular levels of polyamines: α-methylornithine and diaminopropanol, both inhibitors of ornithindecarboxylase. Inhibition of polyamine synthesis in *D. discoideum* significantly reduces the intracellular methylation of particular nucleosides in tRNA at concentrations that had almost no effect on the incorporation of labeled precursors into DNA and protein. The incorporation of uridine into total RNA was inhibited by about 20%, but the incorporation of radioactivity from methionine into total RNA was reduced by about 50%. Nucleoside analysis of the purified tRNA showed that the incorporation of radioactive methyl groups into almost all of the methylated nucleosides was considerably reduced in tRNAs from cells treated with the inhibitor. The effect of the inhibitor on the methylation of specific nucleosides in tRNA was found to be most pronounced for ribosylthimine and N^2,N^2-dimethylguanosine (40% inhibition). These experiments clearly showed that the methylation of tRNA in vivo is dependent on polyamines. From our experiments we obtained further evidence that there is a correlation between polyamine levels and tRNA methylation during differentiation of *D. discoideum*. The polyamine content of the cells 8 h after induction of development is about half that in vegetative cells. At the same time the incorporation of methyl groups from radioactive methionine into newly synthesized tRNA is decreased. Nucleoside analysis revealed that predominantly ribosylthimine and N^2,N^2-dimethylguanosine are affected (see Kersten, this volume pp. 255–263). In vitro, optimal overall tRNA methyltransferase activities were observed in the presence of 1–2 m*M* spermidine or 10 m*M* putrescine. These are exactly the intracellular concentrations of polyamines in growing amoebae. A combination of both polyamines does not further increase the overall enzyme activity. Diaminopropane does not activate the tRNA methyltransferases at physiological concentration (Mach et al. 1982).

It has been suggested for several years that a correlation might exist between polyamine levels and tRNA methyltransferase activities in various tissues, underlying growth changes, differentiation, or neoplastic transformation. From our experiments we obtained clear evidence of a strong correlation between polyamine levels and tRNA methyltransferase activities during differentiation of *D. discoideum*. Our further efforts are directed at finding a similar relationship in tumor cells.

Polyamine Excretion

Ten years have passed since Russel (1971) described elevated levels of polyamines in hydrolyzed urine samples of patients with malignant diseases. Since then polyamine

Table 1. Normal values of polyamine excretion in children (nmol/mg creatinine)

	Male (n = 26)	Female (n = 25)
Acetyl putrescine	38.9 ± 25.8	22.9 ± 13.0
Acetyl spermidine	10.9 ± 3.7	13.1 ± 4.3
Putrescine	1.2 ± 0.9	1.1 ± 0.5

analyses in various body fluids have been performed to find out whether polyamines can be used as markers for early detection of cancer, for the determination of tumor mass, or for the evaluation of the efficiency of anticancer treatment (for review see Jänne et al. 1978). This research was stimulated when it was found that levels of ornithindecarboxylase, the first enzyme in the biosynthetic pathway of the polyamines, rose markedly during carcinogenesis (for review see Bachrach 1980). Increased excretion of polyamines was observed not only in people with hematological and solid tumors, but also in some patients with cirrhosis, active hepatitis, viral and bacterial infections of the lung, and many other diseases (Desser 1980). The combined determination of various markers helps to predict the disease status of patients with breast carcinoma (Woo et al. 1978).

Children with ALL were incurable until the 1960s, but this disease can now be treated with intensive multimodal chemotherapy. Different groups reporting on specific therapy regimens have suggested a recovery rate of 60%–80% (Riehm et al. 1977, Miller et al. 1980). Since the intensity of the therapy has to be adjusted as exactly as possible to the tolerance of each individual patient, pediatricians have sought markers to indicate the effect of the therapy and possibly detect recurrences early. No careful study of polyamine excretion in children with ALL has yet been published. Abdel-Monem (1975) first showed that a major portion of the urinary putrescine and spermidine is excreted in the form of monoacetyl derivatives. We have developed a fast and sensitive method for the quantitative determination of free and acetylated polyamines (Mach et al. 1981). Using this method, we have investigated the daily polyamine excretion in the urine of children with ALL or AML over 30–60 days. For comparison we analyzed the urine of three healthy control children daily over a 4-week period (Table 1).

Tsuji et al. (1975) reported values of acetylspermidine of 5–7 nmol/mg creatinine in normal adults. Considering that children have a faster cell proliferation rate, our values correlate well to those reported. They are also in good agreement with those of Seiler and Knödgen (1979), who reported that in normal adults the amount of free putrescine and spermidine comprise less than 10% of the total amines excreted in urine.

Excretion of Polyamines by Children with ALL and AML

On the basis of studies on tumor-bearing animals and human patients it has been proposed that untreated tumor patients excrete high amounts of polyamines due to spontaneous cell loss by the tumor (Russel et al. 1975). Successful chemotherapy or radiotherapy should produce a further temporary increase in the release of polyamines from tumor tissues, and thereafter the polyamine excretion should return to normal

Table 2. Polyamine excretion by children with leukemia before and during chemotherapy. *Ac Put*, acetylputrescine; *Ac Spd*, acetylspermidine

Patient	Sex	Age (years)	Ac Put (nmol/mg creatinine)	Ac Spd (nmol/mg creatinine)			Post-treatment to pretreatment ratio, of Ac Spd level		Leukocytes	Blasts	Disease
				Day 1	Days 3–4	Day 14	Days 3–4 : 1	Day 14 : 1	Day 1	Day 1	
T. L.	F	2	304.5	31.1	361.5	61.2	11.54	1.95	11000	10800	ALL
C. H.	F	3	67.2	211.3	174.5	41.8	0.82	0.19	5100	4845	ALL
K. B.	M	3	52.9	30.8	271.6	14.2	8.80	0.46	15300	10800	ALL
P. R.	F	5	47.9	10.6	52.6	20.2	4.96	1.90	5200	–	ALL
R. K.	M	7	215.9	27.6	36.0	38.2	1.30	1.38	7000	–	AML
K. A.	F	8	72.2	25.3	121.5	38.1	4.80	1.50	9300	5580	ALL
S. G.	F	9	31.9	19.5	48.3	5.5	2.47	0.28	5400	1600	ALL
A. G.	M	9	17.2	22.2	138.8	17.2	6.14	0.76	4800	2880	ALL
A. L.	F	9	137.1	65.9	29.8	22.5	0.45	0.34	215	–	AML
E. M. D.	F	11	538.5	181.6	35.2	31.4	0.19	0.17	4500	3600	ALL
H. St.	M	11	8.5	8.5	45.4	22.2	5.34	2.70	5500	1650	ALL
A. W.	M	14	72.2	15.4	61.1	32.7	3.96	2.12	5400	5350	ALL

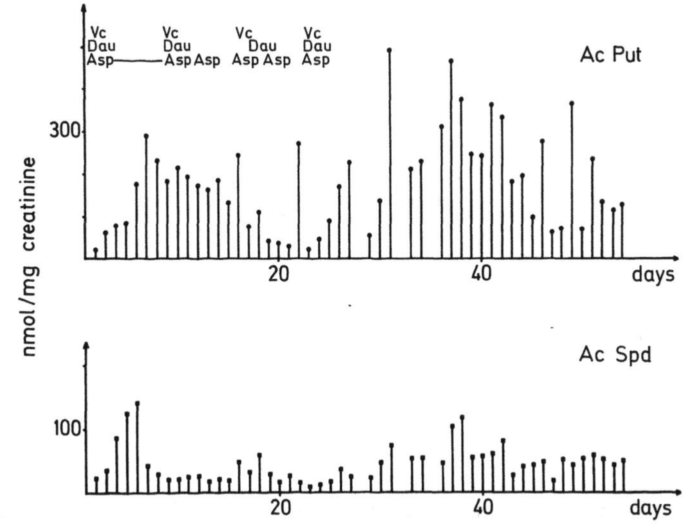

Fig. 1. Polyamine excretion in the urine of a 9-year-old male child (A.G.) with ALL. He was treated with prednisone from day 2 to the end of the observation period. *Dau,* daunorubicine; *Asp,* L-asparaginase; *Vc,* vincristine

levels. Further studies have suggested that spermidine excretion can serve as a marker for destruction of tumor cells, whereas excretion of putrescine should reflect the proliferation of the tumor (Durie et al. 1977; Russel 1977).

In our study we observed elevated polyamine levels in the urine of children with ALL before the onset of chemotherapy, with the exception of two children (Table 2). The elevated polyamine excretion of most patients could be correlated to the risk group of the disease (e.g., number of leukocytes and blasts). This confirms the results of Russel et al. (1977), who examined the polyamine excretion in hydrolyzed urine of adult patients with leukemia and found increased spermidine excretion in most patients.

Acetylputrescine excretion upon onset of chemotherapy increased by a factor of 2–5 within 2–3 days (Fig. 1). Only in those cases where the initial acetylputrescine excretion was very high (patients T.L. and E.M.D., Table 2) did the values not increase further. In no case did acetylputrescine excretion return to normal during the investigation period of 30–60 days, the levels remaining elevated even after suspension of the initial chemotherapy. Since all the children responded well to the therapy, all were in full remission at this time. Therefore we suggest that the prolonged excretion of acetylputrescine reflects the proliferative response of the cells to the drastic chemotherapy. This presumption was supported by the observation that a child treated with vincristine and adriblastine after complete removal of a neuroblastoma showed elevated acetylputrescine levels (Fig. 2). Another child with Crohn's disease who was treated with prednisone also had elevated acetylputrescine excretion (not shown). In both cases the excretion of acetylspermidine was within the normal range. It must be emphasized that continous medication with prednisone is an essential part of the ALL chemotherapy regimen.

Acetylspermidine excretion upon onset of chemotherapy also increased after 3–4 days (Table 2). Here we observed a correlation between the initial leukocyte count or

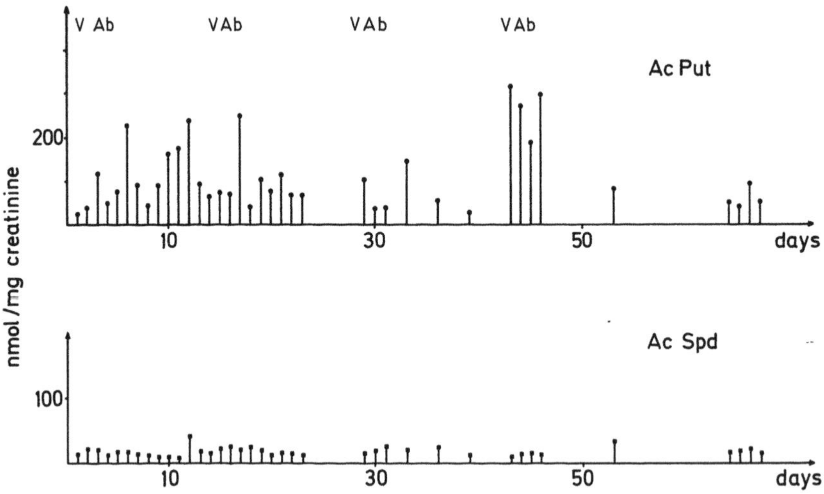

Fig. 2. Drug treatment of a 4-year-old female child (A.St.) after removal of a neuroblastoma. *V*, vincristine; *Ab*, adriblastine

number of peripheral blasts and the increase in the acetylspermidine in urine. The most pronounced elevations of acetylspermidine levels were observed in children with particularly high numbers of blasts. The excretion of acetylspermidine returned to pretreatment values after 10–14 days. The two children with AML did not respond after therapy with an increase of acetylspermidine excretion, whereas the excretion of acetylputrescine increased according to drug treatment. Russel (1977) reported post-treatment to pretreatment spermidine ratios of 1.1–1.5 for nonresponders to the therapy and 4.30 ± 2.5 for responders. The two children in our group with AML had extremely low ratios despite successful remission upon induction therapy. It is well known, however, that patients with AML respond less well to chemotherapy with the progression of the disease.

Conclusion

Free and acetylated polyamines were measured in the urine of normal children and children with AML or ALL. Like adults, children excrete polyamines almost exclusively as the monoacetyl derviatives. The amount of free putrescine and spermidine is below 5% of the total polyamine content. Free spermine was not detectable in the urine of the children studied. In accordance with others (Seiler and Knödgen 1979, Seiler et al. 1981), we observed relatively stable day-to-day excretion of the acetylated polyamines in healthy controls. Cancer patients, however, had great day-to-day variations during chemotherapy.

The levels of acetylputrescine and acetylspermidine were slightly to markedly increased in children with ALL or AML before the onset of chemotherapy. Romano et al. (1980) made the same observations in adult patients with ALL. In our study we could not detect any correlation between pretreatment polyamine excretion and the stage of the disease, e.g., blast number, risk factor, and leukocytes. With the exception of those cases in which acetylputrescine excretion was extremely high before the commencement of therapy, all children displayed dramatic increases in acetylputrescine excretion upon therapy. Since acetylputrescine levels did not return to normal during our observation period, and since all children responded well to the therapy, we have to assume that acetylputrescine excretion is influenced by various other factors. It is known that prednisone stimulates ornithindecarboxylase (Panko and Kenney 1971) and that cyclophosphamide enhances the excretion of acetylated polyamines in the rat (Seiler et al. 1981). Since the children are treated with up to ten different drugs, there might be cumulative side effects.

Since all the children in our group were in full remission after induction therapy, the levels of acetylputrescine in the urine might not reflect the proliferative behavior of the tumor, as suggested by Russel et al. (1975).

Following chemotherapeutic treatment the changes in the urinary acetylspermidine concentration could reflect the success of the therapy. Since we observed a good correlation between the initial leukocyte count and the post-treatment to pretreatment ratios of acetylspermidine excretion, it might be that the response quantitatively reflects the success of the therapy. Since we had no child unresponsive to the therapy, such a hypothesis needs further investigation. One hint, however, comes from the two children with AML, who had extremely low post-treatment to pretreatment ratios. AML is known to respond poorly to the therapy.

In conclusion, urinary polyamine levels may be useful markers of tumor kinetics during therapy. The relationship observed between the cytological and polyamine data confirms the validity of the test and indicates that it might be particularly useful in tumors that have very few measurable data, thus allowing an objective evaluation of the response to the therapy.

Summary

Evidence is presented showing a relation between polyamine concentration and the methylation of tRNA in vitro and in vivo. Polyamine excretion in urine of children with ALL and AML is slightly elevated before the commencement of chemotherapy. Immediately thereafter, excretion of acetylputrescine increases drastically over a period of at least 30–60 days. The elevation seems to be caused by different factors, e.g., destruction of tumor cells, induction of ornithindecarboxylase, and cell recovery after termination of chemotherapy. Acetylspermidine excretion also increases 3–4 days after the beginning of chemotherapy. A positive correlation exists between leukocyte counts and excretion of acetylspermidine. The ratio of acetylspermidine excretion at days 3–4 of the therapy to that before commencement of chemotherapy could be an indicator of response to the therapy.

References

Abdel-Monem MM, Ohno K, Fortuny IE, Theologides A (1975) Acetylspermidines in human urine. Lancet 2: 1210

Bachrach U (1980) The induction of ornithine decarboxylase in normal and neoplastic cells. In: Gaugas JM (ed) Polyamines in biomedical research. Wiley, New York, pp 81–109

Desser H (1980) Polyamines as markers of malignancy in human leukaemia and in other haematological disorders. In: Gaugas JM (ed) Polyamines in biomedical research. Wiley New York, pp 415–433
Durie BGM, Salmon SE, Russel DH (1977) Polyamines as markers of response and disease activity in cancer chemotherapy. Cancer Res 37: 214–221
Jänne J, Pöso H, Raina A (1978) Polyamines in rapid growth and cancer. Biochim Biophys Acta 473: 241–293
Leboy P (1970) Stimulation of soluble ribonucleic acid methylase activity by polyamines. Biochemistry 12: 1577–1583
Mach M, Kersten H, Kersten W (1981) Measurements of polyamines and their acetylated derivatives in cell extracts and physiological fluids by use of an amino acid analyzer. J Chromatogr 223: 51–57
Mach M, Kersten H, Kersten W (1982) Regulation of tRNA methyltransferase activities by spermidine and putrescine. Biochem J 202: 153–162
Marton LJ, Edwards MS, Levin VA, Lubich WP, Wilson CB (1979) Predictive value of cerebrospinal fluid polyamines in medullablastoma. Cancer Res 39: 993–997
Miller DR, Leikin S, Albo V, Vitale L, Sather P, Coccia P, Nesbit M, Karon M, Hammond D (1980) Use of prognostic factors in improving the design and efficiency of clinical trial in childhood leukaemia. Children's Cancer Study Group Report. Cancer Treatment Reports 64: 381–392
Panko WB, Kenney FT (1971) Hormonal stimulation of hepatic ornithine decarboxylase. Biochem Biophys Res Comm 43: 346–350
Riehm H, Gardener H, Welte K (1977) Die Westberliner Studie zur Behandlung der lymphoblastischen Leukaemie des Kindesalters/Erfahrungsbericht nach 6 Jahren. Klin Paediatr 189: 89–102
Romano M, Cecco L, Cerra M, Montuori R, DeRosa C (1980) Polyamines as biological markers of the effectiveness of therapy in acute leukemia. Tumori 66: 677–687
Russel DH (1971) Increased polyamine concentrations in the urine of human cancer patients. Nature 233: 144
Russel DH, Durie BGM, Salmon SE (1975) Polyamines as predictors of success and failure in cancer chemotherapy. Lancet 2: 797–799
Russel DH (1977) Clinical relevance of polyamines as biochemical markers of tumor kinetics. Clin Chem 13: 22–27
Seiler N, Knödgen B (1979) Determination of the naturally occurring monoacetyl derivatives of di- and polyamines. J Chromatogr 164: 155–168
Seiler N, Koch-Weser J, Knödgen B, Richards W, Tardif C, Bolkenius FN, Schechter P, Tell G, Mamont P, Fozard J, Bachrach U, Grosshans E (1981) The significance of acetylation in the urinary excretion of polyamines. In: Caldarera CM (ed) Advances in polyamine research, vol 3. Raven Press, New York, pp 197–211
Speer J, Gehrke CW, Kuo KC, Waalkes TP, Borek E (1979) tRNA breakdown products as markers for cancer. Cancer 44: 2120–2123
Tabor CW, Tabor H (1976) 1.4 Diaminobutane, spermidine and spermine. Annu Rev Biochem 285–306
Tsuji M, Nakajima T, Sano J (1975) Putrescine, spermidine, N-acetylspermidine and spermine in the urine of patients with leukaemias and tumors. Clin Chim Acta 59: 161–167
Woo KB, Waalkes TP, Ahmann DL, Tormey DC, Gehrke CW, Oliverio VT (1978) A quantitative approach to determining disease response during therapy using multiple biologic markers. Cancer 41: 1685–1703

Subject Index

Recent Results in Cancer Research

Sponsored by the Swiss League against Cancer. Editor in Chief: P. Rentchnick, Genève

For information about Vols. 1–9, please contact your bookseller of Springer-Verlag

10 NELSON, R. S.: Radioactive Phosphorus in the Diagnosis of Gastrointestinal Cancer.
11 FREEMAN, R. G. and J. M. KNOX: Treatment of Skin Cancer.
12 LYNCH, H. T.: Hereditary Factors in Carcinoma.
13 Tumours in Children, 2nd Edition. Edited by H. B. MARSDEN and J. K. STEWARD.
14 ODARTCHENKO, N.: Production Cellulaire Erythropoïétique.
15 SOKOLOFF, B.: Carcinoid and Serotonin.
16 JACOBS, M. L.: Malignant Lymphomas and Their Management.
17 Normal and Malignant Cell Growth. Edited by R. J. M. FRY, M. L. GRIEM, and W. H. KIRSTEN (Symposium).
18 ANGLESIO, E.: The Treatment of Hodgkin's Disease.
19 BANNASCH, P.: The Cytoplasm of Hepatocytes during Carcinogenesis. Electron- and Lightmicroscopical Investigations of the Nitrosomorpholineintoxicated Rat Liver.
20 Rubidomycin. A new Agent against Cancer. Edited by J. BERNARD, R. PAUL, M. BOIRON, C. JACQUILLAT, and R. MARAL.
21 Scientific Basis of Cancer Chemotherapy. Edited by G. MATHÉ (Symposium).
22 KOLDOVSKÝ, P.: Tumor Specific Transplantation Antigen.
23 FUCHS, W. A., J. W. DAVIDSON, and H. W. FISCHER: Lymphography in Cancer. With contributions by G. JANTET AND H. RÖSLER.
24 HAYWARD, J.: Hormones und Human Breast Cancer. An Account of 15 Years Study.
25 ROY-BURMAN, P.: Analogues of Nucleic Acid Components. Mechanisms of Action.
26 Tumors of the Liver. Edited by G. T. PACK and A. H. ISLAMI.
27 SZYMENDERA, J.: Bone Mineral Metabolism in Cancer.
28 MEEK, E. S.: Antitumour and Antiviral Substances of Natural Origin.
29 Aseptic Environments and Cancer Treatment. Edited by G. MATHÉ (Symposium).
30 Advances in the Treatment of Acute (Blastic) Leukemias. Edited by G. MATHÉ (Symposium).
31 DENOIX, P.: Treatment of Malignant Breast Tumors. Indications and Results.
32 NELSON, R. S.: Endoscopy in Gastric Cancer.
33 Experimental and Clinical Effects of L-Asparaginase. Edited by E. GRUNDMANN and H. F. OETTGEN (Symposium).
34 Chemistry and Biological Actions of 4-Nitroquinolin 1-Oxide. Edited by H. ENDO, T. ONO, and T. SUGIMURA.
35 PENN, I.: Malignant Tumors in Organ Transplant Recipients.
36 Current Concepts in the Management of Lymphoma and Leukemia. Edited by J. E. ULTMANN, M. L. GRIEM, W. H. KIRSTEN, and R. W. WISSLER (Symposium).
37 CHIAPPA, S., R. MUSUMECI, and C. USLENGHI: Endolymphatic Radiotherapy in Malignant Lymphomas. With contributions by G. BONADONNA, B. DAMASCELLI, G. FAVA, F. PIZZETTI, U. VERONESI.
38 KOLLER, P. C.: The Role of Chromosomes in Cancer Biology.
39 Current Problems in the Epidemiology of Cancer and Lymphomas. Edited by E. GRUNDMANN and H. TULINIUS (Symposium).
40 LANGLEY, F. A. and A. C. CROMPTON: Epithelial Abnormalities of the Cervix Uteri.
41 Tumours in a Tropical Country. A Survey of Uganda (1964–1968). Edited by A. C. TEMPLETON.
42 Breast Cancer: A Challenging Problem. Edited by M. L. GRIEM, E. V. JENSEN, J. E. ULTMANN, and R. W. WISSLER (Symposium).
43 Nomenclature, Methodology and Results of Clinical Trials in Acute Leukemias. Edited by G. MATHÉ, P. POUILLART, L. SCHWARZENBERG (Symposium).
44 Special Topics in Carcinogenesis. Edited by E. GRUNDMANN (Symposium).
45 KOLDOVSKÝ, P.: Carcinoembryonic Antigens.
46 Diagnosis and Therapy of Malignant Lymphoma. Edited by K. MUSSHOFF (Symposium).
47 Investigation and Stimulation of Immunity in Cancer Patients. Edited by G. MATHÉ and R. WEINER (Symposium).
48 Platinum Coordination Complexes in Cancer Chemotherapy. Edited by T. A. CONNORS and J. J. ROBERTS (Symposium).
49 Complications of Cancer Chemotherapy. Edited by G. MATHÉ and R. K. OLDHAM (Symposium).
50 Cancer Registry, Edited by E. GRUNDMANN and E. PEDERSEN (Symposium).
51 Gliomas. Current Concepts in Biology, Diagnosis and Therapy. Edited by J. HEKMATPANAH (Symposium).

52 The Ambivalence of Cytostatic Therapy. Edited by E. GRUNDMANN and R. GROSS (Symposium).
53 A. CLARYSSE, Y. KENIS, and G. MATHÉ: Cancer Chemotherapy.
54 Malignant Bone Tumors. Edited by E. GRUNDMANN.
55 MATHÉ, G.: Cancer Active Immunotherapy, Immunoprophylaxis, and Immunorestoration.
56 Lymphocytes, Macrophages, and Cancer. Edited by G. MATHÉ, I. FLORENTIN, and M.-C. SIMMLER (Symposium).
57 Breast Cancer: A Multidisciplinary Approach. Edited by G. ST. ARNEAULT, P. BAND, and L. ISRAËL (Symposium).
58 B. S. SCHOENBERG: Multiple Primary Malignant Neoplasms.
59 Selective Heat Sensitivity of Cancer Cells. Edited by A. ROSSI-FANELLI, R. CAVALIERE, B. MONDOVI, and G. MORICCA.
60 Tumors of the Male Genital System. Edited by E. GRUNDMANN and W. VAHLENSIECK (Symposium).
61 D. METCALF: Hemopoietic Colonies.
62 Tactics and Strategy in Cancer Treatment. Edited by G. MATHÉ (Symposium).
63 Antitumor Antibiotics. Edited by S. K. CARTER, H. UMEZAWA, J. DOUROS, and Y. SAKURAI (Symposium).
64 Lymphoid Neoplasias I: Classification, Categorization, Natural History.
65 Lymphoid Neoplasias II: Clinical and Therapeutic Aspects.
Lymphoid Neoplasias I & II. Proceedings of the 1977 CNRS-EORTC International Colloquium. Editors: G. MATHÉ, M. SELIGMANN, M. TUBIANA. Devided into two volumes.
66 Carcinogenic Hormones. Edited by C. H. LINGEMAN.
67/68 Adjuvant Therapies and Markers of Post-Surgical Minimal Residual Disease I & II. Proceedings of the 1978 Annual Plenary Meeting of the EORTC. Editors: G. BONADONNA, G. MATHÉ, S. E. SALMON. Divided into two volumes.
67 Markers and General Problems of Cancer Adjuvant Therapies.
68 Adjuvant Therapies of the Various Primary Tumors.
69 Strategies in Clinical Hematology. Edited by R. GROSS and K.-P. HELLRIEGEL.
70 New Anticancer Drugs. Edited by S. K. CARTER
71 Endocrine Treatment of Breast Cancer. Edited by B. HENNINGSEN, F. LINDER, C. STREICHELE.
72 CAWLEY, J. C., BURNS, G. F., HAYHOE, F. G. J.: Hairy-Cell Leukaemia.
73 Thyroid Cancer. Edited by W. DUNCAN.
74 Cancer Chemo- and Immunopharmacology. 1. Chemopharmacology. Edited by G. MATHÉ and F. M. MUGGIA.
75 Cancer Chemo- and Immunopharmacology. 2. Immunopharmacology, Relations and General Problems. Edited by G. MATHÉ and F. M. MUGGIA.
76 New Drugs in Cancer Chemotherapy. Edited by S. K. CARTER, Y. SAKURAI, H. UMEZAWA
77 K. STANLEY, J. STJERNSWÄRD, M. ISLEY: The Conduct of a Cooperative Clinical Trial.
78 Prostate Cancer. Edited by W. DUNCAN.
79 Chemotherapy and Radiotherapy of Gastrointestinal Tumors. Edited by H. O. KLEIN.
80 Adjuvant Therapies of Cancer. Edited by G. MATHÉ, G. BONADONNA, S. SALMON.
81 H. P. LOHRMANN and W. SCHREML: Cytotoxic Drugs and the Granulopoietic System.
82 Early Detection and Localization of Lung Tumors in High Risk Groups. Edited by P. R. BAND.
83 Colorectal Cancer. Edited by W. DUNCAN.
84 Modified Nucleosides and Cancer. Edited by G. NASS.

MIX
Papier aus verantwortungsvollen Quellen
Paper from responsible sources
FSC® C105338

If you have any concerns about our products,
you can contact us on
ProductSafety@springernature.com

In case Publisher is established outside the EU,
the EU authorized representative is:
Springer Nature Customer Service Center GmbH
Europaplatz 3, 69115 Heidelberg, Germany

Printed by Libri Plureos GmbH
in Hamburg, Germany